BEFORE HIV
Sexuality, Fertility and Mortality in East Africa, 1900–1980

BEFORE HIV
Sexuality, Fertility and Mortality in East Africa 1900–1980

by
Shane Doyle

*A British Academy
Postdoctoral Fellowship Monograph*

Published for THE BRITISH ACADEMY
by OXFORD UNIVERSITY PRESS

Oxford University Press, Great Clarendon Street, Oxford OX2 6DP

First edition published 2013

British Library Cataloguing in Publication Data
Data available

Library of Congress Cataloging in Publication Data
Data available

Typeset by
New Leaf Design, Scarborough, North Yorkshire
Printed in Great Britain by
TJ International Ltd, Padstow, Cornwall

ISBN 978–0–19–726533–8

MIX
Paper from responsible sources
FSC® C013056
FSC
www.fsc.org

For Emma, George and Leah

Contents

Figures

Acknowledgements

My research has benefited from the assistance and advice of a number of individuals, including Adrian Browne, Andrew Burton, Asiimwe Godfrey, Benedict Bigirwamungu, Carol Summers, Charles Kahwa, Charles Otim, Chris Prior, Christine Ninsiima, David Anderson, Derek Peterson, Dr Mussa Ndyeshobora, Dr Pius Okong, Emma Coombs, Felicitas Becker, Gerald Lubega, Hebe Welbourn, Jesse Karugaba, Jim Oeppen, Jo Parish, Jo Sadgrove, John Gooch, John Iliffe, John Lonsdale, John Sutton, Joseph Mutua, Katrina Honeyman, Megan Vaughan, Neil Kodesh, Pam Bingley, Paul Lane, Peter Cooke, Phillip Mbatya, Rebecca Tyler, Rhiannon Stephens, Richard Smith, Ron Atkinson, Ros Davies, Sarah Walters, Simon Dixon, Sister Miriam Duggan, Sunil Amrith, Syridion Rweyendere, Vincent Hiribarren, Wilbert Mwandiki, Will Jackson, Yvonne Swai, the several hundred Ugandans and Tanzanians who were willing to speak of an often painful past, and those students, seminar and conference participants, and readers whose ideas and criticisms have enriched this work.

I should also thank those institutions which enabled me to conduct my research in Tanzania and Uganda, COSTECH, UNCST, the Red Cross, the Ministries of Health, and the local administrations.

I have benefited greatly from the assistance of administrative and archival staff who enabled me to consult the records held at the African Studies Centre, Cambridge; British Library, London; Bukoba Roman Catholic Parish Office; Cambridge University Library; Church Missionary Society Archive, Birmingham; Church of Uganda Archive, Mukono; Entebbe Secretariat Archives; Family Planning Association of Uganda, Kampala; Franciscan Missionary Sisters Archive, Dundalk; Kisubi Roman Catholic Parish Office; Kitagata Hospital Records Store; London School of Economics Archive; Makerere Institute of Social Research Library; Makerere University Library; Masaka Hospital Records Store; Mbarara Hospital Records Store; Mill Hill Missionaries Heritage Centre, Freshfield; Ministry of Health Library, Kampala; Mwanza Provincial Archives; National Archives, London; Nkokonjeru Hospital Record Store; Nsambya Hospital Records Store; Nyamitanga Roman Catholic Parish Office; Rhodes House, Oxford; Royal Commonwealth Society Archive, Cambridge; Rubaga Archives, Kampala; Sir Albert Cook Archive, Mulago; SOAS Archive, London; Tanzania National

Archives, Dar Es Salaam; University of Dar Es Salaam; Wellcome Archive, London; White Fathers Archive, Rome; and the Women's Library, London.

This research could not have been completed without the funding provided by the following organizations: the Arts and Humanities Research Council, the British Academy, the British Institute in Eastern Africa, and the Economic and Social Research Council. I am also extremely appreciative of the support and patience of a number of individuals involved in the British Academy and Oxford University Press's Postdoctoral Fellowship Monographs Series.

Most of all, I am grateful to Emma for her research in Buhaya, for her patience during the long process of writing, and for our two children, George and Leah.

Acronyms

AIDS	Acquired immune deficiency syndrome
CBR	Crude birth rate
CDR	Crude death rate
CMS	Church Missionary Society
EAMS	East African Medical Survey
ESA	Entebbe Secretariat Archives
FGD	Focus group discussion
HIV	Human immunodeficiency virus
IMR	Infant mortality rate
NA	National Archives
RAMC	Royal Army Medical Corps
RHO	Rhodes House Oxford
STD	Sexually transmitted disease
TFR	Total fertility rate
TNA	Tanzania National Archives
VD	Venereal disease
WFA	White Fathers Archive

Glossary

Bakama	Buhaya's kings
Balokole	Born-again Christians
Bisisi	A Haya custom which secured paternity rights for the first man to have sex with a woman after she had given birth
Genitor	Biological father
Grandmultipara	A woman who has given birth five or more times
Hima	Pastoralist
Kabaka	Buganda's king
Kwashiorkor	Protein-energy malnutrition
Mukama	A Haya king
Parity	The number of term births
Pater	Socially acknowledged father
Primipara	A woman giving birth for the first time

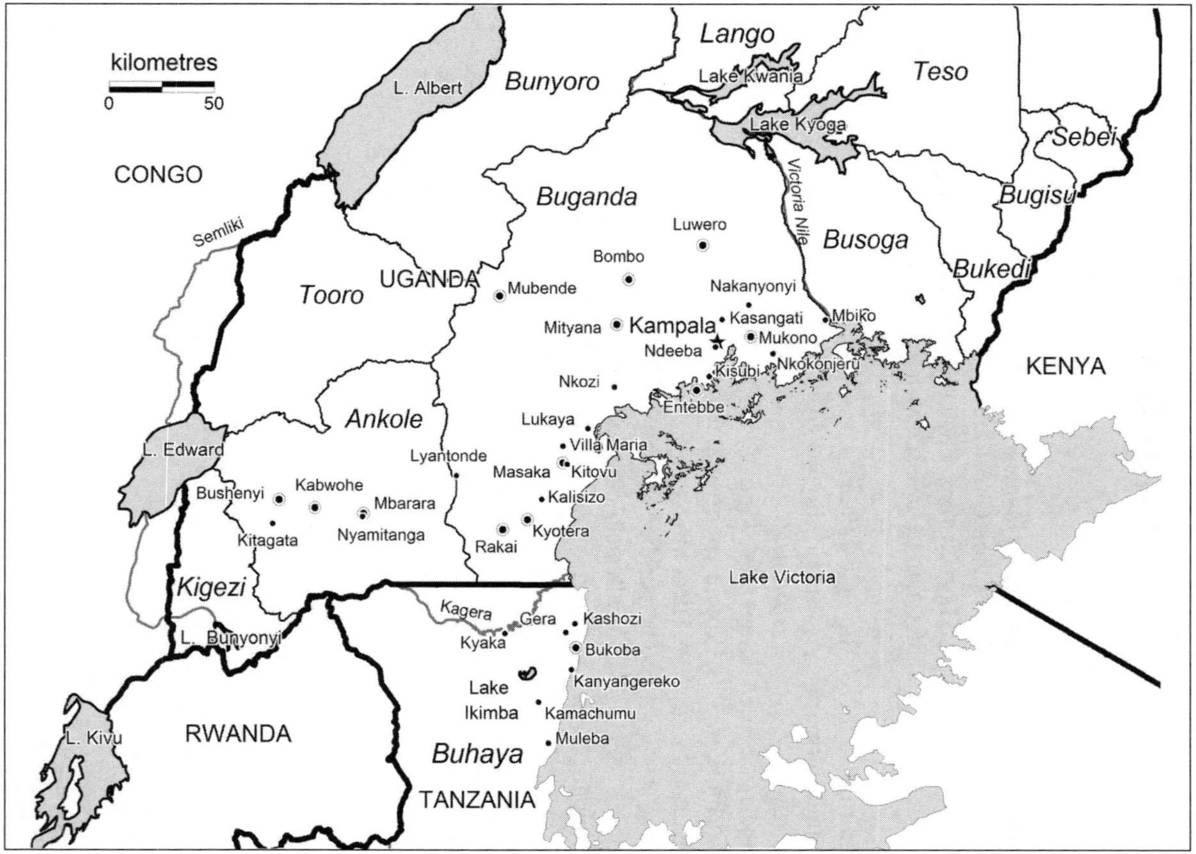

Map 1 Place names

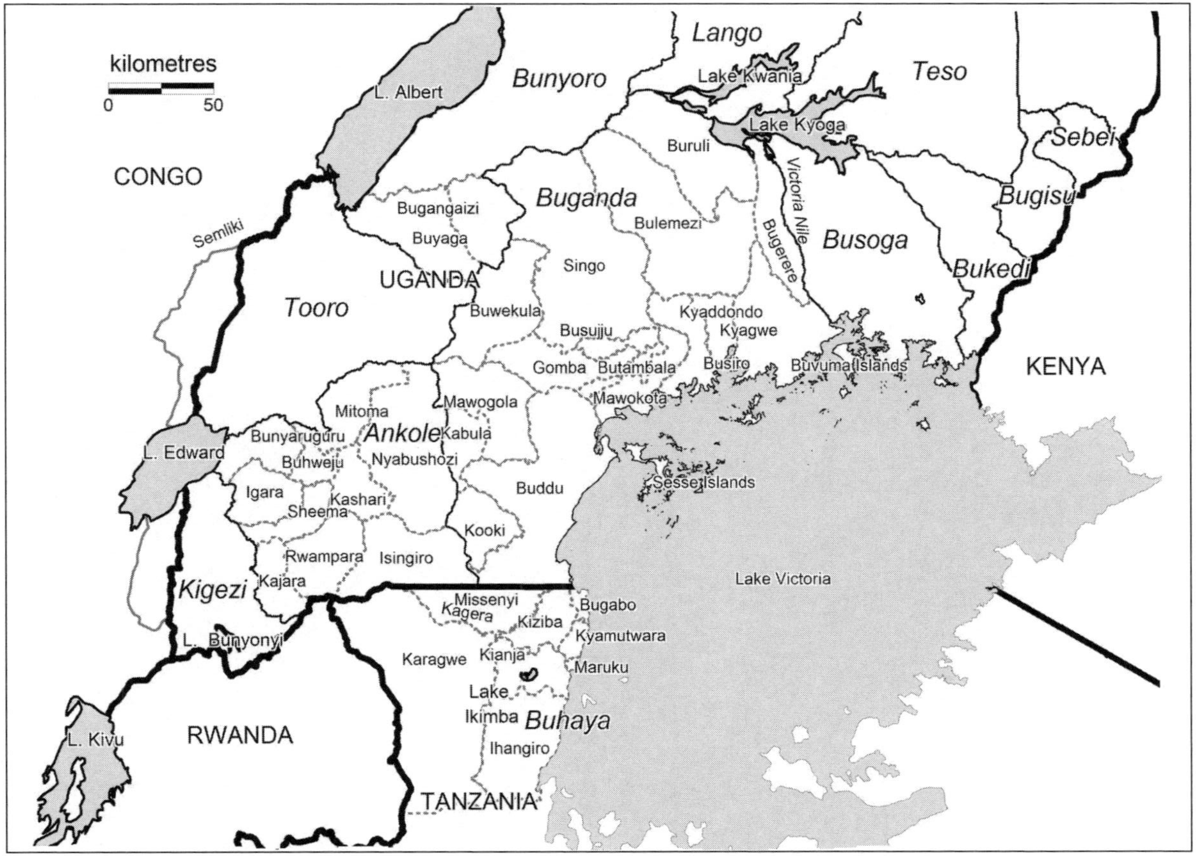

Map 2 Counties and kingdoms

Introduction

THE DEMOGRAPHIC CONTEXT

The scale and rapidity of demographic change in modern Africa is unprecedented in recorded history. The period of conquest towards the end of the nineteenth century brought famine, new diseases, and disruption, so that in the extreme case of the Congo Free State, for example, the population may have halved in a few decades.[1] Given the context of Africa's already low population densities, this was a disastrous introduction to colonial rule. Yet over the course of the twentieth century the estimated total population of the continent increased by around 600%. From the Second World War a sharp rise in birth rates culminated in Kenyan women achieving a remarkable total fertility rate of 8.1 live births in 1980, while death rates declined just as rapidly. Under-five mortality rates in Kenya, for example, fell from 205 per 1,000 in 1960 to 97 per 1,000 in 1990. Towards the end of the century though both fertility and mortality trends underwent a major reversal across much of the continent. Botswana's total fertility rate halved between 1981 and 2001, while AIDS-related mortality caused life expectancy at birth in that country, which had risen from 46 years in 1955 to 65 in 1990, to fall back to 34 by 2005.[2]

The overall experience of immense population growth over the past century conceals many complexities. The causes of much of this change are poorly understood, partly because of the generally poor quality of demographic data, and partly because of the localism of population change. National-level surveys are of great importance in demonstrating how much populations have increased or declined in Africa, but they are not always so useful in helping explain why dramatic changes in fertility or mortality patterns have occurred. It is necessary to shift the focus of analysis to a much lower level to achieve such an understanding, because of the extreme internal heterogeneity of most African countries. Uganda, a country the size of the United Kingdom or Oregon, is made up of fifty-six different indigenous

[1] J. Iliffe, *Africans: the History of a Continent* (Cambridge: Cambridge University Press, 2nd edn, 2007), p. 218.

[2] http://www. unicef. org/sowc03/tables/table9.html; P. Nair, 'Population aging in Botswana: Trends and implications', *Journal of African Studies and Development*, 2, 3 (2010), pp. 58–64; http://www.unicef.org/infobycountry/botswana_statistics.html

ethnic groups.[3] Tanzania, with a territory four times as large, possesses 126.[4] Urbanization, communications, healthcare provision, economic structure, income, education, soil quality, and rainfall vary tremendously from district to district across most African countries. There exists often as much variation in fertility and mortality patterns within countries in contemporary Africa, as there is between different nations. Thus between 1982 and 1995 children from the largest ethnic group in Uganda, the Ganda, were 36.5% less likely to die before the age of five than non-Baganda.[5] Meanwhile, the total fertility of women living in the Ugandan capital Kampala, was less than half that of women from northern districts in 2006, due to the unevenness of fertility decline.[6]

Therefore this study has chosen to focus on three neighbouring societies within the East African Great Lakes region: Ankole,[7] Buganda, and Buhaya,[8] which were historically home to the Nkole,[9] Ganda, and Haya ethnic groups. These societies were selected because of their large size and historical importance, because they were demographically so unusual, and because they shared key geographical and cultural characteristics. Their languages are to varying degrees mutually intelligible; their social relationships have all been shaped by a history of monarchical government; their indigenous religions were based on similar core beliefs and structures; and all three societies have been heavily Christianized over the past century. Methodologically, it seemed best to attempt to explain variations in patterns of sexuality, reproduction, and disease by comparing areas that are culturally and physically alike. That Ankole's population grew by natural increase so much faster than Buganda and Buhaya's during the twentieth century cannot be simply explained by reference to some overriding cultural difference, such as the presence or

[3] As defined by the 1995 Constitution.

[4] East African High Commission, *General African Census, August 1957, Tribal Analysis: Tanganyika* (Nairobi: Government Printer, 1958).

[5] M. Brockerhoff and P. Hewett, 'Inequality of child mortality among ethnic groups in sub-Saharan Africa', *Bulletin of the World Health Organization*, 78, 1 (2000), p. 35. Mortality differentials by ethnicity were even more extreme in Kenya.

[6] Uganda Bureau of Statistics and Macro International Inc., *Uganda Demographic and Health Survey 2006* (Calverton, MD: Macro Int., 2007), p. 52.

[7] The colonial era kingdom of Ankole was created by the amalgamation of the large pre-colonial kingdom of Nkore with a number of smaller polities to the west, which had previously enjoyed varying degrees of independence.

[8] Buhaya consisted in the colonial period of a number of small kingdoms, of which the best known are Karagwe, Kiziba, and Kyamutwara, whose populations were ethnically almost identical.

[9] The Nkole are made up of two sub-groups, the pastoralist Hima, who constituted a small minority of the total population but were nonetheless politically dominant until the era of decolonization, and the agriculturalist majority, known to the Hima by the derogatory term, Iru.

absence of circumcision. It is the fundamental cultural similarity of these societies that makes their demographic divergence so interesting.

The origins of this book lay in my earlier study of Bunyoro, a kingdom situated to the north of Buganda and Ankole, which set out to identify the causes of that society's prolonged population decline during the colonial period.[10] It found that Bunyoro's experience was so extreme that the wider relevance of the case study at first seemed relatively limited. The kingdom suffered repeated invasions by its pre-colonial neighbours, an exceptionally prolonged and destructive war of imperial conquest, discrimination, and then a degree of neglect by the colonial administration, extreme social inequality, radical changes to its disease environment, the near-eradication of its livestock economy, some of the highest divorce rates ever recorded, and the worst nutritional problems in Uganda. Bunyoro did benefit from a high level of cash wealth and medical provision from the 1930s, but still it had endured such a depressing series of misfortunes that it was in the end surprising that its population had not reduced more than it actually did. In fact what was most interesting about Bunyoro's population decline was the realization that this experience seemed to be part of a wider demographic pattern across the entire Great Lakes region. From Bulega in the eastern Congo across to Teso in eastern Uganda and then southwards through Buganda to Buhaya at the southwest of Lake Victoria, a large swathe of East Africa experienced relatively high mortality and unusually low fertility until the last years of colonial rule.

The demographic history of the Great Lakes region of East Africa during the colonial period is striking because this group of societies whose population declined, stagnated or grew slowly neighboured other societies which were experiencing extremely fast rates of demographic increase. Such sharp, localized variations in demographic experience are not exceptional in human history,[11] but the degree of the difference is remarkable. According to census figures, between 1911 and 1959 the numbers of Nyoro in Uganda fell by 10%, while the number of Kiga trebled.[12]

What is most significant though is that the demographic experience of this region does not fit neatly within either of the dominant models, which try

[10] S. Doyle, *Crisis and Decline in Bunyoro: Population and Environment in Western Uganda 1860–1955* (Oxford: James Currey, 2006).

[11] e.g. J. Knodel, *Demographic Behaviour in the Past: a Study of Fourteen German Village Populations in the Eighteenth and Nineteenth Centuries* (Cambridge: Cambridge University Press, 1988); A. Retel-Laurentin, *Un pays à la dérive: une société en régression démographique. Les Nzakara de l'est centrafricain* (Paris: Delarge, 1979).

[12] Uganda Protectorate, *Report on the 1911 Census of the Population of Uganda* (Entebbe: Government Printer, 1912); East African Statistical Department, *Uganda Census 1959* (Nairobi: Government Printer, 1961).

to explain why Africa began to experience dramatic population growth from the 1920s. One school of thought, led by Dennis Cordell and Joel Gregory, argues that colonialism's greatest impact was on fertility, which is thought to have increased as periods of post-partum sexual abstinence and breastfeeding shortened.[13] It is assumed that the reduction of birth intervals occurred earliest where the colonial impact was greatest, among peoples that were most involved in the commercial economy and that enjoyed the best educational, maternal, and child healthcare facilities. Bogumil Jewsiewicki, Gavin Kitching, and Kenneth Swindell, moreover, have suggested that colonial labour demands and cash cropping encouraged earlier marriage and pressured parents to expand the domestic labour supply by increasing the number of children they produced.[14]

This analysis is disputed by scholars such as John Iliffe and Jack Caldwell, who note that there has been little evidence to date of an increase in fertility before the Second World War and therefore place most emphasis on changes in mortality patterns as the driver of demographic growth. They argue that death rates declined from the 1920s due to the wealth derived from newly introduced cash crops, new networks of roads and railways, and the diffusion of western medicine, maternity facilities, missionary activity, and primary education. In their opinion, African fertility had always been relatively high because of an unusually strong demand for human agricultural labour, 'traditional religious pronatalism', and a 'horror of barrenness'.[15] They believe that fertility did increase during the colonial period, but only in its later years, after population growth had already begun. The cause of this later rise in fertility is hypothesized to be a shortening of the durations of post-partum sexual abstinence and lactation after the Second World War related to improving child survival rates, and the spread of Christianity and female education.[16]

[13] D. Cordell and J. Gregory, *African Population and Capitalism: Historical Perspectives* (Boulder, CO: Westview, 1987).

[14] B. Jewsiewicki, 'Towards a historical sociology of population in Zaire: Proposals for the analysis of the demographic regime', in Cordell and Gregory, *African Population*, p. 276; G. Kitching, 'Proto-industrialisation and demographic change: A thesis and some possible African implications', *Journal of African History*, 24, 2 (1983), pp. 229–30; K. Swindell, 'Domestic production, labour mobility and population change in West Africa, 1900–80', in C. Fyfe and D. McMaster (eds), *African Historical Demography, II* (Edinburgh: Centre of African Studies, 1981), pp. 675–83. The influence of E. Wrigley and R. Schofield's *The Population History of England 1541–1871: a Reconstruction* (Cambridge: Cambridge University Press, 1981) is clear.

[15] J. Caldwell, 'The social repercussions of colonial rule: demographic aspects', in A. Adu Boahen (ed.), *UNESCO General History of Africa, VII* (London: UNESCO, 1985), pp. 458, 476–80; Iliffe, *Africans*, pp. 248–52; P. Vimard, 'The decrease in infant mortality on the Dayes plateau, 1930–76' in Fyfe and McMaster, *African Historical Demography II*, pp. 763–70.

[16] R. Lesthaeghe, H. Page and O. Adegbola, 'Child spacing and fertility in Lagos', in H. Page and R. Lesthaeghe (eds.), *Child-spacing in Tropical Africa: Traditions and Change* (London: Heinemann, 1981), p. 163.

Within these opposing points of view there is a large measure of agreement, which is that changes associated with development and modernization, in their various guises, triggered the rapid transition to spectacular demographic increase in twentieth-century Africa. A number of examples from across Africa, the Kikuyu of Kenya, the Chagga of Tanganyika, Salisbury in Southern Rhodesia, Katanga in the Congo, support this correlation. Even in western equatorial Africa, where fertility was significantly lower than the continental average, population growth began earliest in areas of greatest economic and social development.[17]

The experience of the Great Lakes region of East Africa was very different. Areas such as Buganda and Buhaya experienced population decline or only delayed and then slow growth by natural increase, despite having some of the wealthiest populations in colonial Africa, and unusually well-developed administrative, medical, missionary, and educational systems from an early date. Meanwhile districts such as Ankole, which were relatively neglected by the colonial state and whose populations were cash poor, experienced some of the fastest rates of demographic increase ever recorded in human history.[18]

The extent of this demographic divergence, however, began to reduce as the colonial era drew to a close. In the middle of the twentieth century Buganda and then Buhaya experienced a sharp decline in mortality levels, and then a remarkable surge in fertility rates occurred in both societies. If the unexpected delay in the onset of significant population growth is the most intellectually interesting aspect of Buganda and Buhaya's modern demographic history, then the rapidity of the rise in these societies' fertility rates during the 1960s is the most dramatic. But the most original finding of this study is the decline in fertility among Ganda living around the city of Kampala from the mid-1970s. In sub-Saharan Africa around this time fertility levels were only beginning to fall in the most advanced and prosperous societies, first in South Africa, and subsequently in southern Nigeria, southern Ghana, Zimbabwe, Botswana, and Kenya. The decision to limit family size in these areas was influenced by factors such as reductions in the risk of child mortality, high levels of female education, and improving reproductive healthcare. But parental reproductive strategies were also affected by the rising cost of schooling and medical attention, as well as the practical difficulties of bringing up a

[17] Iliffe, *Africans*, pp. 248–52.

[18] East African Statistical Department, *African Population of the Uganda Protectorate 1948: Geographical and Tribal Studies* (Nairobi: Government Printer, 1950); East African Statistical Department, *African Population of Tanganyika Territory 1948: Geographical and Tribal Studies* (Nairobi: Government Printer, 1950); East African Statistical Department, *Uganda Census 1959*; East African High Commission, *Tribal Analysis: Tanganyika 1957*.

large family in an urbanizing, career-focused world.[19] So the onset of fertility decline in these latter African societies was not entirely a product of benign development. But nowhere else in Africa did fertility decline begin in such unpromising conditions as central Buganda during Idi Amin's military dictatorship and Milton Obote's second term in office. Around Kampala fertility started to fall in a context of collapsing living standards, extreme political and physical insecurity, and worsening health and educational services. This final episode in the region's demographic history before the emergence of AIDS reinforces the central argument of this study, that the relationship between demographic change and processes associated with modernization and development in Africa is more complex than has hitherto been assumed.

From its rise to prominence as an academic discipline in the 1930s and 1940s, demography was shaped by theoretical concepts which relied on an evolutionary idea of progress. As the cold war intensified, a global model of demographic change was developed which predicted a series of transitions in population behaviour which would be triggered by definable improvements in economic structure, welfare provision, and technology, all of which were regarded as indicators of modernization. By the late 1960s this consensus began to break down, but, as Simon Szreter has argued, the growing influence of the family planning industry around the world sustained the association between modernization and fertility limitation in the decades that followed.[20] Demographic theory has subsequently shifted away from grand narratives of change, to consider factors such as wealth flows within the household and women's status.[21] Yet as Susan Greenhalgh has observed, this new interest in local cultures and systems is still limited by a focus on structures and the belief that reproduction is driven by timeless, rational, maximizing strategies.[22]

In the region studied for this book, the timing and direction of demographic change have not been predictable, and cannot be easily explained by external models. But this does not mean that none of the processes and concepts associated with modernization were ever of any relevance. Instead the aim of this research has been to examine how and why specific external changes have affected fertility and mortality patterns at particular points in

[19] J. Caldwell, I. Orubuloye, and P. Caldwell, 'Fertility decline in Africa: A new type of transition?', *Population and Development Review*, 18, 2 (1992), pp. 211–42.

[20] S. Szreter, 'The idea of demographic transition and the study of fertility change: A critical intellectual history', *Population and Development Review*, 19, 4 (1993), pp. 685–6.

[21] e.g. J. Caldwell, *Theory of Fertility Decline* (London: Academic Press, 1982); and K. Mason, *The Status of Women: A Review of its Relationships to Fertility and Mortality* (New York: Rockefeller, 1984).

[22] S. Greenhalgh, 'Anthropology theorizes reproduction: Integrating practice, political economic, and feminist perspectives', in S. Greenhalgh (ed.), *Situating Fertility: Anthropology and Demographic Inquiry* (Cambridge: Cambridge University Press, 1995), pp. 19–22.

time. These case studies show that modernizing forces such as the commercialization of agriculture or female education could have contradictory consequences for demographic trends.[23] In part this complexity related to the extent to which modernizing concepts were hybridized and indigenized. Individuals' life stories help explain the often unexpected outcomes of modernizing change because they reveal how some behaviours and beliefs that Ugandans and Tanzanians regarded as entirely modern would not have been recognized as such by contemporary demographers. External ideas were adapted and vernacularized by individuals trying to satisfy old family commitments and social expectations as well as new personal ambitions. People in this region had varying notions of what modernity entailed, and reproductive decisions were not always based on rationality, or were affected by competing strategies of rational self-advancement. Sexual desire, the multiple means by which status could be achieved, and a desire for personal autonomy were just some of the factors which make it necessary to think of fertility in terms of personal agency and ambivalence, and local variation more than macro-theory.

These evolving attitudes and practices shaped the operation of what are known as the proximate determinants of fertility in these societies.[24] The proximate determinants are those fundamental variables, such as the prevalence of contraception or duration of post-partum abstinence, through which behavioural and biological factors function to produce a society's fertility rate. This study will show how different proximate determinants were of greater or lesser significance in different periods, with for example the proportion of women of reproductive age in a stable union and the rate of pathological sterility both falling over time in Buganda. Quantifying the impact of the various proximate determinants is of crucial importance, but the more interesting questions relate to the causes of change within the biological and behavioural context through which the determinants acted.

SEXUALITY AND THE PRE-HISTORY OF HIV

This region's demographic history is significant not just because it will permit a re-evaluation of the origins of Africa's transition to rapid population

[23] While the potential for such contradictory outcomes has long been recognized, attempts to evaluate the impact of a range of external factors have typically focused only on the post-colonial period. Cf. J. Bongaarts, O. Frank, and R. Lesthaeghe, 'The proximate determinants of fertility in sub-Saharan Africa', *Population and Development Review*, 10, 3 (1984), p. 516; R. Lesthaeghe, 'Fertility and its proximate determinants in sub-Saharan Africa: The record of the 1960s and 1970s' (Interuniversity Program in Demography, Working Paper 1984, Vrije Universiteit Brussels, Belgium).

growth. The border between Buhaya and Buganda was the site of the world's first mass rural HIV epidemic. It was here that the disease revealed its capacity to expand rapidly beyond urban sexual networks, an ability that would transform the epidemic in Africa from a crisis to a catastrophe. HIV's emergence as a mass pandemic among a generally heterosexual, non-drug-injecting population has inevitably prompted researchers to ask what was peculiar about Africa in general, and Buganda and Buhaya in particular.

Most researchers have tried to identify key changes that occurred in the 1970s and which could have provided the crucial multiplier effect enabling HIV to become more than just a series of isolated, low-level epidemics. Some of the continent-wide developments that have been emphasized are the growth of urban centres after independence, combined with the increase in unemployment and female poverty after the 1973 oil crisis. In Uganda and Tanzania economic decline took an extreme form from the mid-1970s as a result of Idi Amin's expulsion of the Asian community and Julius Nyerere's villagization programme. Settlements sprang up along the international frontier and the shores of Lake Victoria, where quick money derived from a huge expansion in cross-border black-market trading created an ideal context for rapid sexual partner exchange. An alternative accelerator took the form of the social destabilization, rape, and commercial sex work associated with the Uganda–Tanzania war of 1978–9.[25]

Another hypothesis is that Africa was particularly vulnerable to AIDS because the continent has a unique sexual tradition or inherited pattern of sexual behaviour, which established an enduring culture of frequent partner exchange. The leading proponents of this position are the demographers, Jack and Pat Caldwell and Pat Quiggan, whose main thesis is that African family life has historically centred on the extension and multiplication of the lineage. Given Africa's consistently high levels of mortality, social pressure therefore focused on maximizing fertility, which meant condoning pre-marital and extra-marital affairs. The logic of this line of thought is that traditional African sexual behavioural norms would facilitate the rapid spread of any sexually transmitted disease (STD), including AIDS.[26]

[24] Cf. J. Bongaarts and J. Potter, *Fertility, Biology and Behavior: An Analysis of the Proximate Determinants* (New York: Academic Press, 1983).

[25] e.g. F. Kaijage, 'AIDS control and the burden of history in northwestern Tanzania', *Population and Environment*, 14 (1993), pp. 279–300; C. Obbo, 'HIV transmission through social and geographical networks in Uganda', *Social Science and Medicine*, 36, 1 (1993), pp. 949–55; J. Killewo, L. Dahlgren, and A. Sandström, 'Socio-geographical patterns of HIV-1 transmission in Kagera Region, Tanzania', *Social Science and Medicine*, 38, 1 (1994), pp. 129–34.

[26] J. Caldwell, P. Caldwell, and P. Quiggan, 'The social context of AIDS in sub-Saharan Africa', *Population and Development Review*, 15, 2 (1989), pp. 185–234.

This thesis has been criticized by a number of scholars who object to African sexual behaviour being described in terms that strengthen racist stereotypes about African promiscuity and immorality.[27] Caldwell, Caldwell, and Quiggan's argument though also seems to underestimate the diversity of sexual behaviour across pre-colonial Africa,[28] and ignores the evidence for the existence of heritable landed property in some East African societies.[29] Certainly in many Great Lakes societies, for example, pre-marital sexual activity, particularly among girls, was not condoned in the past. Most fundamentally, the assumption that an ancient African sexual tradition has survived largely intact despite the changes wrought by colonialism, capitalism, and mass conversion to world religions, and that this explains the rapidity of the spread of HIV across modern Africa, is problematic.[30] Jack Caldwell subsequently refined his approach, his main concession to sexual diversity being to separate Africa into circumcizing and non-circumcizing societies, while a new emphasis on the twentieth-century emergence of commercial sex workers and STDs indicated his acceptance of the need to consider historical change.[31] Yet studies of the emergence of AIDS have demonstrated great variation in the nature and popularity of commercial sex work and in the prevalence of STDs across the continent.

A third major approach which tries to explain why Africa has suffered so severely from HIV has focused on the frequency with which Africans have engaged in sustained, concurrent sexual relationships. In recent years, major studies by Helen Epstein and Robert Thornton have argued that Africa's characteristically dense networks of interconnected concurrent sexual

[27] M.-N. Le Blanc, D. Meintel, and V. Piché, 'The African sexual system: Comment on Caldwell et al.', *Population and Development Review*, 17, 3 (1991), pp. 497–505; B. Ahlberg, 'Is there a distinct African sexuality? A critical response to Caldwell', *Africa*, 64, 2 (1994), pp. 220–42; S. Heald, 'The power of sex: Some reflections on the Caldwells' "African sexuality" thesis', *Africa*, 65, 4 (1995), pp. 489–505.

[28] It also overestimates the uniformity of Eurasian sexual cultures. The extreme sexual austerity of the west of Ireland fits the Eurasian model well. J. Messenger, 'Sex and repression in an Irish folk community', in D. Marshall and R. Suggs (eds.), *Human Sexual Behavior: Variations in the ethnographic spectrum* (New York: Basic Books, 1970). Goody's model, however, does not explain why 57% of first births in Germany *c.*1830 were the result of pre-marital sex. Knodel, *Demographic Behaviour*, p. 450.

[29] See for example P. Reining, 'Haya land tenure: landholding and tenancy', *Anthropological Quarterly*, 35, 2, (1962), pp. 58–73; H. Cory and M. Hartnoll, *The Customary Law of the Haya Tribe, Tanganyika Territory* (London: Routledge, 1971 [1945]), p. 20.

[30] See Ahlberg, 'African sexuality', who criticises Quiggan and the Caldwells' ahistoricism, and argues that the high-risk sexual cultures of many modern African societies are the product of missionary Christianity which she believes weakened indigenous systems of moral control and generated sexual double standards, especially among the young.

[31] J. Caldwell, 'Rethinking the African AIDS epidemic', *Population and Development Review*, 26, 1 (2000), pp. 117–36.

partnerships tend to facilitate the transmission of HIV more than the serial monogamy which is so common in western societies, or even serial monogamy combined with occasional high-risk sex. This is because the average chance of HIV infection is low during any individual sex act, and because HIV is highly contagious in the weeks after infection has taken hold. Repeated sex with the same multiple partners maximizes the possibility of transmission, they believe.[32] Epstein asserts that Ugandans do not have more sexual partners over their lifetime than do people in western societies. Rather African vulnerability derived from the nature of their sexual networks, and the often transactional nature of sex, which she believes, fosters infidelity.[33] This thesis has attracted significant criticism, but merits serious consideration, in part because it has become highly influential within African AIDS control programmes.[34]

As this study will show, concurrent long-running relationships were indeed common in Ankole, Buganda, and Buhaya in the past. Over time their nature changed, as polygamy and socially legitimate extra-marital sex declined in acceptability, while, it seems, illegitimate affairs became more common, and often featured some form of material exchange. What the historical record adds is a nuanced sense of how sexual networks evolved and interrelated in the past. For example, Christine Obbo has shown how extensive was the web of sexual contacts within friendship groups maintained since secondary school or university. This was peer-to-peer sex, within income and age groups, with little sense of exploitation or economic pressure. But cross-class sex, it seems, was also common, at least in Buganda, where researchers in the 1960s were struck by how men from all ethnic groups and social classes drank in the same bars, and, often, slept with the same women. Sexual networks, moreover, also appear to have crossed generations with increasing frequency as the twentieth century progressed. But the sexual history of these societies requires a more radical rethinking of the concurrency thesis on two grounds. The first is that a series of surveys between the 1960s and 1980s emphasized that people in this region had a very large number of

[32] H. Epstein, *The Invisible Cure: Africa, The West and the Fight against AIDS* (London: Viking, 2007); R. Thornton, *Unimagined Community: Sex, Networks and AIDS in Uganda and South Africa* (Berkeley: University of California Press, 2008); M. Morris and M. Kretzschmar, 'Concurrent partnerships and the spread of HIV', *AIDS*, 11 (1997), pp. 641–48. See also D. Halperin and H. Epstein, 'Concurrent sexual partnerships help to explain Africa's high HIV prevalence: implications for prevention', *Lancet*, 364, 9428 (2004), pp. 4–6; T. Mah and D. Halperin 'Concurrent sexual partnerships and the HIV epidemics in Africa: evidence to move forward', *AIDS and Behavior,* 14 (2010), pp. 11–14.

[33] Epstein, *Invisible Cure*, pp. 54–79, 159–61, 173–96.

[34] Most powerfully L. Sawers and E. Stillwaggon, 'Concurrent sexual partnerships do not explain the HIV epidemics in Africa: A systematic review of the evidence', *Journal of the International AIDS Society,* 13 (2010), 34.

sexual partners on average, before behaviour changed in response to AIDS. The second is that evidence from the 1950s onwards indicated that a very large proportion of local populations engaged in short-term sexual encounters, and that for some individuals casual or purchased sex occurred with remarkable frequency.[35]

The work of the Caldwells, Quiggan, Epstein, and Thornton has been important in prioritizing the role of sexual behaviour in the spread of HIV, but it demonstrates above all the need for local historical research into sexual behavioural diversity and change. Within the Great Lakes region, the AIDS crisis has led a number of scholars to undertake significant research into the history of sexual behaviour and STDs. All were drawn by the striking parallels between the two STD crises that had started and ended the twentieth century, early colonial syphilis and post-colonial HIV. These studies concentrated primarily on the disputes about the problematic diagnosis of STDs before the 1930s and the unmistakable racism and sexism of early colonial discourse.[36] Writers such as Megan Vaughan, Maryinez Lyons, and Carol Summers, for example, have focused on early colonial European and chiefly concerns about female sexuality being unleashed by the unexpected consequences of Christianity, the commercial economy, or new legal protections.[37] With the exception of an important recent article by Jan Kuhanen,

[35] C. Obbo, 'HIV transmission through social and geographical networks in Uganda', *Social Science and Medicine*, 36, 1 (1993), pp. 949–55; M. Robbins and R. Pollnac, 'Drinking patterns and acculturation in rural Buganda', *American Anthropologist*, 71, 2 (Apr., 1969), pp. 276–85; O. Arya and F. Bennett, 'Attitudes of college students in East Africa to sexual activity and venereal disease', *British Journal of Venereal Disease*, 44 (1968), p. 163. For references to sexual behaviour surveys see Chapters 4, 7, 8 and 9. Whether the growing complexity of sexual behaviour also affected same-sex relationships was impossible to discover. Oral informants spoke only of vaginal sex. Survey data from the period covered by this book made no mention of homosexuality. What court case records have survived indicate that convictions for sodomy were extremely infrequent during the colonial period, though whether this indicates social tolerance, effective concealment, or the rarity of homosexual acts is uncertain. Some sources suggest that homosexuality at court and in boarding school at least was relatively common. Cf. List of saza level cases, File 23, PPMS38/Perlman/Box 8, SOAS archive; H. Médard, 'L'homosexualité au Buganda, une acculturation peut en cacher une autre', *Hypothèse*, 1 (1999), pp. 47–52; S. Nannyonga-Tamusuza, *Baakisimba: Gender in the Music and Dance of the Baganda People of Uganda* (New York: Routledge, 2005); C. Summers, '"Subterranean evil" and "tumultuous riot" in Buganda: Authority and alienation at King's College, Budo, 1942', *The Journal of African History*, 47, 1 (2006), pp 93–113.

[36] For the problems of misdiagnosis, see M. Tuck, 'Syphilis, sexuality, and social control: A history of venereal disease in colonial Uganda' (unpublished PhD dissertation, Northwestern University, 1997).

[37] M. Vaughan, *Curing Their Ills: Colonial Power and African Illness* (Cambridge: Polity Press, 1991); M. Lyons, 'Medicine and morality: a review of responses to sexually transmitted diseases in Uganda in the twentieth century', in M. Lyons, M. Lewis, and P. Setel (eds.), *Histories of Sexually Transmitted Diseases and HIV/AIDS in Sub-Saharan Africa* (London: Greenwood, 1999), p. 97; C. Summers, 'Intimate colonialism: The imperial production of reproduction in Uganda, 1907–1925', *Signs*, 16, 4 (1991), pp. 787–807.

little attention, by contrast, has been paid to sexuality between the 1940s and 1960s in the Great Lakes Region, yet the evidence collected for this study indicates that this era of transition from imperial over-rule to independence was the period when the patterns of behaviour which would facilitate the rapid spread of HIV decades later most clearly took shape.[38] Moreover, European discussions of sexuality, looking at the archival sources for the colonial period as a whole, were on balance more concerned with male than female sexuality.[39] And within this male-focused discourse, there was a marked change in generational focus after the Second World War. Before 1945 European commentators were as likely to blame male elders as youths for what was believed to be the high prevalence of STDs in Buganda and Buhaya. Older men were frequently condemned for their predatory and materialistic sexual instincts. Either they were aggressively seeking to acquire young women as junior or replacement wives, in a way which many Europeans regarded as improper, or they were selfishly inflating bridewealth, making it increasingly difficult for young people to marry each other, or they were delaying passing on their wealth to their sons, which encouraged young men to live a life of dissipation.[40] After 1945, Europeans' underlying concern remained focused on the difficulty in effecting real progress in these societies, but the limited success of the new development plans was blamed primarily on young males, who were seen more and more as a socially disruptive influence and as wasting the new economic opportunities available to them. Thus, in Buhaya young men were described as suffering from education and easy money, which were squandered on alcohol and sex workers (see Chapter 5).

African chiefly hierarchies' policies which aimed at controlling sexual misbehaviour, meanwhile, were not invariably misogynistic. Local government laws were drawn up in Buganda and Buhaya which aimed not only at preventing women from travelling without a male escort, or living alone in towns, but also at punishing men who impregnated unmarried women. The enforcement of such laws by indigenous authorities was equally mixed in its

[38] J. Kuhanen, 'Sexualised space, sexual networking and the emergence of AIDS in Rakai, Uganda', *Health and Place*, 16, 2 (2010), pp. 226–35. Other, broader studies which devote significant attention to sexual change in the decades leading up to the pandemic include A. Barnett and A. Whiteside, *AIDS in the Twenty-First Century: Disease and Globalization* (Basingstoke: Palgrave, 2002); and J. Pepin, *The Origins of AIDS* (Cambridge: Cambridge University Press, 2011).

[39] See for example V. Berry (ed.), *The Culwick Papers, 1934–1944: Population, Food and Health in Colonial Tanganika* (London: Academic Books, 1994); Bukoba District Annual Report, 1947, Tanzania National Archives [TNA] 215/2154; H. Cory, 'The Haya tribe and the incidence of venereal disease', (unpublished typescript, 1949, University of Dar es Salaam Library).

[40] e.g. Berry, *Culwick Papers*; Dr. G. A. Macgregor, MO Bukoba, March 1942, 'The incidence of syphilis among ante-natal women attending Kagondo and Bukoba Hospitals' Maternity and Child Welfare centres', Bukoba District Book, TNA.

impact. Urban or migrant women suffered sporadic harassment by police, but little sustained obstruction, while local courts before the 1950s awarded large damages to very many women who accused their former husbands of infecting them with syphilis, and not infrequently granted custody of children to mothers rather than fathers.[41]

Oral histories tell an equally complex story.[42] Interviewees in Ankole, Buganda, and Buhaya reinforced early anthropological accounts which indicate significant local variation in pre-colonial sexual behaviour and attitudes. When the subject of AIDS was raised, however, there was a remarkable similarity in the stories told by these elders. There existed an almost universal tendency among the elderly in each of the three societies to initially blame the rise of HIV on the changes of the 1970s, when a younger generation had engaged in what they perceived to be new, urban forms of socializing and alcohol consumption. But as they were questioned about these issues, informants from Buganda and Buhaya revealed that in fact these changes had started before the 1970s, that rural behavioural patterns had also changed, and that their own sexual behaviour was perhaps no safer than that of the following generation that was decimated by AIDS.[43] Such assertions of moral displeasure and superiority have been made in these latter societies for at least four generations, suggesting that patterns of behaviour have changed gradually over a century or more.

This book then addresses two issues of great significance, each of which could easily have been the subject of a full-length study on its own. But with such an artificial division much of the complex interplay of sexuality and demography in this region would have been lost. As population studies have become more technical, so they have grown increasingly distant from the other social sciences. Yet demography begins with sex. In the Great Lakes region of East Africa it is impossible to understand the anxiety and aggression with which sexuality was discussed and monitored without an appreciation of the degree of concern which existed about a perceived crisis of

[41] e.g. Cory, 'Venereal disease'; W. Laurie and H. Trant, *East African Medical Survey, Monograph no.2, A Health Survey in Bukoba District, Tanganyika* (Nairobi: Government Printer, 1954); Marriage files, Melvin Perlman papers, School of Oriental and African Studies Archive, GB 0102 PP MS 38; G. Kyomuhendo and M. McIntosh, *Women, Work and Domestic Virtue in Uganda, 1900–2003* (Oxford: James Currey, 2006), p. 70.

[42] Ethical approval for this project was received from the University of Leeds and the Tanzanian and Ugandan national research councils.

[43] e.g. 2000 Buhaya Ints. AK; 2004 Buganda FGDs 79 and 53, and Ints. 41 and 46. Cf. K. Stewart, 'Toward a historical perspective on sexuality in Uganda: The reproductive lifeline technique for grandmothers and their daughters', *Africa Today*, 47, 3/4 (2000), pp. 123–48. Kearsley Stewart's data show that the female age at sexual debut in Bunyoro was already low in the 1960s and 1970s at 16 years and declined only marginally to 15.4 years by the 1990s.

sub-fertility and excess mortality before 1960, and the new threat posed by birth control in the years after independence. Nor can the sharp increase in levels of fertility in Buganda during the middle decades of the twentieth century be analysed fully without an appreciation of the transformation of marriage and family life that facilitated a sharp increase in female pre- and post-marital sex. The interrelationship between sexuality and population change has become distressingly obvious in the age of AIDS, but it is an association that has been recognized in East Africa for more than a century.

CHAPTER SUMMARIES

The first chapter of this book addresses the debate about the universalist traditions of African sexuality directly, by examining what is known about the sexual behaviour of Ankole, Buganda, and Buhaya before colonial rule. It will demonstrate that while some similarities existed, this small geographical region was characterized in regard to sexuality and reproduction more by the diversity of its attitudes and practices in relation to pre-marital sexuality and pregnancy, wife-sharing, legitimate and illegitimate extra-marital sex, ritualized sex, the duration of breastfeeding, and ideal family size. These ethnic differences were shaped by locally distinct patterns of clanship, inheritance, marriage, and moral politics.

The second chapter attempts to explain the high levels of morbidity and mortality experienced in all three societies between 1860 and 1924, a period associated with severe famine, heightened conflict, and the introduction or emergence of new epidemic diseases. The intensification of long-distance trade from the 1860s had an uneven impact on the Great Lakes region. Buganda's attempt to dominate the new regional commerce ultimately contributed to her favoured political and economic status under British overrule, but at great demographic cost. Buhaya, located as she was on the main trade route from the East African coast, is likely to have also suffered population loss in this period due to contagion, famine, succession wars, and slave trading, though, with the possible exception of Karagwe, not on the scale of her larger neighbour. By contrast, with the exception of the great rinderpest cattle plague of the 1890s, Ankole's economic peripherality and political weakness seem to have protected her from the most destructive effects of the regional transformation of the late nineteenth century. The colonial takeover quickly reduced the incidence of war-related deaths, but in the first two decades of the twentieth century did little to affect the late-nineteenth-century pattern of mortality. In part this reflected the fixation with syphilis which dominated the early colonial health system, prompting the development of an unusually intensive, though ultimately ineffective, system of coercive monitoring and treatment. The tendency for new epidemics to affect Buganda more severely than the other case study areas was seen especially clearly with the regional outbreak of sleeping sickness. Early curative interventions had little impact on trypanosomiasis, but coercive disease control measures prevented new infections on a major scale, a pattern which was typical of colonial medicine before the 1920s. By that point though the colonial state had begun to exert a degree of control over crisis mortality. This process is exceptionally well documented in Buganda, where early hospital data appear to corroborate the trends revealed in vital registration records, indicating that child survival had improved significantly by the early 1920s, due to a rise in birthweight, investment in sanitation, and the cumulative impact of mass inoculation campaigns against major epidemic diseases. Buganda led the way in the prevention of crisis mortality, but its example was quickly replicated in Ankole and Buhaya. By the mid-1920s medical data on cause of death revealed the emerging dominance of endemic diseases, a pattern that would survive, with some variation, until the emergence of AIDS.

Chapter 3 will examine why Buganda and Buhaya's population crisis was regarded by European observers as resulting much more from sub-fertility rather than excess mortality. This perception provoked a series of interventions aimed at reforming marriage, gender relations, and sexual behaviour, and so curbing syphilis, the presumed cause of these societies' low birth rates and high miscarriage and stillbirth rates. Rather than constituting a hegemonic programme of patriarchal control, in policy and practice there existed significant differences between colonial state, chiefs, and missionaries; men were the subject of moral criticism almost as much as women; and reforms were marked above all by ambiguity and inconsistency. In Buganda, for example, the codification of customary law on marriage attempted to impose an ideal as a norm, and tension between indigenous and colonial legal principles ultimately undermined the institution that each aimed to support. The actions of church and state may have lacked coherence, but the early twentieth century was nonetheless defined by conservative concerns about the role of urbanization, the cash economy, Christianity, and the legal protection of women's rights in discouraging the young from marrying and undermining sexual restraint. Moreover, in Ankole, where the forces of modernization were much less developed, it seems that the chiefly hierarchy was relatively successful in its attempt to stabilize marriage and maximize fertility.

The next three chapters will examine how sexual behaviour and attitudes changed to a much greater extent in Buganda and Buhaya than in Ankole between the late 1920s and the 1960s. The transformation in Ganda and Haya sexuality derived primarily from these societies' rapid development of cash crop economies. This created a regional economic system which survived largely intact until the 1960s, in which temporary migrants from newly peripheralized societies like Ankole satisfied the seasonal surges in demand for labour around Lake Victoria. But cash cropping increased domestic workloads as well, a burden that was largely borne by wives, while husbands retained most of the profits. Generational as well as gender stresses were heightened by cash cropping. As the value of female labour increased, so did the amount of bridewealth demanded by parents. High divorce rates and, for some, delayed marriage were the most obvious results. Such tensions and outcomes were relatively common across Africa. However, the responses to these problems in Buganda and Buhaya were atypical in their detail, reflecting each society's particular history.

Chapter 4 discusses how in Buganda it was the relative openness of mid-colonial society that facilitated a loosening of sexual constraints. New opportunities for women to leave their husbands and set themselves up as independent householders accompanied the reform of tenancy regulations and the gradual development of towns and small trading centres. Widows enjoyed greater sexual freedom as colonial protection enabled many bereaved women to live on alone in their marital homes. While fewer Ganda women became professional sex workers than was the case in Buhaya, there developed a complex range of relationships, which varied subtly but importantly in terms of respectability, profitability, and duration. The overall trend was for sex to become increasingly commercialized over time, most explicitly in the bars and nightclubs which opened up in semi-urban settings throughout Buganda from the 1940s. These new forms of socializing provided Ganda of all ages with opportunities to acquire new sexual partners, increasingly across generations, fostered a growing tolerance of non-marital sex, and facilitated ever wider urban-rural sexual networks. The sexuality of the young changed fastest, due to the freedom from supervision that arose from schooling and parental employment, and the development of a new culture of adolescence, fuelled by western notions of dating, pre-marital experimentation, and marriage as a love match, and resentment at excessive bridewealth demands. It was during the middle decades of the twentieth century that the pattern of sexual behaviour that shaped the AIDS epidemic in Buganda mainly emerged.

Chapter 5 details how in Buhaya during the colonial period, the scarcity of land suitable for coffee farming enriched elders, delayed the establishment of new households by young men, and heightened further the pressure to secure an heir. Marriage was delayed and destabilized, sexual affairs grew increasingly commodified, and divorcees migrated in remarkably large numbers to East Africa's cities, where they dominated the region's sex trade, seeking to repay their bridewealth and then secure autonomy from spousal and paternal control. From the 1940s many of the women who returned from the cities continued to accept money for sex when they reentered village life. This early development of a rural network of sex workers was fuelled by local men's desire to access these women's make-up, gramophones, and bedsheets, the exotic luxuries of urban modernity. Meanwhile many of the changes in sexual culture seen in Buganda also affected Buhaya, though the sexuality of young unmarried women remained carefully controlled until near independence. These changes in behaviour unsurprisingly were the subject of repeated criticism and attempted regulation. The new sexual freedom undermined fathers and husbands' authority, diverted investment away from the land, added to the already heavy burden of court cases, embarrassed nationalist leaders, ancient and modern, and made a mockery of local churches' position as flagships of the Christianization of Africa. A consensus developed that modernity was to blame for the apparent decline in morality, but authorities disagreed on which aspect of modernity to emphasize. African political leaders tended to be the most inclusive, typically castigating the uncritical aping of western habits. Missionaries complained about a new materialism. Colonial officials worried about rising levels of education and prosperity. Few of the interventions that resulted had a lasting impact.

Chapter 6 explains why, compared to Buganda and Buhaya, sex and marriage in Ankole before the 1970s were characterized by stability and restraint. Local ethnic rivalry, a greater fear of violent repercussions, and the enduring power of ritual punishment ensured that extra-marital affairs were associated with danger and dishonour, and post- and, until the 1950s, pre-marital sex remained heavily regulated. As independence approached though mixed schooling and growing prosperity led to new kinds of social encounters, and the 1960s brought a major expansion of the road network and a slow spread of modern bars and dance clubs. Labour migration did introduce some changes in sexual behaviour, and integrated Ankole intimately with the Ganda, accelerating the openness and homogenization of sexual culture across the region. But economic migration seems to have destabilized marriage and systems of sexual control less than did cash crop farming, a surprising finding given the frequency with which labour migrants have been identified as the bearers of STDs to the African countryside over the past century.

Chapter 7 attempts to explain why the experience of these societies between 1925 and 1969 does not fit comfortably with existing explanations of the transition to higher fertility in modern Africa, all of which associate this development with particular aspects of modernization. Ankole's fertility increase occurred decades earlier than that of Buganda and Buhaya, yet colonial Ankole was a much poorer society, with inferior medical and educational services, and a far lower rate of conversion to Christianity. Much of its adult male population, moreover, was frequently absent due to labour migration. Buganda and Buhaya's higher level of reported STD prevalence only partly explains the apparent exceptionalism of this region. The evidence gathered for this study does not strongly support the neo-Marxist position that falling marriage age and heightened pressure for larger families stimulated the rise in colonial fertility. Neither cash cropping nor labour migration reduced male marriage ages, while female marriage age in Ankole and Buganda rose due to schooling and missionary pressure. An economic desire for increased family labour does seem to have reinforced Ankole's pre-existing pro-natalism, but in Buganda and Buhaya greater cash wealth enabled farmers to secure more immediate benefits by marrying extra wives or recruiting migrant labour. Much more important in Ankole and Buhaya was an increase in the proportion of women who were married, associated with a decline in the incidence of divorce, whereas in Buganda it was the increasing willingness of women to have children outside marriage that proved significant. Higher fertility seems to have been driven by an increase in the duration of women's reproductive lives, partly linked with changes associated with marriage but, more importantly, consequent on improvements in women's health, due to better maternal nutrition, the declining impact of STDs and post-partum infections on female fecundity due to penicillin, and a reduction in the reproductive damage associated with premature marriage. The final factor which was of major importance was the shortening of birth intervals, which began in Buganda in the 1920s, in Ankole in the 1930s, and Buhaya in the 1940s. The decline in birth spacing was the result of improving health, the shortening of the period of breastfeeding, due to female schooling and employment, and growing parental confidence in the likelihood of child survival.

As Chapter 8 shows, the basic trajectory of mortality change between 1925 and 1969 in this region is well known. Major epidemics and famines were largely contained by the mid-1920s, but high levels of endemic disease still caused severe mortality, particularly among the very young. Medical improvements after the Second World War offered new hope to victims of the most common diseases such as malaria. While mortality levels fell at different times for different age groups in the three case study areas, what is most surprising about the pattern of morbidity and mortality in this region is that life expectancy in Ankole seems to have improved as fast as in the other societies. Yet Buganda and Buhaya enjoyed huge advantages in terms of medical and educational provision, and cash income. The case of Ankole emphasizes the significance of livestock, relative equality, preventive medicine, and low levels of malaria in offsetting the demographic effects of cash poverty and peripherality in colonial Africa, while the examples of Buganda and Buhaya illustrate the negative consequences of modernization, especially for child health, in the form of high levels of divorce, fostering, and bottle-feeding. These societies were unusual also in that female education seems to have had less impact on child mortality rates than in many other areas. Paternal education was highly significant here, indicating that fathers played a central role in maintaining the health of their family. Moreover, it appears that where curative care, maternity and child welfare services, and health information were sufficiently ubiquitous, the children of poor and uneducated women benefited almost as much as those whose mothers were literate and wealthy. Finally, this chapter will argue that the tendency of the colonial state to focus its energies on discrete medical campaigns was less destructive in this region than has often been assumed. Pressure on women to give birth in hospital exposed them to periods of intense health education relating to hygiene and nutrition which impacted on subsequent infant and child mortality. Buhaya's STD campaign transformed the nature of rural healthcare, resulting in dramatic improvements in preventive medicine and the treatment of endemic complaints. The kwashiorkor scare in late-colonial Buganda brought broad-ranging improvements in child survival, not just due to better dietary practices, but also associated with improved sanitation, so that gastro-enteritis declined sharply in the 1960s.

Chapter 9 brings the various strands of this study together. Previous studies of the 1970s have tended to emphasize the grimmest aspects of life during this decade, shaped as they generally have been by the imperative to document the worst excesses of Idi Amin's regime, the negative consequences of Tanzanian socialism, or to understand the immediate context of the emergence of HIV. Without doubt poverty and inequality increased during the 1970s in this region, as did urban squalor and the incidence of many childhood diseases. The quality of medical care and, in Uganda, the efficacy of government deteriorated significantly. But the immediate demographic impact of these problems appears to have been rather modest, as missionary institutions expanded their services to compensate for the weakening of state provision, and relatively few people in these societies seem to have been absolutely destitute until the end of the 1970s. The worst period of economic collapse and political insecurity occurred after HIV had already become established. Moreover, the changes in sexual culture and behaviour seen in the 1970s were to a large extent a continuation of trends which had begun many decades previously, ensuring that patterns which had been initially associated with urban contexts dispersed far into the regions' rural communities. Where it is possible to identify a distinct shift in attitudes and practices, it would be as easy to argue that this occurred in the late 1960s as it would be the mid- to late 1970s. What was new in the 1970s was as much the result of aspiration as desperation. Certainly the resurgence in STD incidence following the decline associated with the introduction of penicillin first began in the late 1960s, slowed somewhat thereafter and then resumed a decade later. The final issue addressed by this chapter is perhaps the most surprising, the onset of fertility decline in central Buganda. This had begun in the 1960s but accelerated through the 1970s as people attempted to maintain existing standards of living as Uganda's economy collapsed around them. It is not only the earliness with which birth rates began to fall, nor the exceptionally negative social context in which they did so, which is so significant, but also the role apparently played by postponing and stopping as well as spacing behaviour in this society. This region once again does not fit perfectly with widely accepted theories about African demographic change.

The final chapter is both conclusion and epilogue, considering the role of long-term changes in patterns of fertility, mortality, and STDs in the emergence and control of HIV in this region. Whereas previous scholarship has generally concentrated on the key high-risk groups which accelerated the transmission of the disease, this study is more concerned with the rapidity with which HIV then became a mass epidemic in a largely rural context, hence its focus on the long history of changes in marriage, adolescent sexuality, leisure, materialism, and perceptions of risk. Equally, the remarkable success of AIDS control programmes in both southern Uganda and Buhaya was due in large part to the openness with which sexual matters could be discussed. Yet sex has not always been a suitable subject for public discussion in this region, and it seems unlikely that the unusual frankness that set these societies apart was purely a reaction to AIDS mortality. Buganda and Buhaya were subject to a series of campaigns to improve public morality from the early twentieth century through the period of independence. None of these may have changed sexual behaviour very much, but they must have helped legitimize sex as a topic of serious debate. Finally, the Conclusion also examines the role played by the HIV/AIDS epidemic, now part of the East African experience for three decades, in causing remarkable social change as well as immense mortality and misery. Ideas of the nature of disease and death have become both more scientific and more Christianized. Fear of witchcraft rose then fell then rose again. Concepts of human rights have been widely accepted, with particular significance for the young and women. And the intimate relationship between fertility and mortality in Africa has become clearer.

A NOTE ON SOURCES AND METHODOLOGY

The secondary sources on this region are, for much of the period covered by this book, relatively rich. Nineteenth-century descriptions of each of the three societies were published by various explorers, early missionaries, and imperialists.[44] Late Victorians' initial fascination with these isolated, large,

[44] See e.g. G. Schweinfurth et al. (eds.), *Emin Pasha in Central Africa: Being a Collection of His Letters and Journals* (London: George Philip, 1888); C. Peters, *New Light on Dark Africa* (London: Ward, Lock and Co., 1891); J. Speke, *Journal of the Discovery of the Source of the Nile* (London: Blackwood, 1863); P. Kollmann, *Der Nordwesten unserer ostafrikanischen Kolonie* (Berlin: Schall, 1898).

hierarchical societies was heightened by accounts of the martyrdom of Christian converts, the travails of the Emin Pasha Relief Expedition, the competition to map and then lay claim to the Nile, and the mutinies, rebellions, and civil wars of the 1880s and 1890s.[45] In the twentieth century the tension between ancient tradition and intense, self-conscious modernization produced a remarkable series of ethnographic accounts. The best early European-authored works were by missionaries such as John Roscoe,[46] but more valuable still were the early descriptions of their own changing societies by chiefly intellectuals like Apollo Kaggwa.[47] Professionally trained anthropologists from the 1930s then drew attention to matters of growing contemporary concern such as changes in marriage, the social impact of labour migration, and new gender and generational tensions.[48] Meanwhile, the development of Mulago medical school in Kampala produced research of global significance from the 1940s on a wide range of topics including STDs and malnutrition.[49] The instability of the 1970s and early 1980s impeded new social and medical science research in Uganda, though the Haya were the subject of a large number of studies, mostly on problems of economic development and social inequality, but also on the history of commercial sex work.[50] The return of peace to Uganda coincided with the emergence of AIDS on its

[45] e.g. G. Mackay, *A Life of A. M. Mackay of Uganda* (London: Sunday School Union, 1893); G. Portal, *The British Mission to Uganda in 1893* (London: Arnold, 1893); H. Stanley, *In Darkest Africa* (New York: Sampson Low, 1890).

[46] Most famously, *The Baganda: An Account of Their Native Customs and Beliefs* (London: Macmillan, 1911).

[47] A. Kaggwa, *Basekabaka be Buganda* (TS of English translation by S. Musoke, Africana Collection, Makerere University Library); F. Lwamgira, *Amakuru ka Kiziba na Abakama Bamu* (unpublished TS of English translation); A. Katate and L. Kamugungunu, *Abagabe b'Ankole* (Nairobi: EALB, 1967 [1947]). See also ethnographic works by administrators such as H. Johnston, *The Uganda Protectorate* (London: Hutchinson, 1902).

[48] e.g. L. Mair, *An African People in the Twentieth Century* (London: Routledge, 1934); A. Southall and P. Gutkind, *Townsmen in the Making: Kampala and Its Suburbs* (Kampala: EAISR, 1957); P. Reining, 'The Haya: The agrarian system of a sedentary people' (unpublished PhD dissertation, University of Chicago, 1965); M. Kisekka, 'The Baganda of central Uganda', in A. Molnos (ed.), *Cultural Source Materials for Population Planning in East Africa, vol. III, Beliefs and Practices* (Nairobi: EAPH, 1973), pp. 148–62.

[49] E. Muwazi, H. Trowell and J. Davies, 'Congenital syphilis in Uganda', *East African Medical Journal*, 24 (1947), pp. 152–70; J. Davies, 'A history of syphilis in Uganda', *Bulletin of the World Health Organisation*, 4 (1956), pp. 1042–59; L. Musoke, 'An analysis of admissions to the paediatric division, Mulago Hospital in 1959', *Archives of Disease in Childhood*, 36 (1961), pp. 305–15; O. Arya and F. Bennett, 'Venereal disease in an elite group (university students) in East Africa', *British Journal of Venereal Diseases*, 43, 4 (1967), pp. 275–79.

[50] e.g. P. Raikes, *Coffee Production in West Lake Region, Tanzania* (Copenhagen: IDR, 1976); B. Larsson, *Conversion to Greater Freedom? Women, Church and Social Change in. Northwestern Tanzania under Colonial Rule* (Uppsala: Uppsala University Press, 1991); L. White, *The Comforts of Home: Prostitution in Colonial Nairobi* (Chicago: Chicago University Press, 1990).

border with Buhaya. This area's leading position in the emergence and then the control of HIV produced an immense body of work on modern patterns of sexual behaviour and attitudes, and also new attention to the pre-colonial and colonial history of STDs, sexuality, and gender relations.[51] This study then has benefited from the insights of several generations of commentators and scholars, though inevitably the work they produced is of uneven reliability. Most obviously, some early European accounts of local sexual culture seem to have been influenced by a desire to exoticize or moralize, while late colonial social science research was at times constrained by preconceptions derived from theoretical frameworks that had been shaped by western experience.[52]

This previous scholarship, moreover, is uneven in its coverage. Most obviously, it is heavily biased geographically towards Buganda, with Ankole having been particularly neglected. Thematically, little has been written before on the historical demography of this region. And even where topics have been studied in real depth, still major gaps remain. To give just one example, almost all of the writing on gender and reproduction in this region has focused on women. Historians have argued that pre-colonial religion and healing centred on what they consider female concerns about fertility and child-rearing. They have emphasized the marginalization of elite royal and ritually powerful women after 1900 by a patriarchal alliance of colonial administrators and local Christian chiefs. They have suggested that this alliance went on to reconstruct customary law in ways that advantaged men, and utilized concerns about STDs as an opportunity to limit female freedoms of movement and employment. These entrenched systems of patriarchy have been used to explain why so many women became commercial sex workers during this period. Meanwhile, contemporary writing on HIV has, with good reason, focused on the vulnerability of young women to infection by older men, and of wives to infection by their husbands.[53] But this concentration on the evolving dis-

[51] e.g. J. Iliffe, *The African AIDS Epidemic: a History* (Oxford: James Currey, 2006) for the literature on HIV; C. Summers, 'Intimate colonialism: the imperial production of reproduction in Uganda, 1907–1925', *Signs*, 16, 4 (1991), pp. 787–807; M. Lyons, 'Sexually-transmitted diseases in the history of Uganda', *Genitourinary Medicine*, 79 (1994), pp. 138–45; B. Weiss, *The Making and Unmaking of the Haya Lived World: Consumption, Commoditization and Everyday Practice* (Durham, NC: Duke University Press, 1996); J. Kuhanen, *Poverty, Health and Reproduction in Early Colonial Uganda* (Joensuun: Joensuun University Press, 2005); H. Médard, *Le royaume du Buganda au XIXe siècle. Mutations politiques et religieuses d'un grand état d'Afrique de l'Est* (Paris: Karthala, 2007).

[52] See for example, R. Ashe, *Two Kings of Uganda* (London: Sampson, Low, 1889); M. Ainsworth, *Infancy in Uganda* (Baltimore: Johns Hopkins, 1967).

[53] I. Berger, 'Fertility as power: spirit mediums, priestesses and the pre-colonial state in interlacustrine east Africa', in D. Anderson and D. Johnson (eds.), *Revealing Prophets: Prophecy in Eastern African History* (London: James Currey, 1995) pp. 65–82; H. Hanson, *Landed Obligation: The Practice of Power in Buganda* (Portsmouth, NH: Heinemann, 2003); N. Musisi,

advantages suffered by women has weakened our overall understanding of sexuality in this region. This study will emphasize that infertility and child mortality were of concern to both men and women throughout this period. It will explain how the twentieth century offered women new protection and opportunities for status and income even while it closed down and criminalized other routes to honour, autonomy, and wealth. It will consider the role of the male consumer in the rise of commercialized sex in the region. And it will try to explain not just why women after 1980 were so vulnerable to HIV infection, but also how a sexual culture had developed whereby it was so common for men to have multiple sexual partners.

In its attempt to tell a more complete story, this book has used a wide range of primary sources. Many of these are highly conventional, such as government correspondence and reports archived in Britain, Kenya, Tanzania, and Uganda, missionary letters, diaries and reports, and newspapers in English and vernacular languages. Local newspapers were particularly important in the attempt to reconstruct and periodize changes in public discussion about and attitudes towards sexual behaviour. Changes in the tone and subject of letters to the editor, editorials, and journalistic articles were highly revealing, as were the emergence of sexualized marketing and photographic reportage in the 1950s, advertisements for soft pornography and the introduction of highly popular, sexually amoral cartoons in the late 1960s, and in the 1970s the appearance of horoscopes which advised readers when to avoid extra-marital affairs and the development of a genre of serialized works of fiction which idealized the materialistic sexuality of the urban young.[54]

The book is also based in part on the private papers of various anthropologists, which contain vital, unpublished material on court cases relating to marriage, the gradual integration of immigrants into Ganda sexual and

---

'Morality as identity: The missionary moral agenda in Buganda,1877-1945', *Journal of Religious History* 23, 1 (1999), pp. 51–74; P. Davis, 'On the sexuality of "town women" in Kampala', *Africa Today*, 47, 3/4, (2000), pp. 28–60; C. Obbo, 'HIV transmission: men are the solution', in S. James and A. Busia (eds.), *Theorizing Black Feminisms: The Visionary Pragmatism of Black Women* (London: Routledge, 1993), pp. 160–81.

[54] The analysis of variations in newspaper content as a means of tracing wider social change is not without its problems. Journalists to some degree shaped the terms of the moral debate in this region, they chose which letters to the editor should be published, and, in the 1970s, seemed increasingly wary of publishing anything resembling news, which presumably created space for serialized fiction that would not normally have existed. Nonetheless, the changes in the way in which sexuality was discussed and reported were so striking that they cannot safely be ignored; the periodization of change fits well with informants' personal memories; and, significantly, at times the content of newspapers provided a powerful corrective to supposed government policy on sexual probity. Journalists for example reported how moralizing government ministers' business cards were found in the possession of sex workers, while Idi Amin's decrees against sexual indecency caused only a temporary reversal to the growing hedonism of Uganda's state-sponsored press in the 1970s.

marital networks, and the role of labour migration in facilitating marriage in Ankole. The papers of numerous administrators and healthworkers, housed mainly in Rhodes House and the Wellcome archive, have also been consulted, as have relevant dissertations in Dar es Salaam and Makerere University libraries. In addition, vital registration data, demographic health surveys and censuses have also been analysed, with the unpublished sample censuses from 1948 and 1959 proving particularly useful. Such sources though still left many questions unanswered, so this study has relied heavily on oral interviews and also on the acquisition and analysis of raw demographic data.

Around 250 interviews and focus group discussions with elderly people were held in a number of locations in Ankole, Buganda, and Buhaya.[55] Individuals who were selected for one-on-one interviews typically possessed some particular expertise or specialist knowledge, such as chiefs, clergy, magistrates, commercial sex workers, traditional healers, doctors, nurses, and midwives. Invitations to group discussions were deliberately less discriminate, in an attempt to speak to people from all social classes. Slightly more women than men participated in the interviews and discussions. A few interviews were conducted in English, but most people preferred speaking in their vernacular, and so the discussion was led by a research assistant.

Interviewees were remarkably forthcoming about changes in health, sexuality, social relationships, and reproductive and child-rearing practices. To some degree this openness was structured by the relative absence of restraint associated with sexual discussion between non-contiguous generations. My research assistants and, generously, myself, were categorized by interviewees as honorary grandchildren, seeking knowledge about the past. The willingness to talk about sex though was also in large part a consequence of the intensity with which these societies have been researched since the outbreak of HIV. Few communities in the world can be so familiar with the operation of the focus group. The downside of working with such expert informants is that the repeated public discussion of sexual issues had tended to entrench certain tropes, so that, for example, interviewees repeatedly emphasized how the behaviour of the younger generation was so much worse than in their day. In order to move beyond this received wisdom, the focus of interviews was always on individuals' life histories, a technique which provided new insights into the tragedy of sterility and child loss, the excitement of pre-marital sex, and the logic of fertility limitation, among other matters. The emphasis on personal experience also revealed that many elders had in fact themselves indulged in the behaviours they had earlier condemned as signs of the incivility of modern youth. It provided a means of enabling

[55] Interview transcripts are in the possession of the author, but are available to other researchers.

women to reveal, sometimes inadvertently, that their formalized adherence to gendered expectations of submissiveness and passivity often concealed strategic attempts to reshape marital and sexual relationships, achieve economic autonomy, and control their own fertility. And it showed that when people talked about sex, they were thinking not just about lust and love, or reproduction and lineage. Sex, and discussions of sex, were also a means of renegotiating relationships with chiefs and elders, working out how Christianity could fit with enduring notions of status and advancement, ordering a world of increasing ethnic complexity, profiting from cash cropping and labour migration, holding together lives split between town and country, and understanding what it meant to be modern. Personal testimonies were, it seems, shaped in part by the ways in which sex was useful, and therefore memorable. But if interviewees' memories of the past were to some degree about their own youthful attempts to secure power and security, it is likely that they were also influenced by what some clearly viewed as their disenfranchisement in the modern era. The sense that elders' authority was no longer recognized, by state or society, was pervasive. One aspect of this declining power was the reduced role played by paternal aunts and grandparents in shaping the sexual development of the young, but it seems that a more generalized resentment at their social and political marginalization may have exaggerated elders' sense of how sharply sexual morality had changed in recent decades. These concerns do not mean that the interviews are unusable as an historical source, but they require that they be interpreted carefully. The body of testimony as a whole is perhaps most reliable when viewed comparatively, as accounts of sexual and reproductive experience varied so sharply from one society to another.[56]

Oral histories provided new qualitative information for this book, but just as important was obtaining new demographic and medical data. National and district-level information on disease incidence becomes very patchy from the mid-1960s, while many of the region's censuses during the period under study are inadequate. All the pre-1948 censuses are extremely limited, and in Uganda part of the 1948 census data, and almost the entirety of the 1980 census records, were lost prior to analysis. Some of these gaps can be partially filled by the analysis of church registers of baptism and marriage, which moreover permit highly detailed analysis due to the availability of individual-level data. Parish registers started before the first census occurred in the region; they were of largely consistent quality throughout

[56] For insightful analysis of the problems involved in the oral history of sexuality see the introductions to K. Fisher, *Birth Control, Sex, and Marriage in Britain 1918–1960* (Oxford: Oxford University Press, 2006); and S. Szreter and K. Fisher, *Sex Before the Sexual Revolution: Intimate Life in England 1918–1963* (Cambridge, Cambridge University Press, 2010). Thanks to Carol Summers and Jo Sadgrove for their comments on this theme.

the period; they offer information on demographic factors that were ignored in the censuses; and they permit a more precise dating of shifts in demographic behaviour. One parish was selected from each of the case study areas, Nyamitanga for Ankole, Kisubi for Buganda, and Bukoba for Buhaya. These parishes were selected because of their age, central location, large size, and relative ethnic homogeneity. Ideally a larger, random sample of parishes would have been utilized but the reluctance of many local clergy to participate in the project as well as the expense and time involved in the entry of unusually difficult data prevented this. Catholic registers were used simply because other churches were unwilling to allow their parishioners' personal details to be copied. This was not obviously disadvantageous given that Catholicism was the largest denomination in this region, and its parishes were established so early. The three registers begin in the late nineteenth or very early twentieth century. The Bukoba datasets end in the mid-1950s, as better census information becomes available, while the loss of the 1980 census in Uganda meant that the Kisubi and Nyamitanga datasets were taken through to that year. The limitations and complexities of analysis of these records will be discussed in detail in subsequent chapters, but two issues are so important that they should be emphasized from the start. The most significant weakness of the parish registers used in this study is that only 623 dates of death were recorded, compared to over 53,000 dates of birth and 16,000 dates of marriage. With such small numbers of death dates, full family reconstitution and the calculation of demographic rates was impossible. Nonetheless the analysis of over 71,000 life events before 1980 is a substantial contribution to African historical demography, and has permitted highly significant changes in age at first marriage and birth intervals to be tracked.

Still, the overall value of these parish datasets depends to a large extent on the question of how representative these Catholic communities were of the populations of Ankole, Buganda, and Buhaya as a whole. Christianity is, after all, viewed as one of the key avenues towards the adoption of new attitudes about health and reproduction. To what extent then will a focus on three Catholic sub-populations skew the overall sense of demographic change in this region? The first point to note is that the size of these datasets compensate for many of their inevitable inadequacies. Bukoba, Kisubi, and Nyamitanga parishes were geographically very large. Nyamitanga, for example, encompassed most of central Ankole during the colonial period, an area of several thousand square miles. The number of Catholics within these parishes' total population increased rapidly, such that by the mid-1930s more than 500 infant baptisms per annum were recorded in the Bukoba register, which constitutes a very substantial sample of the reproductive experience of the entire Heya population. The registered population of these three African parishes was equivalent to that of perhaps fifty pre-1801 English parishes.[57]

While Catholics came to form the majority within these three societies during our period, it is still necessary to recognize that they would have differed to some extent from followers of other religions in terms of their worldview, education, and perhaps level of income and social class. Muslims may have constituted only around 10% of the region's population through the twentieth century, but a much larger number of people retained their beliefs in indigenous spirits until the mid-colonial period. Meanwhile Lutherans in Buhaya and Anglicans in Uganda constituted a very large and wealthy minority, with almost none of Ankole's Hima pastoralist elite, for example, joining the Catholic faith. Catholics were largely excluded from political power in colonial Uganda, with Catholicism being condemned by the Protestant elite as the religion of peasants. It seems reasonably safe then to assume that Catholics as a group fell somewhere in the middle of colonial Ugandan society, wealthier and better educated than Muslims and traditionalists, but behind Anglicans. In Buhaya the picture was more complicated, but still Catholics' political dominance did not translate into obvious economic pre-eminence. These concerns about Catholics' representativeness lose some of their significance when it is remembered how frequently missionaries in this region complained of the lack of orthodoxy among their parishioners. Converts were repeatedly criticized for their reluctance to marry in church, devotion to polygamy, and adherence to other unchristian beliefs and practices. It is worth noting though that as the Catholic community matured, and as the church encouraged mass involvement in organizations like the Legion of Mary and Catholic Action, so people grew more likely to adopt a specifically Catholic social identity.

The value of family reconstitution from parish registers is reasonably well recognized in African demographic history.[58] The potential of hospital maternity registers as a demographic source, by contrast, has not been fully appreciated. To a large extent this reflects the greater emphasis placed on records management by the church in Africa compared to medical facilities. Certainly the majority of hospitals I visited in the region had no medical records of more than twenty years of age. Mulago hospital in Uganda had a carefully maintained system of destroying all medical records on a five year rotation,

[57] Compare E. Wrigley, R. Davies, J. Oeppen, and R. Schofield, *English Population History from Family Reconstitution, 1560–1837* (Cambridge: Cambridge University Press, 1997).

[58] Cf. e.g. V. Notkola, I. Timaeus and H. Siiskonen, 'Mortality transition in the Ovamboland region of Namibia, 1930–1990', *Population Studies*, 54 (2000), pp. 153–67; C. Thibon, *Histoire démographique du Burundi* (Paris: Karthala, 2004).

simply because of a lack of storage space, and I was unable to obtain pre-1980 records from any hospital in Buhaya. Fortunately mission hospitals had suffered less from cutbacks of funding and support staff during the 1970s and 1980s. In Kampala, Mengo hospital, which was established by the Church Missionary Society in 1897, donated its early colonial medical records to the Mulago Medical Library many decades ago. A small number of maternity registers before 1940 survived and are publically available. Just as the Mengo records came to an end, so another Kampala hospital archive began. From 1939 Nsambya hospital, which was set up by the Roman Catholic Franciscan Missionary Sisters for Africa, retained the maternity records of its general and private wards in an excellent archive. Nsambya became so successful that it was necessary to take a sample of the registers. Combining the Mengo and Nsambya records has produced a run of maternity data lasting from 1919 to 1984, with the records from every fifth year being entered. In rural Buganda, another Franciscan hospital, Nkokonjeru, had kept records dating back to 1955, so the registers from 1955, 1959, 1964, 1969, 1974, 1979 and 1984 were copied. State hospitals' archives were not so well kept. Patchy records were found from the 1960s through to the 1980s in Mbarara and Kitagata hospitals in Ankole and Masaka district hospital in southern Buganda. In total the details of around 18,000 births were recorded in these various hospitals.

All the maternity registers noted the outcome of the delivery, the birth-weight, and sex of the baby, and the parity or gravidity[59] of the mother. The richest registers were those of Mengo hospital, which also recorded the outcome of the expectant mothers' previous births, the survival of their previous children, and whether or not they or their husbands had or had ever had syphilis. The later registers, particularly from Nsambya, were not quite so detailed but the provision of private maternity facilities permitted an analysis of variations in birthweight and outcomes by income group. Moreover, the maternity registers, because they identify the mothers by name, enable patients' ethnic identities to be established with a high degree of confidence.[60] Thus the fertility of the host community can be compared with that of women from other, immigrant ethnic groups. This helps compensate for the failure of the 1969 and 1980 Uganda censuses to measure the fertility of different ethnic groups, which left unresolved the possibility that the increase in fertility which

[59] Gravidity is defined as the number of times that a woman has been pregnant, parity the number of full-term births.

[60] Unfortunately very few of the women who gave birth in these Kampala hospitals were resident in Kisubi parish, so no useful linkage between the medical and church registers could be made. Kisubi had its own hospital but unfortunately had not retained maternity records from the period under study. It should be noted that some women who possessed Ganda names may have been immigrants who adopted the ethnic identity of the host community.

occurred in Buganda in the 1950s and 1960s was largely due to the higher fertility of immigrants from other areas.

These maternity records then are potentially extremely important. But they share many of the weaknesses of the parish registers. Most fundamentally, the representativeness of these women who gave birth in hospital must be questioned. Three automatic assumptions are made about them. Either they were women who had a history of miscarriages or difficult or unsuccessful labours. Or they were women who were identified as high-risk and referred to a hospital by an ante-natal clinic because of a problem such as high blood pressure or disproportion. Or these women were inclined towards a medicalized delivery because of their high status, education, or closeness to the church. There is some evidence to support the first two assumptions in the early data. The shocking frequency of previous miscarriage, stillbirth, and neo-natal death, and the high levels of obstructed delivery recorded in the first decades of the registers suggests that the hospital records may over-represent problem cases. Notes on the patient files occasionally refer to such a process of selection. But the social status of most women is difficult to identify, and the records of patients' religion in the Mengo registers reveal that a large proportion of patients in this Anglican hospital were Catholics, Muslims, and believers in indigenous religion. Moreover, the forenames of patients at Nsambya hospital indicate that many Protestants and Muslims attended this Catholic institution. Concerns about the representativeness of the deliveries in hospital, though, reduce after the Second World War, when the scale of hospital maternity work increased enormously. By the mid-1950s over 600 women were giving birth each year in Nsambya, which was only one of four major maternity hospitals within Kampala.

The issue of how representative those who gave birth in hospital were of all pregnant women, then, is difficult to estimate before 1950, so some caution is necessary in evaluating the older data, and in establishing trends from the earlier to the later period. A more fundamental problem of course is that maternity registers must to some degree provide a skewed image of overall fertility levels as inevitably infertile women did not appear in the registers. Thus maternity registers from two different societies might present the same levels of average parity, even if one society had a much higher rate of sterility than the other. Another universal problem with data on child survival and the outcome of previous pregnancies is that of memory. Demographic researchers have found that women sometimes forget or choose not to mention deaths of young children, stillbirths, and miscarriages, particularly if they occurred some time in the past. Again, it is necessary to expect that the data on parity, gravidity, and child death will underestimate the true figures.

The last major source that can be employed for demographic historical research in this region takes the form of village, parish, or sub-county surveys that were conducted during our period by a wide range of specialists: anthropologists, administrators, public health workers, and agricultural officers. Inevitably the limited size of some of the samples affect the usefulness of such surveys, and while the researchers often claimed that they had selected their survey sites because they were locally regarded as being typical of an area or of a certain type of community, questions must remain about their representativeness. Nonetheless, even if the survey populations were often too small for any measures of demographic significance to be obtained, the data recorded in this way do provide useful statistical support for qualitative information obtained from interviews and archival documents. For example, some surveys record the role of labour migration in male marriage strategies. Others offer insights into the relationship between parental education and experience of child survival. Others again simply record the severity of specific problems, such as divorce, malnutrition, or STD prevalence within the community under study. Particularly useful surveys were those which examined several communities concurrently, or which returned to an area that had been the object of research in the past, because these reinforce the key theme of this book, that patterns of sexuality, reproduction, and health varied dramatically in this region over space and time. The most valuable local studies of all, such as Culwick's survey of Kanyangereko, produced data on fertility which correlated closely with the data contained in the Bukoba parish registers. As Bruce Fetter has observed, progress in African demographic history must inevitably rely on the accumulation of imperfect, but nonetheless significant, evidence.[61]

[61] B. Fetter (ed.), *Demography from Scanty Evidence: Central Africa in the Colonial Era* (Boulder: Lynne Rienner, 1990).

1
Sexuality and Fertility in the Pre-Colonial Period

INTRODUCTION

The three case study areas selected for this comparative study, Ankole, Buganda, and Buhaya, have much in common. The Bantu languages spoken by their inhabitants possess largely identical core vocabularies. Their pre-colonial spiritual beliefs equally clearly belonged to the same religious family. Many of the major deities which had particular influence over specific phenomena, such as rainfall, plague, or war were shared, the natural environment in each area was guarded by the spirits of rivers, hills, and lakes, and family life everywhere was regulated by the veneration or appeasement of the ancestors. In addition all three societies were governed by kings who presided over complex chiefly hierarchies.[1] These similarities provide much of the logic for the methodological approach adopted for the pre-colonial element of this project. If significant differences in sexual and reproductive attitudes and behaviour existed between these three neighbouring societies, whose histories and cultures were so interconnected, then the idea that sub-Saharan Africa as a whole entered the twentieth century in possession of one ancient sexually permissive, pro-natalist tradition becomes difficult to sustain.[2]

It was the rapidity and severity of the spread of HIV across Africa which intensified scholars' interest in trying to identify a universalistic pattern of sub-Saharan high-risk sexual behaviour. The need to explain what they identified as an enduring continent-wide culture of frequent partner exchange led Jack Caldwell and his associates in 1989 to adapt the theory of the anthropologist Jack Goody that the world has historically been divided into two

[1] D. Schoenbrun, *A Green Place, a Good Place: Agrarian Change, Gender, and Social Identity in the Great Lakes Region to the Fifteenth Century* (Portsmouth, NH: Heinemann, 1998); J.-P. Chrétien, *The Great Lakes of Africa: Two Thousand Years of History* (New York: Zone, 2003, trans. S. Strauss).

[2] Cf. J. Caldwell, P. Caldwell and P. Quiggan, 'The social context of AIDS in sub-Saharan Africa', *Population and Development Review*, 15, 2 (1989), pp. 185–234.

basic types of social systems, the African and the Eurasian.[3] According to Goody, Africa was not historically characterized by settled agriculture, the production of large surpluses, major social differentiation or monotheistic religion. Consequently, African social life was not focused on the safe transfer of property within the family by ensuring stable marriages between spouses of similar social class. Goody argues that Eurasian marital stability, and the safe transfer of property within the family, relied on the restriction of pre-marital and extra-marital sexual activity, especially by females, and this restriction was bolstered by the moral codes of monotheistic religion. Caldwell, Caldwell, and Quiggan hypothesize that instead African family life has focused on the expansion of the lineage. In the context of Africa's exceptionally high levels of mortality, cultural norms therefore centred on maximizing fertility, and so tolerating sex before and outside marriage.[4]

This chapter will challenge both the universalism and some of the detail of this theory. It will demonstrate that the social systems and sexual norms of Ankole, Buganda, and Buhaya, despite the fundamental similarity of these three cultures, not only varied significantly one from the other, but also that local patterns of property inheritance and pre-marital sexuality could appear more 'Eurasian' than 'African'. To explain why these societies do not fit comfortably into the Goody-Caldwell paradigm, it will be necessary to examine in more detail their political structures, systems of land tenure, and attitudes towards marriage and fertility.

POLITICAL AND GEOGRAPHICAL CONTEXT

While all three case study areas were monarchical societies, they differed markedly in terms of scale, unity, and political culture. By the late nineteenth century Buganda was one of the largest kingdoms in East Africa, notable for the remarkably centralized nature of its royal government. A series of civil wars in the eighteenth century had provided the impetus for the replacement of hereditary territorial chiefs and powerful princes by a new administrative system whose staff were promoted and retained on the basis of their competence and personal loyalty to the king or *kabaka*.[5] Buganda's success in regional wars and trade, her rich agricultural base, large population, and heavy taxation of the peasantry permitted the development of a royal capital

[3] Jack Goody's theory has been stated most famously in *Production and Reproduction: A Comparative Study of the Domestic Domain* (Cambridge: Cambridge University Press, 1976).
[4] Caldwell, Caldwell and Quiggan, 'The social context'.
[5] H. Médard, *Le royaume du Buganda au XIXe siècle: mutations politiques et religieuses d'un grand état d'Afrique de l'est* (Paris: Karthala, 2007), p. 11.

of unusual size and sophistication for East Africa. Her achievement of regional pre-eminence by the mid-nineteenth century coincided with the development of a strong ethnic chauvinism, which encouraged the indigenous population of incorporated territories to swiftly adopt a Ganda identity.[6]

Ankole and Buhaya by contrast were not only smaller in scale (each covering approximately 15,000 square kilometres), but consisted of a number of autonomous kingdoms of varying size. Nkore made up only around two-thirds of the territory that would become the colonial-era kingdom of Ankole, only finally being able to incorporate a number of small tributary states to the west such as Buhweju and Igara with the aid of British firepower at the end of the nineteenth century.[7] By contrast Karagwe, the largest kingdom in Buhaya, instead of subsuming its fellow Haya states during the period of conquest, imploded, so that the eight Haya kingdoms, Bugabo, Bukara, Ihangiro, Karagwe, Kianja, Kiziba, Kyamutwara, and Missenyi, entered colonial rule in a semi-federal relationship.[8] This lack of political unity, combined with greater geographical diversity, ensured the survival of more variation in attitudes and behaviour among the populations of Ankole and Buhaya than existed in Buganda. Within Buhaya, for example, Kiziba was heavily influenced by both its proximity to Buganda and its close dynastic ties to Bunyoro, while Karagwe, the driest part of Buhaya, shared some of the characteristics of the neighbouring cattle kingdoms of Rwanda and Nkore. The division between a Hima pastoralist elite and what they derogatorily typically referred to as their Iru or servants, the agriculturalist majority, was sharper in Ankole than Buhaya, presumably because the cattle economy was so much larger in the former society. In Buganda, by contrast, livestock disease marginalized pastoralists. While Hima pastoralists formed a large, dominant minority in Nkore proper, they were fewer in number in the petty kingdoms to the west, where heavy rainfall and richer soil permitted intensive cultivation. It was here that resentment against Hima exploitation and arrogance reached its greatest intensity, with pastoralist mockery of Iru sweat and stupidity being met with a quiet glorification of agriculturalists' closeness

[6] S. Doyle, 'Immigrants and indigenes: the Lost Counties dispute and the evolution of ethnic identity in colonial Buganda', *Journal of Eastern African Studies*, 3, 2 (2009), pp. 284–302.

[7] E. Steinhart, *Conflict and Collaboration: The Kingdoms of Western Uganda, 1890–1907* (Princeton: Princeton University Press, 1977).

[8] R. Austen, *Northwest Tanzania under German and British Rule: Colonial Policy and Tribal Politics, 1889–1939* (New Haven: Yale University Press, 1968). The notional equality of all of Buhaya's kingdoms concealed Kianja and Kiziba's primacy during the colonial period, gained through a close alliance with the colonial state and early enthusiasm for western education respectively.

to the land, industry, and self-control, explicitly contrasting with cattle-keepers' idleness, rootlessness, and sexual profligacy.[9]

BUHAYA

Pre-colonial population densities varied sharply across the Great Lakes region because of variations in levels of soil fertility and rainfall, but nowhere was this so extreme as within Buhaya. When Europeans first arrived among the eastern Haya, they described a sea of grass interspersed with large islands of settlement along the ridges that ran parallel to the western shore of Lake Victoria.[10] Elsewhere in East Africa such villages typically emerged in the nineteenth century as a defensive response to the heightened violence that accompanied the arrival of firearms and a more commercialized slave trade.[11] But in Buhaya ethnographic and archaeological evidence indicates that its villages were of much greater antiquity.[12] This unusual settlement geography, which distinguished pre-colonial Buhaya from what Goody defined as the African norm, derived from the infertility of most of the area's ancient soils. The research of the eminent archaeologist, Peter Schmidt, tells a story of

[9] J. Iliffe, *A Modern History of Tanganyika* (Cambridge: Cambridge University Press, 1979), p. 24; M. Mulokozi, 'The Nanga bards of Tanzania: are they epic artists?', *Research in African Literatures*, 14, 3 (1983), p. 297; M. Doornbos, 'Images and reality of stratification in pre-colonial Nkore', *Canadian Journal of African Studies*, 7, 3 (1973), pp. 477–95; Male Focus Group Discussion (FGD) Nyamitanga, 19 Aug. 2004; Int. RNT, 9 Aug. 2004, Mbarara, M. Hima stereotypes of cultivators were just as negative in Buhaya as Ankole. A praise poem from Karagwe about the crushing of a commoner rebellion emphasized the rebel leader's closeness to the soil: 'He was caked with dirt about the buttocks. You know, it emitted such a stench!' Mulokozi, 'The Nanga Bards', p. 297. S. Karugire, *History of the Kingdom of Nkore in Western Uganda to 1896* (Oxford: Oxford University Press, 1971), pp. 79–80 notes that the historic division between pastoralist and cultivator was not absolute. Justin Willis, like Karugire, emphasizes that cultivators and pastoralists were tied together by networks of patronage, but presents a less benign picture of the pre-colonial relationship. J. Willis, 'Clan and history in western Uganda: a new perspective on the origins of pastoral dominance', *The International Journal of African Historical Studies*, 30, 3 (1997), pp. 583–600.

[10] e.g. P. Kollman, *The Victoria Nyanza: The Land, the Races and their Customs, with Specimens of some of the Dialects* (London: Swan Sonnenschein, 1899), p. 67; H. Stanley, *Through the Dark Continent: Or, the Sources of the Nile around the Great Lakes of Equatorial Africa and Down the Livingstone River to the Atlantic Ocean* (London: Sampson, Low, 1890), pp. 142–3.

[11] K. Fosbrooke, 'The defensive measure of certain tribes in North-Eastern Tanganyika, Part 2', *Tanganyika Notes and Records*, 36 (1954) pp. 36, 50–7.

[12] P. Schmidt, 'A new look at interpretations of the early iron age in East Africa', *History in Africa*, 2 (1975), p. 129; H. Rehse, *Kiziba: Land und Leute* (Stuttgart: Strecker und Schröder, 1910, translated by Mrs Donne, UDSM, CORY 369), Ch.1, p. 2; Int. FKK, 29 Aug. 1999, Kaishemarwa-Katoma, M; Int. PK, 6 Sept. 1999, Rubafu, M; Int. SN, 25 Aug. 1999 Katoma, M: Informants such as these claimed that their plots had been farmed by their families for five to eleven generations.

environmental degradation following the arrival of pastoralists and iron-working agriculturalists several millennia ago.[13] Schmidt describes how centuries of livestock browsing, bushburning, and removal of wood for fuel and construction allowed the 1900 mm of rain that swept across from Lake Victoria every year to slowly leach exposed land, so that soil samples taken by colonial agronomists investigating the poor productivity of Buhaya's grasslands revealed some of the lowest levels of organic matter and nutrients ever recorded.[14] Yet the impoverishment of Buhaya's forests and grasslands was in part a function of a deliberate strategy of environmental management. Over the centuries cultivators had reinforced subtle variations in soil productivity by investing in the more fertile and defensible land along the ridgetops, carrying in soil, planting nitrogen-fixing trees, and carefully mulching and fertilizing their farms with recycled resources extracted from the lowlands, such as wood-ash, livestock manure, and the grass used to thatch and carpet their homes.[15] The introduction of the plantain or cooking banana a millennium or more ago permitted the development of dense, semi-permanent settlements, as a banana plant could fruit for a number of years, the crop was rotated on a decades-long cycle, and the canopy of foliage and carpet of banana-trash

[13] P. Schmidt, *Historical Archaeology: A Structural Approach in an African Culture* (Westport: Greenwood Press, 1978), p. 280.

[14] D. McMaster, 'Change of regional balance in the Bukoba District of Tanzania', *Tanganyika Notes and Records*, 56 (1961), p. 79; G. Milne, 'Bukoba: High and low fertility on a laterised soil', *The East African Agricultural Journal*, 4 (1938), pp. 15–20; A. Evans and H. Mitchell, 1961. 'Soil fertility studies in Tanganyika. Improvement of crop and grass production on a leached sandy soil in Bukoba', *East African Agricultural and Forestry Journal*, 27 (1962), p. 189; F. Baijukya and V. Mwita (eds.), 'Participatory planning and management: an agenda for equity and sustainable use of 'Rweya' grassland in Kagera Region, Tanzania' in F. Baijukya and V. Mwita (eds.), *Proceedings of the 'Rweya' Workshop, Bukoba* (Bukoba: KAEMP, 2000), pp. 32–6; E. Kabwoto, 'Cases of decline in major crop production in Bukoba: banana, coffee and tea' (unpublished MA dissertation, 1976, UDSM). Soil samples taken from the grasslands of eastern Buhaya were acidic, lacking in calcium, chlorine, magnesium, nitrogen, potassium and sodium, and containing almost no organic matter. Around seventy inches or two hundred centimetres of rain falls each year at Bukoba.

[15] W. Allen, *The African Husbandman* (London: Oliver and Boyd, 1965), pp. 172–5; McMaster, 'Change', p. 87; Schmidt, *Historical*, p. 22; Kollman, *Victoria*, p. 69; Int. ZR, 22 June 2000, Karwoshe, M; Int. SPM, 24 June 2000, Gera-Kashambya, M; Int. PK, 6 Sept. 1999, Rubafu, M; Int. FB, 9 Sept. 1999, Maruku, M; M. Schmidt's depiction of late nineteenth-century Buhaya's environment as 'beleaguered' derives from his analyses of pollen and charcoal, which suggest a steady reduction in the range of trees present in Buhaya due to centuries of ironworking and farming. But Haya villages contained large numbers of trees which were planted or protected because they improved soil fertility, provided medicine, or marked boundaries. Many of these trees are leguminous and so their history is not revealed in pollen samples, while they may have been too valuable to be used regularly as charcoal. Schmidt's assumption that *Maesopsis eminii* which were to be found across Buhaya were forest remnants, and thus evidence of long-term deforestation, is questionable given that this was one of the trees most commonly planted by Haya.

mulch softened the impact of rainfall.[16] The sustainability and remarkable productivity of these lush, perennial banana gardens made them the most valuable property in this society, and the politically powerful worked hard to ensure that their heirs would inherit their positions as landowners and landlords, while the poor struggled to maintain and pass on their rights of usufruct, faced with the elite's reserved rights of appropriation.[17]

Early European descriptions of the villages that ran along Buhaya's eastern ridges convey a sense of approval, an appreciation of the familiarity of this intensively cultivated landscape. Surpluses were produced, food was easily acquired, village paths were shaded and cleanly kept, huts were large and built to last, and each plot was separated from its neighbours by tall, carefully maintained hedges.[18] These hedgerows projected an aura of peace and order, but in Haya culture their existence reflected underlying tensions. This is revealed by the names and physical nature of the two species which Haya used to defend their property rights. *Mulinzi* (*Erythrina abyssinica*) was a tough, thorny tree, whose name meant 'the guard'. If it failed to deter an aggressor from tearing down the hedge, then *Mulamula* (*Dracaena fragrans*), 'the arbitrator', would ensure that the true boundary could be re-established. *Mulamula* created a fence-like barrier above the surface, but more importantly its roots were so difficult to remove that the original line of the hedge could always be traced.[19] The space and energy that these carefully maintained hedges consumed signified the exceptional value of the land they protected. They shielded individuals from the greed or jealousy of their neighbours. But they were no defence against the acquisitiveness of kings and their favourites.

According to John Iliffe, Buhaya was pre-colonial Tanzania's most stratified and authoritarian society.[20] Royal power here rested ultimately on control over the land, and the ability to allocate, and remove, estates was the best guarantee of the loyalty of princes and chiefs. Kings, claiming ultimate ownership of all the land in their territory, gradually acquired banana gardens

[16] D. Schoenbrun (1993). 'Cattle herds and banana gardens: the historical geography of the western Great Lakes region, ca AD 800–1500', *The African Archaeological Review*, 11 (1993), pp. 50–3. B. Lejju, P. Robertshaw and D. Taylor, 'Africa's earliest bananas?', *Journal of Archaeological Science*, 33, 1 (2006), pp. 102–13 suggest that the plantain may have arrived in this region at a much earlier date.

[17] See for example P. Reining, 'Haya land tenure: landholding and tenancy', *Anthropological Quarterly*, 35, 2, (1962), pp. 58–73; H. Cory and M. Hartnoll, *The Customary Law of the Haya Tribe, Tanganyika Territory* (London: Cass, 1971 [1945]), p. 20.

[18] Kollman, *Victoria*, p. 68; Rehse, *Kiziba*, Ch.1, p. 2.

[19] Int. SPM, 24 June 2000, Gera-Kashambya, M; Int. MM B, 26 Aug. 1999, Katoma-Irogero, M. *Mulamula* and *Mulinzi* were also used as boundary markers because they served a useful function beyond their natural advantages as a hedging plant, improving soil fertility and providing excellent timber, respectively.

[20] Iliffe, *Tanganyika*, p. 24.

from clans and individuals. Defining the practice of burying people on their own farms as ritually dangerous, they were able to separate clanship from landholding.[21] When an individual landholder died, his children had to seek official permission to inherit. Given the extreme difficulty of establishing a new garden, this society then became one in which the poor had to maintain the goodwill of their superiors, whether monarch or landlord.[22] Over time, more and more Haya became tenants of their kingdom's great men, who were rewarded for success in war or administration with a grant of an estate or *nyarubanja* [big farm]. A *nyarubanja* was usually created by arbitrarily grouping together a small group of individual, contiguous banana gardens, with the occupiers having the choice of becoming tenants or moving off to find some free, cultivable land. Tenancy involved the payment of rent and labour tribute, in exchange for which the landlord might allow access to a share of his cattle's manure, so crucial to gardens' continued fertility.[23] Landlords and peasants alike had limited security of tenure, for the loss of favour would always threaten eviction. Possession of land through several generations tended to entrench land rights, whereas dying without a son guaranteed the loss of family land to the monarch, and might condemn the widow and orphaned girls to enslavement in the royal court.[24] This intimate relationship between reproduction and the land dominated Haya attitudes towards marriage, sex, and fertility.

Buhaya was hardly unique within the Great Lakes region for appearing more 'Eurasian' than 'African', in Goody and Caldwell's terms, with its marked social differentiation, settled agriculture, large surpluses, and concern with family inheritance. Its peculiar ecology though meant that these phenomena were, perhaps, more fully developed than elsewhere. On the surface, it could seem that Haya sexual culture was equally "Eurasian" with its emphasis on marital stability and the avoidance of pre-marital pregnancy. But an examination of what happened within marriage reveals that Haya norms permitted an exceptionally broad spectrum of legitimated extra-marital sexual behaviour, all justified by the need to ensure marital fertility

[21] Int. HL, 17 June 2000, Maruku, M. 'The chiefs used to say that if you buried people in the land you were burying different types of spirits there which should be kept in one place. Only the chiefs should be buried in the land . . . If you were buried in the *kibanja* you owned it . . . you are likely to stay there forever.'

[22] Int. FM, 21 July 1998, Rubya, M.

[23] A. Culwick and G. Culwick, edited by V. Berry, *The Culwick Papers 1934–1944: Population, Food and Health in Colonial Tanganika* (London: Academic Books, 1994), pp. 125, 182–3; P. Schmidt, 'An investigation of early and late iron age cultures through oral tradition and archaeology: an interdisciplinary case study in Buhaya, Tanzania' (PhD Northwestern University, 1974), pp. 48–52.

[24] Cory and Hartnoll, *Customary Law*, pp. 19, 76; Culwick, Culwick and Berry, *Population*, p. 186; Int. N, 23 July 1998, Katongo, M; Int. MK, 19 Aug. 2000, Kanyigo, M.

and thus the continuation of the lineage. This was not a society torn between two competing value systems, one focused on family inheritance, the other on lineage extension, for the ambitions of family and lineage intersected. Both were sustained by inheritance and reproduction.

The most striking aspect of Haya sexual culture was the traditional belief that unmarried girls who fell pregnant should be ritually executed by her family, either by drowning, having a metal peg driven through her skull, or the insertion of a red-hot iron into her vagina. This practice was referred to by all informants, though none knew of any individuals who had suffered such a fate. Still the purpose of the tradition was to deter young girls from having a pre-marital pregnancy, and it seems that this goal was generally achieved, according to oral and ethnographic evidence. The standard explanation for such severe penalties was the ritual danger and shame that such misbehaviour brought the family, but the observation of the German administrator Hermann Rehse in 1910 that girls 'are guarded, as they represent capital which is certain' emphasizes the challenge posed by pre-marital sex to parental authority and elders' control of the process of inheritance. Marriage here was a family investment aimed at securing a legitimate, socially recognized heir.[25] Some informants acknowledged that sex did occur before marriage, and that the extreme rarity of pre-marital pregnancy derived in part from the use of abortifacients.[26] Nonetheless, the restrictions imposed on adolescent sexuality stand in marked contrast to the rules of legitimate sexual behaviour after marriage.

In many African societies custom granted a man's close relatives, usually his brothers, sexual access to his wife. Often this phenomenon has been explained by the need to discreetly satisfy the sexual needs of unmarried young men.[27] But another explanation was that the practice enabled the wife

[25] e.g. Int. AM, 24 June 2000, Kashambya, F; Int. SK, 21 June 2000, Rubya, M; Int. RK, 16 June 2000, Kanyangereko, F; P. Reining, 'The Haya of north-western Tanzania', in A. Molnos (ed.), *Cultural Source Materials for Population Planning in East Africa, Vol. 3, Beliefs and Practices* (Nairobi: EAPH, 1973), p. 217; Rehse, *Kiziba*, ch.7, p. 14; A. Ishumi, *Kiziba: The Cultural Heritage of an Old African Kingdom* (Syracuse University, Maxwell School of Citizenship and Public Affairs, 1980), p. 70. In 1905 Cunningham referred to the 'dreadful penalties', typically drowning, suffered by Haya guilty of pre-marital sex. J. Cunningham, *Uganda and its Peoples: Notes on the Protectorate of Uganda, Especially the Anthropology and Ethnology of its Indigenous Races* (London: Hutchinson, 1905), pp. 284–93.

[26] e.g. Int. SK, 21 June 2000, Rubya, M; see also Rehse, *Kiziba*, Ch.7, p. 11; Reining, 'The Haya of north-western Tanzania', p. 221; Culwick, Culwick and Berry, *Population*, p. 125. An early source on Karagwe's pastoralists emphasized that pre-marital pregnancy, not sex per se, warranted punishment. 'Karagwe: the state', Bukoba District Book, TNA (Tanzania National Archives, Dar es Salaam).

[27] e.g. Caldwell, 'Rethinking', p. 119.

of an infertile man to be impregnated by one of his relatives, so that the lineage would be strengthened. In Buhaya, the scale of this sexual openness was greater than the norm, because of the severity of the repercussions of childlessness. For Haya in the past 'having no children was regarded as a curse and barren women were treated with contempt and despised.' The absolute necessity of securing an heir explains why Haya men were legally required to allow any member of their clan to sleep with their wives. The power of the lineage was particularly strong here because household heads were not merely the descendants of their forefathers, they were also the guardians of rights over specific plots of valuable land which had to be passed on to the next generation. Inheritance was of exceptional importance for Bahaya which helps explain why in some clans, particularly in southern Buhaya, a bride might be required to have her first sexual intercourse with her father-in-law, if he was the one who had given away his lineage's property in the form of bridewealth. This custom would have been regarded as akin to incest in most Great Lakes societies. In Buhaya it was euphemistically referred to as *kutera telerome* – 'clearing the morning dew from the grass'.[28]

A man who lacked sons would marry additional wives if he was wealthy enough, but if he suspected that the problem lay with himself several other options were available to him. In Buhaya, unlike Ankole and Buganda, the possibility that childlessness might be due to male sterility was widely acknowledged, presumably because the stakes were too high for self-deception. Informants reported that a sonless man might encourage his wife to have an affair with a neighbour who had produced many sons, though more often it was his mother who would suggest this course of action.[29] The most extreme response to the anxiety associated with heirlessness was the unique institution of *bisisi*, which emerged at some point in the nineteenth century. *Bisisi* may have evolved out of an older belief, common to many Great Lakes societies, that pregnancies did not necessarily last for nine months. They could be suspended, described as 'going to the back', and then reactivated simply by fate, or by the skilful use of medicine at a more convenient moment.[30] Traditional accounts trace the origins of *bisisi* back to the death of the only son and heir of a king of Karagwe, Ruhinda Ikungurabishake, several centuries ago. Ruhinda had previously sent the child's mother away, and she had remarried and borne a son by her new husband. Ruhinda claimed that the second boy was in fact his, and identified him as his new heir.[31] From this one episode developed a widely accepted custom that the first man to have sex with a

[28] Int. WR, 21 June 2000, Rubya, M; Int. RMR, 13 Aug. 2000, Byabusha, Busindi, M.

[29] Int. WR, 21 June 2000, Rubya, M; Int. MPM, 10 Aug. 2000, Ibare, F.

[30] Cf. e.g. M. Kisekka, 'The Baganda of central Uganda', in Molnos, *Cultural Source Materials III*, p. 157.

[31] Int. RMR, 13 Aug. 2000, Byabusha, Busindi, M.

woman who was a virgin or who had just given birth was the true father of the next child that this woman produced, no matter how far in the future this child was born.[32] *Bisisi* literally means glowing embers, and the metaphor is that the owner of a fire is the man who lit it, not the man who found it later and brought it back to life. The *bisisi* law was designed to enable an infertile man to claim a child that he had not in reality fathered, on the tenuous grounds that he was its genitor. The custom made it more likely that a childless man would divorce his wife, in the hope of securing an heir by proxy. A further development, often reported by informants, was that an heirless man, with witnesses, would bribe a newly delivered woman to have sex with him before returning to her husband's bed, or would wait for a woman to go to wash herself in a river after childbirth, and then ejaculate into the water upstream, shouting 'I have begotten a child, you should bring my child to me, it is mine.' Such actions frequently caused conflict, but they were legal methods of obtaining a child.[33]

Buhaya then had unusually generous opportunities for legitimate extramarital sex. The sources on illegitimate affairs, although rather sparse for the pre-colonial period, indicate that constraints on the sexuality of married people were also relatively limited. It is likely that the semi-urban population densities created by the ecological obstacles to dispersed settlement would have been particularly conducive to sexual affairs. While scattered settlements may have granted greater privacy, the sociability of village life provided greater opportunities and temptations. Widows with children, who were often allowed to live alone, were particularly identified as being free to have affairs if they wished.[34] Sexual exchange was most extensive at the courts of Buhaya's kings. Women flowed towards the capital, due to family debt, enslavement, or royal acquisitiveness. Some became wives of the king or, more frequently, of his clients. Most worked as servants, vulnerable to the demands of courtiers and visitors. One informant recalled hearing of royal feasts where the king would announce to his drunken guests 'let anyone who comes across maize [women] reap it.'[35] Princesses were categorized as men, and were allowed to

[32] Reining, 'The Haya of north-western Tanzania', p. 220; H. Lapioche, 'Table d'enquête sur les moeurs et coutumes indigènes, Diocese de Bukoba', 1956, p. 58, White Fathers Archive, Rome [WFA].

[33] e.g. Int. RMR, 13 Aug. 2000, Byabusha, Busindi, M; Int. WBK, 27 July 1998, Bugabo, M; Int. YS, 10 Aug. 2000, Bukoba, F. Cf. Cory and Hartnoll, *Customary*, p. 36. Some informants stated that men urinated rather than ejaculated into the river, but suggested that urine might contain sperm.

[34] Rehse, *Kiziba*, Ch.11, pp. 4–8; 'Karagwe: the state', Bukoba District Book, TNA; Cory and Hartnoll, *Customary*, p. 94; Cunningham, *Uganda*, pp. 290–3.

[35] Rehse, *Kiziba*, Ch.11, p. 9; Int. LM, 27 Aug. 1999, Katoma-Karwoshe, M; Int. SK, 21 June 2000, Rubya, M; Int. FKK, 29 Aug. 1999, Kaishemarwa-Katoma, M; Int. KK, 15 June 2000, Bibanja, F.

have various lovers, but were forbidden from giving birth, lest the security of the dynasty be threatened. This combination of sexual freedom and restricted fertility, which resulted in their habitual use of apparently effective abortifacients, symbolized their society's fixation with socially appropriate, controlled reproduction.[36] Haya culture demanded an heir but, given the difficulty of opening up new land, did not particularly value extremely large families. Mothers were encouraged to breastfeed for up to four years. Women who fell pregnant too soon after giving birth were sent away to their parents after the next child was born to prevent another short birth interval.[37] This was a culture that encouraged caution in childbearing.

ANKOLE

The antagonism between pastoralists and agriculturalists that defined many pre-colonial Great Lakes societies reached a relatively extreme form in Ankole. One aspect of this divide was that her cultivators possessed one of the most pro-natalist, sexually closed cultures in the region, while Hima pastoralists tolerated a remarkably wide network of sexual contacts and displayed an ambivalence towards female reproduction. As the anthropologist Yitzchak Elam has noted, the enlargement of the family, and particularly the securing of sons, while desirable, was also a source of anxiety for cattlekeepers as it threatened the sustainability of the herd by diverting milk from calves to children.[38] Female fertility's destabilizing power was expressed in various rituals, while anxieties about sustenance and inheritance ensured that reproduction was just as carefully managed among Ankole's Hima as among the Haya. Early sources reported exceptionally long periods of breastfeeding and post-partum abstinence of three years. Moreover, procreation for the Hima was primarily associated with youth. Widows and divorcees, referred to as 'secondhand women', struggled to remarry, even if they were still of reproductive age. In contrast to many East African cultures, prosperous household heads often chose not to take additional wives, preferring instead to save their

[36] Culwick, Culwick and Berry, *Population*, p. 125.

[37] Reining, 'The Haya of north-western Tanzania', pp. 218–20; G. Rwegelera, 'Tribal customs in infant feeding I: Among the Haya', *East Africa Medical Journal*, 40 (1963), pp. 366–9; Int. WBK, 27 July 1998, Bugabo, M; Int. N, 23 July 1998, Katongo, M.

[38] Y. Elam, *The Social and Sexual Roles of Hima Women: A Study of Nomadic Cattle Breeders in Nyabushozi County, Ankole, Uganda* (Manchester: Manchester University Press, 1973), pp. 53, 66.

bridewealth cattle until their sons were old enough to marry, as a means of retaining their labour and loyalty.[39]

The origins of the Hima's sexual and reproductive practices lay in the precarious nature of the cattle economy. Ankole was, by African standards, a rich environment for pastoralism, one that made a more or less exclusive milk diet possible, but this created cultural pressure to maintain a very high cattle: human ratio. Family heads therefore depended on the assistance of friends and relatives to ensure that their herds throve, and had to ensure that the equilibrium between the size of the household and the size of the herd was maintained. The maintenance of the Hima way of life fostered a remarkably strategic attitude to sex. Pre-marital pregnancy, 'that awful thing', was extremely rare not only because of the shame it brought on the family. It would also 'kill the cows', by bringing an extra mouth to feed and closing down an opportunity to enlarge the family herd by bringing in bridewealth. The traditional penalty for unmarried girls who fell pregnant was to be expelled from Hima society and so forced to take refuge, and marry, among agriculturalists, or to be murdered. Adolescent males were also disincentivized from seducing their female peers by Hima society's construction of the unmarried woman as thin, underdeveloped, and thus sexually unattractive. Girls worked hard in the Hima economy, whereas wives were deliberately kept overfed and idle. Elam claimed that this sexual aesthetic was so widely accepted that the constant monitoring of girls' behaviour and whereabouts, so prominent in other Great Lakes societies, was unnecessary here. Elam though may have overestimated how discriminating adolescent males were and it is likely that a more important factor was that the sexual energies of male youths were diverted to the household's married women, who were encouraged to welcome nephews and stepsons into their beds in order to keep them away from those of the girls.[40]

Wives could control the demands placed on their bodies to a degree, but still the breadth of the networks of sexual interchange which they were expected by their husbands to maintain was quite remarkable. Refusal to sleep with any of her husband's friends or relatives, on both paternal and maternal sides, was grounds for divorce, though a beating was a more likely

[39] J. Roscoe, *The Soul of Central Africa: a General Account of the Mackie Ethnological Expedition* (New York: Negro University Press, 1969 [1922]), p. 91; Elam, *Social and Sexual*, pp. 147, 150–2, 174, 186–7. Elam though found much shorter periods of breastfeeding and abstinence in the 1970s.

[40] Elam, *Social and Sexual*, pp. 54–8, 84–8. Pre-marital pregnancy though might, with the connivance of the girl's mother, result in abortion or swiftly arranged marriage. It should be noted that very few sources on Hima practices date from the period prior to the devastating rinderpest epizootic of the 1890s. It is possible that the attempt to rebuild Hima society after rinderpest involved a degree of essentialization of pastoralist culture.

outcome. Rejecting her father-in-law, whose cattle had brought her into the family, was particularly shocking, and could lead to disinheritance or the immediate expulsion of the son and his wife from the camp, and their only means of livelihood. The cooperative nature of cattle herding, and the need for cattle to be milked during their owners' absence, explains why female sexuality was used to reinforce male bonds. Domestic stability and prosperity depended on camp solidarity. Husbands were not immune to sexual jealousy, but questions about paternity never arose, as the father of a child was always its *pater* rather than its *genitor* in this society. Infertility was regarded as a female problem, and would usually result in divorce and remarriage by the husband, as dying childless meant that a man's cattle went to the king for redistribution. In many Great Lakes societies divorce due to apparent barrenness resulted in the return of bridewealth by the wife's family, but Hima prioritization of social networking meant that such women were sent home with a heifer in order to maintain good relations between the families.[41] The sexual availability of married women depended on a level of female subordination greater than that found in Buganda or Buhaya. During the wedding ceremony the bride was instructed by the groom's mother on the nature of married life: 'A woman keeps quiet! A woman is mistreated [and does not complain]. A woman is beaten!' A Hima wife's ties to her natal family were weak, she was excluded from any significant status-enhancing economic activity, she remained veiled throughout her adult life, while movement outside the camp branded her a promiscuous 'woman of the thigh', daring to assert rights over her own sexuality.[42] Hima sexual networks were not completely open. Sexual contact with agriculturalists, while not unheard of, was referred to with disgust or mockery, and most affairs that were regarded as legitimate occurred within the camp. Yet Hima male culture was profoundly sociable. Visiting friends and distant relatives at other camps, which usually involved sexual encounters, was a necessary means of securing access to waterpoints or loans of cattle or labour. This pattern of interconnected nodes of intense sexual exchange would prove ideal for the transmission of STDs.[43]

[41] Elam, *Social and Sexual*, pp. 159–95, 147; J. Roscoe, 'The Bahima: a cow tribe of Enkole in the Uganda Protectorate', *Journal of the Royal Anthropological Institute*, p. 103; P. Nicolet, 'Table d'enquête sur les moeurs et coutumes indigènes, Vicariat Apostolique de Rwenzori: Tribu des Hamites Abahima et Bantu Abairu de l'Ankole', 1951, pp. 15–16, WFA.

[42] Elam, *Social and Sexual*, pp. 76, 107, 123, 150–1, 181, 231; Alex Mugisha Kagume, 'Church and society in Ankole, Uganda: an analysis of the impact of evangelical African Christianity on ethnic and gender relations in Ankole, 1901–1961' (unpublished PhD dissertation, University of Bristol, 1993), p. 23; Roscoe, 'Bahima', p. 105.

[43] Elam, *Social and Sexual*, p. 6; J. Gorju, *Entre le Victoria, l'Albert et l'Edouard* (Rennes, 1920, translated by Ralph Butler, 1957, A. Richards papers, LSE archive), p. 15; Roscoe, 'Bahima', p. 105; Int. RNT, 9 Aug. 2004, Mbarara, M. Moreover, according to Cunningham, penalties for illegitimate extra-marital affairs were minimal. Cunningham, *Uganda*, p. 18.

Ankole's agriculturalists, despite their constructed antagonism, shared some of the same beliefs as Hima pastoralists. Pre-marital pregnancy was described by informants as 'a taboo', which would result in the murder or expulsion of the girl, and permanent disgrace for her mother. Marriage, because it involved the transfer of family wealth, implicitly granted sexual rights over a new bride to the groom's relatives. And women were very much the weaker partner in a marriage. A bride was told by her new husband during the wedding ceremony: 'You say one word and I will say two.'[44] Yet these similarities disguise a fundamental difference in the culture of sexuality and reproduction, for Nkole cultivators valued both sexual restraint and fertility maximization.

Agriculturalist society encouraged early, stable marriage. Parents strove to marry off their children during their adolescence, bridewealth permitting. Wedding rituals emphasized women's duty to produce many children and work hard, with the bride being presented with a hoe. In marked contrast to Buhaya where physical attractiveness was prioritized, the prime qualities sought in a wife were physical strength and membership of a 'good' family with *amara marungi*, good insides, which had a record of producing numerous, healthy children.[45] Divorce was unusually difficult to achieve for Ankole's cultivators, except in cases of infertility, with elders taking their role as counsellors and arbitrators particularly seriously. Moreover, the pressure placed on widows and divorcees to remarry was exceptionally strong. Unmarried women were regarded as a potential source of conflict and shame, and as a waste of reproductive potential.[46]

Women were encouraged to produce children for as long as they were capable. In contrast to many African societies, there was no requirement that a mother's reproductive life should end when her daughters began their own families. According to the sociologist Musa Mushanga, cultivators expected that a woman's lastborn should be of an age with the first children of her third born.[47] Barrenness, a tragedy in any African society, was regarded as an

[44] Int. RNT, 9 Aug. 2004, Mbarara, M; I. Gateley, 'The traditional education of women and girls in Uganda' (unpublished PhD dissertation, University of London, 1968), p. 60; Anon., 'How the Banyankole live', D. Stenning Papers, Cambridge University, ADD 7916, B1, p. 13. A traditional song about unmarried girls who became pregnant contained the lyrics: 'Some fathers are cutting a headdress for marriage, but this one is cutting banana leaves (to burn his daughter to death)'.
[45] B. Mwesiga, 'Traditional marriage among the Banyankole' (unpublished BA Fine Arts dissertation, MUK, 1976–7), pp. 9, 27; M. Mushanga, 'The Nkole of south-western Uganda', in Molnos, *Cultural Source Materials III*, p. 179; Anon., 'How the Banyankole live', D. Stenning Papers, Cambridge University, ADD 7916, B1, p. 29. See Rehse, *Kiziba*, Ch.12, p. 2 for Buhaya.
[46] James Ntozi and John Kabera, 'Marriage patterns in Ankole, South-Western Uganda', African Demography Working Papers no. 16, University of Pennsylvania, August 1988, pp. 24, 28.
[47] Mushanga, 'Nkole', p. 179.

especially terrible curse in Ankole. Women who failed to conceive would often return to their families of their own volition, driven by shame, rather than wait to be divorced.[48] A sense of the scale of this society's pro-natalism is given by the belief that a marriage did not formally exist until the birth of the first child, and that a family with only one child was incomplete.[49] Informants' explanations for the intensity of the pressure to produce as many children as possible included the usual factors such as high child mortality, but strikingly prioritized concerns about physical security. One asked '[suppose someone] has more than five wives. Each has five children. So if you come with your two children, would you attack such a man?' Another observed 'when you produced, relatives would be happy that the clan has been enlarged. During the time of the clan wars, they would be proud because they would be having a number of soldiers to fight.' The particular value of children as a source of protection presumably derived from recurrent Hima aggression and the extreme instability of western Ankole, where a number of small, weak states struggled to mediate local disputes and retain some measure of autonomy from Nkore's persistent expansionism, and occasional intervention by Rwanda, Bunyoro, and Buganda.[50]

High fertility was achieved not just through a high marriage rate but also by means of relatively short birth intervals and high coital frequency. Parents were expected to resume sex four days after the birth of a child, in part to alleviate suspicions that the husband might be having an affair, in part because Banyankole believed in the healing power of sperm. In practice many couples waited until the woman was fully recovered from the delivery, but still a survey of men born in the first half of the twentieth century found that almost all had resumed sex with their wives less than a month after childbirth. Again the cultural norm was that the next child would be conceived before the newborn had cut its teeth, which would have resulted in birth intervals of only fourteen to fifteen months. The demographer James Ntozi recorded thirty-three separate occasions when Nkole were supposed to practice ritual sex. As late as the 1980s, despite the impact of Christianity, a majority of couples still followed these customary requirements, which must have increased the

[48] Male FGD Nyamitanga, 19 Aug. 2004.

[49] P. Kanyadago, *Evangelizing Polygamous Families: Canonical and African Approaches* (Gaba: AMACEA, 1991), p. 15; Mushanga, 'Nkole', p. 180; A. Kamugisha, 'Beliefs and customs connected with childbirth among the Banyankole, with special reference to utilisation of modern medical services' (unpublished BA Social Work and Social Administration dissertation, Makerere University Kampala, 1980), p. 40. Catholic missionaries in Ankole had to seek special guidance from their superiors on how to implement the practice of Pauline Privilege in a culture where a marriage which was childless technically was not a marriage. Compare Buhaya's much more modest fertility expectations. Reining, 'The Haya of north-western Tanzania', p. 217.

[50] Male FGD Nyamitanga, 19 Aug. 2004; Steinhart, *Conflict*, pp. 191–9.

frequency of conception overall within this community.[51] And yet traditional expectations that maximum family size would be between twelve to fourteen live births implied birth intervals of around twenty-four months.[52] Elderly male informants related that their wives managed their fertility to maintain their health and that of their children. 'Sometimes they limit themselves not to have unspaced children or when she is not yet ready to give birth... she would trick you . . . she would refuse if she knew that she could get pregnant.' Various methods of contraception were known, not all of which were likely to be effective. But the use of medicinal herbs with abortifacient properties and the rhythm method, as well as the fertility-suppressing effects of breast-feeding, would have helped women space out their births. Male informants emphasized the inferiority of women, but acknowledged that they possessed significant power within the household, not least over reproduction. 'When she wanted to conceive, she would wait until after her period and try hard to get you into having sex with her. Usually it is her wish to conceive.'[53]

Marriage required the transfer of clan property which explains why family aspirations regarding marital fertility were so explicit. Much more implicit was the sense in some clans that a man's brothers should enjoy some sexual access to the new bride. Anthropological sources and oral informants emphasized that these rights should be exercized with discretion. It should be done 'silently', 'in secrecy', 'privately'. The unease with which this practice was viewed in agriculturalist society was indicated by informants' insistence that only biological brothers possessed such rights, and surveys in the 1980s which revealed that only 8% of women admitted to having sex with their brothers-in-law, whereas 41% of men claimed to have had sex with their sisters-in-law.[54] Beyond this, and a feeling that male virginity at marriage was not necessarily appropriate, agriculturalists' sexual norms were highly conservative. Female pre-marital chastity was bolstered by rituals, with, for example, a mother sealing a newborn girl's vagina with breastmilk. Affairs were discussed using more negative language than in the other case study areas: 'infidelity was not common and it was not acceptable.' 'Men never wanted children outside their

[51] Mushanga, 'Nkole', p. 178; E. and F. Van de Walle, 'Post-partum abstinence in tropical Africa' in R. Gray, H. Leridon and A. Spira (eds.), *Biomedical and Demographic Determinants of Reproduction* (Oxford: Oxford University Press, 1993), p. 450; J. Ntozi, *The Role of Men in Determining Fertility among the Banyankore of Southwestern Uganda* (Kampala: Marianum Press, 1993), pp. 67, 71.

[52] This estimate does not take into account the effect of miscarriage and stillbirth.

[53] Mushanga, 'Nkole', pp. 174–80; Male FGD Nyamitanga, 19 Aug. 2004; Male FGD Ruti, 19 Aug. 2004; Kiyungi FGD Female, 21 Aug. 2004; Kamugisha, 'Beliefs', pp. 42–4.

[54] Mwesiga, 'Traditional marriage', p. 5; Ntozi and Kabera, 'Marriage patterns', pp. 28–34; Male FGD Nyamitanga, 19 Aug. 2004; Int. RNT, 9 Aug. 2004, Mbarara, M; Ntozi, *The Role of Men*, pp. 73–5.

marriages. These children would cause chaos.' And the possible consequences of unfaithfulness during pregnancy and breastfeeding were more severe than in other Great Lakes societies. Such behaviour might result in spiritual retribution in the form of miscarriage, stillbirth, infertility, or the child suffering from a particular respiratory illness called *amkire*, being unable to walk or talk, or dying. Sex before and outside marriage occurred, but this was a culture where immorality was constrained by the belief that marital stability produced large families, by pervasive insecurity, and by the desire to resist Hima assertions of agriculturalists' inferiority.[55]

BUGANDA

Lineage and inheritance were of real importance in Buganda, but they did not shape the character of sexual and reproductive life in the way that they did in Ankole and Buhaya. Instead, the dominant forces in Ganda society were meritocracy, mobility, and competitiveness. Buganda's clans weakened in power through the eighteenth century, undermined by rapid territorial expansion and royal centralization, so that by the nineteenth century chiefly patrons rivalled clan leaders as a source of wives. Chiefs, ambitious for promotion, strove to attract both male and female followers, to enhance their status and improve their capacity to meet royal demands. Clients' willingness to shift their loyalties to a neighbouring chief who offered better terms, and to follow a generous patron who had been transferred to another part of the kingdom, meant that Buganda possessed a remarkably unstable population given the near permanence of its banana gardens. Key to this mobility was the plentiful availability of land, as Buganda was largely free from the limitations on soil fertility that defined Buhaya.[56] This then was a society dominated by a particularly interventionist state, by East African standards, but energized by personal ambition and individual choice.

One individual's strategic advancement though often came at the expense of another's freedom. The early twentieth-century missionary-ethnographer Julien Gorju recorded nine different forms of sexual or marital relationship as having existed in pre-colonial Buganda, which underlines the kingdom's

[55] Mushanga, 'Nkole', pp. 178, 181; Male FGD Nyamitanga, 19 Aug. 2004; Bumbire (Bushenyi) FGD Female, 2004; F. Rubega-Baryakere, 'A study of divorce rate in Igara county, Bushenyi district' (unpublished BA Dip. Ed. dissertation, MUK, 1995), p. 36; Kiyungu Shema FGD Male, 21 Aug. 2004; Anon., 'How the Banyankole live', D. Stenning Papers, Cambridge University, ADD 7916, B1, p. 12.

[56] H. Médard, 'Introduction', in H. Médard and S. Doyle (eds.), *Slavery in the Great Lakes Region of East Africa* (Oxford: James Currey, 2007), pp. 27–30; H. Hanson, *Landed Obligation: The Practice of Power in Buganda* (Portsmouth, NH: Heinemann, 2003), p. 180.

social complexity. These relationships were associated with varying status, rights, and equality between the partners. Freedom of choice was enjoyed more by males than females, and six of these categories involved the transfer of authority over women from one man to another. Women could be brought into a relationship following their enslavement or abduction, to settle a family debt, to enable chiefs to satisfy their male clients, to win favour with a friend or patron, or to sustain a marriage following the death of one of its partners. A widow might be inherited by a relative of her late husband, theoretically for her and her children's protection, while the sister of a widower's late wife might be given as a substitute, to maintain good relations between two families. But three forms of relationship did require the consent of both parties: remarriage after divorce, living together without any formal ceremony, and 'marriage based on love between the parties'. This latter form, *obwamateeka* [of law] or *obwesimire* [of consent], was described as the standard form of marriage in Buganda, 'a proper legal marriage', where a woman 'makes her choice' of a marriage partner, or accepts a suitor's proposal, and full bridewealth was paid.[57] Often these marriages were engineered by the couple's families, though either partner could theoretically veto the arrangement. But the emphasis on sexual attraction, the giving of gifts to the woman before the betrothal, the practice of elopement, and references to love potions suggest that marriage could evolve out of romantic love, much more than was the case in Ankole or even Buhaya. Full bridewealth was the guarantor of a high status wedding, but social recognition of a marriage in Buganda was also secured by consent and, as Gorju observed, this could evolve with time. Originally coercive relationships could develop mutual respect and dependence, and might thus become acknowledged as true marriages.[58]

[57] J. Gorju, *Entre le Victoria, l'Albert et l'Edouard* (Rennes, 1920, translated by Ralph Butler, 1957, A. Richards papers, LSE archive, 6/23), pp. 397–409. See also Uganda Government, 'Report of the Commission on Marriage, Divorce and the Status of Women, 1965' (Entebbe, 1965), p. 10; N. Musisi, 'Women, "elite polygyny" and Buganda state formation', *Signs*, 16, 4, (1991), pp. 783–4; A. Mickleburgh, 'The relevance of marriage for Ganda women in Bwaise, Kampala, Uganda' (unpublished PhD dissertation, University of Cambridge, 1998), p. 93.

[58] Mickleburgh, 'The relevance', p. 96; F.-X. Kyewalyanga, *Traditional Religion, Custom and Christianity in Uganda: As Illustrated by the Ganda with Some References to other African Cultures and Islam* (Freiburg: Renner, 1976), pp. 49, 56; A. Kagwa, *The Customs of the Baganda* (translated by E. Kalibala, edited by M. Edel, New York: Columbia University Press, 1934), p. 172; L. Mair, *An African People in the Twentieth Century* (London: Routledge, 1965 [1934]), p. 79; J. Roscoe, *The Baganda: An Account of their Native Customs and Beliefs* (London: Macmillan, 1911), pp. 14, 87; J. Gorju, *Entre le Victoria, l'Albert et l'Edouard* (Rennes, 1920, translated by Ralph Butler, 1957, A. Richards papers, LSE archive, 6/23), pp. 397–8. That marrying was a process rather than an event can be further demonstrated by the practice of allowing poor men to defer bridewealth payment until after the ceremony which marked the point at which a couple began to live together. The failure of a man to complete the transfer of goods to his wife's family by a specified date was legitimate grounds for her to leave him. Wesigaba of Kitukulwe, 26 Jan. 1904, Marriage files, Mill Hill Fathers' Archive, Bishop's House, Jinja.

This was particularly likely if the relationship produced a child, because in Buganda any of a man's sons from any of his wives or lovers could become his heir. This stood in marked contrast to closely related societies to the east where only a son born to a man's first wife, or borne on her behalf, could inherit. As Rhiannon Stephens has observed, this potential for female upward mobility within a household was acknowledged in various proverbs, such as *Ddungu ayizze, ng'omuzaana azaalidde nyinimu ddenzi* ('The god of hunting has brought home his catch, says the slave woman who has given birth to a son for her master') and *Ndifiira ku biggya bya baze, nga y'azaala omusika* ('I will die at my husband's graveside, says the woman who gave birth to the heir').[59] Stephens' historical linguistic analysis showed that this prioritization of biological motherhood was one of several innovations which formed Ganda society's unique solution to the universal problem of childlessness. Ganda also insisted that men must be the genitor of their sons, and so developed various legitimacy tests to uphold biological fatherhood. According to Stephens, this shift towards an emphasis on biological parenthood and a more exclusive patrilineal system of inheritance partly derived from growing competition for control over the most fertile plots of land and their perennial banana plantations. Yet while, according to most sources, Ganda believed that only women could be infertile, they could hardly deny the existence of male impotence, one factor which would have sustained collateral succession, enabling a sonless man's brothers or brothers' sons to be his heirs.[60]

The varying categories of marriage carried differing rights of divorce. Women who were acquired without their consent were regarded as being akin to their husband's property and had little chance of leaving, no matter how overworked or illtreated. Such a woman was known as *omukazi wensimo* (wife of the worn out hoe). Women who had entered a marriage freely, by contrast, enjoyed more rights than in neighbouring societies, and could leave their husbands on a number of grounds, such as being poorly clothed, sexually unfulfilled, or being in love with another man.[61] But with few exceptions

[59] E. Haydon, *Law and Justice in Buganda* (London: Butterworths, 1960), pp. 82–3; R. Stephens, 'A history of motherhood, food procurement and politics in east-central Uganda to the nineteenth century' (unpublished PhD, Northwestern University, 2007), pp. 78–9. According to H. Johnston, *The Uganda Protectorate*, vol. II (London: Hutchinson, 1902), p. 642 'In former days, the [B]Uganda women being so frequently barren, it was the custom of the men . . . to raid the neighbouring countries . . . for wives, or to obtain large numbers of women by the slave trade.' For another example of slaves becoming wives in this region see S. Doyle, 'Bunyoro and the demography of slavery debate: fertility, kinship and assimilation', in H. Médard and S. D. Doyle (eds.), *Slavery in the Great Lakes Region of East Africa* (Oxford: James Currey, 2007), p. 240.

[60] Stephens, 'A history', pp. 74–5, 95; R. Stephens, 'Lineage and society in precolonial Uganda', *Journal of African History*, 50, 2 (2009), pp. 203–21; Haydon, *Law*, pp. 107, 218.

[61] A. Richards papers, LSE, 7/16, Mawokota, 16 June 1954; N. Musisi, 'Transformations of Baganda women: from the earliest times to the demise of the kingdom in 1966' (unpublished PhD dissertation, University of Toronto, 1991), pp. 103–4, 213.

bridewealth had to be repaid, and so unhappy women had to secure the support of their families. Men, meanwhile, often chose to neglect an ill-regarded wife rather than go to the trouble of formally ending their relationship. Hence divorce may not have been as common as the wide range of legal grounds would suggest. Yet it was frequent enough for laws regarding divorced women's access to land to have evolved, and certainly descriptions of chiefly courts indicate that powerful men often offered refuge to women whose marriages had failed.[62]

Julien Gorju wrote in 1920 that reproduction played an exceptionally large role in marriage in Buganda. The link between the two was so explicit in some clans that menarche was referred to as marriage and a pubescent girl as a wife, while the Luganda word for marriage, *kuwasa*, derives from the verb which means 'to copulate; to make pregnant'.[63] New brides hoped to fall pregnant immediately on marriage, and their mothers-in-law ritually encouraged them to produce as many children as there were fish in Lake Victoria.[64] The unhappiness and jealousy of the childless woman meanwhile was a common theme of songs and proverbs. Roscoe referred to the barren wife as 'despised . . . the slave and drudge of the household'. Women feared barrenness not only because of the ostracism it brought in their lifetime, but also because they knew they would be forgotten when they died. As one song put it, '*To die childless, when I die, I will be quite lost*.'[65]

And yet, despite this social pressure to reproduce, this was not a society constructed around pro-natalism in the way that agriculturalist Ankole was. While having some children was highly valued, women who had very large families were regarded, by society at large if not by their in-laws, as lacking self-control. Proverbs referred to such women as reproducing 'like a dog' or to giving birth as 'a deadly thing'.[66] New wives, unless they had married a chief, were not treated with the indulgence that brides experienced in neighbouring societies. A Ganda woman was kept secluded, fed, and free from

[62] Hansen, *Landed Obligation*, p. 55. Sources which suggested divorce was common include Kagwa, *Customs*, p. 176; Mair, *African People*, pp. 96–7; Kyewalyanga, *Traditional Religion*, p. 69. Contrast Roscoe, *The Baganda*, p. 97; J. Gorju, *Entre le Victoria, l'Albert et l'Edouard* (Rennes, 1920, translated by Ralph Butler, 1957, A. Richards papers, LSE archive, 6/23), p. 407.

[63] J. Gorju, *Entre le Victoria, l'Albert et l'Edouard* (Rennes, 1920, translated by Ralph Butler, 1957, A. Richards papers, LSE archive, 6/23), p. 438; Kyewalyanga, *Traditional Religion*, p. 46; Musisi, 'Women', p. 767.

[64] Roscoe, *The Baganda*, pp. 46, 64.

[65] Int. CNSM, 28 Aug. 2004, Butanga, M; Kisekka, 'The Baganda', III, p. 161; Roscoe, *The Baganda*, p. 46; '*Omusango gw'abalere*—The case of the flutists', http://myweb.tiscali.co.uk/petercooke/websiteDownloads/SSEMPEKE!.pdf

[66] Kisekka, 'The Baganda of central Uganda', in A. Molnos (ed.), *Cultural Source Materials for Population Planning in East Africa, Vol. II, Innovations and Communication* (Nairobi: EAPH, 1972), p. 167.

work for just nine days after her wedding, rather than four months in Ankole and nine to twelve months in Buhaya.[67] Moreover, Médard has argued that the frequency with which children were fostered out to relatives was an indication that they played a less central role in the family than in most African cultures. This may have been connected to the competing rights over a child which were enjoyed by the father and the mother's families. This conflict was one of the factors which left the clan membership of a new baby unclear until it was formally named, and required a man who had not paid full bridewealth to make an additional payment to his father-in-law to redeem his children from his wife's family. Médard also suggests that the model of womanhood emanating from Buganda's royal and chiefly courts gave little weight to reproduction. The huge harems of the kabaka and his senior chiefs inevitably produced relatively few children per woman, while the queen-mother, queen-sister, and two of the king's most important wives were forbidden from giving birth, a prohibition that also applied to all princesses until the mid-nineteenth century.[68]

In addition, there were a number of Ganda practices and beliefs which must have directly and indirectly reduced birth rates across the population. Women aimed for very long birth intervals, ideally breastfeeding for up to three and half years, and attempting to avoid conceiving before their last child was fully weaned. The relative ease of divorce and lack of pressure to remarry after separation meant that many women's reproductive potential was unfulfilled. Widowhood also limited Ganda women's average fertility, for although childless women were inherited, wives with children were not expected to remarry.[69] More unusual was the extent to which reproduction in pre-colonial Buganda was medicalized, due to the management of fertility being a matter of great anxiety and women competing with their in-laws for control of their bodies. The need for royal women to avoid giving birth encouraged the development of medical expertise in this field, which is likely

[67] J. Gorju, *Entre le Victoria, l'Albert et l'Edouard* (Rennes, 1920, translated by Ralph Butler, 1957, A. Richards papers, LSE archive, 6/23), p. 435. For Ankole see Mwesiga, 'Traditional marriage', p. 41; for Buhaya see Culwick, Culwick and Berry, *Population*, p. 124; M. Moller, 'Bahaya customs and beliefs in connection with pregnancy and childbirth', *Tanganyika Notes and Records*, 50, 1 (1958), p. 112.

[68] H. Médard, 'Croissance et crises de la royauté du Buganda au XIXe siècle' (unpublished PhD thesis, University of Paris 1, 2001), pp. 85–6; A. Richards papers, LSE, 6/19, Kinship, Mukwaya, 8 Apr. 1951; A. Richards papers, LSE, 7/16, Mawokota, 16 June 1954; Musisi, 'Transformations', pp. 74, 91. Some princesses did reproduce despite the ban but their children were not socially recognized. See N. Kodesh, 'Beyond the royal gaze: Ganda clans and the construction of an African metahistory' (unpublished PhD thesis, Northwestern University, 2005), p. 297.

[69] Richards papers, 7/16, Birth customs, Maryamu, Kisozi village, 20 Oct. 1954; Roscoe, *The Baganda*, pp. 96, 270; Haydon, *Law*, p. 217. Widows with children could remarry if they could persuade their clan to refund their bridewealth to their late husband's family.

to have spread beyond the court. Certainly early commentators noted that the use of abortifacients in cases of 'shameful' pregnancy or unhappy marriage was widespread in Buganda. Some women actively sought to limit their fertility in a less secretive manner, by avoiding sex during the days when they believed they were fecund, by using herbs believed to have contraceptive properties, or by persuading their husbands to sacrifice a goat to ritually bring a close to their reproductive lives.[70]

This tendency towards interventionism also applied when a pregnancy was desired. Herbs were commonly used to aid conception, and almost universally taken to smooth the course of a pregnancy and then to reduce the duration and pain of delivery. The use of oxytocic drugs to stimulate contractions derived partly from the frequency with which Ganda women, famous for their narrow pelvises, suffered obstructed labour due to disproportion, and partly from the belief that prolonged childbirth was proof of adultery. The effects of the herbal medicines taken during pregnancy have not been investigated, but the oxytocics have been blamed by modern medical researchers for contributing to high rates of ruptured uterus and subsequent stillbirth and maternal mortality.[71] The risk of maternal exhaustion must also have been high, given that traditional birth attendants tried to stop women from resting, eating, or sleeping during delivery. The frequency with which miscarriage, stillbirth, and neo-natal mortality occurred in pre-colonial times often seems to have encouraged a focus on pregnant women's blameworthy behaviour. Husbands' families responded to these beliefs by narrowing Ganda women's already limited diet still further by forbidding a variety of foods during pregnancy. The excluded items were often some of the most nutritious available, such as certain types of fruit, fish, and greens, as well as salt, a lack of which during pregnancy may result in malnutrition of the unborn child and hypertension and toxaemia in the mother. Anxiety about sub-fertility

[70] Roscoe, *The Baganda*, p. 237; Médard, 'Croissance', pp. 85–6; Int. CNSM, 28 Aug. 2004, Butanga, M; Female FGD, Bukoto, 24 Aug. 2004; Int. MGK, 26 Aug. 2004, Takajjunge, F; Int. PLGS, 31 Aug. 2004, Kitala, Busiro, M; A. Cook, *A Medical Vocabulary and Phrase Book in Luganda* (Kampala, 1921 edn. [1903]); Testimony of Yakobo Bazanye before Fr Mathews, 31 July 1903, Marriage files, Mill Hill Fathers' Archive, Bishop's House, Jinja. Thanks to Henri Médard for this reference. Barrenness was also understood in more medical terms than in neighbouring societies, as the result for example of a couple's blood being incompatible, or a woman suffering from cervical incompetence or an obstruction in her uterus. Mickleburgh, 'The relevance', p. 238; C. Olayiwola Akerele, 'Review of present M.C.H. services in West Mengo' (unpublished DPH dissertation, MUK, 1971, p. 17; Int. FKW, 31 Aug. 2004, Kitala, M.

[71] Kyewalyanga, *Traditional Religion*, pp. 20, 26; Roscoe, *The Baganda*, pp. 48, 55; E. Elsden papers, Rhodes House Oxford [RHO], MSS.Afr.s.1872 (49).

and resultant intervention in the reproductive process then may have formed something of a vicious circle.[72]

Sexuality in Buganda was similarly heavily regulated, though more by the state than the family, given its potential to provoke violence and disrespect for social status. Ganda writers have challenged early colonial criticisms of Buganda's licentiousness by emphasizing the complexity of the rules and punishments that governed sexual behaviour. Most sources emphasize that the socially sanctioned extra-marital sex that was so prominent in Ankole and Buhaya did not feature in Buganda. 'That Sodom did not exist', as one biblically minded informant put it.[73] But sexually explicit language and behaviour featured more prominently in Ganda culture than in its neighbours', pre-marital sex was less heavily penalized, and affairs based on individual choice were relatively common.

Ganda mores looked askance at displays or discussions of sexuality in normal public situations, but certain individuals were free from the usual restraints. The birth of twins, a dangerous blessing, required a family celebration that involved particularly lewd rites and dances, and the parents of twins were thereafter permitted to use language that would be condemned in other contexts. In addition, the recently bereaved were ritually freed from normal restrictions on non-marital sex.[74] Court life at Buganda's capital, one of the largest urban spaces in East Africa, also had its own rules of conduct. Princesses were particularly notorious for the freedom with which they spoke and behaved, minstrels sang 'impure and obscene' ditties, and descriptions of

[72] Kisekka, 'The Baganda of central Uganda', III, p. 157; Kyewalyanga, *Traditional Religion*, pp. 24, 28; Roscoe, *The Baganda*, pp. 49, 102; C. Olayiwola Akerele, 'Review of present M.C.H. services in West Mengo' (unpublished DPH dissertation, MUK, 1971, p. 17; Médard, Croissance, p. 68. Normal rock salt was forbidden, but salt made from vegetable ash was permitted. The burgeoning of research on Harmful Traditional Practices (HTP) has had the unintended consequence of reinforcing preconceptions of African backwardness. It is important to note that customs which negatively affected fertility or child survival were common to many cultures in the past. The avoidance of breastfeeding in many German societies in the eighteenth and nineteenth centuries resulted in catastrophic infant mortality rates, for example. Cf. S. Arnfred, 'Introduction', in S. Arnfred (ed.), *Re-thinking Sexualities in Africa* (Uppsala: Nordic Africa Institute, 2004), p. 13; Knodel, J., *Demographic Behaviour in the Past: a Study of Fourteen German Village Populations in the Eighteenth and Nineteenth Centuries* (Cambridge: Cambridge University Press, 1988).

[73] M. Mutyaba and P. Namukadde, 'Chwa II ne Muteesa II' (no date, *c.*1911), pp. 103–8; N. Musisi, 'Morality as identity: the missionary moral agenda in Buganda,1877–1945', *Journal of Religious History*, 23, 1 (1999), p. 70; Int. SKKG, 25 Aug. 2004, Kabonera, M. For one exception see Rubaga mission diary, 30 Oct. 1880, WFA. 'We learn that brothers, when they are together, live in a sort of communism of wives.'

[74] S. Nannyonga-Tamusuza, *Baakisimba: Gender in the Music and Dance of the Baganda People of Uganda* (New York: Routledge, 2005), p. 69; Haydon, *Law*, pp. 117–8; S. Nyanzi, J. Nassimbwa, V. Kayizzi and S. Kabanda, 'African sex is dangerous! Renegotiating "ritual sex" in contemporary Masaka District', *Africa*, 78, 4 (2008), pp. 525–9.

the court with its numerous neglected but heavily guarded wives and highly ambitious, status-conscious, risk-taking pages convey a strong sense of sexual intrigue and danger.[75] In all Ganda communities, events such as weddings or the arrival of the new moon were celebrated with dancing in a style which was perhaps the most heavily sexualized in the region. As Sylvia Nannyonga-Tamusuza has observed, the purpose of female dancing, which emphasized the flexibility of the dancer's waist and her quivering buttocks, was 'to leave all men in the audience aroused'. The verb to dance, *okuzina*, carries the deeper meaning of having sexual intercourse. All Baganda, moreover, were trained for married life in a manner which gave unusual attention to sexual performance. Male endurance was emphasized to grooms, linked presumably to the Ganda horror of impotence, while brides were taught a particular language of lovemaking, how to allure men by wearing beads around the waist, and in some cases how to use medicinal herbs for lubrication or tightness. Preparations for marriage began for girls at puberty, when they were required to elongate their labia, to enhance their future husbands' sexual pleasure. This then was a culture with an explicit, if mostly private, eroticism.[76]

Pre-marital pregnancy was no light matter in pre-colonial Buganda. For a girl to conceive while living under her father's roof was *amawemukirano* (an abomination), which threatened his life and disrupted the natural order of reproduction. Sex before marriage was also condemned, and a bride who was not found to be a virgin brought shame on her family. Yet the usual response to these breaches of proper behaviour lacked the fury reported in Ankole and Buhaya. Some informants mentioned that unmarried girls who fell pregnant used to be drowned, but on being questioned further, this punishment had more of a mythical quality than in neighbouring societies. 'In our clan, it never happened', as one informant put it, and if it occurred in other clans, then it was 'in the 1700s', in the pre-historical past. Other informants, meanwhile, had only heard of such drastic penalties being imposed in other ethnic groups. Interviewees rarely claimed that sex before marriage was an essentially modern corruption. 'In our culture it was not permitted . . . But as you know, they used to rebel and do it.' 'Even though they were not allowed, they did it. Because me I have my grandparent who produced children before marriage and even others.' This relative tolerance extended to the standard treatment of unmarried pregnant girls, who suffered only a partial banishment with the promise of rehabilitation. The disgraced family would either

[75] Roscoe, *The Baganda*, pp. 10, 34–5; J. Speke, *Journal of the Discovery of the Nile* (London: Blackwood, 1863), pp. 282, 339; Musisi, 'Women', pp. 757–86.

[76] Nannyonga-Tamusuza, *Baakisimba*, pp. 148–64; Kisekka, The Baganda', III, pp. 49–50. See also M. Southwold, 'The Baganda of Central Uganda' in Molnos, *Cultural Source Materials III*, p. 167.

send the girl to live with her seducer's family, or build a small hut on the edge of their banana garden, where the girl would have to live and eat alone, until the child was born. Then if the seducer brought a goat to be eaten by the girl's family, and the girl was ritually cleansed, the curse would be removed, and, if all were willing, the couple could move towards marriage. The parental response though might not be so benign if they were on bad terms with the boy's family, and more severe reprisals could be sought through the local chief.[77] Yet on the whole efforts to prevent pre-marital sex were not so intense as in Ankole or Buhaya, with sources referring to youngsters meeting while collecting water, herding goats, or participating in dances. Nor was pre-marital pregnancy a serious impediment to marriage, unless parents hoped to marry their daughter off to a chief.[78] This pattern of generally moderate penalties, a willingness to allow wrongdoers to rectify their mistakes, and an acceptance that rules would at times be broken would continue to characterize Ganda sexuality after marriage as well.

In contrast to Ankole and Buhaya, extra-marital affairs were regarded more negatively in Buganda than sex before marriage. Adultery was referred to as theft, as an adulterer was assumed to be planning to run away with his lover, or as murder because he either wished for the death of her husband or destabilized his household, causing his protective spirits to abandon him. Officially the penalty for adultery was death or mutilation, though this was often reduced to a heavy fine, which might never be paid in full. Affairs which took place during pregnancy or the post-partum period were particularly dangerous for the mother and her child. Yet the emphasis in the ethnographic literature was not on the results of such adulterous acts, but on the wide range of the prohibitions, and the accompanying methods of averting the negative consequences of misbehaviour or of cleansing the guilty party of the various

[77] D. Sempungu, 'Punishment of sin in Baganda traditional religion and in Christianity: an anthropological and biblico-moral study' (unpublished PhD dissertation, Lateran University, Rome, 1985), pp. 163–5; F. Bisase, 'The story of marriage in Buganda' (unpublished BA Fine Arts dissertation, MUK, 1976), pp. 14, 63; Int. AN, 25 Aug. 2004, Kagezi, F; Int. IST, 21 August 2004, Kagezi village, Masaka, M; Female FGD, Kagezi, 25 Aug. 2004; Int. NNFW, 28 Aug. 2004, Kaswa, F; Banaba Lwanga, Mawokota, 16 June 1954, A. Richards papers, LSE, 7/16; Roscoe, *The Baganda*, p. 263. Kagwa, *Customs*, pp. 98–101 mentions that an attempt by Ssuna II in the mid-nineteenth century to discourage pre-marital pregnancy by executing offenders lasted only a few years.

[78] Roscoe, *The Baganda*, pp. 24, 79; Banaba Lwanga, Mawokota, 16 June 1954, A. Richards papers, LSE, 7/16; Musisi, 'Transformations', p. 73. There is some evidence that homosexual sex was not uncommon among unmarried young men in Buganda in the 1880s. Missionaries, the main source on this issue, blamed Arabs for introducing the practice in recent decades, though the evidence for such assertions was rather dubious. Rubaga mission diary, 6 Aug. 1882, WFA. See H. Médard, 'L'homosexualité au Buganda, une acculturation peut en cacher une autre', *Hypothèse*, 1 (1999), pp. 47–52.

sins, through the use of prophylactic herbal medicine or confession and sacrifice. Affairs were dangerous and formally regarded with disapproval, yet Kisekka notes that they were 'recognised as almost an essential part of masculinity: a man who is faithful to his wife only is suspected of having little sexual strength'. The differing gendered expectations about continence were further demonstrated in the Ganda marriage vows, where the bride swore to be faithful to her husband, while the groom promised only not to desert his wife.[79]

The structure of Ganda society facilitated affairs in several ways. Its dispersed villages and the value attached to socializing made clandestine meetings easy to achieve. The power and wealth of the Ganda state brought courtly culture into the countryside, in a modified form, for high and middle ranking chiefs' 'enormous enclosures' attracted young men seeking administrative training and *Banakyeyombekedde* (independent women) who either lacked relatives or sought protection from them. Some widows and divorcees became chiefs' concubines, but it was more usual for them to become servants to the chiefs' wives, having affairs as they chose. And finally the mobility and ambition which so struck outsiders created space for the *Bakirese* (restless people), who moved from contact to contact, seeking material wealth from friends and lovers without being willing to commit to a long-term relationship. Overall, sexuality in Buganda was more complex than in Ankole and Buhaya, because the state here was so much larger and more interventionist.[80] The royal government undermined clan control of marriage and sexual behaviour, displacing it with relatively pervasive regulation and arbitration. But this legalism contributed to the development of means of averting the negative consequences of sexual impropriety. Similarly, the overt submissiveness of Ganda women concealed the fact that they had more rights than wives in most interlacustrine societies, if they enjoyed a full, legal marriage: a wife may have been expected to speak to her husband as though he was her patron,

[79] J. Gorju, *Entre le Victoria, l'Albert et l'Edouard* (Rennes, 1920, translated by Ralph Butler, 1957, A. Richards papers, LSE archive, 6/23), pp. 440–9, 460; Kyewalyanga, *Traditional Religion*, pp. 21–2, 29–32, 61; Kisekka, 'The Baganda of central Uganda', III, pp. 153, 156; Roscoe, *Baganda*, pp. 17, 72, 101–2, 262. The danger associated with adultery was the subject of a number of Ganda proverbs, such as *Mulungi tansukka, bye biwanga by' okumakubo*: 'People who do not allow beautiful women to pass by, are those whose skulls we see by the roadsides.' A. Kiyimba, 'Gendering social destiny in the proverbs of the Baganda: Reflections on boys and girls becoming men and women', *Journal of African Cultural Studies*, 17, 2 (2005), p. 263.

[80] Roscoe, *The Baganda*, p. 13; C. Obbo, 'Town migration is not for women' (unpublished PhD dissertation, University of Wisconsin-Madison, 1977), pp. 172–4; P. Davis, 'On the sexuality of "town women" in Kampala', *Africa Today*, 47.3/4 (2000), pp. 32–5; A. Hastings, *Christian Marriage in Africa, Being a Report Commissioned by the Archbishops of Cape Town, Central Africa, Kenya, Tanzania, and Uganda* (London: SPCK, 1973), p. 50. That materialism did influence some pre-colonial sexual relationships is indicated by the song *Gganga Alula*, which compared women to highly nutritious flying ants, for both 'can be enticed out after being covered with bark cloth'. http://myweb.tiscali.co.uk/petercooke/websiteDownloads/SSEMPEKE!.pdf

but like all clients in Buganda wives developed knowledge of 'the art of being ruled', as Audrey Richards put it, and might transfer her loyalty should she be excessively neglected.[81] Finally, the Ganda aversion to displays of sexuality in public went side by side with an unusual commitment to sexual fulfilment.

CONCLUSION

The primary purpose of this chapter was to test the assumption that pre-colonial sexual behaviour in sub-Saharan Africa was characterized by an unchanging, uniform fixation with the extension of the lineage, which required a tolerance of sex outside marriage. The descriptions of the three case study areas highlighted a series of major differences in sexual and reproductive attitudes and practices across neighbouring ethnic groups. But the strongest challenge to the aggregating aspect of Goody-Caldwell thesis came from within one of the case studies, Ankole, as its agriculturalist majority were the most pro-natalist and sexually austere community examined, while Ankole's Hima pastoralist elite combined a remarkably wide range of legitimate extra-marital sexual opportunities with an anxiety that the fertility of a household's wives should not outstrip that of its cattle. Buhaya, meanwhile, did not fit with Goody and Caldwell and his associates' belief that sub-Saharan societies prioritized maximized fertility over sexual probity, for its long-established villages, fixation with landed property, social differentiation, concern with family inheritance, and intense efforts to prevent pre-marital pregnancy were classically 'Eurasian', to use their terminology, whereas the Haya tolerance of extra-marital sex to ensure the production of a male heir was stereotypically 'African'. Buganda, finally, provides the best evidence of pre-colonial change in social norms, linked to the rapid expansion and increasing interventionism of the state and the decline of the clans, while it also demonstrates the need to consider the role of social class in the evolution of sexual behaviour.

The arguments presented in this chapter have attempted to show complexity and variation, but the limitations of the sources have nonetheless tended to produce normative, apparently environmentally deterministic explanations for diversity.[82] Later chapters will be able to tell a more detailed,

[81] A. Richards, 'Authority patterns in traditional Buganda', in L. Fallers (ed.), *The King's Men: Leadership and Status in Buganda on the Eve of Independence* (New York: Oxford University Press, 1964), pp. 257–8. For an important study of Ganda marriage as a form of patronage see Carol Summers' forthcoming book, *Restless Tongues*.

[82] This chapter has at some points, for the sake of clarity, elided differences in beliefs within each case study area. Some clans in each society had distinct traditions regarding fertility and sexuality, while within Buhaya the practice of *bisisi* for example was not recognized in Kiziba. This is an inevitable problem affecting comparative history in Africa, but if anything it further undermines the unitary thesis of African sexuality.

cultural story, but the significance of the environmental context of social change should not be easily dismissed, for it was key to the development of distinct local settlement patterns and rules of inheritance, which in turn were crucial influences over patterns of sexuality and rules of marriage in the pre-colonial past.

2
Disease and Mortality, 1860–1924

INTRODUCTION

Variations in sexual and reproductive attitudes and practices across the Great Lakes region are relatively easy to discern for the pre-colonial period. Levels of morbidity and mortality, and the beliefs that different peoples held about these phenomena, are more elusive. Even for the early colonial period conclusions drawn from comparative analysis, with few exceptions, must be tentative, for the medical systems of Uganda and Tanganyika during the first quarter of the twentieth century recorded data of very uneven quantity and value, and early ethnographies rarely explored indigenous concepts of disease and death in great detail. Yet much can still be said. Later anthropological and medical investigations contained information that can be extrapolated back to the pre-colonial era, particularly regarding disease ecology. The diaries and correspondence of missionaries in Buganda's capital, which marked out time between the 1870s and 1890s by recording wars, famines, and epidemics give an overwhelming sense of the intensity of the demographic crisis that befell that kingdom in the final decades of its independence. Certain diseases such as sleeping sickness and syphilis posed such a threat to the viability of the colonial project in its infancy that sustained research into their causation and impact was undertaken. One consequence of the determination to quantify and reduce the impact of syphilis on pregnancy loss, infant mortality, and neo-natal morbidity was the early establishment of maternity clinics whose remarkably detailed registers provide a unique, if geographically restricted, resource.

These sources have relatively little to say about variations in disease and mortality patterns between the three case study areas before the middle of the nineteenth century, though it is reasonable to assume, from twentieth-century evidence, that malaria was then a more severe problem in Buganda and Buhaya than in Ankole. Moreover the impact of long-distance commerce from the East African coast was much greater in Buhaya and especially Buganda than in Ankole, with proximity to major trade routes bringing not only new sources of power and wealth, but also heightened conflict, enslavement, epidemic, and famine. The instability associated with the population movements which accompanied the spiralling violence of the 1880s and 1890s and then the imposition of colonial rule disturbed local disease ecologies across the region, culminating in a devastating sleeping sickness pandemic at the start of the twentieth century. Simultaneously the end of Great Lakes societies' relative isolation from the outside world exposed local populations to a myriad of new pathogens, ultimately ensuring that contagious infections would come to rival vector-borne environmental diseases as a source of ill-health.

CONTEXT

Climatic conditions vary significantly across the Great Lakes region, with the heaviest, most regular rainfall occurring on Buganda and Buhaya's Lake Victoria shoreline. Moving westwards away from the lake, annual precipitation gradually declines from a maximum of around 2600mm to a minimum of around 800mm in central Buhaya, western Buganda, and eastern Ankole, before increasing again with altitude in Karagwe and Ankole's western hills to around 1250mm. Rainfall and topography influenced the distribution of a number of diseases, most obviously malaria. Mid-twentieth-century research found that malaria was highly endemic in the wettest areas, prone to erupt in occasional epidemics in areas of moderate rainfall, and generally absent in the highest or driest areas. These variations in transmission translated into distinct patterns of morbidity and mortality, with the greatest impact in the wetter, holoendemic zone being experienced by infants and small children who suffered severe, repeated, and often fatal attacks, while in the mesoendemic areas, which tended to suffer epidemics after unusually severe rainy seasons, infection and death were much less frequent overall, but were likely to occur among older children and adults as well as the very young.[1] More people in Buganda and Buhaya than in Ankole lived in close proximity to a source of water, which greatly increased the risk of malarial infection, but, as partial compensation, permitted a higher level of personal hygiene. Western observers were impressed by the cleanliness of methods of food preparation among the Ganda and Haya, and noted that everyone was expected to wash

[1] EAMS, *Annual Report 1952* (Nairobi: Government Printer, 1953), p. 19; R. Cook, 'Child health in Ankole, Uganda: a programme of immunization and health education and its evaluation' (unpublished DMed dissertation, University of Oxford, n/d [*c*.1968]), p. 19; H. Welbourn, 'A comparison between children attending child welfare clinics in 1950 and in 1955', *East African Medical Journal*, 34, 2 (1957), p. 51. Patterns of malaria infection and mortality will have varied between the nineteenth and the twentieth centuries, as new kinds of *Anopheles* breeding sites and higher rates of migration were countered by new forms of prevention and treatment.

their hands before eating, and to bathe daily. Only the chiefly elite possessed latrines in Buganda and Buhaya, no doubt inspired by the challenges of their semi-urban lifestyle, but the Ganda also took particular care, it seems, over spring protection. Such fastidiousness does not appear to have been common in Ankole, particularly among the Hima pastoralists, so it is likely that Nkole would have suffered significantly higher rates of diarrhoea and respiratory infections, two of the major causes of under-five mortality in this region, and would also have experienced greater morbidity due to infestation with intestinal worms.[2]

Malnutrition was similarly the product of a combination of both natural and social factors. Protein deficiency was likely to have been a problem across most of this region mainly because of recurrent livestock loss due to trypanosomiasis and East Coast Fever (theileriosis). Only the Hima were able to keep a degree of control over the insect vectors of these diseases due to lower rainfall and intensive range management. But the relative scarcity of cattle across most western areas of pre-colonial Ankole was also due to the Hima's attempts to maintain their political dominance by restricting agriculturalist ownership of productive cows. In Buhaya and Buganda too, cattle ownership among the peasantry was rare, and families often reserved their smallstock for feasts and fines. Here dried fish was the staple source of cheap animal protein, but even this was denied to the poor in Ankole, who shared the pastoralist taboo against eating it. Women in all three case study areas, meanwhile, were nutritionally disadvantaged by being forbidden such high value foods as eggs, goat, grasshoppers, and chicken. Officially this ban related to the danger such foods held for female fertility, though oral informants universally agreed that the real motivation was men's greed.[3]

[2] Int. VK, 27 June 2000, Bukoba, M; M. Weiss, *Die Völkerstämme im Norden Deutsch Ost Afrikas* (Berlin: Carl Marschner, 1910), p. 167; H. Rehse, *Kiziba: Land und Leute* (Stuttgart: Strecker und Schröder, 1910, translated by Mrs Donne, UDSM, Cory 369), Ch.2, p. 4; J. Roscoe, *The Baganda: An Account of their Native Customs and Beliefs* (London: Macmillan, 1911), p. 75, 243, 436, 442, 458–9; A. Culwick and G. Culwick, edited by V. Berry, *The Culwick Papers 1934–1944: Population, Food and Health in Colonial Tanganika* (London: Academic Books, 1994), pp. 109, 163; J. Roscoe, *The Northern Bantu: An Account of some Central African Tribes of the Uganda Protectorate* (London: Cass, 1966 [1915]), p. 103; W. Bazley, 'Reminiscences as a district officer in Uganda, 1951–1953, 1958–1960', RHO MSS Afr. s. 924, p. 78. Roscoe, *The Baganda*, pp. 413–4 notes that Arab traders introduced soap making into Buganda in the later nineteenth century, but it was primarily used for washing clothes.

[3] Rehse, *Kiziba*, Ch.3, pp. 3–5, Ch.7, p. 7, Ch.11, p. 4; E. Chipadza, 'The correlation of socio-economic and educational levels, cultural factors and malnutrition among the Banyankole tribesmen of Uganda' (unpublished PhD dissertation, United States International University, 1982), p. 87; I. Gateley, 'The traditional education of women and girls in Uganda' (unpublished PhD dissertation, University of London, 1968), p. 62; Roscoe, *The Baganda*, p. 391; e.g. Int. AC, 9 Aug. 2000, Rubaa-Rubya, F. The restriction on agriculturalist cattle ownership was by no means absolute. See J. Willis, 'Clan and history in western Uganda: a new perspective on the origins of pastoral dominance', *The International Journal of African Historical Studies,* 30, 3 (1997), pp. 583–600.

The peoples of this region sought to avert and control ill-health in highly complex ways. Attempts were made to control local disease environments, the prophylactic consumption of herbal medications against various diseases was commonplace, and immoral behaviour was associated with specific health problems suffered by the guilty party or an innocent near relative. Public healing, whether as an organized community-wide response to a major epidemic, or at a more intimate level, in the form of divination, confession, and compensation, was one response to individual and communal ill-health. But indigenous healers also possessed impressive pharmacological and surgical skill. Afflictions were categorized by cause, symptom and scale, but a culture of pragmatism, and the existence of distinct specialisms, encouraged experimentation.[4] These were not peoples who were helpless in the face of disease, as imperial propagandists argued during the nineteenth century, yet in Africa, as elsewhere in the world, some practices that were common in the past had negative impacts on health. For example, the extreme vulnerability of the newborn baby was unintentionally accentuated in this region by a number of traditions. Babies tended to be left unwrapped and then bathed very soon after birth, which could result in hypothermia. The umbilical cord was typically cut using a dried reed taken from the thatch of the family hut, and then smeared with ash or herbal medicine, practices which would have exposed the infant to a high risk of neonatal tetanus and sepsis, two of the most common causes of death in the first weeks of life. In addition, the belief that colostrum was dangerous for new babies caused parents to feed the newborn with a variety of prelacteals—millet or water in Ankole, mushroom soup in Buganda, beer in Buhaya—until the mother's milk came in. Not only would this have raised the incidence of diarrhoea in the newborn, it would also have increased the likelihood of postpartum haemorrhage in the mother, as early breastfeeding stimulates uterine contraction, and it deprived the baby of the essential nutrients and immunity-building antibodies that colostrum contains.[5]

[4] See for example S. Doyle, *Crisis and Decline in Bunyoro: Environment and Population in Western Uganda, 1860–1955* (Oxford: James Currey, 2006), pp. 31–4; N. Kodesh, *Beyond the Royal Gaze: Clanship and Public Healing in Buganda* (Charlottesville: University of Virginia Press, 2010).

[5] A. Cook, *A Medical Vocabulary and Phrase Book in Luganda* (Kampala: SPCK, 1921 edn.), p. 53; A. Goulet, *Sur les bords du Victoria, chez les Baganda* (Toulouse: Librairie Missionnaire, 1949), p. 37; G. Rwegelera, 'Tribal customs in infant feeding I: Among the Haya', *East Africa Medical Journal*, 40 (1963), pp. 366–9; A. Kamugisha, 'Beliefs and customs connected with childbirth among the Banyankole, with special reference to utilisation of modern medical services' (unpublished BA Social Work and Social Administration dissertation, Makerere University Kampala, 1980), p. 17; Int. BK, 12 Aug. 2004, Mbarara, F. Rehse, *Land*, ch.12, p. 1 noted that in Kiziba in northern Buhaya, babies born into elite families were cleaned by being rubbed with butter rather than washed, which may have reinforced mortality differentials by class.

LONG-DISTANCE TRADE, DISEASE, AND FAMINE

Buganda

This then was no merrie Africa, but when the first western explorers, James Grant and John Hanning Speke, journeyed through Karagwe in western Buhaya and then Buganda in 1861 and 1862, they were struck by these societies' obvious prosperity and localized high population densities, as well as by the seemingly benign environment in which they lay. The reports of their discovery of such large, complex, ordered kingdoms, located at the source of the Nile, created immense excitement in Europe, partly because their isolation from the outside world tended to be exaggerated. In fact Speke and Grant followed a well-established route, guided by experienced traders from the Swahili coast. Buganda's capital had been the terminus of one of East Africa's major trade routes since the 1840s, while for several generations before that Buganda and other parts of the Great Lakes region had been indirectly connected to global markets and epidemic diseases, via Karagwe, the regional entrepot.[6] The large caravans that meandered over several months through a series of villages carried with them not just beads, guns, and cotton cloth, but also a host of new bacteria and viruses.[7]

The analysis of the impact of long-distance trade will focus first on Buganda for two reasons. The consequences of the new commerce were particularly wide-ranging here, for Ganda society was destabilized not only by new diseases but also by the effects of new religions and weaponry. Moreover the Ganda experience is much better documented than that of the other case studies. Explorers tended to remain in Buganda longer than in most societies they passed through, but crucially European missionaries were resident in its capital almost continuously from 1877, documenting every disease outbreak, war, and famine in great detail. Of all the new diseases, smallpox was the most significant. Although an indigenous strain probably existed in the Great Lakes area long before the eighteenth century, it seems that long-distance traders introduced the more deadly Mediterranean strain, *Variola major*, causing huge mortality over the century that followed. Traditional histories identified smallpox as the cause of death of several kings across the region around 1800, but the historical record becomes richer closer to the arrival of

[6] C. Wrigley, *Kingship and State: The Buganda Dynasty* (Cambridge: Cambridge University Press, 1996), p. 57. The opening up of the Nile Basin from the north, by slave traders and then agents of the Egyptian empire, would have created an additional, albeit less direct, source of new infections.

[7] G. Hartwig, 'Economic consequences of long-distance trade in East Africa: The disease factor', *African Studies Review*, 18, 2 (1975), pp. 63–5; J. Iliffe, *A Modern History of Tanganyika* (Cambridge: Cambridge University Press, 1979), p. 81.

literate witnesses. Three major epidemics occurred during the reign of Buganda's King Ssuuna (*c.*1830–57), the last of which killed him. Smallpox outbreaks increased in frequency between 1870 and 1877, and then recurred almost every year between 1883 and 1894. The medical missionary Robert Felkin was informed in 1879 that smallpox epidemics had very high fatality rates, each 'carrying off thousands of victims', a claim that was supported by accounts of the 1884 outbreak which reportedly caused 10,000 deaths.[8]

The other disease classically linked to the caravan trade was cholera, but the symptoms of this disease are so similar to dysentery that definite identification is difficult to achieve. Very large-scale mortality associated with cholera-like symptoms were reported to have occurred during Ganda military expeditions around 1837 and 1870, dates which coincided with outbreaks of cholera on the Indian Ocean coast. These though may simply have been episodes of dysentery, which was a frequent companion of armies on the march in this region. Other imported epidemics recorded as causing major mortality in late nineteenth-century Buganda include measles in 1885, 1889–90, and 1893, influenza in 1892 and 1899, jiggers in 1892, and possibly yellow fever in 1880.[9]

Buganda's pre-colonial history is one of sustained expansion, initially focusing on territorial aggrandisement, then in the nineteenth century concentrating instead on increasing its ability to raid and extract tribute from its hinterland. The exceptional aggression of the Ganda state was fuelled by the frequency with which it emerged victorious from external wars, due mainly to its ability to put more troops in the field faster than its neighbours, an advantage linked primarily to the benefits of banana cultivation.[10] The few major defeats that are documented tended to follow from epidemics among troops on the march, as for example in 1884 in Bukedi. But even this failure cost the lives of only a hundred or so soldiers.[11]

[8] J. Iliffe, *Africans: The History of a Continent* (Cambridge: Cambridge University Press, 1995), p. 209; J. Kuhanen, *Poverty, Health and Reproduction in Early Colonial Uganda* (Joensuu: University of Joensuu Press, 2005), pp. 119–122; Médard, *Le royaume du Buganda au XIXe siècle: mutations politiques et religieuses d'un grand état d'Afrique de l'est* (Paris: Karthala, 2007), pp. 70–6; C. Wilson. and R. Felkin, *Uganda and the Egyptian Soudan* (London: Sampson Low, 1882), p. 183. As Médard notes, the identification of some epidemics must be tentative, given the lack of medical training of most western observers and the imprecision of aspects of Ganda medical terminology. *Kawumpuli* for example is usually translated as plague, but it could refer to any sudden outbreak of a fatal disease.

[9] Médard, *Royaume*, pp. 72–6; J. Speke, *Journal of the Discovery of the Source of the Nile* (London: Blackwood, 1863), p. 309. J. Brierley and T. Spear, 'Mutesa, the missionaries, and Christian conversion in Buganda', *International Journal of African Historical Studies*, 21, 4 (1988), pp. 608–9 suggest that cholera also broke out in 1859 and 1882.

[10] R. Reid, *Political Power in Pre-colonial Buganda: Economy, Society and Warfare in the Nineteenth Century* (Oxford: James Currey, 2002).

[11] Médard, *Royaume*, p. 82.

By contrast, the civil wars of the late 1880s and 1890s inflicted far greater battle casualties on the Ganda, partly because the efficiency of the Ganda military system was turned against its own people, partly because it was only during these civil wars that the Ganda learnt how to use their thousands of imported firearms to their full potential, and partly because these wars were ideologically inspired. Buganda's various warring parties were fighting not just for control of their own kingdom but also, they believed, for the survival of their religion. These heightened stakes explain the brutality of the massacres that followed particularly crushing victories such as that of October 1888 when several hundred Christians died. Contemporary accounts of civil war battlefields described scenes where 'skulls are as numerous . . . as mushrooms'. Yet still, as Médard observes, the demographic effect of such battlefield losses was negligible for a population so large as Buganda's. It was the indirect impact of warfare that was significant.[12]

Buganda's foreign expeditions had always been vulnerable to outbreaks of infectious disease, due to the congregation of thousands of men and the inadequate sanitation of their temporary encampments. But the civil wars that began when a coalition of young Catholic, Muslim, and Protestant members of the kingdom's elite overthrew King Mwanga in 1888, before turning in on itself, triggered a new kind of population loss. While the initial coup was ostensibly in defence of religious freedom, a series of counter-coups and revolts saw each religious group in succession attempt to monopolize power, the power of the Ganda monarchy gradually undermined, and, ultimately, agents of the British empire enforcing Ganda Protestant dominance. Ganda society experienced an unprecedented level of disruption for much of the period 1888 to 1899. A larger proportion of the Ganda population was under arms than ever before, chiefs and their followers were repeatedly transferred due to the constant shifting of the religious balance of power, and villages emptied as the battlefront moved towards them. Crops were deliberately destroyed, troops denuded the countryside of livestock, and normal cultivation was interrupted. Médard estimates that perhaps a third of Buganda's population was displaced during these wars.[13]

Buganda's traditional history, unlike that of her neighbours, did not depend on famine for much of its chronological framework. Before 1880 only two famines, one in the early 1830s, another in 1856, feature in the story of the nineteenth century. Buganda had long enjoyed exceptional food security for East Africa partly due to its regular rainfall and its perennial, heavy cropping bananas. But Buhaya shared these characteristics, yet suffered regular famine. Buganda enjoyed two further advantages, an almost total

[12] Médard, *Royaume*, pp. 84–5; M Twaddle, *Kakungulu and the Creation of Uganda 1868–1928* (Athens, OH: Ohio University Press, 1993), p. 52.
[13] Médard, *Royaume*, pp. 65–7, 82–8.

freedom from destructive invasion, and the capacity to import food in very large quantities during shortages from its tributary states, typically by canoe. The 1880s brought a drought of such widespread severity to East Africa that even Buganda suffered crop failure, but the crisis deepened once civil war broke out, with famine occurring in 1889–90, 1893–4, 1896–7, and 1899–1902. Even so, relatively few people died of starvation. The real loss to Buganda's population came from the epidemics and emigration which followed famine and conflict. Hunger and demographic instability undoubtedly facilitated the spread of smallpox, but more importantly they provided ideal conditions for the transmission of plague, a disease that was long-established in Buganda, but which seems to have increased in severity in the last decades of the twentieth century as the size of the royal capital increased. Epidemics may have typically originated in the squalor of the urban poor, but the elite were rarely spared. One epidemic in 1881 reportedly included 300 royal wives among its victims. Successive outbreaks around the capital in the years that followed culminated in a devastating episode at the end of the decade which, in combination with other epidemics, was claimed by contemporaries to have caused the deaths of between 7,000 and 40,000 people. In the 1890s plague seems to have been most severe in the previously relatively isolated southern province of Buddu. In late 1893 missionaries reported that a combination of plague, smallpox and famine had resulted in the deaths of 18% of the 600 adults who had been baptized in the parish of Villa Maria in the past six months.[14] At the same time Buganda, which had attracted immigrants for generations, suffered the departure of a significant proportion of its population. Even before the civil war started, the profit potential of the new slave trade to the East African coast had encouraged chiefs to sell off criminals, and husbands to rid themselves of difficult wives. This weakening of Buganda's social contract pushed the kingdom towards civil war, which in turn devalued old concepts of reciprocal obligation and generated new notions of internal enemies. The various warbands plundered the population on an unprecedented scale. According to one account, between 1890 and 1892, 20,000 Ganda slaves were sold by the Muslim faction to the neighbouring kingdom of Bunyoro alone. Buganda was no longer the most attractive place in the Great Lakes to live, and hunger, insecurity, and disease drove tens of thousands of

[14] Médard, *Royaume*; H. Médard, 'Croissance et crises de la royauté du Buganda au XIXe siècle' (unpublished PhD thesis, University of Paris 1, 2001), pp. 748–52; H. Médard, 'La peste et les missionnaires: santé et syncrétisme médical au royaume du Buganda à la fin du 19ème siècle', *Outre-Mer Revue d'Histoire*, 346–347 (2005), pp. 79–102. Some of these famines were relatively localized, and several were worsened by drought and locust attack. It may be that the Villa Maria data give an exaggerated overall mortality rates, if, as was common in the early missions, many people sought baptism because they were near death.

Ganda to seek refuge elsewhere. Missionary sources indicated that one-fifth of Kooki's population left during a famine and epidemic in 1896, though no doubt some would have returned later.[15]

The most controversial aspect of Buganda's precolonial medical experience is the role of long-distance trade in the spread of sexually transmitted diseases (STDs). European observers in the late nineteenth and early twentieth centuries believed that syphilis and gonorrhoea were very common diseases in Buganda, and associated their frequency with the disruptive impact of Arab and Swahili traders from the East African coast. It was thought that Ganda society had not yet had time to adapt to the presence of this new kind of epidemic, so difficult to contain once it had taken hold among the general population, destabilized as it was by new forms of commerce, religion, and violence.[16] These assumptions have been questioned in recent scholarship, with Henri Médard, for example, noting that it was hardly surprising that Muslim merchants should have been held responsible for the spread of STDs, given missionary beliefs about both the immorality of the East and the inability of African cultures to resist its contaminating influence.[17] Moreover, Maryinez Lyons, Michael Tuck, and Megan Vaughan among others have emphasized the role played by preconceptions about African hypersexuality in influencing doctors' tendency to overdiagnose STDs.[18] Yet these assumptions also emerged from Ganda chiefs' attempts to deflect Europeans' moral critique onto the coastal outsider, from regional stereotypes of the immoral

[15] H. Médard, 'Introduction' in H. Médard and S. Doyle (eds.), *Slavery in the Great Lakes Region of East Africa* (Oxford: James Currey, 2007), p. 18; J. Nyakatura, *Anatomy of an African Kingdom: a History of Bunyoro-Kitara* (edited by G. N. Uzoigwe (New York: NOK, 1973), pp. 144–7, 101; Médard, *Royaume*, p. 67.

[16] Wilson and Felkin, *Uganda*, p. 184; R. Felkin, 'Notes on the Waganda tribe of Central Africa', *Proceedings of the Royal Society of Edinburgh*, 13 (1885/86), p. 706; A. Cook, 'Notes on the diseases met within Uganda, Central Africa', *Journal of Tropical Medicine*, 4 (1901), pp. 175–8; F. Lambkin, 'An outbreak of syphilis in a virgin soil: Notes on syphilis in the Uganda Protectorate', in D. Power and J. Murphy (eds.), *A System of Syphilis* (London: Oxford University Press, 1908), p. 339; F. Lambkin, 'Summary of evidence', Dec. 1907, National Archives (NA), CO/536/15. 'Swahili' was employed in Uganda as a generic identifier used to describe anyone from the East African coast who spoke Kiswahili.

[17] Médard, 'Croissance', p. 83.

[18] M. Vaughan, *Curing their Ills: Colonial Power and African Illness* (Cambridge: Polity, 1991), pp. 130–6; M. Lyons, 'Medicine and morality: a review of responses to sexually transmitted diseases in Uganda in the twentieth century' in P. Setel, M. Lewis, and M. Lyons (eds.), *Histories of Sexually Transmitted Diseases and HIV/AIDS in Sub-Saharan Africa* (London: Greenwood, 1999), pp. 97–117; M. Tuck, 'Venereal disease, sexuality, and society in Uganda,' in R. Davidson and L. Hall (eds.), *Sex, Sin and Suffering: Venereal disease and European society since 1870* (London: Routledge, 2001), pp. 191–204.

Ganda, and from westerners' observation of sexual behaviour which seemed ideally suited to the spread of STDs in Buganda.[19]

Before the 1890s Europeans' sense of Ganda mores was shaped by the harems, unattached females, feasts, and dances of the royal capital and chiefly courts.[20] Westerners then acquired the freedom to learn more of village society just as a series of civil wars challenged chiefly authority and undermined marital and community stability. A sense of the growing sexual vulnerability of women during this period has been provided by Michael Tuck's analysis of marriage cases arbitrated by Catholic missionaries at the turn of the century. These revealed how common it had become for women on Buganda's increasingly lawless periphery to be kidnapped from their families by individuals, and then how frequently these slaves were transferred from man to man as their owners fell into debt or saw an opportunity to secure a patron or client.[21] At the same time, other Ganda women, having fled the insecurity of their own society, used their sexuality to try to survive in the communities where they had sought refuge. Haya men at the start of the twentieth century reportedly 'scorned the Baganda women who go about the country as prostitutes, because of the danger of disease'.[22] While Ganda sexual behaviour probably did become more high-risk from the 1880s, it is worth noting that even in the mid-nineteenth century, before Ganda society was dislocated by war, a number of societies across the Great Lakes region had attributed a perceived increase in local STD prevalence to Ganda commercial and military intrusion.[23] It was not unreasonable then for European doctors, having heard of, and then witnessed, what seemed to be high levels of partner exchange affecting sections of Ganda society, to have assumed that a high incidence of STDs must therefore exist.

The medical history of syphilis in Buganda was debated throughout the colonial period and will be discussed later in this chapter. The earliest report of gonorrhoea in Buganda's traditional history tells us that Kabaka Kamaanya (*c.*1812–*c.*1830) caught the disease early in his reign. If we assume that this diagnosis is accurate, then gonorrhoea reached Buganda at the very latest a few decades in advance of the coastal merchants. It is of course possible that the disease had been present for centuries before Kamaanya's misfortune, and the linguistic historian Chris Ehret has indeed argued that gonorrhoea is of

[19] F. Lambkin, 'Summary of evidence', Dec. 1907, NA, CO/536/15; M. Tuck, 'Syphilis, sexuality, and social control: a history of venereal disease in colonial Uganda' (unpublished PhD, dissertation, Northwestern University, 1997), pp. 123–4.

[20] Wilson and Felkin, *Uganda*, p. 269; Speke, *Journal*, pp. 300–76.

[21] M. Tuck, 'Women's experiences of enslavement and slavery in late nineteenth- and early twentieth-century Uganda', in Médard and Doyle, *Slavery*, pp. 174–86.

[22] Rehse, *Kiziba*, Ch.11, pp. 7–8.

[23] Médard, *Royaume*, p. 80.

considerable antiquity in East Africa. Although Ehret's linguistic evidence did not derive specifically from Great Lakes societies, the great variety of terms for this disease which can be found in the various Great Lakes languages probably does indicate long familiarity with gonorrhoea in the region. Yet given the large number of wives and concubines Buganda's kings had access to, it seems likely that earlier royal infections would have been mentioned, had the disease been present in the kingdom before the time of Kamaanya.[24] While it is probably safe to assume that gonorrhoea arrived in Buganda at the latest in the late eighteenth century through its trading links with Karagwe, the regional entrepot for long-distance commerce, it is likely that the disease remained relatively uncommon in the general population until the later nineteenth century, as it was regarded before the mid-nineteenth century as an indicator of promiscuity. That gonorrhoea was originally viewed negatively is indicated by linguistic evidence which suggests that the most common Luganda term for the disease, *nziku*, was derived from a verb (*–zika*) which meant to 'go out of cultivation; be overgrown'. Whether *nziku* was conceptually linked to infertility, mortality or a retreat from civilization is unclear, but any of these connotations would have been damaging. According to various accounts, the growing association of gonorrhoea with royalty transformed perceptions of the disease. The Ganda chronicler, Apolo Kaggwa, records that both of Kamaanya's successors, Ssuuna (*c.*1830–*c.*1857) and Muteesa (*c.*1856–1884), also suffered gonococcal infection, Muteesa dying due to complications from his second bout of the disease. Initially considered unclean, now members of the court endeavoured to catch it in imitation of the king. Oral informants reported that the infected 'would call themselves the brave men', for they endured 'the disease of heroes'. A song from the period stated that 'He is a fool who does not have gonorrhoea, he is a coward who fears this disease.'[25] By the 1890s gonorrhoea had spread beyond the courtly elite at least as far as the royal capital's rural hinterland, according to early medical evidence from Mengo missionary hospital, which catered primarily to Ganda from Kampala and its environs. In 1901 this hospital treated 5% of its inpatients for urethral stricture, one of gonorrhoea's most disabling sequelae, a remarkably high frequency. Research in the 1960s suggested that the period between first gonococcal infection to diagnosis of urethral stricture was fifteen

[24] Médard, *Royaume*, p. 79; C. Fyfe and D. McMaster, 'Introduction', in C. Fyfe and D. McMaster (eds.), *African Historical Demography: Vol. 2* (Edinburgh: University of Edinburgh, Centre of African Studies, 1981), p. 8.

[25] J. Miti, 'A Short History of Buganda, Bunyoro, Busoga, Toro and Ankole' (trans. G. Rock, unpublished microfilm, n/d), p. 132; Int. AN, 25 Aug. 2004, Kagezi, F; Int. FN, 29 Aug. 2004 Butanga, F; Médard, 'Croissance', pp. 83–4; B. Zimbe, 'Buganda and the king: A royal history of Buganda' (TS, n/d, trans. Simon Musoke), p. 62.

to eighteen years in Buganda, though a shorter gap between infection and stricture is indicated by other studies. The 1901 evidence indicates that gonorrhoea had been well established for some years. It is possible that it had begun to be dispersed among the general population before 1888, though no doubt the instability of the civil wars accelerated its spread, and that of sexually transmitted syphilis, contributing to Buganda's evolving crisis of low fertility and high child mortality.[26]

External observers agreed that the combined impact of famine, new epidemics, slave exports, and war caused Buganda's population to decline in the later nineteenth century. Ganda women were believed to be 'very poor breeders' due to the destructive consequences of early marriage and STDs, while death rates were thought to have increased after the 1860s.[27] Roscoe suggests that male mortality had always been much higher than female because men faced a greater risk of meeting a violent death. He perhaps underestimated the risks of childbirth, but other evidence suggests that a sex imbalance in the pattern of mortality may have become more evident as the century progressed. In 1898 a Catholic missionary noted that of 100 converts, almost all male, christened between 1880 and 1885, only 57 were still alive, indicating a high annual death rate of approximately 28.5 per 1000. What is interesting about this group is that they belonged to Buganda's courtly elite. When they were baptized almost all of these converts were aged between fifteen and thirty, a group that would be expected to have had relatively low mortality in most societies. But in the peculiar circumstances of the 1880s and 1890s in Buganda, the life expectancy of chiefs and pages declined rapidly. A series of epidemics that ravaged Buganda's capital between 1882 and 1885 accounted for a third of the deaths affecting this cohort. Then seventeen of the converts were executed by Buganda's king in 1886. The remainder died as a result of the civil wars, either in battle or in exile, where the refugees

[26] J. Davies et al., 'Cancer in an African community, 1897–1956: An analysis of the records of Mengo Hospital, Kampala, Uganda: Part I', *British Medical Journal*, 1, 5378 (1964), p. 261; J. Kibukamusoke, 'Gonorrhoea and urethral stricture', *British Journal of Venereal Diseases*, 41 (1965), p. 135; R. Chambers and B. Baitera, 'The anatomy of the urethral stricture', *British Journal of Urology* (1977), 49, p. 545; R. Moffat, 'Uganda Protectorate: Report for the year ending December 31, 1900', *Journal of Tropical Medicine and Hygiene*, 4 (1901), pp. 326–45; J. Davies, 'The history of syphilis in Uganda', *Bulletin of the World Health Organization*, 15 (1956), p. 1052. Interestingly in 1901 the head of the Ugandan colonial medical service, Robert Moffat, reported that gonorrhoea was common, but one of its most disabling sequelae, urethral stricture, was still 'exceedingly rare'. But Moffat's data, according to his contemporary, the missionary doctor Albert Cook, were unrepresentative of the local population, given that most of the patients treated by the colonial health service in its first years were servants of the state, non-Ganda soldiers, and police.

[27] e.g. Roscoe, *Baganda*, p. 97; H. Johnston, *The Uganda Protectorate*, vol.II (London: Hutchinson, 1902), pp. 641–2.

suffered from exposure to a new disease environment.[28] This group of elite male Catholics constitute a small sample, but their experience is an extreme example of the excess mortality that affected the entirety of Ganda society during these decades.

The extent to which Buganda's population declined in the second half of the nineteenth century, though, was probably overstated by several contemporary commentators. For example, Britain's proconsul Harry Johnston, claimed that 'the kingdom of [Bu]ganda in the time of Muteesa [*c.*1856–1884], though then of smaller extent politically than at the present day, probably numbered 4,000,000 people. In 1901 I was not able to estimate the population at much over 1,000,000.' Early colonial writers were quick to accept data which would justify the British takeover on humanitarian grounds. Thus, according to Johnston, only the civilizing mission could save the Ganda 'from dying out as a race'. Médard has recently argued that the perception of cataclysmic demographic decline partly originated in the desire of some early European writers to justify either bringing the kingdom into the British empire or expanding the scale of the local Christian missions. The deliberate exaggerations of Buganda's former population size that resulted set a benchmark that would subsequently create the impression of extreme demographic decline, when later estimates inevitably produced far lower totals.[29] Reports of Buganda's nineteenth-century population size varied wildly between 150,000 and 4,000,000. One of the higher totals was proposed by John Roscoe, a missionary anthropologist and the best informed European writer from the period. During his research in the early twentieth century Roscoe identified informants who were likely to have observed how the pre-colonial state had recorded both the number of households for taxation purposes and the number of men of fighting age for military planning. Roscoe claimed that Buganda's population in the 1890s had stood at 1,500,000, half of what it had been early in Muteesa's reign, that is *c.*1860.[30] As Médard has observed though, the higher total would indicate a population density similar to that found in Buganda

[28] Roscoe, *Baganda*, p. 97; A. Achte to L. Livinhac, Rubaga, 7 Aug. 1898, no.87, 119, White Fathers Archive, Rome (WFA). Cf. Médard, *Royaume*, p. 89. The calculation of the death rate assumes that the converts were baptized at regular intervals during the period 1880 to 1885. In fact, due to the temporary withdrawal of the White Fathers between November 1882 and July 1885, baptisms were clustered at the start and end of this period.

[29] Johnston, *Uganda*, vol.II, pp. 640–2; Médard, 'Croissance', pp. 748–52; R. Kuczynski, *Demographic Survey of the British Colonial Empire, Vol. II* (Oxford: Institute of International Affairs, 1949), pp. 120–1.

[30] Médard, 'Croissance', pp. 748–82; Roscoe, *Baganda*, p. 6; Wilson and Felkin, Uganda, II, p. 20. Supposedly all chiefs were required to send a shell representing each hut in their province to the treasury, while the king used different coloured pegs to record troop numbers in the various chiefdoms.

today, which seems rather unlikely. The most reliable contemporary observer was Henry Morton Stanley, who travelled more widely through pre-colonial Buganda than any other European. Stanley, having accompanied one of Buganda's military expeditions, claimed to have an accurate sense of the number of Buganda's warriors, and the ratio of civilians to soldiers. His 1876 estimate of 870,000 for Buganda's total population seems plausible, if perhaps a little low.[31] An accurate picture of Buganda's demographic situation before the colonial takeover is impossible to provide. The first count of Buganda's population in 1906, which seems to have been carried out with reasonable precision, reported that the population of those areas which had belonged to Buganda in the middle of the nineteenth century totalled around 500,000. Given that the frequency and severity of famine, epidemic, and conflict within the kingdom increased so dramatically in the later nineteenth and early twentieth centuries, it is likely that Buganda's population had formerly been substantially greater.[32]

Buhaya

Buganda may have been transformed by long-distance trade from the East African coast more comprehensively than any of its neighbours, but it is possible that western Buhaya suffered more from the demographic impact of imported military technology, a more intensive slave trade, and new diseases than any other interlacustrine society. The caravans which served the great lakes had terminated at Karagwe for several generations before Buganda supplanted it as the regional entrepôt in the middle of the nineteenth century. But trading parties to and from Buganda and its neighbours continued to pass through Karagwe until the 1890s. Karagwe's exposure to the new commerce was not only of longer duration than Buganda's, but it may also have been more intense, as its rulers were less able to limit traders' influence. For decades, communities of coastal traders were resident at Kafuro, near the royal capital, and Kitengule, on the Buganda border, where they formed the nucleus of villages that grew to substantial size. The close relationship between the merchants and Karagwe's elite though came under strain as Buganda grew ever more interventionist in its attempts to secure access to the outside world. These pressures came to a head when the long-serving, entrepreneurial monarch, Rumanyika, died in 1878, prompting a series of succession wars, during one of which several coastal traders were murdered. With Karagwe no

[31] H. Stanley, *Through the Dark Continent* (London: Simpson Low, Marston, Searle, and Rivington, 1878), vol. I, pp. 196, 384.

[32] A. Rendle, Buganda population 1906–07, enclosure in F. Lambkin, Report, Uganda 1908–54, Women's Library, London, 3AMS/D/49. Demographic decline may have been offset before the 1880s by slave imports, but would have been substantial thereafter.

longer able to guarantee their security, traders looked increasingly to eastern Buhaya and then Lake Victoria as alternative routes to Buganda. Karagwe sank into decline, as its elite conflicted over declining profits and their kingdom's growing dependence on its northern neighbour.[33]

One of the most destructive consequences of the new trade for the Haya states was the role it played in encouraging greater Ganda interference in their affairs. The status of kingdoms like Karagwe and Kiziba oscillated between tributary and ally, while smaller states like Bugabo were forced to allow Buganda control of its lakeshore trade. Most damaging of all was the frequency with which Buganda raided across its southern border and along Buhaya's shoreline seeking slaves and depleting local food reserves.[34] But even the commercial aspects of Buhaya's ever closer relationship with Buganda had demographic implications, with outbreaks of plague that started in Buganda frequently spreading south.[35] In addition Buhaya suffered all the new epidemics associated with the new commerce. The great colonial chief F.X. Lwamgira's history of the Kiziba kingdom emphasized the exceptional severity of famine and disease in the later nineteenth century: 'Disease stayed in Kiziba for two generations and all that time people continually died.' Buhaya's crisis came to a head in the early 1890s, beginning with the great rinderpest panzootic which killed most of the region's livestock, having its greatest impact in the cattle kingdom of Karagwe. A smallpox epidemic followed so closely that it was believed to be the human form of the same contagion, though it probably did result from the disruption which accompanied the sudden loss of people's livelihoods. Soon afterwards large numbers were killed or disabled by the arrival of the South American jigger flea, and then a major famine brought widespread mortality. Finally, Germany's colonial takeover prompted a series of wars between the Haya states, as local rulers sought to turn the immense power of European weaponry against their neighbours.[36]

The impact of the new commerce was not entirely negative for Buhaya. The wealth that was created permitted Haya to import significant numbers of slaves from Buganda in the 1880s, and improving communications probably accelerated the uptake of exotic crops like sweet potatoes, which would have

[33] I. Katoke, *The Karagwe Kingdom: A History of the Abanyambo of North-west Tanzania* (Nairobi: EAPH, 1975), pp. 70–104.

[34] Médard, *Royaume*, p. 143; Rehse, *Land*, Ch.3, p. 4.

[35] Rehse, *Land*, Ch.13.

[36] Lwamgira, 'Kiziba', pp. 78–92; J. Ford and R. Hall, 'The history of Karagwe (Bukoba District', *Tanganyika Notes and Records*, 24 (1947), pp. 3–27 pp. 19–23; Rehse, Land, Ch.7, p. 8, Ch.14, p. 5; S. Kachuchuru, 'A historical survey of Banyambo economy in Karagwe district, 1860–1960' (unpublished MA (History) dissertation, UDSM, 1975), p. 61; Iliffe, *Tanganyika*, pp. 104–5.

compensated to some extent for the increase in conflict-related famine. But what evidence exists suggests that the late nineteenth-century crisis had adverse demographic consequences overall, particularly for western and central Buhaya. Eastern Buhaya's compact villages would have facilitated the spread of new epidemic diseases, but the sources are too sparse to provide any sense of change over time. In Karagwe, however, early European writers created an impression of substantially greater population density than was recorded in the first decades of the twentieth century.[37]

Ankole

While most Great Lakes societies embraced the opportunities presented by the new commerce of the nineteenth century, others attempted to isolate themselves, fearing the instability that might follow the introduction of new sources of wealth and power. Societies such as Rwanda and Burundi, which attempted to close their borders to long-distance traders, delayed their full integration into global disease networks, and so appear to have limited the extent and duration of the increase in mortality that affected the entire region between around 1850 and 1924.[38] The kingdom of Nkore followed an inconsistent policy, usually but not always refusing to allow coastal caravans to travel across its territory, and at times stopping the Swahili from entering the kingdom at all. No doubt such vacillation would have limited the Ankole region's exposure to new communicable diseases, but only to a degree. Local traders remained free to purchase and distribute coastal merchandise from Karagwe, using the commercial networks that for generations had brought salt from Lake Katwe across Nkore and the petty kingdoms to its west on to Buganda, Buhaya, and Rwanda. Still the long-distance trade route through Nkore was of distinctly secondary importance, and the rarity of references to new epidemics in local traditional histories before the 1890s presumably reflects the indirect and infrequent nature of Ankole's contact with coastal commerce.[39]

[37] F. Stuhlmann, *Mit Emin Pascha ins Herz von Afrika* (Berlin: Reimer, 1894), pp. 712, 726; Rehse, *Land*, Ch.3, p. 4, Ch.1, p. 2; Kachuchuru, 'Historical', p. 1; Ford and Hall, 'Karagwe', pp. 19–23; Culwick, Culwick and Berry 'Population', p. 177.
[38] J.-P. Chrétien, *The Great Lakes of Africa: Two Thousand Years of History* (New York: Zone, 2003, trans. S. Strauss), pp. 139–201; C. Thibon, 'Un siècle de croissance démographique au Burundi (1850–1950)', *Cahiers d'Études Africaines*, 27, 105/106 (1987), pp. 61–81.
[39] G. Schweinfurth et al., *Emin Pasha in Central Africa: Being A Collection of His Letters and Journals* (London: G. Philip, 1888), p. 489.

Ankole's fortunes began to change when civil war broke out in Buganda in 1888, prompting the Christian Ganda to seek refuge in Kabula on the Nkore border. While this alliance would bring diplomatic rewards in the future, in the short term the Ganda arrival was associated with sickness and violence. The disruption brought by the Ganda though was of minor significance compared to the impact of the rinderpest panzootic which destroyed not only the great majority of the area's livestock, but most of its game as well. Frederick Lugard in 1891 found pastoralist Nkore devastated: 'large numbers of the people . . . had died, unable to procure food, or to accommodate themselves to an unwonted diet. The remnant are thin and half-starved.'[40] Soon afterwards a severe outbreak of smallpox caused further mortality, particularly among the ruling elite, possibly, according to Ford and Hall, because famine had reduced Hima resistance, or more likely because, as Marc Dawson has suggested in relation to Kenya, hunger tended to drive pastoralists into closer contact with agriculturalists, among whom smallpox had been able to become an endemic disease due to their greater population density.[41] Nkore then attempted to regain its strength by recruiting Ganda gunmen into its army, and using them to raid cattle from its southern neighbours. This hubristic assault on Rwanda, now the most powerful state in the region, prompted a retaliatory invasion in 1894, which resulted in the evacuation of Nkore's capital, significant mortality, and the loss of many of Nkore's remaining cattle. The heirless death of Ntare, Nkore's king, in 1895 then brought four years of internecine and occasionally bloody conflict, Ntare's only son having died during the 1892 smallpox epidemic.[42]

The consequences of long-distance trade seem not to have been particularly severe in Ankole until the decade-long crisis at the end of the nineteenth century. Even then, the western parts of the area that would become Ankole seemingly were less affected by disease and the violence that followed it. Lugard, having witnessed the misery of the pastoralist Hima in Nkore, was surprised to see the prosperity of the agricultural communities to the west, 'a country densely populated, and with enormous areas of cultivation'.[43] Population estimates around the turn of the century confirmed that population density was higher in the west of Ankole than the east. This had probably

[40] F. Lugard, *The Rise of Our East African Empire: Early efforts in Nyasaland and Uganda* (Edinburgh and London: William Blackwood and Sons, 1893), vol.II, p. 159; R. Mettam, 'A short history of rinderpest with special reference to Africa', *Uganda Journal*, 5, 1 (1937), pp. 22–6.

[41] Ford and Hall, 'Karagwe', p. 21; M. Dawson, 'Socioeconomic change and disease: smallpox in colonial Kenya, 1880–1920', in S. Feierman and J. Janzen, *The Social Basis of Health and Healing in Africa* (Berkeley: University of California Press, 1992), p. 94.

[42] Steinhart, *Conflict and Collaboration* (Kampala: Fountain, 1999 [1977]), pp. 134–40.

[43] Lugard, *Rise*, II, p. 162.

long been true, as pastoralism does not tend to allow for heavy settlement, and limited evidence suggests that STDs may have been long-established among the Hima. A seemingly traditional admonition to a new bride warned her not to catch syphilis before her husband. Nonetheless, the differential became more extreme in the 1890s, if Hima claims in 1901 that their population had fallen by two-thirds since the rinderpest were at all accurate. Early estimates of the total population of the area were almost certainly gross overestimates. Stanley for example believed Ntare to have 200,000 spearmen. Estimates for the whole of Ankole at the start of the colonial period ranged from 250,000 to 600,000, while the 1911 census, which should not be considered particularly reliable, reported a total of 229,000. It is likely that the population would have been substantially higher than this figure before the disasters of the late nineteenth century.[44]

THE COLONIAL TAKEOVER

Sleeping Sickness

Pro-empire propagandists in the late nineteenth century made much of the population loss that they believed had resulted from uncontrolled war, slave raiding, epidemic, and famine in their attempt to persuade often unenthusiastic European governments of the merits of a proposed colonial takeover in East Africa. In the event, crisis mortality would remain at a high level until the mid-1920s across much of the region. The colonial takeover did reduce the incidence of war-related deaths dramatically, even though significant numbers of Ganda died in the German East African campaign of the First

[44] J. Willis, *Mengo Notes*, 2, 7 (1901), p. 88; Johnston, *Uganda*, II, pp. 615, 626; Y. Elam, *The Social and Sexual Roles of Hima Women: A Study of Nomadic Cattle Breeders in Nyabushozi County, Ankole, Uganda* (Manchester: Manchester University Press, 1973), pp. 121–2; H. Stanley, *In Darkest Africa, or the Quest, Rescue, and Retreat of Emin, Governor of Equatoria* (London: Sampson Low, Marston, Searle & Rivington, 1890) I, p. 33; vol. 2 p. 331; A. Tucker, *Eighteen Years in Uganda and East Africa* (Westport, CN, Negro Universities Press, 1970 [1911]), II, p. 232; J. Meldon, 'Notes on the Bahima of Ankole', *Journal of the Africa Society*, 6, 22 (1907); Uganda Protectorate, *1911 Census Returns* (Entebbe: Government Printer, 1912). The assumption that STDs were more common among the Hima than local agriculturalists is based on ethnographic evidence indicating a wider range of sexual contacts among the former than the latter, and suggesting that affairs between members of the two groups were not common, and usually involved dependent agriculturalist men or women, who were it seems largely isolated from their communities of origin. Intermarriage between the two communities occurred in the past but does not seem to have been frequent. Yet as the following chapter will show, there is some evidence of high agriculturalist secondary sterility in the early colonial period, and suggestions that moral codes were tightened around the same time. STDs therefore may have been more common among the pre-colonial agriculturalist population than the normative stereotypes of the twentieth century would indicate.

World War. Evidence of the slave trade, moreover, disappeared very rapidly from British records in Uganda after 1900. German tolerance of the institution of slavery ensured that Buhaya's experience was rather different, but still, missionary criticism ensured that slave exports on any serious scale quickly became impossible.[45] Yet the colonial takeover at first only added to the instability that had characterized the region for decades. The acquisition of Ankole, Buganda, and Buhaya all saw the destructive power of imperial forces being employed on behalf of their local allies against rival kingdoms or religious groups. Then the establishment of colonial control introduced unprecedented levels of taxation and labour extraction, prompting significant migration, both temporary and permanent. This upheaval was magnified in Buganda by the establishment of *mailo* land tenure following the 1900 Agreement, which awarded the best farmland in Buganda as freehold estates to the kingdom's elite. A series of evictions and voluntary resettlements followed, 'until the whole population was at movement. Streams of men, women and children going east with all their household goods, cattle, sheep, goats, and fowls, met similar streams going west.'[46]

This was the context in which a devastating epidemic of sleeping sickness broke out, first along the shores of Lake Victoria around 1898 and then a decade later in the western Rift Valley, on Ankole's western border. Some observers portrayed sleeping sickness or human trypanosomiasis as the ultimate symbol of Africa's anarchic nature, its scattered, uncontrolled population helpless against an equally undisciplined environment.[47] For other European witnesses, though, the suffering brought by the epidemic inspired feelings of guilt, not condemnation, as sleeping sickness was viewed as the ultimate colonial disease. They believed that sleeping sickness, though long resident in West Africa, had never been present in East Africa before the European arrival. Most early colonial researchers seeking the origin of the outbreak held that *Trypanosoma brucei gambiense* had been recently introduced from the eastern Congo or southern Sudan, blaming the 'opening up of equatorial Africa' and British proto-imperialists' relocation of Sudanese soldiers from Egypt's Equatoria empire.[48] Others focused less on the method of importation of the infection, and emphasized instead the series of crises of

[45] J.-P. Chrétien, 'The slave trade in Burundi and Rwanda at the beginning of German colonisation', in Médard and Doyle, *Slavery*, pp. 210–27; Médard, 'Introduction', p. 3.

[46] Tucker, *Eighteen Years*, II, pp. 261–2.

[47] e.g. A. Swynnerton, *Report on the Control of Elephants in Uganda, 6 Nov. 1923* (Entebbe: Government Printer, 1924), pp. 9–15.

[48] e.g. Moffat to commissioner, 17 June 1902, NA, FO/2/591. See K. Morris, 'The movement of sleeping sickness across central Africa', *The Journal of Tropical Medicine and Hygiene*, 66 (1963), pp. 59–76 for an expanded version of this thesis. Cf. M. Lyons, *The Colonial Disease: A Social History of Sleeping Sickness in Northern Zaire* (Cambridge: Cambridge University Press, 1992).

the 1890s which followed the European arrival: the rinderpest epizootic, Kabaka Mwanga's rebellion in 1897, the mutiny of Britain's Sudanese troops, a succession of epidemics, and shocking scenes of famine.[49] This perspective became dominant once John Ford published his research in 1971 on the ability of African communities to live in equilibrium with the trypanosomes and their vector, the tsetse fly. Ford and a number of other environmental and medical historians have argued that pre-colonial African societies were sufficiently stable for a degree of resistance to sleeping sickness to be achieved through intermittent, unintentional inoculation. But this long-standing endemic situation was upset in the 1890s, according to Ford. The rinderpest panzootic initially reduced tsetse numbers due to the disappearance of so many of their hosts, but then the tsetse population rebounded as its bushland habitat expanded due to the absence of game and livestock. Environmental change thus exposed human communities to unprecedented levels of contact with dense colonies of tsetse, overcoming the limited resistance that people had previously acquired, and triggering epidemics.[50]

Recent research though has offered some refinement to the Fordian thesis. It seems significant that the initial focus of the outbreak, southern Busoga, had been subject to Ganda slave raids long before the disruption of the 1890s, so the extent to which people enjoyed some kind of harmonious relationship with their local disease environment is doubtful. Secondly, a review of the early clinical descriptions of sleeping sickness in Uganda found that the rapidity with which these cases died did not fit with the usual slow progression of *T. b. gambiense*, a chronic if ultimately fatal disease. One possible explanation for this anomaly is that greatly increased fly–human contact would have enabled acute epidemics of sleeping sickness to occur, as trypanosomes were passed quickly through the human population by direct mechanical inoculation. Sleeping sickness contracted in this manner proves fatal in a short time. Increased contact, it should be noted, did not necessarily require heavy tsetse populations. Descriptions of some local epidemics instead found that conflict, smallpox, drought, and famine in the late 1890s had forced local communities for prolonged periods into areas inhabited by tsetse. The bush contained more people, not necessarily more tsetse. An alternative hypothesis is that the Lake Victoria epidemic was not in fact caused by *T. b. gambiense* at all, but by *T. b. rhodesiense*, which causes the most acute form of sleeping

[49] e.g. A. Hodges, 'Sleeping sickness report, Jan. 1902', NA, FO/2/589.

[50] J. Ford, *The Role of the Trypanosomiases in African Ecology* (Oxford: Oxford University Press, 1971), pp. 243, 250; Lyons, *Colonial*, pp. 47, 226–7; H. Kjekshus, *Ecology Control and Economic Development in East African History* (London: Heinemann, 1977), p. 25; H. Soff, 'A history of sleeping sickness in Uganda: administrative responses, 1900–1970' (unpublished Ph.D. dissertation, Syracuse University, 1971), pp. 10–12; Lyons, *Colonial*, pp. 54–6.

sickness. *T. b. rhodesiense* was first identified in Northern Rhodesia in 1910 and then found in Busoga following a sleeping sickness outbreak in the 1940s, when it was assumed to have spread from southern Africa in the interwar years. Recently though *T. b. rhodesiense* in Uganda has been shown to be genetically distinct from the southern African community, and appears to have been very long established. As Fèvre and his associates have argued, because *T. b. rhodesiense* is a zoonosis whose reservoir is principally domestic cattle, it may be that the sleeping sickness outbreaks of 1898–1920 were triggered by intense restocking efforts following the rinderpest panzootic. As cattle were raided and traded with unprecedented urgency across the entire region after 1891, trypanosomes may have been introduced into a series of previously uninfected tsetse communities, creating the conditions for a regional pandemic.[51] This thesis though does not explain why the epidemic began in the established endemic area of Busoga, reinforcing the significance of the unusual opportunities for trypanosomal transmission created by the instability of the 1890s.

Whatever the colonial role in the origins of the great sleeping sickness epidemic, the colonial state felt compelled to respond rapidly to the danger presented by the outbreak. Perhaps 250,000 people died during the great Ugandan outbreak, with the majority of recorded cases occurring in Buganda. Mortality was on a lesser scale in German East Africa, with hundreds rather than thousands of victims in Bukoba. In the early years, scientists anticipated that the scale of mortality might be much greater. Before its epidemiology was fully understood, it was feared that there was 'nothing to prevent this disease spreading down the Nile or to Mombasa and eventually to India'.[52] This combination of danger and ignorance resulted in some of Britain and Germany's leading medical researchers such as David Bruce, Aldo Castellani, and Robert Koch being dispatched to the region, but their political masters quickly lost patience with the lack of practical results emanating from the

[51] Pearson to Wright, 29 Sept. 1879, Church Missionary Society Archives, Birmingham (CMS), CA6/019/13; Pearson to Mackay, 29 July 1880, CMS G3 A6/0 1881/22; Doyle, *Crisis and Decline*, pp. 146–50; G. Carpenter, 'Some of the problems connected with sleeping sickness', 9 Aug. 1926, ESA (Entebbe Secretariat Archives), A46/193; A. Hodges, Diaries, 1–3 Jan. 1905, MS, RHO, MSS. Afr. s. 1782 noted that tsetse numbers had not yet recovered to pre-rinderpest levels in the Bunyoro epidemic area; Fiske, 'A history of sleeping sickness and reclamation', 6 May 1926, NA, CO/536/140; T. Koerne, P. de Raadt, I. Maudlin, 'The Uganda sleeping sickness epidemic revisited: a case of mistaken identity?', *Parasitology Today,* 11, 8 (1995), pp. 303–306; E. Fèvre, P. Coleman, S. Welburn and I. Maudlin, 'Reanalyzing the 1900–1920 sleeping sickness epidemic in Uganda', *Emerging Infectious Diseases*, 10, 4 (2004), pp. 567–73.

[52] W. Eckart, 'Medical experiments at the colonial periphery: the fight against sleeping sickness in German East Africa and Togo', in V. Roelcke and G. Maio (eds.), *Twentieth Century Ethics of Human Subjects Research: Historical Perspectives on Values, Practices, and Regulations* (Stuttgart: Franz Steiner Verlag, 2004), p. 73; Sadler to Lansdowne, 5 June 1902, NA, FO/2/590.

laboratories. The death of several Europeans in the colonial capital further undermined research into the aetiology of sleeping sickness in Uganda. The governor, Hayes Sadler, with 'the fear of death in him' decided that in the absence of a cure, 'there is no course but to let the epidemic . . . work itself out,' and devoted his energies into trying to relocate the sleeping sickness research station away from his headquarters in Entebbe. The laboratory finally closed in 1906 when one of the researchers died from the disease he was studying.[53] Later that year a new governor, Hesketh Bell, proposed a strategy of evacuation and relocation. Bell was driven to this policy partly by a desire to alleviate the suffering he witnessed in a sleeping sickness hospital soon after his arrival, partly by the need to shift the Protectorate's focus from disease to economic progress.[54]

By this time the Colonial Office had come to the conclusion that British research had been 'in no sense, first class'.[55] The most able scientists sent by the Royal Society had long gone, and the careful observations of the ecology of the disease by Protectorate medical officers had resulted in proposals that seemed neither exciting nor cheap. Localized bush clearance, the removal of the sick, and education on tsetse avoidance for the healthy would, decades later, become standard elements in Uganda's tsetse control programmes.[56] But in 1906 a more attractive alternative emerged from German East Africa, where an experiment involving the mass evacuation of tsetse-infested habitats was being trialled. Its mastermind, Robert Koch, convinced Bell and the Colonial Office of the need to remove the entire Ugandan population from the vicinity of the lake by claiming that 'nearly every soul now remaining in the islands is infected, and that . . . all must assuredly die within a year or two.' Koch hoped that depopulating the tsetse-infested areas would deprive the vectors of their source of infection, so that within 'a comparatively short period, the insects would no longer be capable of transmitting the disease'. Meanwhile, the segregation of the sick in lazarets inland would facilitate their

[53] Soff, 'History of sleeping sickness', pp. 43–5, 104, 106; Moffat to Greig, 16 May 1905, Bruce papers, Albert Cook Library, Kampala; W. Foster, *The Early History of Scientific Medicine in Uganda* (Nairobi: EALB, 1970), pp. 101–3; Sadler to Lansdowne, 28 July 1904, NA, FO/2/858.

[54] H. Bell, 'Uganda Diary 1906–09', 3 May 1906, 24 June 1906, Royal Commonwealth Society Archive, Cambridge. Bell had hoped that through evacuation 'the Government would be relieved of thc great cost that was involved in dealing with this problem', as 'all who had already been infected would either have been cured by some medical remedy or would be dead.' In 1909 Bell was distressed to find that 'though cures are not being effected, medical measures are keeping alive a lot of people upon whose disappearance we had calculated.' Bell to Crewe, 6 Jan. 1909, NA, CO/536/25.

[55] Minute by Read, 23 Jan. 1907, NA, CO/536/8.

[56] Will to Chief Secretary, 22 Nov. 1906, NA, CO/536/8; Hodges to Will, 31 Oct. 1906, NA, CO/536/8.

treatment with atoxyl, a drug that, according to Koch, held out the promise of a cure.[57] In fact Koch had arrived at his estimate of the prevalence of the disease by testing only the sick, and the effectiveness and safety of atoxyl were equally exaggerated, so that its use was discontinued in Uganda in 1908.[58] Nonetheless, evacuation did result in a rapid decline in new infections in Ankole, Buganda, and Buhaya, so that sleeping sickness quickly lost its place as the disease that dominated all others.[59]

Sleeping sickness's legacy though would remain significant for several decades. The evacuation and relocation of the population of a large proportion of these territories had depended on the active support of the local chiefly hierarchies. Their success convinced colonial authorities of the need to work through African administrative structures in the implementation of public health measures in the future. It took some time before European officials realized that the remarkable success of the sleeping sickness evacuation would not easily be replicated in all future health campaigns. Sleeping sickness, after all, had broken out in the more peripheral and troublesome parts of these territories, and chiefs would be less enthusiastic about enforcing intrusive regulations in the core of their societies. Equally, the evacuations, like the successful mass vaccination programmes which soon followed, required a temporary imposition of administrative will. The more difficult and unpopular task of changing health-related behaviour in a sustained manner was beyond the early colonial state, European and African. The sleeping sickness experience was typical of colonial healthcare before the 1920s. It was energized as much by economic concerns and by the desire to avoid offending metropolitan public opinion as by humanitarianism. Coercive disease control measures prevented new disease outbreaks on a major scale after 1910, but curative efforts had little success before the 1920s. This same pattern of coercion, chiefly involvement, and inadequate chemotherapy would also shape the colonial response to syphilis, the disease that displaced sleeping sickness as the dominant threat to health in the Great Lakes area after 1906.

[57] Minutes of meeting of the Reichs-Gesundheitsrat on measures to control sleeping sickness, 10 Dec. 1910, 'Scientific Correspondence of the Institut für Seuchenbekaempfung', TNA (Tanzania National Archives, Dar es Salaam), G 5/16, Vol. 1 1907–1910; Bell to Elgin, 23 Nov. 1906, NA, CO/536/8. The programme ultimately effected in German East Africa was in fact more comprehensive, and expensive, than that adopted by Bell, as it involved bush clearance and game culling as well as population relocation and treatment.

[58] Soff, 'History of sleeping sickness', pp. 111–14; Gray, Report for quarter ending 29 Feb. 1908, NA, CO/536/20.

[59] For a recent study of the ongoing scientific importance of sleeping sickness, see H. Tilley, *Africa as a Living Laboratory: Empire, Development, and the Problem of Scientific Knowledge, 1870–1950* (Chicago: University of Chicago Press, 2011), pp. 169–216.

Syphilis

In 1907 Governor Bell asked the Colonial Office to send an STD specialist to set up a syphilis control programme in Uganda. Bell had been convinced by Albert Cook, the great missionary doctor, and by Buganda's leading chiefs that syphilis threatened to complete what sleeping sickness had started, the destruction of the Ganda ethnic group. Cook was not the first western observer to suggest that syphilis was a common affliction in Buganda, but his moralistic fervour combined with unparalleled medical authority added a new urgency to discussions of the disease. Cook's position as East Africa's leading consultant physician and his ability to support his assertions with statistical evidence ensured that his warnings about the dangers of syphilis would be taken seriously by senior colonial administrators. Mengo hospital, established by Cook in 1897, was remarkable not only for its popularity among the Ganda—it treated 13,000 new cases in 1908—but also for the detailed nature of the case notes recorded for each patient. It was not until the 1920s that the colonial health system could match Cook's knowledge of the incidence of disease in Buganda.[60] So when Cook asserted 'that between 1897 and 1907 . . . the incidence of syphilis [had] increased rapidly' at Mengo hospital, he was believed.[61] An apparent epidemic of syphilis spoke to a number of audiences. The local church hierarchy was reassured of the relevance of Cook's medical mission by this association of disease with sin. Ganda chiefs found an outlet for their concerns about their weakening social control. And the European administration saw an opportunity to address the demographic decline, which seemed to threaten not only the moral justification for colonial rule, but also its revenue base.[62]

In response to Bell's appeal, Colonel F. J. Lambkin, one of the Royal Army Medical Corps' (RAMC) leading syphilologists, was despatched to Uganda, where he interviewed a number of chiefs, missionaries, administrators, and medical officials. The majority of informants, both European and Ganda, agreed that syphilis had existed in Uganda for centuries but had begun spreading rapidly in the late 1890s, as the Uganda railway intensified the degrading impact of coastal traders, the Pax Britannica permitted 'freer

[60] A. Cook, 'An urgent need in Uganda', *Mercy and Truth*, 12 (1908), pp. 44–50; A. Cook, 'Syphilis in the Uganda Protectorate', *British Medical Journal*, 2, 2502 (1908), pp. 1780–1; Foster, *Early History*, p. 70.

[61] A. Cook, 'The treatment of ante-natal syphilis in Baganda women', a paper read before the Uganda branch of the British Medical Association, 22 Mar. 1929, Albert Cook Library, Kampala.

[62] Vaughan, *Curing*, p. 135; Lambkin, Mission to the Uganda Protectorate on the prevalence of venereal diseases. Summary of evidence, Dec. 1907, NA, CO/536/15; Bell to Elgin, 22 Mar. 1907, CO/536/12, NA.

and wider communication among the people', and European influence began to undermine patriarchal limitations on what were termed the 'naturally immoral proclivities of the Baganda women'. Lambkin's report went beyond this local consensus, claiming that the majority of Ganda and 90% of Nkole were infected with syphilis, that the apparent suddenness with which syphilis became widespread since the late 1890s derived from its 'virgin soil' nature, and that Christianity was to blame for social disintegration and social degeneration, which had unleashed 'female animals with strong passions, to whom unrestricted opportunities for gratifying those passions were suddenly afforded'.[63] Lambkin asserted that the epidemic if unchecked would 'decimate some of [Uganda's] tribes, and the remainder will become so degenerate as to be practically useless'.[64] This cataclysmic analysis persuaded the Colonial Office and the Protectorate government to despatch three RAMC specialists to establish an STD control programme in Uganda, though the campaign would be limited to Buganda due to funding restrictions and the relative weakness of the chiefs in Ankole and other districts.[65]

For Buganda's saza or county chiefs, the syphilis scare was as much an opportunity to secure the obedience of their sub-chiefs as it was a means of reasserting control over their subjects. The chiefly elite had seen their coercive power limited by the imperial takeover, but quickly learned that the colonial government would legitimize their exertion of authority when the key interests of the state were threatened. Public health was an arena where senior chiefs could demonstrate their commitment to Britain's civilizing mission, and so gain official approval for coercive interventions that would not have been tolerated in most other fields of policy. The saza chiefs' enthusiasm for syphilis control was not matched at the lower levels of Buganda's administration, with sub-chiefs recognizing the local unpopularity that would result from requiring a large proportion of their followers to attend one of the new treatment rooms for a course of painful mercury injections lasting up to six months.[66] With the syphilis campaign stalling, the frustration of colonial

[63] F. Lambkin, 'An outbreak of syphilis on virgin soil', *The Lancet* (1908), p. 1022; Lambkin, Mission to the Uganda Protectorate on the prevalence of venereal diseases. Summary of evidence, Dec. 1907, NA, CO/536/15; Vaughan, *Curing*, pp. 132–4; C. Summers, 'Intimate colonialism: The imperial production of reproduction in Uganda, 1907–1925', *Signs*, 16, 4 (1991), p. 800.

[64] Lambkin, Prevalence of venereal disease in the Uganda Protectorate, Dec. 1907, NA, CO/879/99.

[65] Bell to E.E.K., 20 Jan. 1908, NA, CO/536/18; Hodges to Deputy Commissioner, Apr. 1908, NA, CO/536/19.

[66] D. Zeller, 'The establishment of western medicine in Buganda' (unpublished PhD dissertation, Columbia University, 1972), pp. 195–9; cf. D. Arnold, *Colonizing the Body; Imperial Medicine and Indigenous Societies* (Berkeley: University of California Press, 1993) for a similar situation in India.

officials mounted. One complained in 1911 that '[a] declining birth-rate which under present conditions appears to be inevitable means in years to come declining revenue . . . and therefore from a financial point of view apart from a higher motive these people must be prevented from allowing themselves to commit race suicide.' Therefore saza chiefs' suggestion that a new law be passed to compel sub-chiefs to send in their sick was met with enthusiasm, and draft legislation was drawn up by the RAMC officer in charge of the campaign, Lieutenant Keane, who promised that compulsory treatment would enlarge the labour supply by up to 20%.[67] This colonial fixation with declining tax revenues and the recurrent shortage of labour for public works and Uganda's nascent plantations influenced even missionary writing which anticipated STD treatment would convert 'diseased human lives . . . into valuable products'.[68]

In December 1913 the simultaneous publication, after prolonged negotiations, of the Townships (Venereal Diseases) Rules by the Protectorate government and the Law for Preventing Venereal Disease by the Buganda kingdom government symbolized this alliance of revenue and authority. Under this legislation syphilis was declared a dangerous disease, those suspected as being infected could be compulsorily examined, and the infected were required to endure a full course of treatment, during which they could not trade, marry, or have sex. Non-compliance would be punished with heavy fines or imprisonment. Two aspects of this legislation are particularly significant. The first is the heavy, early focus on prostitution, with sex workers targeted for intense supervision by chiefs and police, and their managers required to ensure they did not work if infected. The second is the remarkable degree to which the Ganda population would be monitored by the chiefly hierarchy. Local chiefs and landlords were required to check twice a month among their subjects and tenants if any new infections had occurred, and to ensure that new cases presented for treatment. Sub-county chiefs then had to report to their superiors each month on how many defaulters existed in their areas and what punishments they had received. At last the senior chiefs had found a mechanism that held out the possibility of disciplining their sub-chiefs, and the mass of the people they ruled over.[69] But the system relied on there existing the capacity

[67] Lt. G. Keane, Medical Officer i/c Venereal Disease Investigations to the Provincial Commissioner Buganda, 19 May 1911 in Buganda Annual Report 1910–11, ESA, A46/420.

[68] Mengo CMS Hospital Annual Report 1912–13 (Albert Cook Archive, Mulago Hospital, Kampala), p. 5.

[69] Uganda Protectorate, Annual Medical and Sanitary Report for 1913, p. 21, NA, CO/685/2; Zeller, 'Establishment', pp. 197–201. In general African prostitution was characterized by the absence of pimps, so the reference to prostitutes' managers in Uganda is striking. Later sources though indicate that pimps were not prominent in the selling of sex in this region before 1980. See White, *Comforts*, p. 1 and E. Akyeampong, 'Sexuality and prostitution among the Akan of the Gold Coast *c.* 1650–1950', *Past and Present,* 156 (1997), pp. 144–73 for a discussion of the irrelevance of pimps in colonial Kenya and Gold Coast.

to treat all the patients identified by the authorities, and here the colonial government failed to live up to its promises. Saza chiefs built treatment rooms and staff housing in their counties, but before 1922 the medical department could not find the funds or personnel to operate most of them, so the syphilis campaign remained limited to the immediate neighbourhoods of Buganda's few urban centres.[70]

Yet the campaign, while limited in scope, was intense in its focus. Around towns like Kampala and Masaka, STD specialist officers, supported energetically by the local saza chiefs, organized regular, mass examinations of the populations of entire communities. Local inhabitants were required to stand in a line, lift their clothing, and submit to a cursory, public inspection of their genitalia. Such actions were deeply shameful to the Ganda, so intolerant of public nudity. In addition to these occasional village-level investigations, chiefs were paid for sending in suspected victims of syphilis to one of the venereal disease centres. In either case, the presence of sores which appeared syphilitic in nature resulted in an order to complete a course of treatment, with defaulters tracked down by the local police.[71] The campaign in its early years was shaped by the military background of its RAMC founders, with syphilis treatment being viewed essentially as a form of inoculation, designed to limit further disease transmission, with the greater good of the community outweighing the liberty of the individual. Compulsory intramuscular injections seemed the ideal treatment strategy to the overstretched early colonial health system as they freed the 'patient of all participation in his treatment and the medical officer is independent of his assistance and makes no demands on him'. Over time though, this approach became less extreme, in the face of funding restrictions that dimmed hopes that mass treatment could eradicate syphilis from the entire population, and missionary criticism of a system of treatment that was designed to ensure that 'no responsibility is entrusted to the patient'.[72] At the end of the First World War, Uganda's bishops persuaded the governor of the need to combat 'growing immorality', evidenced by falling marriage rates and the poor example set by chiefs, resulting in new government funding for a campaign of propaganda aimed at instilling a sense of guilt among those infected with STDs, and for a network of maternity centres,

[70] Uganda Protectorate, Annual Medical and Sanitary Report for 1919, p. 8, NA, CO/685/3; Uganda Protectorate, Annual Medical and Sanitary Report for 1920, p. 9, NA, CO/685/4. The First World War inevitably distracted medical attention away from STDs in the civilian population, but shortages had restricted the scale of the programme from the start.

[71] Dr M. Lamont to Dr J. Walker, 1 Jan. 1922, Uganda 1908-54, Women's Library, London, 3AMS/D/49; M. Lyons, 'Sexually transmitted diseases in the history of Uganda', *Genitourinary medicine*, 70 (1994), p. 140.

[72] Report on the treatment of venereal diseases from 27 Jan. 1909 to 31 Mar. 1910, NA, CO/536/33.

one of whose aims was the creation of a new family-oriented morality.[73] Yet only a small proportion of Ganda women used the mission-run maternity clinics before the 1940s, partly because their services were so heavily flavoured with moral criticism, while the association of syphilis with shame was more successful in deterring people from seeking treatment than from becoming infected in the first place.[74]

The dominant form of STD work remained compulsory inspection and treatment until 1922, when a recently arrived venereologist, Dr Lamont, was dismissed from the colonial medical service for complaining about the coercive and degrading mass examination of women. Once back in Britain, she brought her mistreatment and that of the Ganda women to the attention of the suffrage movement, the International Federation of Medical Women and, most importantly, the Association for Moral and Social Hygiene, a pressure group that had long campaigned against STD policies that unfairly victimized women. The ensuing scandal forced the Colonial Office to launch an enquiry. Keane defended his venereal policy strongly, acknowledging that "the compulsory measures of Uganda are the most rigorous and far-reaching" in the world, but emphasizing that such an extreme response was justified by the scale of the crisis, claiming that Uganda suffered 90% STD prevalence, infant mortality of up to 900 per 1,000, and a stillbirth rate of 12%.[75] The Cooks also endorsed the colonial system by referring to the severity of the STD problem in Uganda, their case records showing that 22% of recent outpatients were infected with an STD, while 66% of maternity cases had a current or previous syphilis infection.[76] Policy in Uganda had been driven for fifteen years by such estimates, but only now would they be examined sceptically. A prevalence of 90% was dismissed as ridiculous by the Association for Moral and Social Hygiene, based as it was on the examination of individuals who were suspected by their chiefs of suffering from STDs. The assumption that all stillbirths were caused by syphilis was indefensible, and

[73] Coryndon to Secretary of State, 30 May 1918, NA, CO/536/89; Keane, Report on venereal disease measures, Medical Report 1921, NA, CO/536/119; Coryndon to Secretary of State, 11 Nov. 1920, NA, CO/536/101; H. Hansen, *Mission, Church and State in a Colonial Setting: Uganda 1890–1925* (New York: St. Martin's, 1984), p. 294; A. Cook, *Uganda Memories, 1897–1940* (Kampala: Uganda Society, 1945), p. 342; Vaughan, *Curing*, p. 130.

[74] Webb, Annual report on venereal disease measures, 1922, NA, CO/685/5; A. Cook, Annual letter 1923, CMS, G3/AL/1917–1934. Over ten years, thirty CMS clinics delivered 2,026 live births. Cook, *Memories*, pp. 325–7, 339, 361.

[75] Lyons, 'History', p. 140; G. Keane, Report, in J. Hope Reford, Ag PMO, to National Council for Combating Venereal Diseases, 22 Aug. 1922, 'Uganda 1908–54', Women's Library, 3AMS/D/49.

[76] J. Cook to Mrs Smithett YMCA, 3 Apr. 1922, 'Uganda 1908–54', Women's Library, 3AMS/D/49.

the Colonial Office was reminded that hospital-derived data provided only the incidence of STDs among the sick, not among the general population. Equally, it was reasonable to assume that many women who chose to attend maternity clinics before it became normal to do so had suffered particular health problems in the past. That the reported stillbirth rate among mission maternity cases was almost three times higher than in the general population may indicate that they had had an atypical experience of STDs. Lamont implied that doctors in Uganda overestimated the frequency of STD infection, and complained that laboratory testing was restricted purely on the grounds of expense. Her own inspection of the general female population found evidence of active infection in only 5% of women, though as she was instructed only to examine women's genitalia, and was allowed only one minute per patient, it is likely that her prevalence rate was an underestimate. Taken together, the Association for Moral and Social Hygiene considered that the data indicated that the STD situation in Uganda, with perhaps 10 to 20% prevalence, was probably similar to that in the UK, 'but we don't adopt Ugandan measures'. The National Council for Combating Venereal Diseases similarly considered the panic about STDs in Uganda disproportionate, given that only 5,343 people had been treated for these diseases in government units in 1920. Keane's claims that it was Buganda's chiefs who had demanded such extreme measures, and that coercion was 'relied on solely as an educational measure' were dismissed. Instead the episode was regarded as an example of how the excessive power of the colonial state could be abused.[77]

The Colonial Office, still embarrassed by recent revelations of forced labour in East Africa, quickly ordered the ending of compulsion. The STD campaign lost its autonomous, quasi-military character and was merged with the general work of the medical department. The rhetoric of the medical department towards STDs became less moralistic and less confident. At Mulago hospital in Kampala, Uganda's flagship medical institution, as the 1920s progressed the problems of accurate diagnosis of syphilis in particular were acknowledged more freely than before, laboratory testing became more common, and positive test results were interpreted more cautiously. In 1923 the principal medical officer admitted that differential diagnosis of yaws and

[77] Visit of Mrs Smithett and A. Neilan to A. and K. Cook, n/d [1922], 'Uganda 1908–54', Women's Library, 3AMS/D/49; A. Neilans, AMSH, Some notes on the Memorandum issued by the CO concerning anti-venereal measures in Uganda, 'Uganda 1908–54', Women's Library, 3AMS/D/49; Dr M. Lamont to Dr J. Walker, 1 Jan 1922, 'Uganda 1908–54', Women's Library, 3AMS/D/49; Interview of Webb, 20 Apr. 1922, NA, CO/536/120; Keane, Venereal diseases in Uganda, 1922, NA, CO/536/120; Notes of a conference on anti-venereal measures, 6 Apr. 1922, NA, CO/536/123. Lamont noted that government hospital records showed 15% of patients had acute syphilis.

syphilis was 'extremely difficult' in primary and secondary cases, and 'in many cases impossible' in tertiary cases. Consequently 'the diagnosis . . . [was] very largely a matter of personal convention.'[78]

But the embarrassment resulting from this metropolitan criticism meant that the shift in tone and practice regarding STDs was largely confined to the upper echelons of the government medical system. Little effort appears to have been devoted to reversing decades of medical training and propaganda that had created an enduring belief that syphilis was the most common and dangerous disease in the Protectorate. Administrators, medical missionaries, and rural dispensary staff, the front line of Uganda's colonial health service, were unaware of the loss of diagnostic confidence at Mulago. This was particularly significant because Keane's last act before the Lamont scandal was to secure Colonial Office funding for the establishment of a series of venereal disease centres attached to dispensaries throughout Buganda. Between 1922 and 1926 eighteen of these centres came into service, an impressive achievement which made STD treatment available to the bulk of the Ganda population, but which also entrenched in the rural dispensary system a tendency to overdiagnose syphilis. Thus the number of syphilis cases diagnosed in government medical units increased sevenfold during these years. A recently arrived medical officer was shocked to discover in 1928 that 'any pain not readily diagnosable, tended to be labelled "syphilis"' in rural dispensaries. A few years later another new appointee found that 'often ninety percent of infants were diagnosed as congenital syphilitics' in the countryside, yet 'most of them had scabies, malaria, yaws or kwashiorkor.'[79] Meanwhile, just as the medical department was quietly reducing the role of chiefs in the control of syphilis in Buganda, so in 1926 the Provincial Commissioner was urging Ankole's chiefs 'to exercise more persuasion with their people' to attend the district's dispensaries, whose staff reported, almost certainly erroneously, that 'a great majority of deaths are due to syphilis.' Medical missionaries too sustained pre-1922 diagnostic assumptions long after the shift in thinking within government medical circles. As late as 1932 Albert Cook was still reporting that in Buganda and Ankole 'we are dealing with a highly syphilized population.'[80] Even more remarkably, only months after ordering the repeal of Uganda's STD legislation, the Colonial Office forwarded Keane's 1922 defence of his STD policy to Dar es Salaam, suggesting 'that anti-venereal measures in the Tanganyika

[78] Uganda, Annual report on the medical department, 1923, NA, CO/685/6, pp. 9, 131–2.

[79] Buganda Annual Report 1922, ESA, A46/439; Buganda Annual Report 1926, ESA, A46/428; R. Barrett papers, RHO, MSS.Afr.s.1879(9); H. Trowell, 'The beginning of the kwashiorkor story in Africa', in H. Trowell, J. Davies and R. Dean (eds.), *Kwashiorkor* (London: Arnold, 1982 [1954]), p. xxiv.

[80] Western Province Annual Report, 1926, NA, CO/685/9; Report of the Lady Coryndon Maternity Training School, Namirembe, 1932, Cook Archive, Albert Cook Library, Kampala.

Territory might usefully be directed on the lines which have been found so successful in Uganda'. A similar request meanwhile came to Tanganyika's governor from Buhaya's district commissioner who, reporting that syphilis was the only significant health problem in his district, believed that '[i]t will be necessary . . . to institute a campaign somewhat on the lines of that now being adopted by the Uganda administration . . otherwise this rich and fertile district will . . . become depopulated and revert to bush.'[81] It is ironic that elements of Keane's system were introduced in Buhaya just as Uganda was changing its policy, but it is perhaps not surprising. Missionary perceptions of sexuality and the near universality of syphilis infection among the Haya were very similar to those found across the border, and colonial administrators and senior chiefs were as concerned in Buhaya as they were in Buganda about perceived population decline and a breakdown in social control. The British takeover in Tanganyika at the end of the First World War moreover had intensified contact across the frontier, with the Cooks for example taking the opportunity as early as 1919 to visit Bukoba, Buhaya's district headquarters, and warn of the dangers of STDs.[82]

In practice, the more extreme aspects of Keane's STD policy were not implemented in Tanganyika. Bukoba's administrators' periodic requests for permission to enforce compulsory inspection and treatment were impossible to approve so soon after the Lamont scandal. Instead in 1924 the Tanganyika government followed Keane's revised model of mass, intensive, semi-voluntary inspection and treatment, primarily implemented through a new network of dispensaries staffed by tribal dressers. In Tanganyika though the syphilis campaign was combined with an attempt to eradicate yaws, a closely related illness, as both illnesses responded to the same treatment, bismuth. In most of Tanganyika yaws was regarded as a much more common disease than syphilis and indeed it accounted for 55% of all cases treated in the Territory in 1928. Bukoba was different. Here syphilis was perceived to be the dominant disease, so much so that in 1925 syphilis made up 29% of all cases diagnosed at Bukoba hospital, and yaws just 1%. Bukoba's district report for that year claimed that 90% of the peasantry had been or were infected with an STD. As in Uganda doctors based in the district gradually became more aware of the difficulties of accurate diagnosis of syphilis as the 1920s wore on. Partly this reflected an improvement in the quality of senior personnel, with a fully qualified doctor taking over the running of Bukoba hospital from a sub-assistant surgeon after 1925. The district medical officer acknowledged in

[81] Devonshire to Governor Sir H. Byatt, 4 May 1923, Venereal Disease: Anti-venereal Measures, vol.1, TNA, 19153; Bukoba District Annual Report 1923, TNA, 1733/8 (AB10), p. 18–19.

[82] EAMS, *Annual Report, 1952*, p. 65; TNA 215/77/A Bukoba District Annual Report, 1927; TNA 1733/5 (AB48) Bukoba District Annual Report, 1919, p. 8.

1928 that the 42% of patients treated for syphilis at rural dispensaries in that year probably included many cases of yaws. In reality it is probable that a wide range of conditions were misdiagnosed. But again, as in Uganda, little effort was devoted to the retraining of rural staff. In part this was due to financial considerations, given the impressive scale of rural healthcare in Bukoba district, where, due to chiefly willingness to pay for the construction of dispensaries, Bukoba's campaign affected a much larger proportion of its population than was the case elsewhere in Tanganyika. In part it was because European officials believed that while African dispensers probably exaggerated the prevalence of STDs, diseases of immorality were nonetheless extremely common. Colonial reports consistently emphasized the degradation of the Haya in general, and women in particular. 'The native . . . in no wise thinks it a disgrace to be affected by [STDs].' On top of the Haya innate 'lack of character and personal uncleanliness', the missions' enforcement of monogamy had 'led to illicit intrigue'.[83]

In Uganda from the early 1920s medical officers and administrators became less and less prone to making such moral criticisms of local populations. After the First World War the Protectorate's early investment in African education and welfare and the absence of a significant settler voice created a progressive reputation which became self-reinforcing. A new generation of medical officers, more research-oriented, less constrained by racial preconceptions, were attracted to Uganda in the later 1920s and 1930s, where they tended to adopt a more pragmatic approach to STDs, regarding them as one of a range of preventable diseases, all of which needed a more rigorous understanding of their aetiology if they were be brought under control. One product of this retreat from moralistic pre-judgement was C. J. Hackett's groundbreaking environmental theory, now generally accepted, of the evolution of syphilis and other related diseases, based on his research into yaws in northern Uganda. Hackett argued that the causative agents of these three diseases, *Treponema pertenue*, *T. endemicum* and *T. pallidum*, are all members of the same species, which diverged due to the varying habitats in which humans began to live over the millennia. Yaws (*T. pertenue*) adapted to humid environments where nudity and perspiration facilitated infection through day-to-day skin contact, typically in childhood. Endemic syphilis (*T. endemicum*), which also mainly affected children, emerged in warm but less humid areas

[83] TNA 1733/3:46 (AB40) Bukoba District Annual Report, 1925 (Bukoba sub-dist); Kuczynski, *Demographic*, II, p. 381; Tanganyika Territory, *Annual Medical Report 1928* (Dar es Salaam: Government Printer, 1929); Bukoba District Annual Report, 1924, Appendix 2, TNA 1733/33 (AB105). For missionary critiques of Haya sexual morality see B. Larsson, *Conversion to Greater Freedom? Women, Church and Social Change in North-Western Tanzania under Colonial Rule* (Uppsala: University of Uppsala Press, 1991), pp. 70–99.

with cooler nights, where transmission by skin contact was restricted by the wearing of clothes, so that lesions of the mucous membranes developed ensuring that the disease could spread though the sharing of eating and drinking utensils, pipes, and so on. Finally, when people began to live fully clothed in dense, urban environments then infection through multiple, regular sexual contact became both possible and necessary and led to the evolution of *T. pallidum*.[84]

This then led to the realization that all three versions of treponemal disease—sexually transmitted syphilis, endemic syphilis, and yaws—probably co-existed in Uganda in the nineteenth and twentieth centuries, if not before. In 1956 another medical researcher, J. N. P. Davies, based on a re-analysis of the case notes of early twentieth-century diagnoses of syphilis, argued that for most patients the symptoms recorded in fact indicated endemic syphilis. In Davies' opinion, sexually transmitted syphilis was introduced by coastal traders after 1850, but at first spread slowly due to the partial immunity granted by previous treponemal infection. Sexually transmitted syphilis, he argued, only became dominant around the 1920s after colonial rule had upset local sexual controls and introduced the large-scale use of mercury and arsenical treatment, which caused the rapid decline of endemic syphilis and the cross-immunity it had provided. Davies explained the mass misdiagnosis of the early twentieth century in terms of Albert Cook's fixation with sin and his remarkable persuasive powers, which managed to convince both European officialdom and the Ganda elite that sexually transmitted syphilis had developed into a devastating epidemic.[85]

It still seems remarkable though that early European writers almost universally assumed that Ganda suffering from skin lesions that appeared treponemal in form were suffering from sexually transmitted syphilis, rather than endemic syphilis or yaws. These three diseases after all produce such similar symptoms beyond the early stages, that differential diagnosis, when relying on visible signs or even the laboratory tests available to colonial doctors, is extremely difficult. Lay observers can be excused, and medical training in British universities may not have referred to endemic syphilis, even though this disease of poor living conditions was widespread on Europe's peripheries, and had only disappeared from Scotland and Ireland in the middle of the nineteenth century. Yaws may have been one of the most common tropical diseases, but it was not well known nor understood before

[84] D. Robertson, A. McMillan and H. Young, *Clinical Practice in Sexually Transmissible diseases* (Edinburgh: Churchill Livingstone, 1989), pp. 108–12, 179–81. See also C. Hackett, 'On the origin of the human treponematoses (pinta, yaws, endemic and venereal syphilis', *Bulletin of the World Health Organization*, 29, 1 (1963), pp. 7–41.

[85] Davies, 'History of syphilis', pp. 1052–3. Tuck, 'Syphilis', p. 68, though suggests that endemic syphilis remained predominant longer than Davies allowed for.

the First World War, and it is possible that doctors such as Robert Felkin and Albert Cook would have been unaware of it before their arrival in Africa.[86] Cook though was infected with syphilis a number of times during his career in Uganda, as an unfortunate consequence of manual examination of patients without the protection of surgical gloves. So he would have certainly known that syphilis could be transmitted non-sexually. Yet he regarded such 'syphilis of the innocent' as a tragic side-effect of a predominantly sexually transmitted disease. Transferring one of the recurring motifs of Victorian moral discourse to Uganda, Cook blamed ignorant adults for unwittingly passing on their sexually acquired infections to their children by non-sexual means.[87]

Cook's perception that a sexually driven epidemic had affected the majority of the Ganda population was shaped in part by the shameless manner in which Ganda reported that they had *kabotongo*, which Cook translated as sexually transmitted syphilis.[88] For Ganda though, *kabotongo* described a medical condition believed to have been inherited congenitally or transmitted by direct or indirect, non-sexual contact. Children were given regular doses of preventive medicine to protect them from infection, and people suffering severe symptoms might be quarantined. *Kabotongo* was an unpleasant affliction, but there appears to have been little association of the disease with immorality.[89] As Michael Tuck has observed, none of the many proverbs that relate to *kabotongo* indicate any explicit connection between the disease and sexual activity. References to infection via the lips or buttocks (from using the same eating and drinking vessels and sitting in the same place as a *kabotongo* sufferer) could of course be interpreted as allusions to sexual infection. But this seems unlikely given that proverbs about gonorrhoea were so explicit in connecting that disease with misbehaviour: 'Too great a load of firewood kills the gatherer: gonorrhoea kills the fornicator.'[90] It then becomes necessary to explain why European medical thinking so readily dismissed the evident belief of the Ganda that *kabotongo* was an endemic non-sexual disease.

Beyond the local influences of racial preconceptions, missionary moralism, demographic decline, and patriarchal insecurity, Michael Tuck has demonstrated that the tendency to over-diagnose syphilis was profession-wide at this time, due to the excitement generated by the isolation of *T. pallidum* in 1905,

[86] Hackett, 'On the origins', pp. 23–4.

[87] W. Foster, *Sir Albert Cook: A Missionary Doctor in Uganda* (Newhaven: Newhaven Press, 1978), p. 146; L. Engelstein, *The Keys to Happiness: Sex and the Search for Modernity in Fin-de-siècle Russia* (Ithaca: Cornell University Press, 1992), p. 166. Cook appears not to have been aware of Duncan Bulkley's well-known book, *Syphilis of the Innocent* (New York Bailey and Fairchild: 1894), which associated the endemicity of non-sexually-transmitted syphilis with a lack of civilization.

[88] A. Cook, *A Medical Vocabulary*.

[89] Zeller, 'Establishment', pp. 400–1.

[90] Tuck, 'Syphilis', pp. 52–3; F. Walser, *Luganda Proverbs* (Berlin: Reimer, 1982), proverb 1663.

the development of a diagnostic laboratory test for syphilis in 1906, and the discovery of a reasonably effective cure, the arsenical salvarsan in 1911. This great interest in syphilis, along with its diverse symptoms which caused it to be known as 'the great imitator', encouraged doctors across the world to mistake it for a range of skin conditions. Two further common assumptions would have increased still further the likelihood of doctors in Buganda misdiagnosing cases of yaws or endemic syphilis as sexually transmitted syphilis. The first was that the site of lesions was associated with the mode of infection, so that medical examinations which found genital or anal sores would have tended to result in a diagnosis of sexually transmitted syphilis. Yet subsequent research has shown that lesions around the genitals and anus are common features of endemic syphilis and yaws, especially during drier periods when the *Treponema* are more likely to be found in the more moist areas of the skin. As the dry season was the time of year when doctors tended to tour in rural areas, and also when farmers often had more free time to seek treatment for chronic conditions, then the probability of such misdiagnoses would have been increased. The second predisposing factor was that nineteenth-century writing on syphilis in the west associated syphilis with urbanity, civilization, and individualism and the endemic treponematoses with backwardness. This seems to have preconditioned doctors to expect to find syphilis in Buganda, commonly accepted as the most advanced society in East Africa, and one where literacy, missionization, and war-related upheaval appeared to have released the individual from the authority of chiefs, elders, and the clan. These assumptions were self-reinforcing. As late as 1947 Hackett himself noted that Buganda had always been 'regarded as a "syphilis area"', in contrast to Lango in northern Uganda, a 'yaws area'.[91]

Ever since Davies' article was published in 1956, its historical reconstruction has been generally accepted. Two of the assumptions on which it is based, though, may not be entirely accurate. The first is that Davies followed the received opinion that yaws was essentially absent from Buganda. Yet endemic syphilis is usually a disease of arid and semi-arid climates, whereas yaws is a disease associated with high humidity. The climatic fact that Buganda is actually more humid than northern Uganda's 'yaws area' was ignored because it was assumed that Ganda culture, with its horror of adult nudity and emphasis on personal hygiene, prevented yaws from becoming prevalent.[92] Yet yaws

[91] Tuck, 'Syphilis', pp. 58–9, 65; Robertson, McMillan and Young, *Clinical Practice*, pp. 179–81; Engelstein, *Keys*, pp. 166–9; Hackett, 'Incidence', pp. 88–90.

[92] Hackett, 'Incidence of yaws', pp. 88–90; Hackett, 'Origins', pp. 27–9. Hackett notes that endemic syphilis is typically a disease of arid environments and hypothesizes that Buganda might instead have experienced occasional non-sexual transmission of *T. pallidum*. Tuck, 'Syphilis', p. 68 meanwhile suggests that the colonial Hut Tax, enforced between 1900 and 1910, encouraged overcrowding and the abandonment of traditional quarantining and so helped endemic syphilis to survive.

is primarily a disease of childhood, and children in pre-colonial Buganda typically went naked until puberty, while 'both boys and girls were careless about bathing during their minority.'[93] Despite the ingrained bias towards the diagnosis of syphilis in colonial Buganda, medical records show that cases of yaws among the Ganda were not in fact uncommon.[94] Moreover, Ganda proverbs referred to *nnungu*, painful cracks in the feet, as a common symptom of *kabotongo*, and such cracks are associated much more with yaws than the other treponematoses.[95] The second assumption is that sexually transmitted syphilis was not present in Buganda before 1850. Yet Buganda had strong indirect links with the coastal trading network long before the first caravans arrived in the 1850s, so it is entirely possible that syphilis reached Buganda from the East African coast before a direct trade route was established. Alternatively it may be that syphilis had already been brought to Buganda from the north, as Leo Africanus recorded that as early as the sixteenth century raiders had brought the 'mal de Naples' from Libya to the Bahr-El-Ghazal in central Sudan, only 600 miles from Buganda.[96]

The story of syphilis in Buganda then during this early period is complex. Much of the confusion, it now seems clear, derived from the fact that several treponemal diseases co-existed in the nineteenth and early twentieth centuries. Most Ganda and Europeans, however, initially acknowledged the presence of only one disease, but disagreed on the nature of that disease. *Kabotongo*, according to standard Ganda thinking, had diverse signs and means of transmission, but was non-sexual in origin, whereas Europeans typically observed only syphilis, explaining away the peculiarities of its symptoms and responsiveness to treatment by referring to the possible impact of race, climate, or malarial fever.[97] It is likely, but unproven, that sexually transmitted syphilis, like gonorrhoea, was present in Uganda at the start of the nineteenth century. It is also likely that it was not until the early twentieth century that most treponemal infections were sexual in origin.

It is impossible now to reconstruct a precise chronology of the changing pattern of sexually transmitted syphilis in Buganda. Certainly the disease was common by the 1940s, judging by autopsy reports and the results of careful testing and cautious diagnosis at Mulago.[98] It seems reasonable to assume

[93] Roscoe, *Baganda*, pp. 75–9.

[94] e.g. Hackett, 'Incidence of yaws', pp. 88–90; Johnston, *Uganda*, II, p. 644.

[95] Tuck, 'Syphilis', p. 50.

[96] A. Retel-Laurentin, *Causes de l'infécondité dans la Volta Noire* (Paris: INED, 1979), p. 60. Admittedly the local terrain would have tended to isolate the Bahr-El-Ghazal.

[97] Davies, 'History of syphilis', p. 1048. The educated Ganda elite came to accept the European belief that sexually transmitted syphilis had become epidemic in their society, but it is unlikely that they entirely abandoned traditional ideas about *kabotongo*.

[98] J. Davies, 'Pathology of central African natives: Mulago Hospital post mortem studies', *East African Medical Journal*, 24, 8 (1947), pp. 289–303.

that syphilis would have followed a similar trajectory to gonorrhoea, since both diseases were usually transmitted in the same manner. Gonorrhoea moreover is a useful proxy for levels of syphilis as accurate diagnosis of gonococcal infection was more straightforward.[99] While it is much easier to transmit sexually than syphilis, gonorrhoea is also much less affected by aquired immunity.[100] Medical reports indicate that gonorrhoea was very frequently encountered by Uganda's doctors in the early colonial period. One recorded in 1907 that it 'exists to a fearful extent and no doubt is the main cause of abortion and sterility'. An RAMC officer, using the typically extreme language of the military specialists, claimed in 1910 that the disease was 'universal' in Buganda. Such overblown comments sit uneasily with medical records from this period which typically show that gonorrhoea made up only around 2% of new cases at Buganda's dispensaries. Yet such disease incidence data were inevitably skewed by the limited ability of medical personnel at this time to cure gonorrhoea. A better sense of infection levels comes from a 1922 report that retention of urine as a complication of gonorrhoea caused 'a very high mortality' among the Ganda, and from a 1933 survey in northwest Buganda which found that while victims of the disease rarely troubled dispensary staff, untreated gonorrhoea affected 13% of the adult population, a remarkably high proportion.[101] Certainly then patterns of sexual behaviour that would have permitted the transmission of sexually transmitted syphilis throughout Ganda society did exist by the early decades of the twentieth century.

[99] Admittedly in the early decades of the twentieth century a diagnosis of gonorrhoea was usually based solely on the presence of a characteristic discharge and history, unsupported by laboratory tests. But it is likely that most discharges in this period that were not gonococcal in nature would have been caused by other sexually transmitted infections. Tuck, 'Syphilis', p. 230.

[100] D. Barlow, *Sexually Transmitted Infections: the Facts* (Oxford: Oxford University Press, 2006), p. 40; L. Thompson, J. Ryden and J. McGregor, 'Vaginitis and Sexually-Transmitted Diseases', in J. Ryden and P. Blumenthal (eds.), *Practical Gynecology* (Philadelphia, PA: ACP, 2002), p. 225; J. Zenilman and C. Deal, 'Gonorrhea: epidemiology, control and prevention', in L. Stanberry and D. Bernstein (eds.), *Sexually Transmitted Diseases: Vaccines, Prevention and Control* (Cambridge: Academic Press, 2000), p. 370; A. Mindel and C. Estcourt, 'Syphilis', in Stanberry and Bernstein, *Sexually Transmitted Diseases*, p. 405; Robertson, McMillan and Young, *Clinical Practice*, p. 177.

[101] Hodges in Lambkin, 'Mission to the Uganda Protectorate on the prevalence of venereal diseases. Summary of evidence', Dec. 1907, NA, CO/536/15; Report on the treatment of venereal diseases from 27 Jan. 1909 to 31 Mar. 1910, 1 May 1910, NA, CO/536/33; Buganda Annual Report 1927, ESA A46/433; J. Hope Reford, Ag PMO, to National Council for Combating Venereal Diseases, 22 Aug. 1922, 'Uganda 1908-54', Women's Library, 3AMS/D/49; A. Williams, 'Report on an investigation into the prevalence of serious disease in Buyaga county, Mubende district', Sept. 1933, RHO, Mss.Afr.s.1872/xxxix.

EARLY COLONIAL HEALTHCARE AND FAMINE CONTROL

Colonial medicine concentrated in its early years on ensuring, perhaps unsurprisingly, the survival of the imperial project, by focusing limited resources on maintaining the health of European officials, their servants, and local soldiers and police. Where the colonial state did move to reduce African ill-health, this has often been regarded as in part a self-interested, responsive series of isolated actions, aimed at limiting the danger to European personnel and the loss of revenue inherent in uncontrolled epidemics. Yet the medical responses to sleeping sickness and syphilis can also be seen as forerunners of the type of interventionist healthcare that would characterize the mature colonial state of the 1940s and 1950s. Sleeping sickness stimulated an ongoing interest in public health among the chiefly class of this region that was quite distinct, and would prove significant in its demographic impact in later decades.[102] The syphilis campaign, meanwhile, evolved remarkably between 1908 and 1924. Initially a militaristic imposition of unexplained, external medical knowledge, the STD programme over time incorporated serious, albeit imperfect, attempts at health information provision, and, crucially, stimulated the development of large-scale medical training of African staff and the delivery of medical care to the mass of the rural population. The apocalyptic tone of much European discourse on STDs in this period had destructive consequences in several ways, but it did secure enhanced funding which permitted the rapid expansion of a network of dispensaries and aid posts in Buganda, Buhaya and to a lesser extent Ankole. The realization that African staff with substantial medical training would be needed if a serious impact was to be made on patterns of disease resulted in sustained investment in medical education. The introduction of a new training programme in 1923 soon resulted in the development of a small number of assistant medical officers, a larger group of medical attendants who could run local medical sub-centres, and around 800 junior attendants with some hospital training. The great majority of these individuals remained within Uganda. As most of them before the 1940s were Ganda, and as the heaviest concentration of medical facilities was in Buganda, this programme resulted in a significant indigenization of medical services at a remarkably early stage.[103]

[102] Kuczynski, *Demographic*, II, pp. 381–2; Zeller, 'Establishment', pp. 163, 178–6. Cf. Vaughan, *Curing*, pp. 36–40. Uganda's early colonial annual medical reports are dominated by concerns about European health, and detail in particular the immense efforts devoted to limiting the impact of malaria on the white community; e.g. Annual Medical Report for Uganda, 1908, NA, CO/685/1.

[103] Zeller, 'Establishment', pp. 225–41. Cf. D. Arnold, *Imperial Medicine and Indigenous Societies* (Manchester: Manchester University Press, 1988), p. 20.

The impact of this change in tone and personnel on health only began to be noticed in the mid-1920s. In the first years of European rule the pre-colonial pattern of recurring epidemics, holding no regard for wealth or status, continued to haunt these societies. A sense of the horror and helplessness of sudden sickness in these years is provided by one senior chief's final communications with Apollo Kaggwa, Buganda's prime minister. On 18 June 1908 the Kawaulo thanked Kaggwa for his note of sympathy:

> When the letter arrived already five people had died in my house . . . when I got to the doctor's my remaining wife died . . . Old friend Apollo, my death has been a most horrible one. The plague germs started with the thigh bones, but did not show any exterior symptoms. I can neither sit nor stand . . . We shall meet in Heaven. Tell the Lukiiko [Buganda's governing council] all about me.

The next day he reported that his entire household had been devastated. 'Dear friends mine has been a bad death. Europeans have taken away all the people who used to serve me. . . I am guarded by six Askaris. Six more people have died and six more ill. It is all very miserable.'[104]

Policies adopted by the early colonial state inevitably facilitated the spread of a number of diseases. The establishment of a system of labour migration from isolated societies like Ankole and Rwanda towards the nascent cash cropping centres of Buganda and Buhaya enabled the rapid transmission of communicable infections such as smallpox across the region. The concentration of these travellers in ill-maintained designated rest camps along the migration routes provided ideal conditions for tick-borne relapsing fever to increase in frequency. Migrants then faced new threats once they arrived at their destinations, with the unsanitary nature of their housing resulting in recurrent outbreaks of dysentery. Uganda's major cash crop, cotton, meanwhile provided an ideal breeding ground for plague-bearing rats, while the construction of the Uganda railway and the rapid movement of troops during the First World War ensured that the region would not escape the influenza pandemics of 1900 and 1918, nor meningitis which burnt through Uganda's garrison towns in 1916. Colonial demands for tax and labour undermined household food security so that drought in 1899–1905, 1907–08 and 1917–19 resulted in widespread scarcity and isolated clusters of hunger-related deaths. Where possible colonial governments studiously avoided using the term famine to describe this suffering, but it was impossible to deny the association between scarcity of food and outbreaks of smallpox. In 1918 Uganda's annual medical report noted that hunger aided the spread of

[104] P. Sebugulu, Kawaulo to Sir Apolo Kagwa, 18 and 19 June 1908, Buganda Lukiiko Archives, 1894–1918 (translated for John Rowe in the 1960s and made available to me by Holly Hanson. A copy exists in Makerere University Library.)

smallpox through 'depressed vitality and the necessity of people travelling long distances in search of food'.[105]

The response of colonial medicine to this sustained epidemic assault reflected the coercive approach to healthcare, and the limitations of funds and personnel, that also characterized sleeping sickness and STD control in the first two decades of the twentieth century. Enforced mass smallpox vaccination was only partially successful in containing the disease before the 1920s, despite local legislation in Buganda requiring parents to ensure their children were inoculated, because effective lymph was in such short supply. Attempts to eradicate plague in Uganda in 1913 by paying individuals to kill rats, controlling the movement of cotton and people out of plague-affected areas, and relocating cotton storage and processing facilities away from residential and commercial areas had limited impact, and it required mass inoculation and health education in the early 1920s to significantly reduce the mortality it caused. Efforts to improve sanitation and so reduce dysentery and relapsing fever similarly had only a degree of success before the 1920s because the focus of sanitary work remained fixed on protecting Europeans' health. Nonetheless, outbreaks of plague, smallpox and dysentery no longer had the cataclysmic character of the epidemics described in the late nineteenth century. It seems unlikely that a wide range of diseases should have become less virulent at the same time, so the achievement of the early colonial medical system in lowering the peaks of mortality should be recognized.

Similarly, early colonial interventions in times of famine appear entirely inadequate at first glance. Little in the way of systematic intervention was attempted in Buhaya during the German period. Some colonial innovations if anything increased food insecurity. Hut tax was imposed universally across southern Uganda at the start of the twentieth century, even in areas suffering severe famine.[106] Uganda's governor in 1905 went to some lengths to reassure the Colonial Office that levels of food scarcity recorded at that time were entirely usual, even though, as Jan Kuhanen has observed, his subordinates had recently reported extreme hunger in western Buganda.[107] In 1907 little was done to prevent famine migration from the relatively dry borderlands of Buganda, and in 1917 food requisition for military purposes contributed to famine across Uganda. Nonetheless, the catastrophic famines that devastated the region in the late nineteenth century largely disappeared with the British takeover. Partly this reflected the rapid widening of food markets, but more important was the provision of food relief to severely affected areas from

[105] Kuhanen, *Poverty*, pp. 265–74; Uganda Protectorate, Annual Medical Reports, NA, CO/685/1–7.
[106] e.g. Doyle, *Crisis*, p. 97.
[107] Kuhanen, *Poverty*, p. 222.

1908, even though this only contained rather than eliminated mortality at first. The 1908 famine control effort began too late and was underfunded, yet it marked a commitment that would see Uganda achieve freedom from severe famine earlier than much of colonial Africa. The model of relief which emerged in 1908—large-scale food imports from surplus areas, the use of wheeled transport to bring grain rapidly to central depots, the provision of food stations at dozens of points throughout the affected locality—would be maintained throughout the colonial period. So was the determination to avert future famines through the establishment of local famine reserves in the most vulnerable regions, and the institution of a monitoring system that would trigger the importation of additional food supplies before market prices escalated excessively.[108] This system of famine aversion limited suffering in 1917–18, but proved so expensive to the colonial state, and ultimately to the local taxpayer, that legislation requiring more rigorous prevention and more localized, and therefore cheaper, relief, was passed in 1919. Now local governments were required to ensure that all households grew famine crops like cassava, while plans for emergency public works and controls on food prices were instituted.[109] This new system was not without its costs, as dietary habits adjusted to the constant availability of drought-resistant but less nutritious crops, but the horror of widespread starvation receded. Death was becoming an individual tragedy rather than a mass trauma.

The demographic impact of this reduction in the severity of famine and epidemic are difficult to evaluate from traditional sources. Uganda's censuses in 1911 and 1921 are of limited value, as they provide little more than an indication of total population size, ethnicity, sex ratio, and the proportion of children in each community. Over this decade Buganda's population increased from 705,615 to 774,753, largely it seems because of immigration, while Ankole's population rose slightly from 228,700 to 251,156. Tanganyika's censuses were more limited still, revealing little more than that the estimated population of Bukoba District fell from 270,500 in 1913 to 255,730 in 1921.[110] At least in Ankole and Buganda some additional light can be shed on patterns of mortality before 1925 by these districts' vital registration records. From

[108] D. Chwa et al. to Milner, 8 May 1919, in Coryndon to Colonial Secretary, 30 June 1919, NA, CO/536/94; Wallis to Colonial Secretary, 7 Aug. 1914, NA, CO/536/70; Kuhanen, *Poverty*, p. 239. See J. Iliffe, *The African Poor: A History* (Cambridge: Cambridge University Press, 1987), pp. 157–9 for a full discussion of the colonial management of famine, modelled on the Indian Famine Codes.

[109] Uganda Protectorate, Famine Relief Ordinance 1919 and Native Foodstuffs Ordinance 1919, NA, CO/684/2.

[110] Uganda, 1911 Census; Uganda Protectorate, *1921 Census Returns* (Entebbe: Government Printer, 1922); Uganda Protectorate, *1931 Census Returns* (Entebbe: Government Printer, 1932).

1910 chiefs in 'advanced' districts in Uganda were required to send in annual totals of births, deaths, and still-births for the district commissioner to compile. Little effort was devoted to training the chiefs or supervising their data collection, however, and the returns were weakened by recurrent problems of definition. It seems that some babies who died soon after birth may have been recorded as still-births, many deaths in infancy were probably never recorded at all, and child deaths over the age of one may have been included in the infant mortality returns. In general it seems that a large proportion of all vital events went unrecorded.[111] Medical and administrative officers viewed these annual totals with some scepticism, but typically concluded that while an individual year's data should not be assumed to be accurate, the figures gave 'an idea of the general trend of things'.[112] During the years 1910 to 1924, the average crude death rate per 1,000 calculated from vital registration was 18.4 in Buganda and 21.2 in Ankole (see Figure 2.1). Over this same period, 8.8% of all births were stillborn in Buganda, and 11.1% in Ankole. Only from the mid-1920s were data on infant mortality collected, with the rate per 1,000 in 1926 being 150 in Buganda, almost certainly too low, and 370 in Ankole, which is high but not at all impossible for tropical Africa during the early twentieth century.[113]

Crude death rates fluctuated much more from year to year in Ankole than Buganda in the early colonial period, which perhaps indicates that the more intensive colonial administration experienced in Buganda may have reduced crisis mortality more than in neighbouring societies, though it may simply reflect greater consistency in data recording.[114] Little else can be detected from the standard data sources that could help identify and explain demographic change during the early colonial period. In Buganda though large mission-run hospitals existed from the late nineteenth century, characterized by their popularity among the local Ganda population and by the care with which case histories were obtained and archived. Albert Cook established a system of data recording at the Church Missionary Society's Mengo hospital from its inception in 1897 that survived for decades. At first maternity records were scattered through the general case files, but from 1919 a separate maternity register was maintained which ensured greater consistency in case recording.[115]

[111] Annual medical report, 20 June 1911, NA, CO/536/42.

[112] Annual medical report, 1912, NA, CO/685/1.

[113] Uganda Protectorate, Annual Medical Reports 1911–1926, NA, CO/685/1-9.

[114] The standard deviation was 1.5 for Buganda and 3.9 in Ankole.

[115] Kuhanen, *Poverty*, pp. 309-12 has discussed Mengo's maternity records from earlier years. His data are not directly comparable, but they show clearly how high maternal and infant mortality was at the start of the twentieth century.

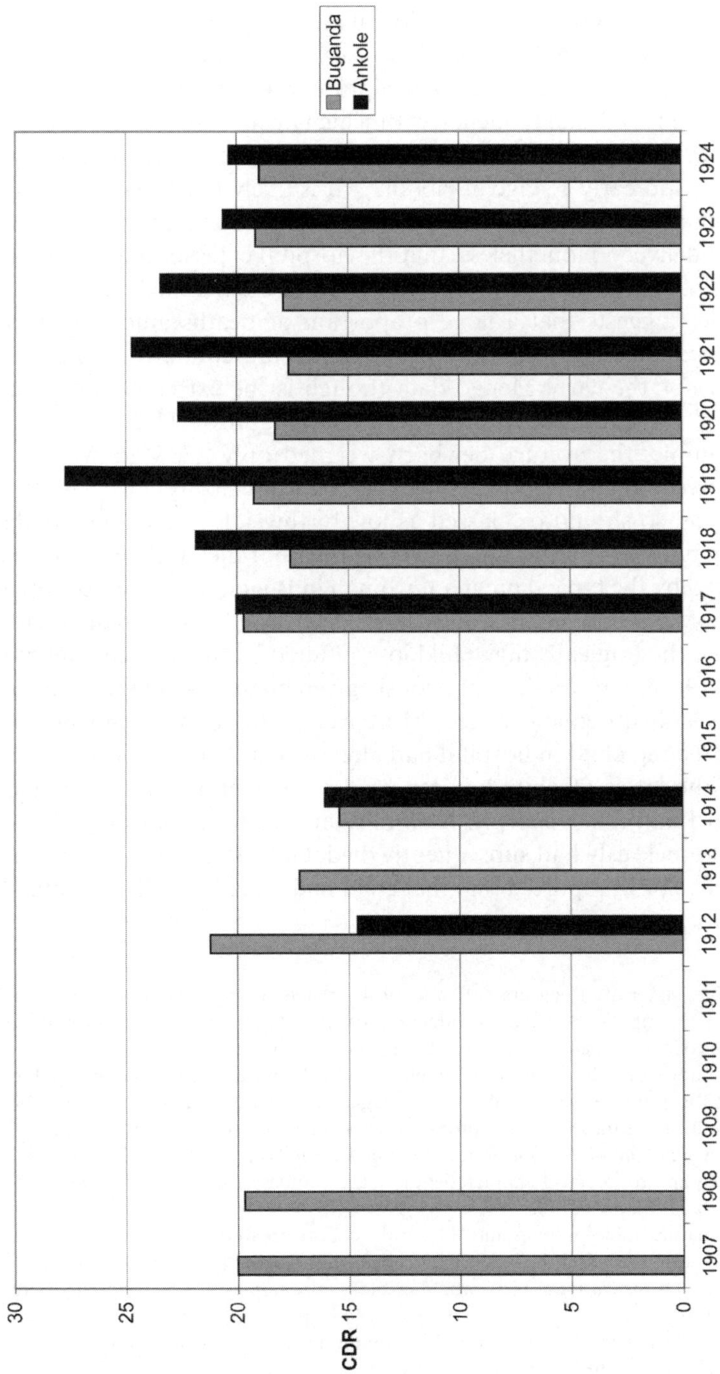

Figure 2.1 Crude death rate per 1,000 in Ankole and Buganda 1907–24, from vital registration records

The analysis of the Mengo maternity records from 1919 and 1924 adds new depth to our understanding of early colonial mortality.[116]

One of the medical problems for which the Ganda would become famous was obstructed delivery, and consequent rupture of the uterus. Various medical reports emphasized the frequency with which death resulted, especially if women resorted to the use of powerful oxytocic herbal medicines to strengthen contractions at too early a stage in labour.[117] It is likely that Mengo's admissions included a disproportionate number of women with a previous history of obstructed delivery. Nonetheless, that the hospital experienced a maternal mortality rate as high as 43 per 1,000 in 1919, despite the medical interventions available, suggests that a large proportion of deaths among younger women in Buganda more generally occurred during childbirth. The most striking aspect of the early Mengo data though is the extremely low mean birthweight of the babies born in hospital (see Figures 7.11 and 7.12). In 1924, for example, the average newborn weighed only 2785 grams, or six pounds and two ounces. The proportion of babies who weighed less than 2500 grams, and so should be classed as low birthweight, was a remarkably high 27.9% in both 1919 and 1924, reflecting the poor diet and heavy disease burden suffered by the typical pregnant woman in Buganda.[118] This extremely small average weight at birth would have been one of the main factors contributing to the tragically high child loss suffered by the women attending Mengo. In 1919 women who had previously given birth reported that 55% of their children had subsequently died. Moreover, 60.6% of women who gave birth to their second child in hospital had already lost their firstborn.[119]

By 1924, the levels of child loss reported by women attending Mengo's maternity ward had fallen sharply. Now mothers reported that only 30% of children born previously had subsequently died. Only 45.2% of mothers with one previous live birth reported that that child had already died, a reasonably

[116] Mengo Hospital Maternity Registers 1919 and 1924, Mengo Hospital Archive, Albert Cook Library, Mulago, Kampala. See the introduction of this book for a discussion of the representativeness of the women who gave birth in maternity wards.

[117] Report of the Lady Coryndon Maternity Training School, Namirembe, 1932 (Cook Archive); C. Rendle-Short, 'Rupture of the gravid uterus in Uganda', *Obstetrics and Gynecology*, 79, 6 (1960), pp. 1114–20; D. Allbrook, 'Some problems associated with pelvic form and size in the Ganda of East Africa', *Journal of the Royal Anthropological Institute*, 42 (1962), pp. 102–14; S. Zivanovic, 'The anthropological characteristics of the Ganda pelvis', *East African Medical Journal*, 45, 2 (Feb. 1968), pp. 68–70.

[118] Twins and premature babies were excluded from the cohort because changes over time in the incidence of premature birth and the increasing tendency for women pregnant with twins to be encouraged to have an institutional birth would create a false impression of changing average birthweight over time.

[119] This did not reflect particularly high mortality among primiparae or first-time mothers as child loss was almost as common at higher parities.

strong indication that this improvement was relatively recent.[120] It is possible that this change in reported child mortality simply reflected the widening appeal of western maternity care. The number of women admitted in 1924 had more than doubled since 1919 to 327. It could be argued that as Mengo grew more widely popular, then high risk individuals would comprise a much smaller proportion of the women admitted. Undoubtedly over time hospital delivery in Buganda did become extremely common among women with no expectation of particular complications. But that change occurred most obviously in the 1930s and 1940s. The expansion of Mengo's activities by 1924 is likely to have reflected the impact of recent investment in rural maternity centres as much as the Church Missionary Society's propaganda efforts from 1921 to promote maternity care as the route to social purity and a truly Christian family life.[121] The midwives who were sent into the Buganda countryside to spread the gospel of modern maternity care were trained by the Cooks to identify women with potential complications or a poor obstetric history during ante-natal checks for referral to Mengo. Certainly the consistency in average birthweight and the slight rise in rates of stillbirth (to 10.5%) and neo-natal mortality (to 6.5%) between 1919 and 1924 does not suggest that the nature of the cohort had changed dramatically over these years. The possibility remains that child mortality had indeed fallen due to investment in sanitation around Kampala and especially because of the cumulative impact of mass inoculation campaigns against major epidemic diseases such as smallpox.

CONCLUSION

Anything written about morbidity and mortality in East Africa before the 1940s must be tentative given the limitations of both data and ethnographic observation. It does seem clear however that none of the three case study areas was especially disfavoured by the ecological conditions in which these societies lived. Ankole though did suffer less than Buganda and Buhaya from the new epidemics, conflict and social upheaval associated with long-distance trade in the nineteenth century. Buganda suffered most from the violence that accompanied colonial conquest, and from the outbreak of sleeping sickness

[120] A very large reduction in child spacing theoretically could have achieved the same results but while the Kisubi parish baptism register data indicate that birth intervals did indeed fall significantly in the early 1920s, the reduction from 36 to 32.5 months would not have been sufficient to produce a decline in reported child mortality of the scale recorded.

[121] A. R. Cook, Report of the Lady Coryndon Maternity Training School, Namirembe, 1931; Cook, *Memories*, pp. 325–7, 339, 361.

that was almost certainly triggered by the imperial takeover. But the intensity of Buganda's encounter with globalization began to work in her favour as the colonial state gradually moved beyond the mere achievement of control and financial stability. Indeed Buganda is one of the best-evidenced examples of the early colonial state's gradual achievement of control of epidemic disease and famine in Africa. Buganda led the way in the prevention of crisis mortality, but its example was quickly replicated in Ankole and Buhaya. By 1924 the annual compilation of statistics on cause of death throughout the region revealed the emerging dominance of endemic diseases, a pattern that would survive, with some variation, until the age of AIDS. This though was only a partial success, for endemic conditions, most importantly malaria and pulmonary and intestinal infections, accounted for very heavy morbidity and mortality in most years. Early colonial healthcare was largely incapable of making an impact on these most common ailments, in either a preventive or a curative sense.[122] Only from the mid-colonial period would this situation change.

[122] See for example A. R. Cook, Report of the Lady Coryndon Maternity Training School, Namirembe, 1931; Cook, *Memories*, pp. 325–7, 339, 361.

3

Early Colonial Sexuality and Fertility

INTRODUCTION

Except during the worst years of the sleeping sickness epidemic, demographic concerns during the first quarter of the twentieth century focused much more heavily on fertility than mortality. This was largely because sub-fertility was typically associated with sexual misbehaviour, sexually transmitted diseases, changing gender relations, and a crisis in marriage. This chapter will explore the relationship between morality, social change, and reproduction, and examine the subtle differences in the attitudes of chiefs, missions, and colonial administrators, whose public statements seemed so frequently to coincide. Whereas previous scholarship has tended to prioritize rhetorical and legislative attempts to exert control over women, this chapter will emphasize that interventions in the sphere of sex, marriage, and reproduction were frequently gender-neutral or focused on male behaviour, that reforms often resulted in ambiguity and confusion, and that the application of new regulations was characterized above all by inconsistency.[1] It is difficult to detect a hegemonic patriarchal agenda shaping the gender politics of this region, particularly in Buganda. Undeniably though, this was a period defined by conservative concerns about the impact of the new freedoms granted to women and the young. It is striking how early in the colonial period it was that complaints were made in Buhaya and especially Buganda about the role of the commercial economy, Christianity, the legal protection of female rights, and urbanity in discouraging the youth from marrying and undermining sexual constraints. In Ankole by contrast, partly because the factors associated with modernization were much less developed, the chiefly elite appears to have been able to engineer a strengthening of the institution of marriage, which seems likely to have contributed to the relatively high levels of fertility enjoyed in that society.

[1] Some important studies of the patriarchal tendencies of the mission churches and the colonial and indigenous states in this period include P. Davis, 'On the sexuality of "town women" in Kampala', *Africa Today*, 47, 3/4 (2000), pp. 28–60; N. Musisi, 'Morality as identity: the missionary moral agenda in Buganda, 1877–1945', *Journal of Religious History*, 23, 1 (1999), pp. 51–74; M. Tuck, 'Syphilis, sexuality, and social control: A history of venereal disease in colonial Uganda' (unpublished PhD dissertation, Northwestern University, 1997).

For the Ganda and Haya, the sense that unsanctioned sexual relationships and divorce were on the rise, despite the efforts of missions and state, contributed to the perception that birth rates were falling and that these societies were suffering a demographic crisis. In reality the early colonial period was a time of broad demographic stability in these three societies. It was after 1925 that the demographic trajectories of Ankole, Buganda, and Buhaya would diverge significantly.

MARRIAGE AND DIVORCE

During the early colonial period in Uganda and northwest Tanganyika chiefs, missionaries, and European officials intervened repeatedly in the realm of gender and marital relations. In part this interference was inspired by anxieties about demographic decline, but it also reflected growing concerns about the conflict between enduring norms of behaviour dictated by family and clan, and what were perceived as the progressive but destabilizing forces of commercialization, Christianity, and westernization.[2] Marriage became one of the most complex elements in this debate about the dangers presented by competing cultural ideals. In its various forms marriage was alternately viewed as the traditional guarantor of social stability or a mechanism which would enable Africans to demonstrate their commitment to modernity and a truly Christian lifestyle.[3] The response to the contradictory potential of such diverse goals was to formally create three separate marital codes through regulation. Africans in the early twentieth century were required to choose whether to marry in the village according to customary law, in a registrar's office according to the colonial Marriage Ordinance, or in a place of worship, which was regulated by both the Marriage Ordinance and the laws of Islam or one of the Christian churches.[4]

Complications arose because many individuals wanted to marry under more than one code over their lifetimes. Conversion to Christianity presented few problems for a couple who had been married according to customary law, if they had a monogamous relationship, as their existing union could simply

[2] See e.g. D. Chwa, 'Education, civilization and foreignisation', in D. Low (ed.), *The Mind of Buganda: Documents of the Modern History of an African Kingdom* (Berkeley: University of California Press, 1971), pp. 104–8.

[3] Musisi, 'Morality', pp. 64–5; N. Musisi, 'Transformations of Baganda women: from the earliest times to the demise of the kingdom in 1966' (unpublished PhD dissertation, University of Toronto, 1991), p. 202.

[4] Uganda Marriage Ordinances of 1902, 1903 and 1904 in Uganda Protectorate, *Laws of Uganda* (Entebbe: Government Printer, 1935); Tanganyika Territory, *Ordinances under the Tanganyika Order in Council, 1920* (London: HMSO, 1923), no. 12; Tanganyika Territory, *Ordinances Enacted during the Year 1923* (Dar es Salaam: Government Printer, 1924), no. 17.

be blessed in church. But sometimes one partner in a relationship converted and then wished to marry another convert in church, having decided to leave their original spouse because of the latter's refusal to abandon their old religion. Such a course of action seemed entirely logical to some African clergy, but was generally opposed by missionaries who insisted on the basic validity of pre-existing customary marriages.[5] However, where a woman claimed to have been married against her will, some clerics were happy to dissolve what they regarded as substandard marriages. Such interventions naturally caused unrest, prompting the church hierarchy to require evidence of resistance before and after a marriage ceremony, rather than the mere absence of consent. In one 1915 case the request of a woman that her marriage be annulled was rejected due to the testimony of her father that her objections prior to the wedding ceremony were 'but disinclination . . . Had she really refused, he said he would have beaten her.'[6]

The complexities of marriage reform can be demonstrated with particular clarity in Buganda because laws passed by the Kingdom and Protectorate governments as well as records of marriage disputes adjudicated by both the churches and Buganda's parliament, the *Lukiiko*, have survived.[7] The early years of British overrule saw the greatest enthusiasm of Buganda's modernizing chiefs for wholehearted westernization, as they, with the support of colonial officials and missionaries, passed laws which, for example, outlawed wife-beating and allowed polygamously married wives to leave their husbands if they wished to be baptized.[8] But over time this unity of purpose evaporated, as the colonial state came to regard the undermining of customary marriage as a threat to social stability and an affront to natural justice, and as the personal circumstances of the Ganda elite became more complicated due to their increasing age and personal wealth. Daudi Chwa and Apollo Kaggwa, Buganda's king and prime minister, and the leading lay members of the Native Anglican Church, for example, fathered children through a number of simultaneous relationships in the early decades of the twentieth century.[9] Such well-known, if largely unpublicized, misdemeanours forced church and

[5] Owen to Bishop, 26 Aug. 1915, Marriage files, Namirembe Church of Uganda Archive, Mukono; J. Willis, 'Reflections on Uganda' (TS, n/d), RHO, MSS. Afr. S. 1792 Box 38.

[6] Musisi, 'Morality', p. 60; Owen to Bishop, 20 Nov. 1915, Marriage files, Namirembe Church of Uganda Archive, Mukono.

[7] Cf. M. Tuck and J. Rowe, 'Phoenix from the ashes: Rediscovery of the lost Lukiiko archives', *History in Africa*, 32 (2005), pp. 403–14.

[8] Buganda Lukiiko Archives, 1894–1918 (translated for John Rowe in the 1960s and made available to me by Holly Hanson. A copy exists in Makerere University Library), Buganda Laws, 9 July 1895; Musisi, 'Transformations', p. 206.

[9] Musisi, 'Morality', p. 60; Marriage, [Kawalya] Kagwa, 18 Feb. 1956, A. Richards papers, LSE, 7/16.

state into a series of uncomfortable compromises. Admittedly both Catholic and Protestant missions frequently expressed generalized condemnation of the backsliding of the first generation of converts and the tokenistic belief of the second. Missionaries, moreover, refused to administer the sacraments to a significant proportion of local congregations due to various marital offences and demanded that the colonial administration enforce the bigamy laws, with particularly enthusiastic clergy seeking the conviction of minor chiefs under the Marriage Ordinance for marrying a second wife by customary contract.[10] But it is telling that the church hierarchies were nervous of publicly humiliating Buganda's highest chiefs, and that the sharpest criticism directed by the missions towards the colonial government over the polygamy issue resulted from the British Chief Justice's willingness in 1920 to set out clearly what his understanding of the essential elements of existing marriage legislation actually was. Bishop Tucker of the Church Missionary Society (CMS) complained that the government had thus informed Africans 'how far they may go in the matter of free marriage'.[11]

Ambiguity also seems to have characterized Buganda's chiefly elite's marriage policy. When Buganda's senior judge, Stanislaus Mugwanya, advised the *Lukiiko* in 1919 that customary unions entered into by Christians were not legally recognizable marriages, it is possible that he did so simply in order to re-emphasize the primacy of church marriage.[12] It seems more likely though that this was instead an indirect solution to the threat of conviction for bigamy. This interpretation is supported by the statements of Apollo Kaggwa and Ham Mukasa, two of the most powerful members of the *Lukiiko*, to the 1920 Uganda Development Commission. 'We do not see why action should be taken against a Christian man who takes a wife by native religion. If his wife wishes to take action, she can do so but it is no one else's business.' Certainly the colonial government took Mugwanya's judgement as an opportunity to avoid the potential embarrassment of high profile bigamy cases, by confirming that where Christians had previously married in church, any subsequent customary marriage was invalid. By defining a Christian's customarily married second wife as a concubine the colonial government

[10] H. Hansen, *Mission, Church and State in a Colonial Setting: Uganda 1890-1925* (New York: St. Martin's, 1984); P. Kanyadago, *Evangelizing Polygamous Families: Canonical and African Approaches* (Gaba: AMECEA, 1991), p. 15; Owen to DC, 10 May 1915 and Owen to Bishop, 10 Mar. 1916, Marriage files, Namirembe Church of Uganda Archive, Mukono.

[11] Tucker to Coryndon, 13 Mar. 1920, Marriage questions: legal opinions and memoranda, Namirembe Church of Uganda Archive, Mukono. Daudi Chwa's various sexual indiscretions left the Church of Uganda with little choice but to refuse him communion but his position protected him from the full application of church discipline. Musisi, 'Morality', pp. 65–9.

[12] C. Obbo, 'Town migration is not for women' (unpublished PhD dissertation, University of Wisconsin-Madison, 1977), p. 44.

ensured that it would no longer have to prosecute Ugandan men for breaches of the Marriage Ordinance. In 1923 the Protectorate High Court went further and fully upheld Mugwanya's 1919 opinion, ruling that Christians could only marry legally under the Marriage Ordinance, thus defining even Christians' monogamous customary marriages as extra-marital liaisons. Recognizing the dangers inherent in such a baldly stated policy, the Protectorate government declared that customary marriages should be governed by customary law, leaving the question of how to categorize customary marriages entered into by Christians deliberately unsettled.[13] According to Hastings, such uncertainty made many Ganda men worry that if their marriage dissolved they would be unable to recover their bridewealth: 'This appears to have encouraged many poorer people to reject both church and customary marriage.'[14]

This was not the only way in which early colonial reformers threatened the integrity of customary marriage across this region. The church offered refuge to female converts who refused to be married polygamously or to a non-Christian, thus helping to undermine the role of family networks not only in selecting spouses but also in negotiating the terms of marriage and resolving subsequent marital disagreements. The Catholic mission in Buhaya was particularly welcoming to women who were unhappy with the marriages into which they were being forced. In just one month in 1911, seven young women sought refuge with the White Fathers' mission at Kashozi rather than marry a non-Christian. By 1916, 132 women lived with the White Sisters at Kashozi, though some of these were only temporary escapees from cruel or unfaithful husbands, for in general the churches favoured reconciliation over long-term refuge for monogamously married women.[15] Across the region, meanwhile, polygamously married men who converted were allowed to retain only one 'ring' wife. The churches' insistence that the remaining wives should be discarded but maintained by their ex-husband until they died or remarried

[13] Musisi, 'Transformations', pp. 223, 230–2. Apparently unaware of the events of 1919–23, a subsequent Chief Justice in 1933 informed missionaries that Christians who married in church and then by custom were indeed guilty of bigamy, but it is unclear whether any prosecutions followed. Correspondence between Rev. P. Brazier and Bishop Willis, 2 Nov. 1932 and 15 Feb. 1933, Marriage questions: legal opinions and memoranda, Namirembe Church of Uganda Archive, Mukono.

[14] A. Hastings, *Christian Marriage in Africa, Being a Report Commissioned by the Archbishops of Cape Town, Central Africa, Kenya, Tanzania, and Uganda* (London, SPCK, 1973), pp. 168–70. See also A. Mickleburgh, 'The relevance of marriage for Ganda women in Bwaise, Kampala, Uganda' (unpublished PhD dissertation, University of Cambridge, 1998), p. 114.

[15] Musisi, 'Transformations', pp. 176, 206; B. Larsson, *Conversion to Greater Freedom? Women, Church and Social Change in North-Western Tanzania under Colonial Rule* (Uppsala: University of Uppsala, 1991), pp. 33–7, 66–7. Some of the women at Kashozi may also have been runaway *Bazaana* slaves.

appears to have been honoured relatively rarely in these societies. Women who lived on land owned by their former husbands, especially if they continued to care for their small children, were not regarded as having fully divorced according to customary law, and it seems often illicitly resumed their former relationships. Many men though refused to support their ex-wives and sent them back to their families. As bridewealth was not returned in these circumstances, again such women had not formally been divorced.[16] Such situations became still more complicated on the death of the husband, when the contradictions between the marriage law of custom and church were most at odds. This was because inheritance was governed by customary law, which held that a child born to one of the rejected wives could be named as the primary heir, with the right to evict the 'ring' wife from her marital home. Alternatively, one of the late husband's brothers could be legally appointed guardian of the 'ring' wife's children, meaning that if she wished to remain with them, she would have to consent to becoming her brother-in-law's wife, potentially in a polygamous union.[17]

The institution of marriage was also undermined by broader changes arising from the colonial takeover. The introduction of regular, ungraduated taxation and heavy labour demands meant that the status of full adulthood was viewed with little enthusiasm by some young men, who reportedly chose to avoid the new responsibilities that came with marriage and heading a household.[18] In Ankole the decision by the early colonial government to develop western Uganda as a source of labour migrants rather than cash crops resulted in many wives being abandoned for prolonged periods, putting marriages under a new form of strain.[19] Moreover, the early commercializa-

[16] O. Beaudoin to Michaud, 26 Mar. 1933 in E. Michaud, 'Enquêtes sur les conditions morales dans le vicariat de l'Uganda, 1933', Rubaga archives, 904.1; Musisi, 'Morality', pp. 64–5; J. Willis, 'Reflections on Uganda' (TS, n/d), RHO, MSS. Afr. S. 1792 Box 38, pp. 135–7; Larsson, Conversion, pp. 118–21. The churches' encouragement of converts to discard their excess wives drew on a general disdain for polygamous marriage and the perceived cultural superiority of the west. Bishop Willis, for example, believed that 'the hardship is probably very much less keenly felt than it would be in a more advanced and civilized people. The dismissal is probably the lesser of two evils.' Polygamy was 'the mark of a primitive and still immature people'.

[17] Musisi, 'Transformations', p. 209; H. Banks to Bishop Willis, 18 Mar. 1921 and Guthrie Smith to Bishop, 22 Apr. 1921, Marriage questions: legal opinions and memoranda, Namirembe Church of Uganda Archive, Mukono.

[18] H. Hanson, *Landed Obligation: The Practice of Power in Buganda* (Portsmouth, NH: Heinemann, 2003), p. 180; Mubendi District Annual Report, 1910–11, ESA (Entebbe Secretariat Archives) A46/420; J. Cunningham, *Uganda and its Peoples : Notes on the Protectorate of Uganda, Especially the Anthropology and Ethnology of its Indigenous Races* (London: Hutchinson, 1905), pp. 148–69.

[19] D. Stenning, 'A note on migrant labour from the Muko area (Ndunguru)', Derrick Stenning Papers, University of Cambridge archive, D12 migrant labour; O. Beaudoin to Michaud, 26 Mar. 1933 in E. Michaud, 'Enquêtes sur les conditions morales dans le vicariat de l'Uganda, 1933', Rubaga archives, 904.1.

tion of the economy in Buganda and Buhaya enhanced the financial value of female labour, triggering an increase in bridewealth demands which was thought to have delayed marriage for many poorer men. This tendency was heightened by bridewealth in these societies becoming monetized, and thus individualized, so early. Poor young men were even less likely than their predecessors in earlier generations to obtain contributions to their bridewealth payments from family and clan, now that the payment was to be made in cash rather than livestock.[20] In Buhaya the onset of British rule coincided with a remarkable expansion of coffee production, which saw 2 million Robusta trees being planted in 1923 alone. By the following year, typical bridewealth demands had risen from a pre-war range of 6 to 20 shillings to between 400 and 600, equivalent to a lifetime's poll tax. Only male elders who possessed substantial coffee-producing land could afford such rates, but they did not necessarily rush to facilitate their sons' marriages.[21] Meanwhile, women's exemption from tax and some labour levies in Buganda opened up for them new alternatives to remaining in an unhappy marriage, because divorcees' low official outgoings encouraged some landowners to allow them to settle on their estates, on the basis that female tenants could thus be asked to pay higher rent.[22] In Buhaya marriage was destabilized by the growing tendency for fathers to marry off their daughters to wealthy older men who demanded unprecedented levels of labour from their new wives in compensation for the huge cost of bridewealth. Reports from as early as 1925 claimed that as a result a significant number of women were leaving their marriages and travelling by bus and ferry to become sex workers in Kampala and Nairobi.[23]

Secular and religious authorities responded to these developments by attempting to remove some of the obstacles to marriage and reduce the ease with which divorce could be obtained. Missionaries endeavoured to ensure that the state capped bridewealth at an affordable level, but found to their frustration that such regulations were easy to evade. Chiefly councils in Buganda and Buhaya passed laws which tried to impose new controls on independent women. And new divorce laws in both Uganda and Tanganyika

[20] Musisi, 'Transformations', pp. 195, 214. A. Southall and P. Gutkind, *Townsmen in the Making: Kampala and its Suburbs* (Kampala: East African Institute if Social Research, 1957), pp. 82–3 suggest that higher bridewealth also resulted from churches' insistence that marriage must be permanent and monogamous.

[21] Larsson, *Conversion*, p. 95; Bukoba District Annual Report 1924, TNA (Tanzania National Archives, Dar es Salaam) 1733/33 (AB105), Appendix 2, pp. 3–4.

[22] Hanson, *Landed*, p. 180.

[23] Bukoba District Annual Report 1925 (Bukoba sub-dist), TNA 1733/3:46 (AB40), p. 25; Southall and Gutkind, *Townsmen*, pp. 82–3. This issue will be further discussed later in this chapter.

removed many of the traditional justifications for ending a customary marriage, and made legal separation almost impossible within Christian marriage.[24] As several scholars have previously noted, the early enthusiasm for protecting women's rights within marriage in Buganda quickly fell away as they were charged with taking unfair advantage of reformers' generosity. As early as 1896 one CMS missionary wrote that:

> There is danger of the freedom and liberty granted to the women becoming licence and laziness . . . there must be some control over the women, they cannot be allowed to wander about from home to home just as they like . . . there are numbers of women who refuse to be married . . . If a man brings any pressure to bear on the woman of his household, he is afraid of being charged with introducing slavery again.[25]

Chiefs' concern about female autonomy and their rejection of marriage was expressed sporadically throughout the early colonial period. The opinions of Buganda's elite were stated particularly clearly during Lambkin's investigation into the causes of syphilis in 1907, but popular antagonism to independent women, at least as evidenced by male letter writers to vernacular newspapers, appears not to have been particularly strong before the 1920s. As Kyomuhendo and McIntosh show, it was only in that decade that complaints about the numbers of Ganda women living and growing cotton on their own became significant. Even then the focus of their irritation was on chiefs' willingness to provide women with land and failure to enforce the laws restricting women's movement.[26]

Such restrictions and criticisms were inevitably deeply resented, with some Ganda women expressing their dissatisfaction with becoming 'prisoners' within Christian marriage by giving themselves or their children names such

[24] On Buganda see N. Musisi, 'Gender and the cultural construction of "bad women" in the development of Kampala-Kibuga, 1900–1962', in D. Hodgson and S. McCurdy (eds.), *'Wicked Women' and the Reconfiguration of Gender in Africa* (Oxford: James Currey, 2001), p. 179; Musisi, 'Transformations', pp. 195, 214, 246–7; Marriage enquiry: government questionnaire and answers, 1932–8, Archdeacon of Uganda comments, n/d, Rubaga archives 49.6; H. Morris, 'Marriage and divorce in Uganda' (lecture given to the Uganda Society, 22 Apr. 1959), Marriage questions: the Uganda Council of Women, 1952–61, Namirembe Church of Uganda Archive, Mukono; Cunningham, *Uganda*, pp. 64–7. On Buhaya see Bukoba District Annual Report 1925, TNA 1733/3:46 (AB40), p. 3; Larsson, *Conversion*, p. 103.

[25] Walker to family, 25 October 1896, CMSA, A7/G3 letter 337 quoted in Musisi, 'Transformations', pp. 177–8. See J. Roscoe, *Twenty-Five Years in East Africa* (Cambridge: Cambridge University Press, 1921), pp. 170, 179 for further missionary criticism of female independence, considered by this respected ethnographer to be undermining Buganda's economy, morality, and social stability.

[26] Lambkin, Mission to the Uganda Protectorate on the prevalence of venereal diseases. Summary of evidence, Dec. 1907, PRO, CO/536/15; see also Mubendi District Annual Report, 1910–11, ESA A46/420; G. Kyomuhendo and M. McIntosh, *Women, Work and Domestic Virtue in Uganda, 1900–2003* (Oxford: James Currey, 2006), p. 73.

as Sirinagyendida (I will have nowhere to return) and Bwakwegayirira (marriage is a struggle of begging). While Ganda men composed new songs bemoaning the new freedoms demanded by women, so female Ganda responded with songs such as *Ssamanyirira*, 'I never knew'.

> I repent, I repent, but I have repented too late.
> I am fed up with the Christian marriage.
> I detest him who found this man for me.
> I hate my brother who presented this man to me.
> I dislike my parents for it.
> I can no longer manage. Goodbye.[27]

These lyrics suggest above all that attempts to enforce female submission were only partially successful. Women were still able to leave unhappy marriages, and now in Buganda and Buhaya had options after separation beyond a return to a natal family which would encourage an unwanted reconciliation. Moreover, while legislation in Buganda and Buhaya may have become increasingly patriarchal in nature, the actual arbitration of cases before local courts revealed that the letter of the law was not consistently applied. Runaway women were not always forced to return to their husbands, female resistance to spousal mistreatment was regarded as reasonable, and when a woman became pregnant before full bridewealth was paid, it was the man who was punished.[28]

More than this, some regulatory innovations were quietly forgotten, or proved unenforceable. In 1918 Archdeacon Owen of the CMS campaigned for a law to require the registration of customary marriage in Buganda to make it harder to separate informally and re-marry, entirely unaware that such a law had been passed by the *Lukiiko* in 1896.[29] The most obvious conclusion to be drawn from the frequency with which Buganda's *Lukiiko* passed resolutions aimed at preventing wives from abandoning their marriages is that such regulatory activity was not particularly successful.[30] Christine Obbo has argued that while the 1917 Adultery and Fornication Laws seemed to suggest that Buganda's chiefs intended to intervene in a sustained manner in the private lives of Ganda subjects, in fact 'bridewealth, adultery and divorce

[27] J. Waliggo, 'The Catholic Church in the Buddu Province of Buganda, 1879–1925' (unpublished PhD dissertation, 1976), pp. 283, 291; Musisi, 'Gender', p. 176; Musisi, 'Transformations', pp. 175–7, 181.
[28] Kyomuhendo and McIntosh, *Women*, pp. 69–70; Buganda Lukiiko Archives, 1894–1918, 19 June 1905, 15 May 1905, 13 Mar. 1916, 16 Mar. 1916; Report of the Sultan of Kiziba, Bukoba, Oct–Dec 1913, TNA, G34/1.
[29] W. Owen to the Bishop of Uganda, July 1918, Marriage files, Namirembe Church of Uganda Archive, Mukono; Buganda Lukiiko Archives, 1894–1918, 28 January 1896.
[30] Musisi, 'Gender', p. 179.

became private family matters because chiefs publicly frowned upon and discouraged the hearing of cases on such matters in the courts.'[31] It is striking that when Buganda's Provincial Commissioner consulted the regents in 1912 about the unfortunate consequences of converts divorcing excess wives, the kingdom's three senior chiefs downplayed the risks of motherless children or increased prostitution.[32] Moreover, in the surviving *Lukiiko* records, issues such as land, economic affairs, the maladministration of chiefs and theft were discussed and arbitrated much more frequently than sexuality, marriage, and gender.[33] Buganda's great chiefs, it seems, were not particularly enthusiastic about enforcing the various regulations they had passed.

Unfortunately Tanganyika's early censuses provide us with no statistical data which could help contextualize the evolving debates about marriage. By contrast Uganda's are quite revealing. The 1911 and 1921 censuses suggest that marriage has not always been as universal in Ankole as some later ethnographies have argued.[34] In 1911 a lower proportion of adults were married in Ankole than in Buganda, but the marriage rate increased sharply in Ankole over the following decade, from 73.2% for men to 78.1% and from 74.4% for women to 76.3%. This change was driven primarily by a sharp decline in the incidence of widowhood, presumably due to chiefly encouragement of remarriage after the death of a spouse. Over this same period in Buganda there occurred a significant decline in the percentage of adults, and especially women, who were married, adding credence to the contemporary belief that Buganda was experiencing a moral crisis and a weakening of the institution of marriage. The proportion of men who were single and widowed had increased by 1.75% and 0.83% respectively, while for women, the proportion who were single and widowed had increased by 2.1% and 2.6%. By 1921 more than 30% of women in Buganda were unmarried. This change was not a function of growing immigration, as the data, which were broken down by ethnicity in 1921, show that the marital status of the Ganda ethnic group almost exactly replicated that of the Province of Buganda as a whole.[35]

What links these two societies' diverging marital trajectories was a decline in the recorded frequency of polygamy associated with the widening and deepening of Christianization in southern Uganda. The proportion of women

[31] Obbo, 'Town', pp. 44–5.

[32] PC Buganda to Chief Secretary, 27 Nov. 1912, Marriage files, Namirembe Church of Uganda Archive, Mukono.

[33] Buganda Lukiiko Archives, 1894–1918.

[34] e.g. J. Ntozi and J. Kabera, 'Marriage patterns in Ankole, South-Western Uganda' (African Demography Working Papers no.16, University of Pennsylvania, August 1988), pp. 128.

[35] Uganda Protectorate, *1911 Census Returns* (Entebbe: Government Printer, 1912); Uganda Protectorate, *1921 Census Returns* (Entebbe: Government Printer, 1922). These censuses defined men as being aged eighteen and over and women as being fifteen and over.

who were polygamously married in Ankole declined by 3.2% over this decade, which largely explains why the male marriage rate had increased much faster than the female in this district. In Buganda, where more than half the population were Christian by 1921, the number of women defined as being polygamously married had fallen from 18% to 7.8% since 1911. It may of course simply have been the case that the chiefs who took the census in Buganda followed the legal ruling that Christian men could not be polygamists, or that polygamists became more likely to conceal their marital arrangements. Alternatively, the incidence of polygamy may truly have fallen due to missionary pressure on men not to seek additional wives, and as a result of women refusing to become a second or third wife, reflecting a growing association of polygamy with low status as much as moral impurity. Certainly the tendency for the polygamy rate to decline in Buganda over the rest of the colonial period, and into the post-colonial era, long after the abandonment of the non-recognition of Christian polygamy, suggests that the change between 1911 and 1921 may have reflected actual behaviour rather than legal fiction.[36]

Sexual Behaviour

What documentary evidence survives from early colonial Ankole offers no indication that sexual behaviour was significantly affected by colonization and missionization. This is perhaps unsurprising given that the colonial presence in Ankole was so light in this period, the Nkole were only marginally integrated into the colonial economy, and both Catholic and Protestant missionaries continued to concentrate their resources in Buganda and Buhaya. John Roscoe's ethnographic descriptions of Nkole society just after the First World War emphasize the continued, or possibly intensified, strength of Hima disdain for local agriculturalists, such that only a Hima girl who had fallen pregnant before marriage could marry a cultivator. Roscoe noted though the extreme rarity of such an occurrence, for girls still lived by 'a high code of morality', with pre-marital pregnancy usually being punished by death. By contrast, Roscoe found that local norms of Hima hospitality meant that guests were invited to share a bed with the host's wife.[37] Oral informants agreed that ritualized execution resulting from pre-marital pregnancy persisted into the colonial period among the cultivating population as well,

[36] Musisi, 'Transformations', p. 176. In 1921 10.5% of Ankole's population were Christian. Malakites, who supported polygamy, were not defined as Christians in the census.

[37] Roscoe wrote about Ankole in the ethnographic present, so that at times it is uncertain whether he is describing pre-colonial customs or current conditions, but this section seems quite clearly to report contemporary practice. J. Roscoe, *The Soul of Central Africa: a General Account of the Mackie Ethnological Expedition* (New York, 1969 [1922]), pp. vii–x, 62–5.

albeit rarely, naming close relatives who died in this manner. But more typically the consequence was shame and banishment rather than death. Even young girls who were the victims of incest or rape by boys in the village would be sent away, for the presence of any resulting baby would threaten misfortune or further violence. Elderly female interviewees in Ankole emphasized the moral and physical dangers inherent in pre-marital sex much more than their contemporaries in Buganda and Buhaya. Equally striking was the absence of any reference to the state in relation to the policing of sexuality in this society, suggesting that chiefs and European administrators were much less active in passing and enforcing laws regulating their subjects' private lives. Even the outlawing of honour killings was associated in popular memory with the arrival of Christianity in rural communities between the wars, rather than government intervention.[38]

Buhaya's early colonial experience was very different from that of Ankole. While non-intervention largely characterized German rule in Buhaya, largely due to the fixation with social stability that followed the Maji Maji uprising, the British takeover in 1916 marked a new willingness to criticize and attempt to reform Haya behaviour. According to Ralph Austen, moreover, the missions in Buhaya, especially that of the Catholic church, constituted a third force rivalling colonial and chiefly authority. In addition, Haya participated enthusiastically first in labour migration and then, with spectacular results, in the colonial cash crop economy, setting the district on its way to becoming one of the richest parts of East Africa. The ease with which coffee could be integrated into the farming system of eastern Buhaya meant that almost all the land which supported bananas was quickly intercropped with Robusta. The sudden wealth which landholders enjoyed from the early 1920s devalued chiefly patronage, delayed the transfer of resources to the younger generation, and created new inequalities within marital relationships. By the mid-1920s discussion about these emerging sources of social tension had coalesced around one peculiarly emotive issue, sexual behaviour. This was because Buhaya was becoming as famous for exporting sex workers as coffee. Anxieties about prostitution energized debates about sexuality with an air of crisis

[38] e.g. Female Focus Group Discussion (FGD) Nyamitanga, 19 Aug. 2004; Female FGD Kiyungi, 21 Aug. 2004. The churches also seem to have been less interventionist in Ankole than in the other societies. One minor exception was the largely unsuccessful attempt by Bishop Willis of the CMS to force female Hima converts to abandon the veil, an indirect assault on Hima wives' 'lifelong seclusion and idleness', which facilitated their being made sexually available to their husbands' relatives and guests. J. Willis, 'Reflections on Uganda' (TS, n/d), RHO, MSS. Afr. S. 1792 Box 38, p. 132.

which was sustained by evolving moral, economic, and political debates right through to independence.[39]

Why Haya women should have become involved in sex work across East Africa so early and in such numbers has been investigated by a number of scholars. Attempts to identify pre-colonial causes of the twentieth-century development of prostitution have focused attention on the role of various factors which interfered with 'normal' patterns of marriage. During the lifetime of their father, the king, Buhaya's princesses were forbidden from marrying, but not from having sex. One of Birgitta Larsson's informants told her, 'They certainly had a number of men, but the fact that they had property made them independent of any man. They were like men.' At the other end of the social scale there existed the *bazaana*, female household slaves. Whereas the princesses could be presented as a model of female sexual autonomy which was later imitated on a commercial scale, the *bazaana* seemed to constitute an extreme example of the commodified nature of Haya female sexuality. Some *bazaana* were presented to Buhaya's kings and great chiefs in payment of debt, others were simply taken from their families due to their exceptional beauty. Though regarded as concubines of their owner the *bazaana* could be allocated to guests or clients as lovers and wives, on the understanding that any ensuing female offspring would belong to the original owner.[40] In reality, the sexual situation of princesses and royal slaves in pre-colonial Buhaya differed little from that reported from a range of neighbouring societies.[41] What was distinctive perhaps was that the numbers and function of *bazaana* were sustained in Buhaya for so long. German officials feared the consequences of depriving Buhaya's kings of a hundred or so members of their harems, and while the British quickly abolished the institution of female slavery after their takeover in 1916, *bazaana* continued to exist, albeit in a less public manner. Young women were still offered in lieu of debts owing to local rulers, *bazaana* could be concealed among the women who were required to perform labour service at the royal capitals, and local chiefs were encouraged to round up divorcees and widows living independently in their communities, described as *bijuju* (parasites) or *malaya vijijini* (village

[39] R. Austen, *Northwest Tanzania under German and British Rule: Colonial Policy and Tribal Politics, 1889–1939* (New Haven: Yale University Press, 1968); Larsson, *Conversion*, pp. 92–114. Coffee was far from new to the Haya, being sold in significant quantities in pre-colonial times, and under the Germans, but the scale of production was transformed in the 1920s by governmental pressure combined with rising prices.

[40] Larsson, *Conversion*, pp. 34–6, 112; M.-L. Swantz, *Women in Development: a Creative Role Denied. The Case of Tanzania* (London: Hurst, 1985), pp. 49–52.

[41] Médard, 'Croissance', pp. 85–6; G. Schweinfurth et al., *Emin Pasha in Central Africa: Being A Collection of His Letters and Journals* (London: G. Philip, 1888), pp. 87, 117.

prostitutes), and send them to their king.[42] A further, and more widespread, situation in which female sexual services were redistributed derived from the relatively common practice of husbands allowing their male relatives to have sex with their wives, something which missionaries in the early twentieth century strove energetically to discourage.[43] Finally, the exchange value of the sexual act had long been accepted due to the law of *bisisi*. The rule of *bisisi* meant that the *genitor* of a child was the first man to have sex with a woman after she had given birth, which reportedly resulted frequently in an infertile man paying another man's wife to allow him to have sex with her soon after childbirth so that he could claim her next child.[44]

Such pre-determining factors are no doubt significant, and certainly local missionaries considered Haya culture to be particularly sexually immoral, but more emphasis must be placed on colonial-era developments.[45] One suggested innovation was the emergence of a new sense of comparative aesthetics, with some colonial commentators believing that Haya women were particularly attractive to men outside of Buhaya because of their light skin colour. However, relatively pale skin was a characteristic shared across western Uganda, Rwanda, and Burundi. What was perhaps more unusual was the extent to which Haya culture prioritized a woman's beauty when measuring the attractiveness of a bride, an attitude which contrasted with that of many ethnic groups such as the Nkole and Kiga, where obedience and, above all, industry were emphasized. Certainly the care with which Haya women cultivated their physical appeal was appreciated by the officials and soldiers of German East Africa.[46] Most important of all though was the impact of the new commercialism of Haya society due to the success of the coffee industry. According to Southall and Gutkind, the ensuing inflation of bridewealth

[42] Larsson, *Conversion*, p. 113; B. Weiss, *Sacred Trees, Bitter Harvests: Globalizing Coffee in Northwest Tanzania* (Heinemann: Portsmouth, NH, 2003), p. 189. The practice of arresting unmarried women was formalized by a decree of 1908, despite missionary criticism that such women would be redistributed among the kings' clients, a practice described as akin to prostitution.

[43] Larsson, *Conversion*, pp. 58–9.

[44] Bukoba District Annual Report 1925 (Bukoba sub-dist), TNA 1733/3:46 (AB40), p. 55.

[45] B. Sundkler, *Bara Bukoba: Church and Community in Tanzania* (London: Hurst, 1980), pp. 1–3; Larsson, *Conversion*, p. 98.

[46] A. Southall and P. Gutkind, *Townsmen in the Making: Kampala and its Suburbs* (Kampala: East African Institute of Social Research, 1957), pp. 82–3; H. Rehse, *Kiziba: Land und Leute* (Stuttgart: Strecker und Schröder, 1910, translated by Mrs Donne, UDSM, Cory 369), Ch.12, p. 2; Austen, *Northwest*, p. 41; Int. YK, 19 Aug. 2000, Kikukwe, F; Male FGD Nyamitanga, 19 Aug. 2004; M. Edel, *The Chiga of Uganda* (New Brunswick, NJ: Transaction, 1996 [1957]), pp. 59, 185. Catholic missionaries in Buhaya recorded with relish accusations of German officials' sexual misadventures with local women, though their willingness to believe such rumours no doubt reflected the generally strained relations between church and state in this period. See for example Kashozi mission diary, 8 June 1894, White Fathers Archive.

made husbands behave to their wives 'as headmen rather than as lovers, keeping them slaving to make up for the expense incurred to get them'.[47] Colonial officials believed that wives, influenced in part by Christianity and education, in turn demanded practical recognition of their increased value as labourers. By the 1920s village women were aware of the 'silk, perfume and high heeled shoes' worn by the mistresses of Indian merchants and colonial officials in Bukoba, and began to demand such luxuries for themselves. Husbandly neglect supposedly created an opportunity for unmarried younger men, 'who by gifts of clothes and money render the women independent of their husbands'. It is noticeable here that European condemnation of Haya sexual behaviour is not particularly patriarchal in tone. The 1925 district annual report referred to women 'proceeding to Nairobi and Kampala rather than submitting to the old social order of things in Bukoba' as the logical outcome of elders' greed, the unsatisfactory nature of Haya marriage, and the 'idleness and promiscuous immorality of the younger men'.[48] Yet the sympathy felt for women was limited by the consequences of declining fidelity and marital stability. The impact of sexually transmitted disease on health and fertility was discussed in Buhaya explicitly as a threat to tax revenues, so crucial given the absence of significant economic development across so much of Tanganyika.[49] This interlinkage of coffee and sex would shape responses to STDs for decades to come.

Buganda shared many of the characteristics of Buhaya in its early colonial experience of sexual behavioural change. The Ganda were also pioneers of cash cropping by African landholders, they were perhaps even more heavily influenced by politically powerful missionary bodies, and discussions of sexuality were equally fixated on the problem of STDs. Yet the trajectory of change differed significantly in Buganda for several reasons. Buganda's *Lukiiko* was an exceptionally active and centralizing legislative body and the influence of Mengo and Mulago hospitals ensured that debates about sexuality in early colonial Buganda would be exceptionally medicalized, while the existence of the city of Kampala permitted the development of new forms of relationships and, along with the kingdom's unique land tenure system, created new opportunities for women to live independently of men.

Previous writing on early colonial sexuality in Buganda has suggested that a patriarchal alliance of the colonial administration, the missions, and senior chiefs used the apparent threat of an upsurge in sexual immorality to

[47] Southall and Gutkind, *Townsmen*, pp. 82–3.

[48] M. Koku and M. Ngaiza, 'The life history of a housewife: her life, work, income and property ownership', in M. Ngaiza and B. Koda (eds.), *Unsung Heroines: Women's Life Histories from Tanzania* (Dar es Salaam: WRDP, 1991), p. 92; Bukoba District Annual Report 1925, TNA 1733/3:46 (AB40), p. 3.

[49] Bukoba District Annual Report 1923, TNA 1733/8 (AB10).

re-exert control over Ganda women.[50] This approach can draw on some substantial evidence in its support. The Divorce Ordinance imposed harsher penalties on female adultery than that of men in divorce proceedings. As was noted in the previous chapter, the report of a major commission of enquiry into syphilis in Buganda referred to Ganda women as 'female animals' whose sexual urges had been 'unleashed' by the forces of modernity. In 1918 and 1919 the Catholic and Protestant bishops requested that secular authorities impose restrictions on women's movement, to prevent them leaving their husbands. In 1921 the leading European authority on Ganda culture, the missionary ethnographer John Roscoe, bemoaned the inability of Ganda women to become true helpmeets of male converts. 'When they were liberated from their old status of drudgery and slavery as a heathen wife and an attempt was made to raise them to a higher level as wives of Christian men, in accordance to Christian ideas, they took unfair advantage of their freedom.' Women were not, he continued, 'strong enough in the faith of the new religion to resist sensual desires, and they were not prepared to live pure and upright lives without the strong arm of primitive custom and law, or the fear of the husband which they had lost.' Such concerns resonated with some Ganda men, with Apollo Kaggwa, Buganda's prime minister, ordering the arrest of divorcees living independently, and the emergence as early as 1920 of a popular male critique of wives' new avariciousness, focusing particularly on their coveting of expensive dresses, a theme that would run through the rest of the colonial period.[51]

It may be, however, that the strength of this patriarchal alliance has been overestimated. Hardly any Ganda actually sought a divorce under the colonial Ordinance because of the expense involved in such a formal procedure. Lambkin's syphilis report received a hostile reception within Uganda, and the medical policy which was adopted in its wake was equally offensive to both sexes. Roscoe's opinions on sexuality were taken less seriously than those of the missionary doctor, Albert Cook, whose criticism of current behaviour

[50] Tuck, 'Syphilis', pp. 17, 87; Musisi, 'Morality', pp. 60–73. Musisi does note several occasions when the colonial government refused to support the more extreme policies of the missions and *Lukiiko*.

[51] Uganda Divorce Ordinance 1904 in Uganda Protectorate, *Laws of Uganda* (Entebbe: Government Printer, 1935); Lambkin, Mission to the Uganda Protectorate on the prevalence of venereal diseases. Summary of evidence, Dec. 1907, NA, CO/536/15; Musisi, 'Morality', pp. 64–5; J. Roscoe, *Twenty-five Years in East Africa* (Cambridge: Cambridge University Press, 1921), p. 179; Musisi, 'Gender', p. 179; 'Ebye Roma', *Munno*, Feb. 1920. For important studies relating to western imagery of black female sexuality see S. Gilman, *Difference and Pathology: Stereotypes of Sexuality, Race, and Madness* (New York: Cornell UP, 1985), pp. 81–83; A. McClintock, *Imperial Leather: Race, Gender and Sexuality in the Colonial Contest* (London: Routledge, 1995), pp. 41–42.

was generally gender-neutral, emphasizing 'the entire absence of a national conscience against sins of immorality'. Pre-colonial Ganda behaviour had been constrained, he argued, 'by harsh, deterrent responses to adultery or illicit sex, such as enslavement or death', while the colonial abolition of such offensive penalties combined with the only partial adoption of Christian norms of behaviour had left the Ganda 'confused amid moral anarchy'. Rather than emphasizing the dangers of female liberation, Cook's rhetoric instead identified productivity, population decline, and patriotism as the issues most likely to stimulate moral reform and colonial and chiefly investment in missionary medicine. The Mengo Hospital report from 1913 observed that 'if even sewage can be used as the finest fertilizing agent that agriculture knows of, there need surely be no waste products of human lives considered too foul to be reclaimed, or so contaminated as to be useless.' Cook's social purity campaign in 1921 told the Ganda that 'a strong prosperous nation is a land where there are numerous healthy families, in which the population is growing year by year.' Buganda, 'a dying nation', could only be saved by early marriage, acceptance of STD treatment, and parental and public encouragement of self-control among the young.[52]

Cook was representative of broader missionary fears that Ganda spirituality had regressed since the martyrdoms, religious wars, and revival of the 1880s and 1890s. The churches' efforts to reinflame the fervour of the early church and cleanse their converts of unchristian influence brought new emphasis on discipline and redemption. The Church of Uganda under the reforming Bishop Willis, for example, set out the grounds for excommunication, ruled against the baptism of illegitimates, and discouraged drinking, naming ceremonies, and traditional music and dancing in an attempt to limit parishioners' exposure to sexual temptation.[53] Such innovations affected men as much as women, and there is evidence that church authorities at the local level also viewed population decline and rising levels of STD infection as problems requiring general moral reform. The Nakanyonyi Church of Uganda parish council reported in 1920 that education offered the best hope for repentance, but only if it included the poor and especially females. The council's opinion that 'it is the girls who can conquer bad manners by rejecting

[52] A. Cook, 'An urgent need in Uganda', *Mercy and Truth*, 12 (1908), pp. 44–50; CMS Mengo Hospital Annual Report 1912–13 (Albert Cook Archive, Mulago Hospital, Kampala), p. 5; A. Cook, 'A social purity campaign in Uganda', *Mercy and Truth*, 25 (1921), pp. 271–98; C. Summers, 'Intimate colonialism: The imperial production of reproduction in Uganda, 1907–1925', *Signs*, 16, 4 (1991), p. 796. Cf. P. Brantlinger, *Dark Vanishings: Discourse on the Extinction of Primitive Races, 1800–1930* (Ithaca: Cornell UP, 2003). Admittedly women appear to have resented genital examination in public more than men, but that was not the intention behind the policy.

[53] A. Kagume, 'Church and society in Ankole, Uganda: an analysis of the impact of evangelical African Christianity on ethnic and gender relations in Ankole, 1901–1961' (unpublished PhD dissertation, University of Bristol, 1993), pp. 140–1.

them; then the boys also will reject them' was indicative of a belief that females possessed superior natural moral purity and that sexual self-control was particularly problematic for male adolescents.[54]

Similarly, the bulk of the morality-focused legislation passed by Buganda's ruling council was gender neutral in its intent. The *Lukiiko*'s Adultery and Fornication Law of 1918, which aimed to be a definitive set of guidelines on all aspects of sexual morality, set out equal penalties for men and women for most transgressions, except where a man had sex with a betrothed woman, in which case only the man was punished.[55] Moreover, it seems that Buganda's courts tended to regard men as the guiltier partners in any adulterous affair. Missionaries in 1916 demanded that the Lukiiko pass a law which punished adulterous men and women equally, unaware that such a law had in fact been passed in 1895 but not consistently enforced. The transcript of one 1905 case tried by the *Lukiiko* court certainly suggests that the ascription of guilt did not always follow the letter of the law. One Bulazi was brought to the court accused of biting off his wife, Tereza's, ear, due to his anger at her having had an affair with another man, Kagondo. While Bulazi was imprisoned for a year, Tereza was found guilty but left unpunished, perhaps because she had already suffered enough. The treatment of Kagondo though suggests that adultery in itself was not regarded very seriously by judicial authorities. Kagondo's chief crime was in challenging Bulazi's position within his own home. 'He went beyond reasonable limits when he actually entered Bulazi's house, gave money to his wife, and had two well prepared meals washed down with simsim soup.'[56]

For the colonial state, sexuality was a realm in which it had little desire to intervene. Mission requests that the colonial government should control female movement and clear the streets of sex workers were typically refused, or passed on to the Buganda government.[57] The apparent excess of deaths over births however was a source of embarrassment as well as declining

[54] H. Stanton, 'A picture of Uganda in the 1960s. A tribute to Makerere University College and to African women', RHO, MSS. Afr. s. 2285, n/d [*c.*1980], Ch.3, pp. 8–9.

[55] *The Native Laws of Buganda* (Kampala, 1947), pp. 2–6.

[56] Musisi, 'Morality', pp. 64–5; Buganda Lukiiko Archives, 1894–1918, 19 June 1905.

[57] Musisi, 'Gender', p. 180; Musisi, 'Morality', pp. 64–5. It may be that this non-interventionism stemmed from an awareness of the possibility that the colonial administration might be accused of hypocrisy. European officials appear to have maintained local mistresses in a less than discreet manner well into the 1920s. Dr M. Lamont to Dr June Walker, 1 Jan 1922, Uganda 1908–54, Women's Library, London, 3AMS/D/49. The Crewe Memorandum from 1909 warning colonial officials of the penalties for such 'gravely improper conduct' was circulated again among all officers in the Uganda service in 1923. An isolated piece of evidence from 1903 indicates that some Ganda men procured women to provide sex for Europeans during their itinerations. IM to Reverend Father, 4 June 1903, Marriage files, Mill Hill Fathers' Archive, Bishop's House, Jinja. Thanks to Henri Médard for this reference.

revenue, and encouraged a policy of limited regulation to protect fertility. This was the context for the remarkably intrusive policy of mass STD examination and treatment adopted following Lambkin's report, but, as Carol Summers has pointed out, Uganda differed from standard British practice in that here more men than women were subjected to medical investigation. Even the law to regulate prostitution criminalized sex work only when an individual was infected with an STD, and even then culpability was shared between the sex worker and her employer.[58] The colonial administration may have been concerned about the growing independence of women, but attempts to control women were constrained by a sense that sexual misbehaviour was far from a predominantly female problem, and by a compulsion to restrict the harshness with which male discipline over females was enforced. For example the state took away household heads' right to beat their wives and daughters, regarded by Ganda as a key element in their sexual regulation.[59]

The literature on sexuality in early colonial Buganda has focused heavily on legislation by church and state, and has tended to overemphasize the patriarchal nature of new regulations, and underestimate the complexities of enforcement.[60] It is important not to forget though that the pressure to regulate derived in large part from the rapid transformation of Ganda society following the colonial takeover. Voluntarily or involuntarily, many couples separated as a result of the internal conflict of the late nineteenth century, the abolition of slavery, and the huge population movements associated with the introduction of freehold land tenure.[61] The colonial commercialization of the economy created new spaces into which Ganda women could escape on a scale which Buhaya could not match. The 1900 Agreement created thousands of landholders who regarded cash-cropping female tenants as particularly attractive. Buganda's capital seems to have grown rapidly after 1890, drawing in refugees, runaway slaves, and labour migrants, so that by 1911 it and the adjoining city of Kampala had a population of 32,441. Despite the efforts of

[58] Buganda, Annual Report For 1914–1915, ESA, A46/426; Summers, 'Intimate', p. 801; The Townships (Venereal Diseases) Rules 1913 in *The Native Laws of Buganda*.

[59] R. Yeld, 'Continuity and change in Kiga patterns of marriage; an analysis of structural change in Kiga marriage in the 1930s and the 1960s', (UEA Social Science Conference, December 1966), RHO, MSS. Afr. s. 1792/48, 7/23 Continuity and Change, p. 6; Buganda Lukiiko Archives, 1894–1918, Buganda Laws, 9 July 1895.

[60] Early missionary correspondence regarding marriage disputes conveys a strong sense of confusion among clergy trying to deal with individuals who had been married a number of times, through means such as abduction, purchase, and inheritance. One wrote despairingly 'the Baganda are such liars especially when there is any hope of dissolving an unhappy marriage.' T. Matthews to Fr. Biermans, 23 Apr. 1904, Marriage files, Mill Hill Fathers' Archive, Bishop's House, Jinja.

[61] See for example J. Biermans to Bishop Hanlon, 12 Apr. 1904, Marriage files, Mill Hill Fathers' Archive, Bishop's House, Jinja.

the churches and the kingdom government, women were able to move to and around town largely unsupervised. In 1911 43% of the population were female, an unusually high proportion for early colonial Africa. This permitted the development of an evolving model of urban sexuality that would be imitated across Ganda society and beyond as the twentieth century progressed.[62] If Haya sexuality was shaped by coffee, then sexual change in Buganda was driven by independent landholding and the interconnections between the urban and the rural.

Fertility, Sterility, Miscarriage, and Stillbirth

The low birth rates which were recorded across the region during the first decades of colonial rule lent credence and urgency to the sense that marriage, sexuality, and gender roles had drifted out of control. Thus the annual report from Buganda for 1914–15 noted that 'the discrepancy between the number of births and deaths in the country is most alarming . . . Enquiries are being prosecuted with a view to ascertaining whether anything can be done to stop the decline of population. Venereal Diseases account for many deaths and the low birth rate, as does want of restraint amongst women and general immorality.' In Buhaya as in Buganda the apparent decline in the birth rate was regarded as being 'of the utmost importance'. Successive administrative reports emphasized the excess of deaths over births, and associated the resultant population decline with promiscuity and STDs. The 'virtual depopulation' of Karagwe, which suffered both low fertility and emigration, was held to be inevitable unless unspecified steps were taken. Buhaya's missionaries adopted an even more apocalyptic tone, as in this 1913 report. 'We live among a dying people. We always return from the clinic with this impression: sick from top to bottom. Unclean diseases have penetrated the people to a terrifying degree.'[63] Ankole's chiefs meanwhile also reported with concern low birth rates and high levels of syphilis infection in the first decade of the twentieth century. In the years that followed, however, anxieties about a moral crisis in Ankole dissipated, it seems because the district's population began to rise steadily. The context of demographic recovery enabled administrators and

[62] Obbo, 'Town', pp. 174–5; Davis, 'Town', pp. 32–3; Musisi, 'Morality', pp. 62–3; Uganda, *1911 Census*.

[63] Buganda Annual Report for 1914–1915, ESA A46/426; Coryndon to Secretary of State, 30 May 1918, NA, CO/536/89; Buganda: Annual Report for 1917–1918, ESA A46/431; Bukoba District Annual Report 1925, TNA 1733/3:46 (AB40); Larsson, *Conversion*, p. 96. Such predictions of biblical catastrophe were also common among missionaries in Buganda. One wrote in 1907 that due to the twin plagues of syphilis and sleeping sickness 'the decrease by death would if continued at the same rate for twenty years wipe out the whole population.' Walker to Baylis, 1 Dec. 1907, Birmingham, CMS archives, G3/A7/0/1907/190.

medical officers to ignore statistics indicating that during the First World War syphilis was more severe in Ankole than anywhere else in Uganda.[64]

The automatic equation in Uganda of low fertility with syphilis was further undermined during the Lamont scandal when metropolitan STD specialists challenged the tendency towards monocausal explanations of pregnancy loss. 'We do not understand why all stillbirths are ascribed to syphilis.'[65] Before 1922 the great missionary doctor Albert Cook had tended to attribute the 'appallingly frequent' occurrence of miscarriage and the tragedy of successive stillbirths in Buganda above all to the 'almost universal infection with syphilis'. By 1933 syphilis was no longer the primary threat to the fertility of the Ganda, according to Cook. Partly this was due to the extension of mass treatment of syphilis at ante-natal clinics, so that 'in scores of cases disheartened and saddened women who have had five to ten pregnancies ending in miscarriages or stillbirths, have borne healthy children.' But it was also because the target of missionary medical concern was shifting from immorality to ignorance. Cook believed that 18% of Ganda women suffered obstructed labour due to contracted pelvis, the result of poor diet, and a childhood spent carrying heavy burdens. Worse than this poor parenting, though, was 'the immense force of long established custom', which encouraged birth attendants to give women powerful oxytocic herbs to accelerate labour. Miscalculations of dosage and timing resulted in numerous cases of uterine rupture or maternal exhaustion.[66] Each of the network of maternity centres which the Cooks established after 1919, supported by government subsidy, was envisioned as 'a potential centre of light and learning'. The initial emphasis on sexual reform and STDs was not forgotten, but over time the centres came to focus more on waging 'warfare against the forces of ignorance, superstition and dirt'. Ganda were warned that 'the dirty conditions under which most children are born in the *kyalos* [villages] do not give either the mother or the child a fair chance', and that herbal oxytocics were 'always [emphasis in the original] extremely dangerous'. The message that clinics' professional expertise and hygiene gave women a much higher likelihood of successful

[64] Lambkin, 'Mission to the Uganda Protectorate on the prevalence of venereal diseases. Summary of evidence', Dec. 1907, NA, CO/536/15; Annual medical report 1918, NA, CO/536/95.

[65] A. Neilans, Some notes on the Memorandum issued by the Colonial Office concerning anti-venereal measures in Uganda, AMSH, Uganda 1908–54, Women's Library, London, 3AMS/D/49.

[66] A. Cook, 'Obstetric medicine in Uganda', *British Medical Journal*, 1, 2789 (1914), pp. 1281–3; A. Cook, 'Recent history', Cook Archives, Mulago, Kampala, *c.*1933. In 1932 Cook also acknowledged that a 'good many . . . premature births and still-births' were due to malaria and anaemia. Uganda, Annual medical report, 1932, British Library, B.L.SPR.MicB, Group 5, Reel 281.

childbirth seems to have resonated more with the Ganda than the sexual criticism of earlier years, as the number of inpatient deliveries grew rapidly from the 1930s.[67]

Cook's repackaging of maternity care appealed to the colonial state as well as to his Ganda clientele. The medical department hoped to restore its reputation after the syphilis debacle by offering basic healthcare to the masses in the countryside in alliance with the missions. By 1926 Buganda was served by twenty dispensaries and nineteen maternity centres, in addition to the various government and missionary hospitals in Kampala, Entebbe, and Masaka. The following year Buganda's provincial commissioner observed with satisfaction that the excess of births over deaths, first noticed in 1924, was increasing in size, and might 'well be considered to be the result of the increase in Buganda of dispensaries and Maternity Centres'.[68] Maternity care was initially conceived as an opportunity to develop a new kind of Christian family, but was in fact most successful in transmitting a deeper faith in the value of western healthcare. The maternity centres run by Catholic missionaries were regarded as 'quite a triumph' primarily because they were 'the strongest factor in the total acceptance of the "Sisters' Medicine"'.[69] In Tanganyika the medical department had adopted a similar strategy of focusing on reducing infant and child mortality through encouraging women to give birth within health facilities. However, neither in Buhaya nor indeed in Ankole could the state or the missions match the scale of operations seen in Buganda, and local suspicions of medical intentions remained largely untouched in both societies throughout the early colonial period. A maternity centre opened in Ankole in 1921 but closed within the year. Only six deliveries had occurred, two of which resulted in the deaths of both mother and baby. One midwife was dismissed, suffering from gonorrhoea, the other returned to Mengo for further training. Such a lack of success also characterized the efforts of Tanganyika as a whole during these years, with only thirty-one

[67] Summers, 'Intimate', pp. 803–4; A. Cook, Report of the Lady Coryndon Maternity Training School, Namirembe, 1931, Cook Archives, Mulago, Kampala; A. Cook, *Uganda Memories, 1897–1940* (Kampala: Uganda Society, 1945), pp. 325–7, 339, 361.

[68] Buganda Annual Report 1926, ESA A46/428; Buganda Annual Report 1927, ESA A46/433.

[69] 'Our congregation's contribution to medical work in Buganda', n/d, *c.*1968, FMSA (Franciscan Missionary Sisters Archive, Dundalk), Box 12A, pp. 7–9. The Franciscan Sisters opened their own midwifery school in 1921 at Nsambya to rival that of the 'fanatical' Cooks at Mengo. The Sisters however had to rely on lay medical workers until 1936, when the papal prohibition against nuns' involvement in maternity work was lifted, and so their efforts were initially rather limited. See also Buganda Annual Reports 1923, ESA 46/432. Buganda's provincial commissioner believed the maternity centres were bringing 'to the door of every peasant very tangible evidence of the benefits of the British raj'.

births in the entire Territory occurring in a clinic in 1926, compared to 2,000 in Buganda in that same year.[70]

The sense of crisis inspired by the apparent decline in fertility prompted both the colonial and the Ganda state to pass pro-natalist legislation in the early twentieth century. Abortion was criminalized by both governments in 1901 and 1904, though it seems that cases were most likely to come to court in association with suspected adultery. Techniques of abortion were commonly known in Buganda and Buhaya, but by its nature this was an act which was unlikely to be frequently prosecuted, as it was performed in secrecy, and was often understood as suspending rather than terminating an inconvenient pregnancy.[71] More positive interventions were the exemption of pregnant women from public works and men who had five living children with one wife from poll tax and *luwalo*. This latter measure indicated that the low fertility of the Ganda was viewed partly as a deliberate choice, which could be reversed through the provision of material incentives. Interestingly, the colonial state's tax exemption was restricted to men whose oldest child was under the age of ten, a policy which must have appeared to encourage shorter birth intervals than would have been typical in Buganda. It may be though that the intention of this restriction was simply to limit the financial loss to the colonial state. Poll tax returns from 1910–11 indicate that only one in four hundred Ganda men benefited from this exemption, a marker of colonial parsimony as well as Ganda sub-fertility.[72]

Concerns about population decline in this part of Africa were such a prominent element in political discourse in part because more demographic information was available to local governments than was typical for this period. Two population censuses had been held in both Uganda and Tanganyika by 1921, and some form of vital registration was established in the first decade of the twentieth century in all three case study areas. Colonial officials generally accepted that such demographic data gave a reasonable sense of general trends, even if they were sceptical of the accuracy of particular

[70] Western Province Annual Report, 1922, ESA A46/1094; S. Walters, 'Fertility, mortality and marriage in northwest Tanzania, 1920–1970: a demographic study using parish registers' (unpublished PhD dissertation, University of Cambridge, 2008), p. 47; Summers, 'Intimate', pp. 803–4. Around 16,000 live births were registered in Buganda in 1926.

[71] Musisi, 'Transformations', p. 249; Buganda Lukiiko Archives, 1894–1918, Adamu vs Mukubansi, 11 July 1905 and Zakalia Maganga vs Matayo Nsubuga, 24 July 1905; Rehse, *Kiziba*, Ch.11.

[72] Buganda Annual Report For 1917–18, ESA, A46/431; Buganda Lukiiko Archives, 1894–1918, 18 Apr. 1916; Lukiko resolutions passed at the annual meeting held at Mengo during the month of Oct. 1924, ESA, A46/1408; Buganda Annual Report 1910–11, Statement of poll tax payers, A46/420.

returns.[73] Administrators suspected that some chiefs undercounted their populations to 'avoid unpleasant questions as to the decrease of poll tax', while returns of births and deaths from peripheral areas were viewed with great uncertainty given the lesser legitimacy of imported chiefs and the durability of 'superstitions' about the dangers inherent in counting family members. Thus in 1910–11 the county of Buyaga, still very much ruled by Buganda as conquered territory, recorded the unfeasibly low crude birth and death rates of 9.5 and 14.5 per 1000.[74] A sense of the unevenness of early vital registration is provided by Buganda's figures of 1907, the first year in which they were collected. The overall average crude birth rate was a reasonably credible 16.6 per 1000, but individual county returns varied wildly from 8.5 to 56 per 1000. Over time officials in Buganda believed that data collection became more consistent, though it is clear that they were happier to believe in the accuracy of registration from the mid-1920s when the excess of births over deaths could be ascribed to the expansion of European healthcare.[75] The vital registration figures in Uganda show that any clear increase in crude birth rates only began from 1920 in both Ankole and Buganda. That Ankole's average crude birth rate between 1907 and 1924 of 24.7 per 1000 was 63% higher than Buganda's, at 15.1, suggests that the public debate about low fertility in Buganda was perhaps rooted in some degree of reality (see Figure 3.1).

No doubt the relatively low reported fertility levels of both Ugandan societies in this period were partly due to non-universal registration of births, but crude birth rates, it seems, were also suppressed by high levels of stillbirth. In Ankole 11.1% of all full-term babies were recorded as stillborn before 1924, compared to 8.9% in Buganda (see Figure 3.2). It may be that Buganda's earlier and sharper fall in stillbirth rates reflected that society's superior maternity facilities.

Hospital registers of maternity cases offer a depth of detail about fertility which is generally absent from more conventional colonial era sources,

[73] Uganda Protectorate, Annual Medical Report 1912, NA, CO/356/1; Report of the Sultan of Kiziba, Bukoba, Oct.–Dec. 1913, TNA, G34/1. Censuses had occurred in Uganda in 1911 and 1921, and in Tanganyika in 1913 and 1921.

[74] Buganda annual report, 1910–1911, Masaka and Mubendi district reports, ESA A46/420; Buganda annual report, 1915–16, ESA A46/425.

[75] A. Rendle, MO Kampala, Women's Library, London, Uganda 1908–54, 3AMS/D/49; Buganda Annual Report 1927, ESA A46/433. It is tempting to see the excess of births over deaths in Buganda as partly caused by the Buganda Births and Deaths Registration Law of 31 May 1923 which imposed a fine of twenty shillings for failure to register a birth but only one shilling for failing to register a death. *The Native Laws of Buganda* (Kampala, 1947). R. Kuczynski, *Demographic Survey of the British Colonial Empire, Vol. II* (Oxford: Institute of International Affairs, 1949), p. 371 indicated that vital registration in Buhaya was more accurate than the Tanganyikan average.

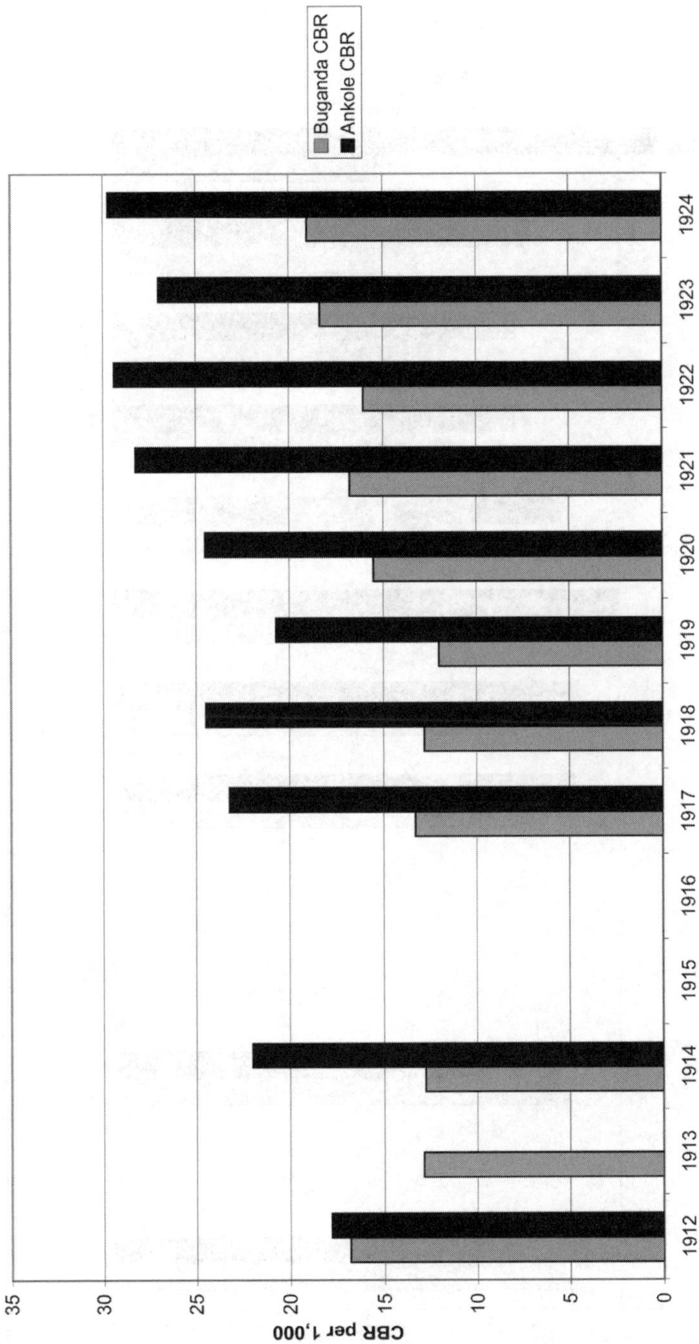

Figure 3.1 Crude birth rate per 1,000 in Ankole and Buganda 1912–24, from vital registration records

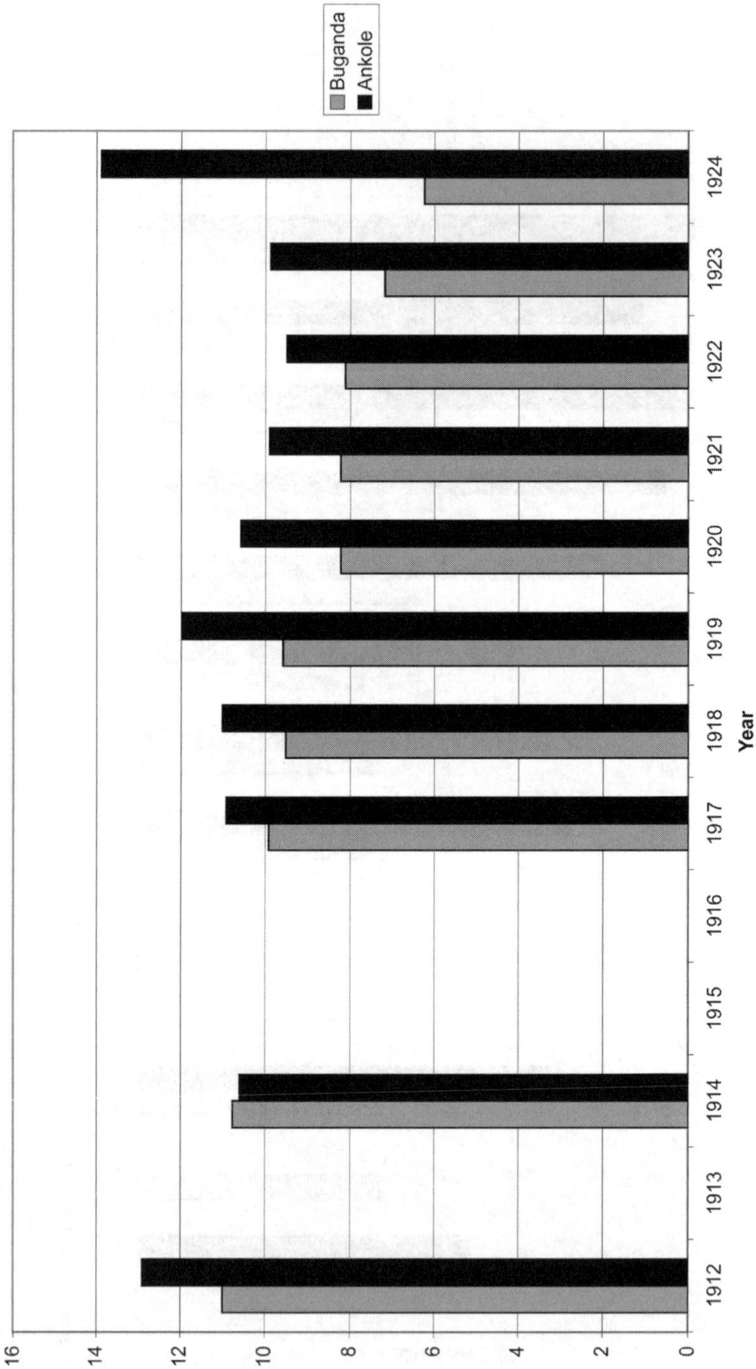

Figure 3.2 Stillbirths as a percentage of all registered births in Ankole and Buganda 1912–24

certainly from the earlier twentieth century. The Mengo hospital registers contain information on parity, history of miscarriages and stillbirths, history of syphilis from both mother and father, whether previous children were still alive, whether herbal medicines had been used to strengthen contractions, the outcome of the current delivery, and the birthweight and sex of the newborn. Occasionally a full narrative of a woman's reproductive history was provided, in addition to the basic statistical data. These registers constitute a remarkable body of material, but they must be used with caution. Like all records of demographic experience, the maternity registers may have suffered from problems of recall and definition. Reports of previous stillbirths may have been confused with miscarriages or neonatal deaths, and any of these unhappy events might not necessarily have been remembered or revealed. Counting children moreover was regarded as a potentially harmful exercise, a hubristic invitation to Death to reduce their number. In addition, it is reasonable to assume that many, perhaps most, of the early beneficiaries of missionary obstetrical expertise were atypical. The most ardent supporters of Mengo's maternity ward were the wives of Buganda's great chiefs, for whom medicalized childbirth was yet another very public demonstration of their devotion both to modernity and to Christianity. In contrast to this elite cohort, presumably the healthiest of all Ganda women, were those women who viewed Mengo as a last resort, driven by desperation. One woman who appeared in the 1919 register had had seven previous pregnancies, all of which had ended in miscarriage. In that year 45.3% of maternity inpatients had a specific reason to come into Mengo, either an immediate crisis such as a threatened miscarriage or obstructed delivery, or a previous history of repeated miscarriages, difficult deliveries, stillbirths, or infant deaths. But between these two extremes of the elite and the tragic lay a large body of women, perhaps half, whose medical notes give no indication that their presence in a maternity ward arose from exceptional circumstances.[76]

As the colonial period progressed, medicalized childbirth became a commonplace in central Buganda. At the same time though, high levels of immigration from across the Great Lakes region meant that an ever increasing proportion of women who appear in the medical records were non-Ganda. Increases in average parity or birthweight and reductions in stillbirth rates might therefore simply derive from the much greater ethnic diversity of Buganda's population. Over the course of the twentieth century, then, women in the maternity registers became more representative of the population of Buganda, but not necessarily of the Ganda ethnic group. Therefore the maternity data have been refined to exclude non-Ganda, in order to achieve

[76] Mengo maternity register for 1919, Mengo Hospital Archive, Albert Cook Library, Mulago, Kampala; Musisi, 'Transformations', p. 358.

some consistency in the sample population over time. In some years the maternity registers recorded the stated ethnicity of each patient, but in other years an ethnic identity has been ascribed to women on the basis of their names. The Ganda have a different system of naming from most Great Lakes societies, with the great majority of names being clan-based, and usually inherited from a remembered ancestor. Names are an imperfect proxy for ethnicity, but less imperfect in Buganda than in most African societies in this region.[77]

Maternity cases were treated at Mengo from the foundation of the hospital in 1897 but complete maternity registers survive only from the interwar period. This study has examined the registers from every fifth year from 1919. The most striking aspect of the fertility data from the two early colonial registers, those of 1919 and 1924, is how consistent they are, reinforcing the sense from other sources that fertility decline in Buganda had bottomed out as the instability of the post-civil war years eased. Average parity in 1919 stood at 2.35, and was only slightly higher in 1924 at 2.43. Unsurprisingly given such low parity levels, in 1919 only 12.8% of women were grand-multiparous (having had five or more full-term deliveries), a rate which had increased only marginally by 1924 to 13%. Obviously these data were obtained from women who had not necessarily finished childbearing, so should not be taken as a proxy for completed family size, but nonetheless they represent an extremely low level of fertility given that infertile women were by definition excluded from the maternity records. The most obvious reason for this low parity was the high level of pregnancy failure reported by women. Just over a quarter of women in both years had suffered at least one miscarriage in the past, and as recurrent pregnancy loss was common, the average number of miscarriages per woman was 0.41.

The high number of babies born dead at Mengo further confirms the scale of the fertility problems facing Ganda women in the early colonial period, with 9.2% of babies registered in 1919 and 10.5% in 1924 being still-born. That these stillbirth rates are even higher than those recorded in the vital registration data for these years can be explained by the self-selection of the Mengo patients. Stillbirths were clustered among women who had unfortunate histories. The sense that Mengo was increasingly regarded as a place where reproductive difficulties could be resolved is indicated by the increase in admissions of women immediately after a problematic home delivery. By 1924, 20% of the stillbirths recorded had actually occurred before admission.

[77] For a fuller discussion of the complexities of naming in this region, see S. Doyle, 'The child of death: Personal names and parental attitudes towards mortality in Bunyoro, Western Uganda, 1900–2005', *The Journal of African History*, 49, 1 (2008), pp. 361–82; S. Doyle, 'Immigrants and indigenes: the Lost Counties dispute and the evolution of ethnic identity in colonial Buganda', *Journal of Eastern African Studies*, 3, 2 (2009), pp. 284–302.

No doubt the skill of Mengo's personnel prevented still further stillbirths but the frequency of surgical intervention during delivery was surprisingly low given the frequency of obstructed labour. Between 1897 and 1913 only 17.1% of deliveries involved some intervention, primarily the use of forceps. Caesarean section was extremely rare, given the danger of sepsis and the universal accompaniment of hysterectomy at this time due to the risk of uncontrolled haemorrhage. All this would change radically in the decades that followed.[78]

The Mengo registers offer a useful series of snapshots of female fertility, but they give no information on completed family size or levels of infertility. Retrospective fertility surveys compensate for these inadequacies, but possess their own weaknesses. The likelihood of forgetting reproductive events would have increased when the objects of enquiry were women who had passed the age of childbearing. Similarly, the risk that grown-up children would not have been included in accounts of parity would have worsened. In 1952 the anthropologists Priscilla Reining and Audrey Richards participated in a fertility study of Buhaya and Buganda, in collaboration with the East African Medical Survey. They found that women aged sixty and over from Buhaya reported an average number of live births over their lifetime of 4.08, compared to 3.21 in Buganda. The reason for this divergence was that 31.3% of women born before 1892 in Buganda had never had a child, compared to just 7% in Buhaya. Ganda women who were fertile though had borne more children than Haya mothers, 4.8 compared to 4.4. Fertility problems would intensify in both societies during the interwar years, but this survey indicates that Buganda's fertility problems were well established by the start of colonial rule, whereas Buhaya's were in large part a product of the twentieth century.[79]

So far the analysis of variation in fertility has focused on the relative severity of a range of reproductive problems. The final major source to be discussed in this chapter provides insights into the mechanisms of reproduction

[78] Mengo maternity registers 1919 and 1924; A. Cook, 'Obstetric medicine in Uganda', *British Medical Journal*, 1, 2789 (1914), pp. 1281–3. The maternity registers have one further weakness, common to many systems of medical record-keeping in the past. Idiosyncrasies in the use of medical terminology mean that records cannot be taken at face value. In particular, the early Mengo records appear to have confused parity, the number of full-term births, and gravidity, the number of pregnancies. What was described as a patient's parity in the early Mengo registers was equal to the number of live births, stillbirths, and miscarriages, i.e. her gravidity. This study has used the total of live births (including the current delivery) plus stillbirths as the equivalent of parity. Usage of these terms is still not fully standardized today in the UK. M. Creinin and H. Simhan, 'Can we communicate gravidity and parity better?', *Obstetrics and Gynecology*, 113, 3 (2009), 709–11. The 1924 register makes this confusion clear by recording the number of past labours as well as the parity of the patient.

[79] A. Richards and P. Reining, 'Report on fertility surveys in Buganda and Buhaya, 1952' (UDSM, Cory 373).

itself. The Christian churches in the Great Lakes region identified their adherents, and measured their success, by recording participation in the sacraments. The resultant registration of baptism, marriage, and burial possesses such great potential for demographic history because it enables individuals to be tracked over the course of their lifetimes, it permits the reconstruction of familial relationships over generations, and it reveals the age at which major life events occurred. The techniques of family reconstitution have been used to significant effect by scholars hoping to compensate for the absence or inadequacy of censuses in Africa before the Second World War.[80] However, unlike historians of early modern Europe, who first developed these techniques, Africanists have had to work with new Christian communities. Many converts entered the church as adults, often already married and in the middle of their reproductive lives. The adoption of a permanent religious identity was rarely immediate, so that individuals might maintain adherence to older indigenous beliefs, or experiment with other world religions. This problem of temporary dissociation was worsened by church discipline against members of the congregation for such offences. The huge physical size of early parishes, moreover, made burial in consecrated ground and the early baptism of infants impractical for converts who lived at some distance from the mission centre. Later, as congregations grew larger, daughter parishes were created, meaning that many families were lost to observation. As time progressed an ever smaller proportion of converts could be followed through to burial for the obvious reason that many parishioners have not yet died. Finally, clerical opposition to polygamy and divorce deterred most adults from marrying in church.[81]

Family reconstitution in Africa then is complicated in many ways by the youthfulness of Christian communities. There is no record of the many babies who must have died before they could be baptized. It is impossible to calculate the interval between marriage date and the first birth for couples who never married in church. Not all children born to a couple were necessarily baptized in the same parish. Converts moreover remained a minority in most societies well into the colonial period, raising concerns about the representativeness of the demographic data which can be extracted from the parish registers. In addition to these problems the ability to track individuals from baptism through marriage and then parenthood relies on their names being

[80] e.g. S. Colwell, 'Infant and child mortality on Kilimanjaro, 1894–1935' (unpublished paper, Harvard School of Public Health, 2001); H. Siiskonen, A. Taskinen and V. Notkola, 'Parish registers: A challenge for African historical demography', *History in Africa*, 32 (2005), pp. 385–402; Walters, 'Fertility'.

[81] For further discussion of the complexities of family reconstitution in Africa see Walters, 'Fertility', Ch.3 and pp. 168–70.

recorded consistently over time. As it was not unusual for people in this region to acquire several vernacular names over their lifetimes, it can only be hoped that individuals would have consistently utilized their church names to avoid the potential for mis-identification. Some people though did adapt their names, most commonly by dropping the diminutive prefix 'ka-' as they reached maturity. The greatest problem arises from the non-standardization of orthography during the colonial period, and the difficulty experienced by European missionaries in recording clausal vernacular names accurately. Thus for example there were over forty variants of the forename John in the Kisubi baptismal register, ranging from Jonasamu to Yovani.[82] These various problems mean that only a small minority of couples can be followed from baptism through their marriage and on to the burial of one of the spouses. Moreover, as none of the parishes used in this study kept a record of parishioners who took communion or attended Easter services, it is impossible to be confident about which couples remained consistently resident within their home parishes.[83]

It is not feasible therefore to create with any degree of confidence age-specific marital fertility rates or total marital fertility rates from these parish registers. Nonetheless, family reconstitution from the Bukoba, Kisubi, and Nyamitanga Catholic parish registers has permitted calculations to be made regarding age at first marriage and birth intervals, two of the key factors contributing to fertility levels. Priests did note where people who had been widowed were remarrying, or where couples who were marrying in church were simply having an existing union blessed. Such marriages have been excluded from the marital age calculations, but it is likely that clergy were not always aware of individuals' marital condition. It is probable therefore that the following data exaggerate the true average age at first marriage, particularly when it is considered that the church opposed girls marrying in their early teens, one of many factors affecting the representativeness of Christian marriage. Nonetheless, as reproduction does still seem to have predominantly taken place within marriage during the early twentieth century, these data which suggest that fertility in these societies was partially suppressed by delayed marriage are of significance. Before 1924 Catholic women married at an average age of 20.4 years in Buhaya, 21.7 in Ankole, and 23.1 in Buganda. The exceptionally late age of female marriage in Buganda must have

[82] Some of these problems are not unique to African contexts, particularly those relating to population mobility and the difficulty of fixing a name to an individual.

[83] Compare the most complex attempt at full family reconstitution in Africa, Sarah Walter's study of Mwanza region. Walters, 'Fertility', pp. 168–70. Even though her parishes had much greater information on time in observation than Bukoba, Kisubi and Nyamitanga, only ninety couples could be identified for whom age-specific fertility calculations could be made.

contributed to elders' concerns about female autonomy and the rejection of marriage by the young. Male marriage age is of much less significance for overall birth rates, but male fertility does decline incrementally from the early twenties, and the risk of widowhood increases with male marital age. Whereas young Catholic men married for the first time at an average age of 23.3 in early colonial Ankole, their peers in Buganda and Buhaya married when they were three years older, perhaps reflecting the economic obstacles to early marriage in these heavily commercialized societies. Just as important as age at marriage though, was what happened after couples married. The average birth interval in Ankole and Buhaya before 1924 was four months shorter than in Buganda (see Figure 7.4). But whereas intervals were increasing steadily in the former societies until the 1930s, in Buganda birth-spacing was already declining quickly by the early 1920s.[84] It seems clear that pre-colonial norms of fertility behaviour were being rapidly reshaped during the early colonial period. So early in the twentieth century it is possible only to hypothesize what the causes of this divergent pattern might have been. Worsening levels of child mortality during the first decades of colonial rule in Ankole and Buhaya may have encouraged mothers to lengthen the period of breastfeeding to increase the chance of infant survival. The suggestive evidence that early colonial Ankole experienced a movement towards moral reform may indicate that social rules regarding post-partum sexual abstinence would have been observed with greater care. Buganda by contrast was not only far in advance of the other societies in terms of Christianization, female education and commercialization, all factors which tended to weaken adherence to social rules regarding breastfeeding and sexual abstinence, but also seems to have experienced a reduction in child mortality before its neighbours (see Chapter 2).[85]

CONCLUSION

The recurring sense of crisis affecting public debates about morality and marriage stemmed from concerns about declining fertility. The nature of the debate in each of the case study areas varied over time. In Ankole, the early fears of demographic decline eased as chiefly pressure reinforced marriage and fertility levels began to recover. In Buganda, the fixation with syphilis as the fundamental cause of low fertility decreased, to be replaced by a new

[84] Individuals whose birth intervals were biologically unlikely (less than nine or more than sixty months) were excluded.

[85] That female education was taken seriously from an early date in Buganda is indicated by the records of Kisubi parish which showed that in 1906 as many girls as boys attended the church's schools. Kisubi parish diary, 6 July 1906, White Fathers Archive.

emphasis on training Ganda to be good mothers. In Buhaya, the sudden prosperity brought by coffee after the First World War focused attention on the inability of the young to marry, and wives' rejection of marriage for the dubious attractions of the colonial city.

Sterility, delayed marriage, miscarriage, and stillbirth featured prominently in all three case study areas during this period, especially in Buganda. In oral interviews elders frequently emphasized how low fertility had been in the past, and the trauma that often resulted. One remembered that in the early twentieth century, 'if a person managed to have a child or two, then he was seen as a boss.' Others told of male relatives who married successive wives in the hope of securing an heir. Some informants bore names such as Mpabuka, which means 'When I was born, children were scarce,' and Mukamutachumwa, 'An only child must be both son and daughter.' Anxieties about low fertility in the early colonial period may have provided opportunities for interventions in the world of sex and marriage, but they should not merely be viewed as convenient justifications for patriarchal interventions.[86]

There are good reasons why so many scholars have emphasized male subjugation of women during the colonial period in this region. Female members of the royal family were excluded from power when Europeans took control of these societies. Some of the rhetoric emanating from missionaries, administrators, and doctors in response to the perceived crises of syphilis and demographic decline in the early twentieth century was profoundly misogynistic. Men benefited far more than women from the enhanced opportunities for material wealth and status created by the economic and educational systems established by the early colonial state. Female public behaviour, meanwhile, despite the occasional outrage at the actions of independent women, continued to be characterized by subservience and silence. However, as this chapter has shown, moralistic diatribes from this era frequently condemned male behaviour as well. The colonial economy would develop spaces for female autonomy and, occasionally, prosperity. Female education developed unusually early in Buganda and Buhaya. Men, with good reason, frequently suspected that they were being manipulated by their wives. And finally, local courts provided women with a surprising degree of protection. Data preserved by Melvin Perlman show that in Buganda, for example, women were much more likely than men to win cases relating to sexual misconduct or marital dispute, whether as plaintiff or defendant. Moreover, the degree to which courts favoured women increased over time. Two aspects of the data seem particularly significant. One is that women won twice as many child

[86] Int. EFC, 23 July 1998, Katongo, F; Int. JM, 12 Aug. 2000, Kanoni, M; Int. MM, 12 Aug. 2000, Kamachumu, F; Int. MPM, 10 Aug. 2000, Ibare, F.

custody disputes as did men, and were particularly likely to be successful if they could demonstrate independent income, even though customary guardianship law gave priority to the family of the father, and officialdom was supposedly antagonistic to displays of female autonomy. The other is that 40% of appeals to higher courts were brought by women. In sum, then, this branch of the apparatus of the state served overall to uphold or even increase women's rights, while women themselves, in contrast to their passive stereotype, were prepared to speak up for themselves in court, and to persist in their quest for justice with a remarkable degree of success. As the three following chapters will show, changes in sexual behaviour and attitudes in the various case study areas would, like those affecting gender relations, also be characterized by ebb and flow. On balance though efforts to exert control over sexual behaviour, male as well as female, were unsuccessful.[87]

[87] List of saza level cases, File 23, PPMS38/Perlman/Box 8, SOAS archive.

4

Marriage and Sexuality in Buganda, 1925–69

INTRODUCTION

Most historical writing which has endeavoured to explain the origins of the HIV epidemic in this region has tended to focus on the early colonial period, dominated as it was by concerns about STDs, population decline, and moral collapse, or the 1970s, the years of violence and corruption during which the virus began to spread rapidly. Yet it was during the middle decades of the twentieth century that the pattern of sexuality that defined the AIDS epidemic in Buganda mostly emerged. This chapter will trace the development across the period 1925 to 1969 of the increasing ease with which pre-marital and extra-marital affairs could be conducted in Buganda, the kingdom's remarkable marital instability, the growing incidence of non-marital sex across generations, its well developed urban-rural sexual networks, and the rise of commercial sex work, bars, and nightclubs. It will focus heavily on the new forms of socializing which provided Ganda of all ages with opportunities to acquire additional sexual partners, but it will also show how sexual behaviour and attitudes evolved in the context of a growing social permissiveness, and the greater legal protection and opportunities for wealth creation enjoyed by youths, widows, and divorcees.

Both the framework of this chapter, and the oral sources which have been used so frequently to illustrate it, may, perhaps naturally, be viewed with some scepticism. People everywhere tend to argue that sexual morality deteriorated over their lifetimes, while the detailing of the emergence at different points during the colonial and early post-colonial periods of various aspects of the sexual culture associated with AIDS may ring of goal-oriented historical reconstruction. However, while it would be possible to read the story of Ganda sexuality as a narrative of gradual declension overall, it should be noted that in the 1950s and 1960s some social developments and sporadic attempts at moral reform complicated this broad trend. Moreover, as the next two chapters show, the direction of change in Ankole and Buhaya was very different. In Buhaya marriage appears to have been stabilized to some degree between the 1950s and early 1970s, while in Ankole sexual conservatism remained dominant until the 1960s. In all three societies oral informants did initially tend to assert that the 1960s and 1970s had ushered in a new kind of sexual promiscuity. But in Buganda and Buhaya, though rarely in Ankole, further questioning revealed that, in fact, during the 1930s, 1940s, and 1950s most elders had themselves participated in the kinds of behaviours that they had initially condemned. What elderly interviewees objected to most about post-colonial behaviour was not that sexual practices had radically changed, but that sexuality in general had become more public, a mark of disrespect towards parents and spouses. Finally, it should be noted that the oral accounts of sexual behavioural change which enrich this chapter are closely supported by exceptionally rich documentary records. Buganda had a vibrant vernacular press, whose editorial policies ranged from the moralistic to the prurient; its culture was carefully analysed by a succession of sensitive ethnographers; the epidemiology of STDs was the subject of increasingly sophisticated medical research; its local government was particularly active; its courts were heavily utilized; and the records of its churches' interventions in the spheres of marriage and morality are unusually detailed. Moreover, the primarily qualitative evidence presented in this chapter should be read in conjunction with the extensive statistical data, which is presented in Chapters 7 and 8 and shows, for example, that both pre- and post-marital female fertility, and the incidence of abortion, rose sharply over time, and that adolescents contributed an increasing proportion of STD infections in the post-Second World War era. The oral evidence then has not been accepted at face value. Informants were pressed to move beyond the recycling of tropes, testimonies were examined for obvious signs of evasion or exaggeration, and individuals' remembering of the past was compared with a range of alternative sources.

MARRIAGE

Marriage in the early colonial period was characterized above all by ambiguity and uncertainty, but several trends began to emerge which would become more significant as the twentieth century progressed: polygamous marriages became less durable, and women found new alternatives to marriage in the region's rapidly growing cash economy. These developments were driven by larger changes in social relations within Great Lakes communities. Women's ability to shape their futures increased overall, and individualism gradually came to rival the demands of clan and lineage in the establishment of new families.

This story of marital change in Buganda will be discussed in more detail than in the other case study areas, for the Ganda were affected earliest and in the most complex ways by the trends that would reshape family life across the entire region. Buganda had become a Christian kingdom in the 1890s, officially at least, through an alliance between missionaries, chiefs, and colonial officials. By the second decade of the twentieth century Ganda society too had been largely Christianized, or at least churched, as hundreds of thousands of Ganda joined the Catholic and Anglican churches, often under the forceful encouragement of their local chief or landlord, but also attracted by an exceptionally generous provision of mission education and healthcare. By the early 1930s this alliance had begun to disintegrate. The missions grew increasingly critical of the chiefly elite, whose inadequacy as role models and guarantors of public morality was associated with their ever more conspicuous polygamy.[1] Unable to reform the chiefs themselves, missionaries demanded that the state should intervene. At the same time, missionaries hoped to revive and purify their congregations by addressing the growing reluctance of converts to marry in church. Religious leaders again wanted the state to ensure that a church marriage would be materially as well as spiritually advantageous. For example, the missions asked that a widow from a Christian marriage should be permitted to remain on her late husband's land as guardian of her children rather than be pressed to marry his heir or driven back to her parents.[2]

By the 1930s, however, the colonial state in Uganda was governed by the principles of indirect rule. Determined to preserve the integrity of indigenous culture and structures of authority, colonial officials became less willing to interfere with those aspects of life which were regulated by customary law. Thus in 1933 Governor Bourdillon refused to make an example of a chief who had been divorced for marrying two women by custom after his church wedding, and then severely beating his church wife, on the grounds that such interventions would undermine the authority of Buganda's king, the kabaka, and the stability of the chiefly system.[3] Bourdillon's successor, Philip Mitchell,

[1] Mission criticism of chiefly misbehaviour was relatively contained by the Anglican church's reluctance to undermine its status as the unofficial state religion, and the Catholic church's acknowledgement that European societies' adoption of a fully Christian lifestyle occurred centuries after formal conversion. K. Ward, '"Obedient rebels": The relationship between the early "Balokole" and the Church of Uganda: The Mukono crisis of 1941', *Journal of Religion in Africa*, 19, 3 (1989), p. 197; Roman Catholic Missions, 'Reply to the questionnaire on the marriage of natives', Rubaga Archives, Kampala, 49.6.

[2] Aissia, 'Suppression of women', *Matalisi*, 9 Oct. 1942, pp. 5–6. So determined was the Anglican church to preserve the primacy of church marriage, that it even complained that customary marriages were 'being celebrated in much the same way as Christian marriage, i.e with bridal garments, bridesmaids, cakes, speeches, feasts etc', and asked what government could do about such unwanted imitation. Bishop to Katikiros, 5 Feb. 1931, Marriage files, Namirembe Church of Uganda Archive, Mukono.

[3] Scott to Willis, 7 Sept. 1932 and Bourdillon to Willis, 23 Jan. 1933, Marriage files, Namirembe Church of Uganda Archive, Mukono; G. Kyomuhendo and M. McIntosh, *Women, Work and*

had formed strong opinions about the incompatibility between the principles of indirect rule and Christian marriage while serving as Chief Secretary in Tanganyika. Writing before his transfer to Uganda, Mitchell observed that customary marriage was 'a civil contract between two families', whose durability depended on the transfer of wealth and the production of children. The family in Africa, he argued, had been undermined by missionaries' introduction of 'two concepts entirely foreign to all Bantu ideas and social organisation: i. That marriage is a contract between two individual persons and ii. that marriage is a sacrament, and so can never be dissolved.' Missionaries' complaints about Christian women being sold to suitors or forcibly deprived of their children following divorce were 'ignorant and bigoted' 'half-truths', while their 'attacks on the social system of the natives, on all that they hold most sacred, on the institutions to which they cling with such devotion', and their attempt to use colonial law to force Africans to follow the European pattern of marriage must be resisted.[4]

In 1936 Mitchell, now governor of Uganda, dismissed missionary allegations that women were being coerced into marriages against their will and forced to return to unhappy marriages. Public opinion and the courts dealt adequately with such rare events, he reported. 'It may be that tribal custom in relation to marriage produces an occasional abuse or injustice, but anything which tends to weaken it may result in far worse evils, for it is not excessive restraint which is the most serious danger for the women of Africa but excessive licence.'[5] Mitchell's government took the view that mission pressure on the state to uphold Christian marriage had had the unwelcome effect of undermining not only customary marriage but morality more widely. In 1937 the governor of Southern Sudan, Martin Parr, was invited to investigate Uganda's marriage system. His report particularly condemned missionary obstruction of attempts to rationalize the illogical situation in Buganda. Ganda Christians who married in church could only obtain a divorce from the High Court, which however had no authority to order the return of bridewealth, the traditional marker of the end of a marriage. Being restricted to the colonial courts, meanwhile, meant that church-married Christians could not make use of the kingdom's laws concerning adultery. To add to the confusion, whereas Christians whose customary marriage failed were unable to sue for a refund of bridewealth, because Ganda courts defined such mar-

Domestic Virtue in Uganda, 1900–2003 (Oxford: James Currey, 2006), p. 71; N. Musisi, 'Morality as identity: the missionary moral agenda in Buganda, 1877–1945', *Journal of Religious History*, 23, 1 (1999), pp. 65–7.

[4] P. Mitchell, 'Female circumcision and the status of women in Tanganyika Territory', 26 Apr. 1930, TNA, 18881.

[5] Mitchell to Colonial Office, 3 Dec. 1936, Native Marriage, CMS archive, Birmingham, Acc. 206, Z1.

riages as invalid, colonial courts refused to prosecute Christian polygamists for bigamy, on the grounds that local opinion did not recognize such marriages as illegal. Parr claimed that the Ganda preferred this 'chaos' to further state intervention, as the colonial laws were so largely ignored as to be irrelevant. Between 1935 and 1938 only four of the 60,000 or so Christian marriages in Buganda were ended by the prohibitively expensive High Court. Local administrators, however, were convinced that the creation of so many obstacles to the penalizing of adultery or the securing of a refund of bridewealth when a wife left her husband undermined marriage. The removal of the expectation that bridewealth might have to be refunded, they argued, reduced familial interest in ensuring the stability and durability of a union.[6] Parr compared Uganda unfavourably with Nyasaland, where Christian marriage was both more common and more stable because it brought no legal rights or penalties. As in France, only marriages officiated by the state were legally recognized, with the church blessing serving only a ceremonial and spiritual function. Parr observed that such a system would legalize polygamy, render the crime of bigamy irrelevant, and establish one universal law of divorce. As a result, Mitchell circulated a questionnaire among the churches and colonial and indigenous administrations, designed to encourage all parties to recognize the contradictory nature of the existing laws, and accept the need for reform.[7]

In this he failed, for his proposals were vehemently criticized by the missions, and crucially by Buganda's chiefly council, the *Lukiiko*, on the grounds that it would undermine Christian marriage. The missions downplayed most of the problems identified by Parr, describing them as 'very rare' or occurring 'in one or two cases', and accused the government of 'proclaiming the superiority of paganism over Christianity'. The Church Missionary Society (CMS) had framed its opposition to the suggested reforms in a manner designed to work on Ganda anxieties. The Archdeacon of Uganda's statement that abandoning the law on bigamy would imply that the Baganda were incapable of achieving a western level of morality, was replicated almost verbatim in the *Lukiiko*'s response to the questionnaire.[8] Mitchell was left with no option

[6] M. Parr, Governor of Equatoria Province, Sudan, Memorandum on the marriage and Divorce of native Christian members of African tribal communities, 2 Jan. 1938, and extract from the Annual Report on the Province of Buganda 1936, CMS archive, Birmingham, Acc. 206, Z1; Digest of replies to questionnaire accompanying Chief Secretary's Circular of 19 Apr. 1938 on the subject of native marriage, and Roman Catholic Missions, 'Reply to the questionnaire on the marriage of natives', Rubaga Archives, 49.6; E. Haydon, *Law and Justice in Buganda* (London: Butterworths, 1960), p. 107.

[7] N. Musisi, 'Transformations of Baganda women: from the earliest times to the demise of the kingdom in 1966' (unpublished PhD dissertation, University of Toronto, 1991), pp. 234–6.

[8] Digest of replies to questionnaire accompanying Chief Secretary's Circular of 19 Apr. 1938 on the subject of native marriage, and Roman Catholic Missions, 'Reply to the questionnaire on the marriage of natives', 49.6, Rubaga Archives, Kampala; A. Hastings, *Christian Marriage in Africa,*

other than to propose a further commission of enquiry, but the outbreak of war and his transfer left the issue to fester until the 1950s, when it revived, due partly to the rise of Ganda ethnic nationalism, partly to the emergence of Uganda's women's rights movement.[9]

In 1956 Buganda's *Lukiiko* passed a new Succession and Wills law confirming the long-established Ganda rule that all sons, legitimate and illegitimate, had an equal claim to inherit their father's property. It also ruled that customary marriages entered into by Christians were legally valid. The muted response of the missions to this affirmation of Ganda traditions reflected the new political context shaped by the return of Kabaka Muteesa II from exile, and the vulnerability of the Anglican church in particular to accusations that it suffered from the same domineering mindset which had caused Governor Cohen to deport Buganda's king in 1953.[10] It could be argued that the Uganda Council of Women (UCW), which directly challenged the *Lukiiko* legislation, was something of a front for the CMS, as it was essentially an offshoot of the Mother's Union, and was heavily influenced by Winifred Brown, wife of Buganda's Anglican Bishop. But the UCW's opposition was driven as much by the concerns of class and gender as religion. The leaders of the UCW were primarily members of the Ganda female educated elite, whose vision of marriage was similar to that found in western societies: a companionate union between near equals, which prioritized the nuclear over the extended family, and aimed to exclude what they considered illegitimate offspring from the line of inheritance. Their concern was that Buganda's male educated elite were still captive to the demands of the clan and the temptations of polygamy, and that men's desire to project their influence beyond the confines of their Christian union would be enhanced after independence. Educated women feared that patriarchy and patriotism would rise together. These anxieties reflected a wider uncertainty about how self-government would shape the conflict between the forces of modernization and tradition. Christian reformers argued that 'as the tempo of urban and industrial life increases social stability will depend to an ever growing extent on the "isolated" family unit.'

Being a Report Commissioned by the Archbishops of Cape Town, Central Africa, Kenya, Tanzania, and Uganda (London: SPCK, 1973), pp. 168–70.

[9] Musisi, 'Transformations', p. 237. In 1948 Buganda's modernizing *katikiro* or prime minister Kawalya Kaggwa persuaded the *Lukiiko* to introduce a variant on the Nyasaland system, so that the kingdom government would be responsible not only for the registration of all marriages, Christian and customary alike, but also the arbitration of all divorce cases. However, the opposition of the Anglican Bishop Stuart—'He told me I was not a Christian katikiro ... He squashed it'—prevented the reform from becoming law. Marriage: [Kawalya] Kagwa, 18 Feb. 1956, A. Richards papers, LSE archive, London, 7/16.

[10] Haydon, *Law*, pp. 100–101; Cabana to Brown, 27 Feb. 1957, and Conference of Bishops and Archdeacons, Feb. 1957, Marriage Cases, Namirembe Church of Uganda Archive, Mukono. The Anglican church was affected particularly directly by the succession issue, as it would potentially have to enthrone a kabaka chosen not from a Christian marriage.

The threat posed by atomism could only be met by the equally modern nuclear family, which had to be legally protected from clan interference immediately, lest 'an upsurge of nationalistic opinion' caused Christian marriage to be 'considered an alien imported system ... [which] might be swept away'.[11] As was typical of late colonial governments presented with highly divisive issues, however, the matter stalled, as the administration delegated responsibility for the matter to local government and a commission of enquiry. Milton Obote's commitment to modernization was sufficient to bring forth yet another commission of enquiry after independence, which did support most of the demands of Christian reformers and women's groups—above all, widows were not to be driven away or inherited, and children from a Christian marriage would take precedence in inheritance. Yet the lack of real government support for either any increase in male responsibilities or weakening of the clans became apparent when the unfortunate commissioner's attempts to read out his report in parliament foundered amidst general hilarity.[12]

The perceived crisis in Christian marriage was to some extent exaggerated, at least in terms of its popularity before the late colonial period. The 1931 census showed that while Christians made up 59% of Buganda's population, 31% of all marriages in the kingdom had taken place in church, a reasonably high rate. Hastings' data show that the proportion of Catholics marrying in church was somewhat lower than would be expected in the late 1930s, but it was only in the late 1940s that the frequency of church marriage showed a significant decline. The rate of Catholic marriage then halved between 1949 and 1969. An investigation in 1938 reported that 39% of Anglicans who married that year did so in church, whereas Taylor's survey of a number of parishes in the late 1950s found that only a quarter of married Anglicans had had a church wedding.[13] So resistance to church marriage was

[11] B. Saben to L. Boyd, 24 Feb. 1957, and Conference of Bishops and Archdeacons, Feb. 1957, Marriage Cases, Namirembe Church of Uganda Archive, Mukono; Uganda Council of Women, 'Memorandum to the commission of enquiry into marriage, divorce and the status of women in Uganda' (unpublished TS, African Studies Centre Library, Cambridge), n/d *c.*1961. Of the many cross-currents complicating the story of marriage, the contrast between Ganda elite women's suspicion of nationalist politicians and their energetic campaigning for the return of the kabaka, depicted as the husband of all Ganda women, was one of the most striking. Pers. comm. Carol Summers.

[12] Uganda Government, *Report of the Commission on Marriage, Divorce and the Status of Women, 1965* (Entebbe: Government Printer, 1965); Kyomuhendo and McIntosh, *Women*, p. 121 For an important recent study of the place of the widow in East African society see D. Cohen and E. Atieno Odhiambo, *Burying SM: The Politics of Knowledge and the Sociology of Power in Africa* (London: James Currey, 1992).

[13] Uganda Protectorate, *1931 Census Returns* (Entebbe: Government Printer, 1932); Hastings, *Christian Marriage*, pp. 141–3; Report of the NAC Committee on Marriage, 1938, Marriage Cases, Namirembe Church of Uganda Archive, Mukono; J. Taylor, Analysis of parishes, CMS archives, ACC. 265 Z5.

significant in the 1930s, but became serious in the 1950s. It seems that a church wedding became associated with prestige, requiring a larger and more elaborate celebration, and often involving a larger bridewealth payment, than was involved in a customary marriage. In an attempt to remove the material obstacles to church marriage, Joseph Kiwanuka, soon after his appointment in 1939 as the first African Catholic bishop in four centuries, forbade any men marrying in church from making a bridewealth payment exceeding 120 shillings. Kiwanuka held immense authority over the Catholic population of southern Buganda, so this was one of the more successful attempts at limiting bridewealth. But several informants remembered 'underground negotiations' leading to 'black market' bridewealth payments being made late on the wedding night, after the local catechist had gone home, while the cost of the accompanying costs of a ring marriage usually far exceeded the actual bridewealth.[14]

Whereas marrying in church was obligatory for the elite and the deeply spiritual, for many couples it was something to aspire to and save for over a number of years, while an increasing majority viewed it with suspicion. The expense of a church marriage was a significant deterrent, but more important was an unwillingness to commit to a union which was particularly difficult to escape. Catholicism, of course, forbade divorce entirely, but even Anglicans divorcing under the Ordinance could not do so on the grounds of infertility or unhappiness, which were accepted as legitimate reasons to end a customary marriage. Unsurprisingly, Shorter found that 'Christians have inherited a highly legalistic picture of the churches' marriage ideal. Christian marriage is seen by them as a series of impossible obligations—monogamy, indissolubility and so forth—stemming not from the nature of human love or of the marriage covenant itself, but from the partisan adherence to a church with a set of unexplained laws and dogmas.' As independence approached, the ability of the clergy to overcome such resentment declined along with their disciplinary power and their knowledge of their ever expanding congregation.[15]

[14] Int. NPNK, 24 Aug. 2004, Kyanakase, F; Int. AN, 25 Aug. 2004, Kagezi, F; Male Focus Group Discussion (FGD), Kisubi Kiwulwe, 4 Sept. 2004; Int. JS, 26 Aug. 2004, Takajjunge, Masaka, M; C. Summers, 'Catholic Action and Ugandan radicalism: Political activism in Buganda, 1930–1950', *Journal of Religion in Africa*, 39, 1 (2009), p. 73; L. Mair, *Native Marriage in Buganda, International Institute of African Languages and Cultures Memorandum XIX* (Oxford: Oxford University Press, 1940), p. 28. Mair's survey of one Ganda village in the early 1930s found that bridewealth paid in Christian marriages was 44% higher than that required in customary unions.

[15] A. Shorter, *East African Societies* (London: Routledge and Kegan Paul, 1974), pp. 72–3; Hastings, *Christian Marriage*, pp. 50–2; Digest of replies to questionnaire accompanying Chief Secretary's Circular of 19 Apr. 1938 on the subject of native marriage, and Roman Catholic Missions, 'Reply to the questionnaire on the marriage of natives', Rubaga Archives, 49.6. An elderly Ganda woman told Gutkind in the early 1950s that her '"Christian marriage was such a difficult thing that she had lived in fear all the time". In a slightly amused manner, she added,

A more direct challenge to church authority than the growing reluctance to commit to a ring wedding, was the frequency with which men ignored the church rules on monogamy. In 1958 John Taylor found that only half of those Ganda Anglicans who had married in church had remained monogamous, and as most Anglicans married outside the church, fully 87% of male Anglicans had been permanently excommunicated. Adrian Hastings' smaller scale post-independence study suggested that the situation in the Catholic church was little better, with 72% of couples falling under church discipline.[16] While some Ganda accepted that adherence to Christianity ruled out polygamy—one informant relating that her father married only once 'because he was a Catholic'—others regarded monogamy as a dispensable aspect of church teaching. A leading chief told Audrey Richards in the 1950s that he did not think 'any African really believes in the Christian rule of marriage. It isn't in the bible,' while an informant defined himself as 'Catholic! Staunch! Baptised from Rubaga, the child of Rome,' yet freely discussed his polygamous marriages. 'A Muganda marries as he finds fit.'[17]

Christianity appears nonetheless to have reduced the durability if not the incidence of polygamous marriages, as religious belief, along with education and a more general aspiration towards a western lifestyle, seems to have been more likely to cause women to leave their husbands on learning that they had married again, than to deter men from contracting multiple marriages in the first place.[18] It is perhaps unsurprising that Christian marriage did not eradicate polygamy, for both were associated with male wealth. One informant's account of his multiple relationships was structured by his career progression. After becoming a court interpreter in 1954 he married in church, did well, and was promoted to Kampala to serve as chief clerk to one of Buganda's first indigenous district commissioners. 'That salary increase caused me a very serious problem. So I decided to get myself another wife.' This second wife accompanied him on various postings, as 'she was mobile, while the first

"my husband died last year and now I feel better".' P. Gutkind, 'A preliminary report of Mulago, Kampala, Uganda, 1954' (TS, ASC, Cambridge), p. 66.

[16] J. Taylor, *The Growth of the Church in Buganda* (London: SCM, 1958, pp. 244, 182; Hastings, *Christian Marriage*, pp. 55–6.

[17] Int. AN, 25 Aug. 2004, Kagezi, F; Marriage, [Kawalya] Kagwa, 18 Feb. 1956, A. Richards papers, LSE, 7/16; Male FGD, Kitala, 1 Sept. 2004. Int. FKW, 31 Aug. 2004, Kitala, M; FKW was one of several informants who quoted the Old Testament in defence of polygamy. 'Now if Jacob had only married Leah, would we have got Joseph?' Another of Richards' informants asked her whether polygamy was forbidden in Europe, and told her 'We Africans … cannot understand this as part of religion. This mixing of religion and business.' Marriage, Sematimba, 25 Jan. 1956, A. Richards papers, LSE, 7/16.

[18] Int. JS, 26 Aug. 2004, Takajjunge, Masaka, M; Int. HGN, 10 Sept. 2004, Kiiso, F; Int. FN, 29 Aug. 2004, Butanga, F; A. Southall and P. Gutkind, *Townsmen in the Making: Kampala and its Suburbs* (Kampala: East African Institute of Social Research, 1957), pp. 88–9.

wife was on standby ... left to take good care of the home in the village'. With further promotions 'money increased. I was then earning 640 shillings. So when the money was enough, and you also know how tempting money is,' he married again. This informant at times referred to his second and third partners as wives, but on being questioned further he stated that he had 'one lawfully wedded wife', and that the others were not married. 'I did have them of course, but they were not in the houses that I built. They stayed outside,' and he did not pay bridewealth for them.[19] The 1919 ruling of the *Lukiiko* that unions entered into by men who had already married in church were not customary marriages, but mere concubinage, came to contain an element of truth, for over time unions of this kind often omitted some of the key elements of the customary marriage ceremony.[20]

It was not only already married men who entered into relationships of uncertain status. Gutkind and Southall's research in the urban communities of 1950s Kampala described a spectrum of attachment lying between the extremes of short-time sex work and full marriage secured by the payment of bridewealth. Some cohabiting arrangements were intentionally temporary, but others were viewed as trial marriages. The subsequent payment of a token bridewealth or even the introducing of a partner to family members would convert such a relationship into a legal customary marriage, but even mere durability or the birth of a child would, it seems, cause it to be socially recognized as a marriage. Eighteen per cent of urban non-casual, monogamous Ganda unions, which had produced children, belonged to this latter 'free marriage' category. Such relationships were a common feature of African cities after the Second World War, but Buganda was unusual in that free marriage was common in rural communities as well.[21] As early as the 1930s Lucy Mair found that it was not unusual for rural Baganda to live together without being married, while Audrey Richards' survey of a village in 1952 found that cohabitations made up 13% of all relationships, almost as many as in the city.[22]

[19] Int. JS, 26 Aug. 2004, Takajjunge, Masaka, M.

[20] See chapter 3. Mair, *Native Marriage*, pp. 23–4 found numerous cases of unions in Ganda villages unsecured by any contract, usually because one of the partners was still tied by a previous Christian marriage.

[21] Southall and Gutkind, *Townsmen*, pp. 71, 89–91; D. Parkin, 'Types of urban African marriage in Kampala', *Africa*, 36, 3 (1966), pp. 272, 279; P. Gutkind, 'African urban family life: comment on and analysis of some rural-urban difference', *Cahiers d'Études Africaines*, 10 (1962), p. 172; Gutkind, 'Preliminary report', pp. 62–5, 76. While Southall and Gutkind, and indeed Christine Obbo some decades later, examined multi-ethnic neighbourhoods in the city, they were in general careful to identify the ethnicity of the individuals they discussed, so that only their material which explicitly related to Ganda, or to urban areas in general, has been utilized. Kampala's ethnic makeup was similar to that of Buganda as a whole.

[22] Mair, *Native Marriage*, pp. 23–8; A. Richards, *Economic Development and Tribal Change: A Study of Immigrant Labour in Buganda*. (Cambridge: Heffer, 1954), p. 384. A Catholic survey of

These relationships of convenience were the product of an unusually well-developed individualism, which also reshaped formal marriage during the colonial period. Ganda marriage had allowed the individual unusual freedom even before the European takeover. Children conceived outside of marriage were fully legitimate in terms of clan membership, succession and inheritance, both parties to an arranged marriage had the right of veto if they disapproved of their families' choice, love matches were tolerated, and divorce was easier to secure than in many pre-colonial East African cultures. By the mid-colonial period, however, the prioritization of individual choice had gone much further, as the concept of free will had become entrenched through exceptionally intense missionization and widespread education, and Buganda's cash crop economy had encouraged a high level of population mobility and undermined clan control of land.[23] Arranged marriage did not disappear, and many informants eulogized it as a means of bringing families together and ensuring the careful choice of a mate on the grounds of character rather than attractiveness. Yet several informants' life stories displayed dissatisfaction with their parents' choice. Some reported simple incompatibility, others complained of their spouses' laziness, alcoholism, serial adultery, and physical abuse.[24] Most informants who had married between the 1930s and 1960s had selected their own partners. Some fulfilled the worst predictions of the older generation, one man rushing to marry an attractive woman he met in town, only to find on his return from a business trip the following year that she had left with their child. 'And how could I look for her? I didn't even know the village from where she had come.' But others, and especially women, made more practical choices. One woman decided on a man because she liked him,

Ganda customs in 1951 reported that 'public opinion seems to have almost lost interest [in the increasing frequency of free marriage] and accepts the fact as being without remedy.' P. Lefebre, 'Table d'enquête sur les moeurs et coutumes indigènes, Vicariat Apostolique de l'Ouganda: Tribu des Baganda', 1951, WFA, p. 23.

[23] Marriage enquiry: govt questionnaire and answers 1932–8, Archdeacon of Uganda, n/d [1938], Rubaga archives 49.6; Paula Davis has objected to previous scholars' definition of the kinds of informal relationships described above as a form of marriage as they deprive women of legal or familial protection, leaving them 'completely vulnerable to the exercise of male hegemony'. This re-emphasis of the ambiguous status of such relationships is helpful, but earlier accounts stress the determination of women to retain their freedom to leave a relationship that might turn sour, and certainly many women were sceptical of the capacity of courts or parents to protect their interests in formal marriage. P. Davis, 'Re-contextualizing the female-headed household: Culture and agency in Uganda', in S. Szreter, H. Sholkamy and A. Dharmalingam (eds.), *Categories and Contexts: Anthropological and Historical Studies in Critical Demography* (Oxford: Oxford University Press, 2004), p. 302.

[24] e.g. Female FGD, Takajunge, 26 Aug. 2004; Int. CNSM, 28 Aug. 2004, Butanga, M; Int. FN, 29 Aug. 2004, Butanga, F; Int. PLGS, 31 Aug. 2004, Kitala, Busiro, M.

but also 'he was educated, and I knew he had a well-paying job that would make us survive.'[25]

It became standard practice to seek parental approval of the choice of marriage partner, which limited marital autonomy to some extent, but the exercising of the parental veto, or even disapproval in the form of a demand for an excessive bridewealth, was increasingly resisted. Elopement was of course a largely strategic manoeuvre, designed to force parents to accept the will of their children, but its growing frequency formed part of an evolving culture of romantic attachment which became prominent in the mid-colonial period.[26] Young women were courted through secret assignations, love letters decorated with flowers and sprayed with scent, and gifts of powder, perfume, bathing soap, and handkerchiefs. Informants remembered that while the gifts acted as 'a symbol of love', the money enclosed in the letters indicated seriousness of intent.[27]

Based on fieldwork in the early 1930s Lucy Mair reported, perhaps with some exaggeration, 'the complete absence of the idea of romantic love' in Ganda customary marriage. Sexual attraction was less important than the partners' productive and reproductive ability in ensuring a successful marriage, she argued. Mair contrasted this tradition with the ideal of Christian marriage, which was presented by missionaries as the true marker of western civilization. Couples being prepared for marriage in the Anglican church were instructed that the sacrament was a 'fulfilment of the Christian law of Love', exclusivist and indissoluble. 'The husband and wife should be companions', which required the 'complete sharing of the married life. This includes wise sharing of work and money.' This new vision of married life seems to have been accepted by some Baganda by the early colonial period. As early as 1916

[25] Male FGD, Kitala, 1 Sept. 2004; Female FGD, Kagezi, 25 Aug. 2004; Digest of replies to questionnaire accompanying Chief Secretary's Circular of 19 Apr. 1938 on the subject of native marriage, and Roman Catholic Missions, 'Reply to the questionnaire on the marriage of natives', Rubaga Archives, 49.6; Parkin, 'Urban African marriage', p. 270. Cf. C. Thibon, *Histoire démographique du Burundi* (Paris: Karthala, 2004), p. 310.

[26] Female FGD, Takajunge, 26 Aug. 2004; Taylor, *Growth of the Church*, p. 183; A. Shorter, *East African Societies* (London: Routledge and Kegan Paul, 1974), p. 74.

[27] Int. BMJ, 29 Aug. 2004, Kyankoole, M; Int. FNN, Wekaaye, Kaswa, 28 Aug. 2004, F; Male FGD, Kisubi Kiwulwe, 4 Sept. 2004; Int. NPNK, 24 Aug. 2004, Kyanakase, F; Haydon, *Law and Justice*, pp. 87–8. Cf. E. Akyeampong, '"Wo pe tam, won pe ba" ("You like cloth but you don't want children"): Urbanization, individualism and gender relations in colonial Ghana *c.*1900–1939', in D. Anderson and R. Rathbone (eds.), *Africa's Urban Past* (Oxford: James Currey, 2000), pp. 222–34. Akyeampong, has described how men in colonial era Gold Coast developed elaborate rituals of romantic love in response to a perceived increase in female materialism. This connection was not made in sources on Buganda, perhaps because the costs of securing a wife remained low. Wives' increasing material demands, however, were often cited as a factor in divorce. Int. JN, 29 Aug. 2004, Butanga, F; Int. KJK, 31 Aug. 2004, Kitala, M; Int. CNSM, 28 Aug. 2004, Butanga, M.

several men wrote to the Luganda newspaper, *Ebifa*, advising their compatriots to view wives as 'our companions', and to love them 'as the most important key in keeping them'. Researchers in the late colonial period suggested that companionate marriage was still only to be found among the deeply religious and the highly educated. Moreover, several informants contrasted a truly Christian marriage, where 'the woman you married would be your friend and yours forever', with customary marriages, where 'a woman was regarded as an object, some thing you would rule over'. However, very few interviewees indicated that the nature of their marital relationship in reality had been fully shaped by either church teaching or custom.[28]

As individuals increasingly came to choose their own spouses, mutual affection featured more prominently in customary marriage. As one informant put it, 'we loved each other, stayed together and produced our children.'[29] Sexual satisfaction, moreover, had it seems long been prioritized within Ganda marriage. Ganda men displayed a high level of anxiety about their sexual performance, while Ganda women were trained before marriage in the use of erotic language, and how to excite their husbands with the beads they wore around their waists. Herbalists reported that treatments to increase sexual potency and enjoyment were among their most popular products, while sexual counselling was one of the key roles played by paternal aunts.[30]

Nakanyike Musisi and Peter Gutkind reported that by the later colonial period discussions among Ganda men about the characteristics of the good wife had amalgamated elements from both traditional and modern ideals. Wives should be educated but still willing to dig, they should continue to be subservient and obedient, but should now also be loving and forgiving. Old ideas of domesticity were reshaped as husbands found new reasons to restrict

[28] Mair, *Native Marriage*, pp. 12–13; Instruction for Christian Marriage, n/d, Marriage 1931–45, Namirembe Church of Uganda Archive, Mukono; Musisi, 'Transformations', pp. 197, 331; C. Byaruhanga, 'Divorce in Uganda sociologically viewed' (unpublished thesis ad lauream, Pontifical Gregorian University, 1954), p. 53; Southall and Gutkind, *Townsmen*, pp. 88–9; Int. NNFW, 28 Aug. 2004, Kaswa, F; Int. AN, 25 Aug. 2004, Kagezi, F; Male FGD, Kitala, 1 Sept. 2004. Marriage among the born again *Balokole* Anglicans allowed wives unusual freedom.

[29] Int. TNN, 3 Aug. 2004, Kitala, F. See also Male FGD, Kisubi Kiwulwe, 4 Sept. 2004. Some Ganda believed that the intimacy of a long-established couple would cause them to come to resemble each other physically. Male FGD, Kitala, 1 Sept. 2004.

[30] J. Nabaitu, C. Bachengana and J. Seeley, 'Marital instability in a rural population in south-west Uganda: Implications for the spread of HIV-1 infection', *Africa*, 64, 2 (1994), pp. 246–7; Int. CNSM, 28 Aug. 2004, Butanga, M; Int. NM, 28 Aug. 2004, Lugazi, Butanga, F. A customary marriage would be rendered void where a man was impotent or a woman had failed to elongate her labia after puberty. Elongated labia were believed to increase male sexual enjoyment. M. Kisekka, 'The Baganda of central Uganda', in A. Molnos, *Cultural Source Materials for Population Planning in East Africa, vol. III, Beliefs and Practices* (Nairobi: EAPH, 1973), p. 149; Int. PLGS, 31 Aug. 2004, Kitala, Busiro, M; C. Obbo, 'Town migration is not for women' (unpublished PhD dissertation, University of Wisconsin-Madison, 1977), p. 48.

their wives to the household. Male anxieties about childlessness, infidelity, and desertion caused men to discourage their wives from making lengthy visits to their kin or from socializing at local drinking clubs. Instead wives should focus on their maternal responsibility for hygiene, nutrition, and childrearing, which had been reified by the teaching of both the church and the medical profession.[31]

Marriage was destabilized above all by changing expectations rather than changing behaviour in itself. Female interviewees repeatedly emphasized that the former relative stability of Ganda marriage had depended on wifely stoicism and subservience. Women 'used to endure and carry the cross of marriage with one heart'.[32] By the mid-colonial period, however, wifely tolerance of what was increasingly seen as mistreatment and disrespect reduced. On a number of issues, male and female interviewees demonstrated profound disagreement about what constituted acceptable husbandly behaviour. While men emphasized the honorific titles bestowed upon the first wife in a polygamous marriage, and the reduction in female workloads which resulted from men marrying further wives, women who found that their husbands had become polygamists expressed anger that their marriage vows had been broken, that their marriage could no longer be viewed as a partnership, and that their aspirations towards modernity had been destroyed.[33] Disagreements also grew on the issue of wife-beating, which a number of men felt was a sign of husbandly love and played a character-forming role in marriage: 'After being beaten the wife would thank you very much, because she knew that she was in the wrong and therefore it was right to correct her.' While male informants acknowledged 'that some men could over-beat', women who married after the 1920s regarded such attitudes as belonging to the past. Divorcees showed their scars in explanation of the ending of their marriage, or talked about their anger at being beaten for petty offences. Other women only consented to return to their marriages on condition that they would never be hit again.[34]

Similarly, most men claimed that their wives had worked much harder than them because 'it was their joy', yet many female informants complained

[31] Musisi, 'Transformations', pp. 197–9; Gutkind, 'Preliminary report', p. 76.

[32] Int. HGN, 10 Sept. 2004, Kiiso, F; Female FGD, Takajunge, 26 Aug. 2004; Int. NPNK, 24 Aug. 2004, Kyanakase, F.

[33] Int. JS, 26 Aug. 2004, Takajjunge, Masaka, M; Male FGD, Takajjunge, 26 Aug. 2004; Int. HGN, 10 Sept. 2004, Kiiso, F. Cf. Obbo, 'Town migration', p. 186; F. Kamoga, 'School leaving as affected by separation of parents in Buganda' (unpublished TS, EAISR seminar paper 1963, African Studies Centre Library, Cambridge), p. 6.

[34] Int. CNSM, 28 Aug. 2004, Butanga, M; Male FGD, Kitala, 1 Sept. 2004; Int. EM, 28 Aug. 2004, Kyansi, M; Female FGD, Bugiri Kiwulwe, 10 Sept. 2004; Female FGD, Kagezi, 25 Aug. 2004; Female FGD, Takajunge, 26 Aug. 2004; Int. ZMN, 28 Aug, 2004, Butanga, F; Int. NNFW, 28 Aug. 2004, Kaswa, F.

bitterly about their husbands' idleness. 'The husbands, the rulers, the governors of women, would just wake up in the morning then go to boozing … Women were the owners of digging and domestic work.' 'Men used to take us as labourers. Sometimes they would not get hold of a hoe.' Nor did women accept the common male justification for extra-marital affairs that infidelity was in men's nature: 'A woman is just there to be conned.' Both men and women acknowledged that accusations of infidelity were as common a cause of divorce as affairs themselves, but female complaints focused especially on the diversion of family resources to lovers.[35] Both sexes did agree that male alcoholism was a common and legitimate cause of divorce, partly because it was often associated with extreme violence, but more because it brought poverty to the home. One informant's father once beat her mother severely when he returned after a drinking session that had lasted several days and found that the food cooked in his absence had all been eaten. Another described her husband as 'an expert in boozing. Indeed this was his best job, his most intimate wife. This was the one area where I should say he was very hard working.' In the end it was her husband's inability to clothe his family that caused her father to fetch her home.[36] Nonetheless, while men accepted that a failure to provide the household with financial stability was an established justification for divorce, they felt that wives over the colonial period had become excessively demanding in material terms: 'A woman loves a man only so long as he has a good job and money.' There is some evidence that wives did become more materialistic. Christine Obbo's female informants told her that in rural Buganda in the 1940s aspirational women threatened to leave their husbands if they were not bought western clothes, high heeled shoes, and a handbag, or if they did not get new dresses at Christmas and Easter. But the driving force behind such demands was women's insistence that the contribution made to household income by their agricultural skill be recognized.[37]

Many male informants concluded that the rise in divorce was ultimately due to the new demanding nature of their wives, which they blamed on 'whites and their human rights'. 'People got so taken up with equality. Women

[35] Male FGD, Kitala, 1 Sept. 2004; Int. SKKG, 25 Aug. 2004, Kabonera, M; Int. JS, 26 Aug. 2004, Takajjunge, Masaka, M; Female FGD, Bugiri Kiwulwe, 10 Sept. 2004; Int. NNFW 28 Aug. 2004, Kaswa, F; Int. FN, 29 Aug. 2004, Butanga, F. Cf. Southall and Gutkind, *Townsmen*, p. 91; M. Southwold, 'The Baganda of Central Uganda', in Molnos, *Cultural Source Materials III*, p. 166.

[36] Int. IST, 21 August 2004, Kagezi village, Masaka, M; Int. JS, 26 Aug. 2004, Takajjunge, Masaka, M; Int. ZMN, 28 Aug, 2004, Butanga, F; Female FGD, Takajunge, 26 Aug. 2004; Int. NPNK, 24 Aug. 2004, Kyanakase, F.

[37] Int. IST, 21 August 2004, Kagezi village, Masaka, M; Int. CNSM, 28 Aug. 2004, Butanga, M; Int. KJK, 31 Aug. 2004, Kitala, M; Obbo, 'Town migration', pp. 186–7. A survey in 1957 found that wealthy men spent 'lavishly' on clothes for their wives. *Uganda Argus*, 4 Jan. 1957, p. 4.

changed and they tended to think that they were equal to men, that they could behave like a man. So in the end husband and wife couldn't be together.'[38] Human rights were held responsible by elderly informants for a range of social ills, serving as a convenient shorthand for the advancement of the individual under a largely gender neutral legal system, a religion that stressed personal salvation, an educational system that gave limited encouragement to freedom of thought, and a market economy that provided women with a new sense of value. The individualization of marriage was seen most clearly in the gradual decline in the significance of dispute mediation by partners' kin groups. As bridewealth became non-refundable, so wives' families' material interest in ensuring the continuation of a marriage reduced. Ganda lineages had in any case become unusually dispersed by mobility, cash cropping, and individual land tenure. The forces that acted to hold Ganda marriage together were very often weaker than those pulling it apart.[39]

Disagreements between husbands and wives about what should be expected from a spouse are hardly unusual, but the daily tensions of married life were exacerbated in Buganda by the pressures created by contradictory colonial and kingdom legislation and the uncompromising enforcement of Christian marriage dogma. The context in which the ideal of marriage was repeatedly debated in Buganda was the perception that marital dissolution was becoming more common, though what few data exist indicate that the frequency of marriage breakdown remained largely unchanged, albeit at a high level, between the 1930s and 1950s. In the early 1930s Lucy Mair found that 36% of householders in one of her survey villages had separated from their first partners. Marrying in church seems to have brought only a marginal increase in stability. In 1938 the Anglican church in Buganda recorded 7,935 weddings and 2,360 cases where church marriages had ended in separation in the past year. Gutkind's study of the Mulago suburb of Kampala in the early 1950s showed that 34% of ever-married adults had broken marriages. Marital instability was a major problem in Buganda from a very early date.[40]

[38] Male FGD, Bukoto, 24 Aug. 2004; Male FGD, Kitala, 1 Sept. 2004; Int. LLS, 21 Aug. 2004, Bukunda, Masaka, M.

[39] Int. HGN, 10 Sept. 2004, Kiiso, F; Male FGD, Bukoto, 24 Aug. 2004; D. Parkin, 'Types of urban African marriage in Kampala', *Africa*, 36, 3 (1966), p. 270. Cf. L. Fallers, 'Some determinants of marriage stability in Busoga, Africa, 27, 2 (1957), pp. 214–21; R. Yeld, 'Continuity and change in Kiga patterns of marriage: An analysis of structural change in Kiga marriage in the 1930s and the 1960s', (UEA Social Science Conference, December 1966), RHO, MSS. Afr. s. 1792/48, 7/23 Continuity and Change, pp. 6–7; Southwold, 'The Baganda', p. 175. Cf. Thibon, *Histoire démographique*, pp. 292–3.

[40] Int. SKKG, 25 Aug. 2004, Kabonera, Masaka District, M; Int. HGN, 10 Sept. 2004, Kiiso, F; Int. IST, 21 August 2004, Kagezi village, Masaka, M; Hastings, *Christian Marriage*, pp. 19–20; Report of the NAC Committee on Marriage, 1938, Marriage Cases, Namirembe Church of Uganda Archive, Mukono; Mair, Native Marriage, p. 24; P. Gutkind, 'A preliminary report of

POST-MARITAL SEXUALITY

Widowhood in colonial Buganda may have been relatively uncommon by African standards, given the narrow gap between male and female age at marriage, the relative decline in polygamy, and the presumed longevity of men who came to maturity after the First World War.[41] Nonetheless, divorce was so frequent that growing social acceptance of post-marital sex would have exposed a very large number of Ganda women to greater risk of infection with STDs. In many African societies such as Ankole, such risk was limited by the intense pressure to remarry which was experienced by women whose marriages had ended, because of the sexual danger associated with unmarried women, the belief that such women were a material burden on their natal families, and, in the case of divorcees, the need to try to recoup the bridewealth which had had to be returned to their first husbands' families. Of course some Ganda women did remarry after their first marriage ended, often after a gap of several years.[42] But widow inheritance was relatively rare in Buganda, because it required the widow's consent, while male relatives of the deceased were frequently unenthusiastic heirs, fearing that such a marriage of convenience would provide little deterrent to wifely infidelity, and often suspecting that the death had resulted from the widow's malign intent.[43]

Instead, for a great many Ganda women, the end of their marriage ushered in a new life of relative autonomy. Some widows secured the right to live on in their late husband's home with their children, assisted by a gradual shift towards naming sons rather than brothers as heirs. Another important trend saw the rule that fathers retained the custody of children being increasingly ignored, especially where women were financially self-sufficient, a change which undermined perhaps the greatest emotional obstacle stopping wives

---

Mulago, Kampala, Uganda, 1954' (TS, ASC, Cambridge), p. 79. P. Gutkind, 'African urban marriage and family life: a note on some social and demographic characteristics from Kampala, Uganda', *Bulletin de l'IFAN*, 25, 3 (1963), pp. 266–87 did not collect data on divorce rates per se, but did show that both urban and 'free' marriages were significantly less stable than other forms.

[41] Data on adult mortality are neither very plentiful nor reliable. However, they indicate a sustained decline from the interwar period (see chapter 8), as after 1918 famine was eradicated, major epidemics were rare, few Ganda were forced to encounter new disease environments through labour migration, public and domestic sanitation was unusually advanced, and curative health provision was exceptionally generous.

[42] Gutkind, 'African urban family', pp. 198–9; Int. FN, 29 Aug. 2004, Butanga, F; Int. AN, 25 Aug. 2004, Kagezi, F.

[43] Male FGD, Kagezi, 25 Aug. 2004; Int. NPNK, 24 Aug. 2004, Kyanakase, F; H. Hanson, *Landed Obligation: The Practice of Power in Buganda* (Portsmouth, NH: Heinemann, 2003), p. 32; Int. IST, 21 August 2004, Kagezi village, Masaka, M. Social convention also held that it was undignified for middle-aged widows to remarry.

leaving an unhappy marriage.[44] This growing social recognition of the ability of women to manage a household independently was related to the new economic opportunities for female emancipation which developed during the colonial period. A significant number of women inherited or bought freehold *mailo* land on which they could live if their marriage broke down.[45] More common was the acquisition of *bibanja* tenancies from chiefs, or the receipt of a plot to farm from a brother. Not only was female landholding unusually easy to achieve in Buganda, but so was its profitable usage. Buganda was one of colonial Africa's great cash cropping success stories, and independent women were among the beneficiaries, for they were unencumbered by tax, they had acquired skills and, illicitly, often capital through coffee and cotton production while married, and agricultural labour was easily obtainable. Buganda's urban centres offered women alternative means of making a living. Chiefly capitals required servants, while most women who went to local trading centres, small towns, and the city of Kampala sold food or alcohol.[46]

As early as 1925 men complained in Luganda newspapers, with a degree of exaggeration, that in some villages there were as many households headed by independent women or *Banakyeyombekedde* as by men. Still, widows and divorcees made up 12% of household heads in a village surveyed by Lucy Mair in the early 1930s, and by the 1950s studies of rural Buganda found that this proportion had risen to between 23 and 51%, while 35% of householders in one Kampala-based study were female.[47] Some of these *Banakyeyombekedde* 'had given up on sex completely', according to informants, but in general Ganda society tolerated female post-marital sex. Widows were expected to

[44] Int. PLGS, 31 Aug. 2004, Kitala, Busiro, M; Int. NPNK, 24 Aug. 2004, Kyanakase, F; Southall and Gutkind, *Townsmen*, p. 70; Kamoga, 'School leaving', p. 2. Of course many widows were still evicted from their marital homes, and, along with divorcees, deprived of their children. Cf. 'Suppression of women', *Matalisi*, 9 Oct. 1942, pp. 5–6; 'How do women feel about sharing their husband's property?', *Munno*, 26 Mar. 1960.

[45] M. Southwold, 'The inheritance of land in Baganda', *Uganda Journal*, 10 (1956), pp. 88–96; A. Mukwaya, *Land Tenure in Buganda: Present Day Tendencies* (Kampala, 1953), p. 31. By 1950 women in Mukwaya's sample made up 10% of landowners and owned 15% of freehold land.

[46] Sematimba's relatives, 1 Sept. 1952, A. Richards papers, LSE, 6/19; Obbo, 'Town', pp. 35, 175; Mair, *Native Marriage*, pp. 32–33, 40, 25; Gutkind, 'African urban family', p. 192; Gutkind, 'Preliminary report', pp. 49, 29. For a less positive view of Ganda women's economic opportunities, see Kyomuhendo and McIntosh, *Women*, p. 73.

[47] Hanson, *Landed Obligation*, pp. 178–9; Mair, *Native Marriage*, p. 23; Obbo, 'Town migration', p. 197; P. Reining and A. Richards, 'Report on fertility surveys in Buganda and Buhaya, 1952', in F. Lorimer et al. (eds.) *Culture and Human Fertility* (Paris: UNESCO, 1954), p. 359; Taylor, *Growth of the Church*, p. 123; A. Richards, 'Kisozi village 1952' (unpublished seminar paper, n/d), A. Richards papers, LSE, 6/19; Southall and Gutkind, *Townsmen*, p. 121. Davis, 'Recontextualizing', pp. 301–2 has questioned the labelling of these women as independent household heads, in that they often remained part of a larger kin-group, though the same could be said of many male household heads.

keep their affairs secret, but interviewees observed that divorcees were free to choose how to live their lives. According to one source, a divorcee's non-marital sexual relationship could even be formally recognized by her brother if her suitor confirmed his interest by presenting him with gifts. Other women had shorter-term relationships, in some cases securing young men's affections with presents.[48]

PREMARITAL SEXUALITY

Q. Was sex before marriage allowed?
R. Not at all.
Q. Even though it wasn't allowed would some people do it?
R. Of course they would.[49]

When elderly Ganda informants talked about pre-marital sex during their youth, they struggled to escape the concerns and language of contemporary Uganda. English-language phrases such as children's rights, sugar daddies or mommies, and defilement repeatedly interrupted the flow of Luganda, usually to emphasize their distaste at what most perceived as a serious decline in sexual morality in society as a whole, and especially among the young. As children, almost all had been instructed by their elders that sex before marriage was ethically wrong and socially dangerous, a message that was reinforced by the teaching of Islam and Christianity. It would have been unsurprising if Ganda interviewees had presented an image of probity and restraint when discussing the sexual behaviour of their younger selves and their peers.[50] Yet most dated the collapse of pre-marital self-control, 'when people started going mad', in the relatively distant past, the 1960s most commonly, but often the 1950s, and sometimes the 1940s. Occasionally this moral decline was associated with a particular event: the euphoria of self-government in 1962, the perceived loss of discipline and cultural integrity that followed the deposition of the kabaka and *ssaza* chiefs in 1966, or the arrival of the first nightclub or modern drinking bar in the local trading centre. But usually the dating of moral corruption coincided with the interviewee's coming to maturity, perhaps

[48] Male FGD, Kagezi, 25 Aug. 2004; Haydon, *Law*, pp. 82–3; Southwold, 'Baganda', p. 168. Interviewees who emphasized divorcees' sexual freedom included Int. FKW, 31 Aug. 2004, Kitala, M; Male FGD, Kitala, 1 Sept. 2004; Int. ZMN, 28 Aug, 2004, Butanga, F.

[49] Female FGD, Kagezi, 25 Aug. 2004.

[50] e.g. Int. NPNK, 24 Aug. 2004, Kyanakase, F; Female FGD, Kagezi, 25 Aug. 2004; Male FGD, Kitala, 1 Sept. 2004.

reflecting personal experience as much as broader change.[51] Certainly a large minority of Ganda informants stated that they, or sometimes parents or siblings, had had sex, or even children, before marriage. One woman remembered that when she and her three oldest sisters married in the 1950s, each time their mother was rewarded with a goat, 'because we were good girls', virgins. But her two youngest sisters, who married in the 1960s, brought no goat home. Many informants who had had pre-marital sex displayed an uncomfortable awareness that they, and many others, had breached a moral code. Sex before marriage 'would be very bad, but it would still be done'. But others indicated no dissonance between sexual attitudes and behaviour, one female interviewee stating that 'people in love should always have sex before getting married.' It was more common for male informants to demonstrate such disregard for inherited norms, perhaps because boys traditionally received little familial guidance about relationships, whereas girls were taught about sexuality and married life by their paternal aunts, though modern education increasingly interfered with this. In addition it may be that the trend towards spousal self-selection undermined the role of the paternal aunt not only as a matchmaker but also as the major source of sex education. A number of men meanwhile stated that they had needed no training, for they believed that sex during adolescence, known in Luganda as 'the stupid years', was natural for boys, that they had been like 'a cock running after a hen'.[52]

While the kingdom authorities viewed the indiscipline of the young with constant disapproval during the colonial period, their efforts to prevent and punish pre-marital sex were somewhat inconsistent. The 1919 law against fornication permitted heavy fines for sex before marriage, especially for a man who seduced a woman betrothed to another. Until the Second World War almost 5% of cases heard in local courts in Buganda related to fornication, a significant proportion. In the 1940s, however, fornication accounted for only 2% of all cases. In the 1950s and early 1960s, perhaps due to the conservative backlash associated with the deportation of the Kabaka, fornication cases rose significantly, to 3% of the total, but never regained the levels found between the wars. Meanwhile, ethnographic and oral accounts note that whereas local elders had the power to fine men who impregnated unmarried women, or to force the

[51] Male FGD, Kitala, 1 Sept. 2004; Int. MMA, 24 Aug. 2004, Kyanakase, F; Int. FN, 29 Aug. 2004, Butanga, F; Int. RK, 26 Aug. 2002, Takajjunge, M; Int. PLGS, 31 Aug. 2004, Kitala, Busiro, M; Male FGD, Kagezi, 25 Aug. 2004; Int. JN, 29 Aug. 2004, Butanga, F.

[52] e.g. Int. NM, 28 Aug. 2004, Lugazi, Butanga, F; Int. AN, 25 Aug. 2004, Kagezi, F; Male FGD, Kitala, 1 Sept. 2004; Int. TNN, 3 Aug. 2004, Kitala, F; Int. NPNK, 24 Aug. 2004, Kyanakase, F; Female FGD, Takajunge, 26 Aug. 2004; Male FGD, Kagezi, 25 Aug. 2004; Int. CNSM, 28 Aug. 2004, Butanga, M. Cf. Rev. J. V. Taylor to M.A.C.W., 24 Jan. 1954, CMS archive, Birmingham, Acc. 265; Mair, *Native Marriage*, p. 66. Mair recorded some advice given by fathers to their sons in the 1930s: 'Do not commit adultery, but love unmarried women who have no husbands.'

couple to marry, such authority was exercised inconsistently, especially by the 1950s.[53]

A factor which was probably more important in facilitating pre-marital sex, as well as increasing its social acceptability, was the weakening of parental discipline. It was still relatively common for young women who fell pregnant before marriage to be beaten and expelled from the family home by their fathers into the 1950s, though the severity of physical punishment was restrained by colonial legislation.[54] But the fear behind such displays of anger, that a previously pregnant woman could not make a good marriage, was gradually lessened by evidence to the contrary. Admittedly such women would be denied a church wedding by the religious authorities, but their demonstration of fecundity proved attractive to many potential husbands, given the anxiety about childlessness within Ganda society during the colonial period. This increase in pre-marital fertility though was limited by another factor which was held to increase female marriageability after the Second World War, education. Several sources indicate that the incidence of abortion increased as girls, usually with the assistance of their mothers, sought to avert expulsion from school, and punishment from their fathers.[55] More important than parental connivance in pre-marital sex was a decline in parental supervision. This had never been absolute—one very elderly informant remembered that while parents of his generation had been very strict, still young lovers met in the bush while herding goats. But as Buganda's economy and state became more complex, so both men and women found themselves working away from home more frequently, and unable to check their children's whereabouts. Accounts of individuals' early sexual lives detail the growing generational autonomy particularly of boys, whose social lives increasingly revolved more around friends than family. The young were more likely to be allowed to walk to markets and water sources unaccompanied by adults and attend social functions such as weddings than in the past. Opportunities for sexual assignations, often encouraged and facilitated by groups of friends, expanded. This new liberty was enjoyed by youths all over Buganda, but as Peter Gutkind found in the early 1950s, it was most extreme in Kampala, where 'older children

[53] Mair, Native Marriage, pp. 7–8; Southall and Gutkind, *Townsmen*, p. 68; Int. CNSM, 28 Aug. 2004, Butanga, M; Int. RK, 26 Aug. 2002, Takajjunge, M; List of saza level cases, File 23, PPMS38/Perlman/Box 8, SOAS archive.

[54] Southall and Gutkind, *Townsmen*, pp. 88–9; Mair, *Native Marriage*, p. 32. Int. FN, 29 Aug. 2004, Butanga, F. Cf. Yeld, 'Continuity and change', p. 6.

[55] Mair, *Native Marriage*, p. 11; Int. SKKG, 25 Aug. 2004, Kabonera, M; Int. FN, 29 Aug. 2004, Butanga, F; Int. AN, 25 Aug. 2004, Kagezi, F. A strict father might refuse to pay bridewealth on behalf of a son who had pre-marital sex, but it seems this again was rare. Cf. Int. EM, 28 Aug. 2004, Kyansi, M.

are expected to provide their own amusement.... [T]he free play of sexual activity is a pleasant and satisfying pastime.'[56]

Education and urbanity provided the context within which a distinct culture of adolescence emerged in 1950s and 1960s Buganda. The growth of schooling, which became almost universal for both sexes after 1945, gave youths unprecedented opportunity to develop relationships unobserved. This was especially true for children sent to boarding school, or to live with town-based relatives whose homes were closer to good secondary schools. But groups of age-mates everywhere travelled to school and studied together, spawning the development of gangs, and increasingly competitive and emulative attitudes to sex. Though schools were generally single-sex, educational facilities for boys and girls usually neighboured each other, and permitted the development of boyfriend/girlfriend relationships of a kind which seem not to have existed before. Boys learnt the arts of seduction from older pupils, girls learnt the language of love from the letters pages of magazines and newspapers, and young lovers verbalized their desires in an exchange of letters. In the early colonial period most youthful sexual encounters with other adolescents were opportunistic, discreet, and sporadic, arising from chance meetings while grazing or fetching water. Mass schooling engendered a more strategic approach among the young. Early sexual relationships were now increasingly preceded by the sustained courtship of a girl, and depended on the repeated transfer of gifts, as Odeybea Morrow's female informants remembered. 'Where boys had bicycles they would always want to give you a ride ... They would buy you soda, buns. That's how they used to start.' Interestingly, although they had acquired more individualistic attitudes to sex and a more explicitly emotional and affectionate language of intimacy, Ganda who had grown up in the late colonial period in fact had more materialistic and less romantic memories of their youthful sexual lives than their more elderly compatriots.[57]

The emergence of adolescent gangs by the end of the colonial period was most marked in town. Here the emerging urban middle class, cinemas, and clubs, and the development of the weekend produced 'the smart teenage set',

[56] Int. SKKG, 25 Aug. 2004, Kabonera, M; P. Gutkind, 'Some problems of African urban family life', *Diogenes*, 10, 37 (1962), p. 95; C. Obbo, *African Women: Their Struggle for Independence* (London: Zed Press, 1980), pp. 26–8; D. Parkin, *Neighbours and Nationals in an African City Ward* (London: Routledge and Kegan Paul, 1969), p. 95.

[57] A. Maleche, 'Sociological and psychological factors favouring or hindering the education of African women in Uganda' (unpublished TS, EAISR seminar paper 1961, African Studies Centre Library, Cambridge), pp. 6–7; Kisubi boys, A. Richards papers, LSE, 6/27; Ndejje School TTC, 27 Jan. 1956, A. Richards papers, LSE, 7/16; Brother Charles, 'Moral conditions in the schools', Rubaga Archives, 904.1; Southall and Gutkind, *Townsmen,* p. 72; O. Morrow, 'Sexual cultures and vulnerability to HIV infection among Baganda youth in Mpigi' (unpublished PhD dissertation, Johns Hopkins University, 2000), p. 280.

the vanguard of adolescent culture, and the subject of frequent newspaper coverage. While editors recognized that photographs of girls in mini-skirts and crop tops dancing the "shake shake" increased sales, journalists emphasized the alienation of the youth, their separateness from the older generation displayed by their distinct, sexualized dress, their willingness to socialize publicly in mixed groups, and their 'modern ideas' culled from 'lurid magazines'. But one of the most important aspects of sexuality in Buganda has been the rapidity with which rural communities have imitated urban developments, shaped partly by the wealth of the countryside, and partly by the rapid expansion of bus routes linking city, town, and village from the 1930s. Nightclubs, already open by the end of the school day, had spread to relatively small trading centres by at least the early 1950s, providing a venue for the young to meet away from their families.[58]

This discussion so far has focused on pre-marital sex between children and young adults in their teenage years. This was, according to informants, the most common form of youthful sexual activity.[59] But interviewees confirmed contemporary newspaper and epidemiological reports that sex between youths and the older generation was also becoming increasingly frequent. Adolescent male adventurism led many boys towards older independent women in their neighbourhoods, attracted by their occasional generosity, and by the lower risks associated with any pregnancy which might result. The material benefits of a sexual relationship with an older person were, it seems, even more important for young girls, but not all inter-generational sex was so consensual.[60] The pressure which schoolgirls experienced from male teachers to agree to sex was one of the few factors which discouraged female education in this society. As early as the 1960s, schoolgirls were sought out by older men because they were thought likely to be free of STDs. Rape was so common in the 1950s that perineal repair of pre-pubescent girls was a regular procedure

[58] *The People*, 3 Feb. 1969, p. 7; 'Kampala teenagers going astray', *The People*, 22 Aug. 1964, p. 11; Mair, *Native Marriage*, p. 33; R. Billington, *A Tune on Black and White Keys. Partnership in Healing: the Story of Mengo Hospital* (London: Janus, 1993), pp. 75–9; Int. AN, 25 Aug. 2004, Kagezi, F; Int. NPNK, 24 Aug. 2004, Kyanakase, F; Int. MMA, 24 Aug. 2004, Kyanakase, F. Cf. Shorter, *East African*, pp. 69–71, 116; J. Caldwell et al., 'The construction of adolescence in a changing world: implications for sexuality, reproduction, and marriage', *Studies in Family Planning*, 29, 2 (1998), pp. 137–53; A. Ivaska, *Cultured States: Youth, Gender and Modern Style in 1960s Dar es Salaam* (Durham, NC: Duke University Press, 2011).

[59] e.g. Int. NM, 28 Aug. 2004, Lugazi, Butanga, F; Female FGD, Kagezi, 25 Aug. 2004; Female FGD, Bukoto, 24 Aug. 2004; Int. JN, 29 Aug. 2004, Butanga, F.

[60] Male FGD, Kagezi, 25 Aug. 2004; Int. NPNK, 24 Aug. 2004, Kyanakase, F; Int. RK, 26 Aug. 2002, Takajjunge, M; Southall and Gutkind, *Townsmen*, p. 88; *Obugagga Bwa Uganda*, 14 Mar. 1956, p. 6; O. Arya and F. Bennett, 'Attitudes of college students in East Africa to sexual activity and venereal disease', *British Journal of Venereal Disease*, 44 (1968), p. 163; O. Luwaga, 'Prostitutes in church parishes: what shall we do to save Buganda?', Letter to the Editor, *Matalisi*, 25 Dec. 1942, p. 2.

at Kampala's Mulago hospital, and one of Uganda's few social workers was reassigned to support rape victims.[61]

Formerly marriage had been the key marker of the shift from childhood to adulthood in this society, such that one early colonial chief had objected to the taxation of unmarried men on the grounds that they were not adults. Precolonial Ganda society had been relatively unusual in its acceptance that readiness for marriage required emotional as well as biological maturity, so that a new couple could cope with the responsibilities and tensions of a marital relationship.[62] But concepts of adulthood were reconfigured over the colonial period, as new avenues to maturity and status such as higher education or a professional career often served to delay formal marriage. Schoolteaching and nursing offered women new opportunities for domestic independence, with unmarried nurses in particular developing a reputation for sexual freedom. University students meanwhile benefited from a growing liberalism among academic staff by the 1950s, some of whom considered 'that a certain opportunity for sowing wild oats is a valuable experience', which would teach the ill-effects of over-indulgence.[63]

Many students though proved to be slow learners. In 1966 Makerere University's medical practice found that 28.3% of 1,200 male undergraduates had been infected with an STD over the previous twelve months. The rate among Ganda students was higher than average, at 36%. Another 5% had asked to be tested, having had sex with a contact perceived to be high-risk, but were uninfected. These were mature men, mainly in their early twenties,

[61] A. Maleche, 'Sociological and psychological factors favouring or hindering the education of African women in Uganda' (unpublished TS, EAISR seminar paper 1961, African Studies Centre Library, Cambridge), pp. 5–6; Interview with Sematimba, 7 Aug. 1952, A. Richards papers, LSE, 6/19; Arya and Bennett, 'Attitudes of college students', p. 163; Dr. W. Sheldon and Dr. P. Evans, 'Report to the Board of Governors of the Hospital for Sick Children, Great Ormond Street, of the visit to Uganda, 24.10.53–21.11.53', P. R. Evans papers, Wellcome CMAC, PP/PRE A.1/2; C. Potts, 'Memorandum on youth projects: juvenile legislation, July 1955', Community Development Reports, Kampala, RHO, MSS. Afr. s. 590; List of saza level cases, File 23, PPMS38/Perlman/Box 8, SOAS archive. Between January and June 1955 eighty-four females under twenty were treated at Mulago Hospital following rape. Twenty-two of the cases were thirteen or younger. Moreover, 6% of all cases heard at Buganda's local courts resulted from rape accusations, with the proportion increasing steadily over the period covered by this chapter.

[62] Mair, *Native Marriage*, p. 13; Int. BMJ, 29 Aug. 2004, Kyankoole, M; Int. NPNK, 24 Aug. 2004, Kyanakase, F.

[63] N. Musisi, 'Colonial and missionary education: Women and domesticity in Uganda, 1900–1945', in K. Hansen (ed.), *African Encounters with Domesticity* (New Brunswick NJ: Rutgers University Press, 1992), p. 178; Uganda Protectorate, *Annual Medical Report 1951* (Entebbe: Government Printer, 1952); D. Mills, 'Life on the hill: students and the social history of Makerere', *Africa*, 76, 2 (2006), p. 256. Musisi relates that in the 1920s young women who trained to be teachers told missionaries that they did not want to marry in the village, 'to spend their lives as other girls they knew, hoeing, cooking or resting without a thought outside the native hut and green bananas in which they lived'.

almost all of whom were still unmarried. The incidence was indeed highest among the freshers, with 23% acquiring an STD in their first six months of college life, but 16% of all students had been infected more than once, 2.5% more than five times. One of the most significant findings was that while students considered their infection to be very much a function of their urban environment, in fact many returned from vacations in their village homes, or from fieldwork in agricultural out-stations, newly infected. Equally important was the discovery that students with previous STD infections and those without had both begun sexual activity at a similarly young age, 22% by fifteen, 79% by twenty. Fifteen per cent first had sex at primary school, 70% at secondary. Only 60% of controls were still virgins. Almost all condemned promiscuity, yet a majority of both cohorts approved of pre-marital sex, regarding it as pleasurable and physically necessary, and, often, as a means of ensuring compatibility with a potential wife. A mere one in five in each group had received sex education from family or school. The groups though differed significantly in the numbers and nature of previous sexual relationships. A relatively high proportion of controls, 40%, had had more than five partners, but the rate among students with a history of STDs was twice as high, and members of the latter group were much more likely to report sexual partners who were described as barmaids, nightclub girls, prostitutes, and pick-ups, and whose affections required some form of payment. Many of the controls had had sex that was literally pre-marital, a prelude to or preparation for marriage, whereas the cases were motivated more by a desire to have new partners, with a majority reporting that they had continued with their high risk patterns of behaviour after their first infection.[64]

Social disapproval of the sexual behaviour of these elite occupational groups was limited by Buganda's highly aspirational and status-conscious culture, by their institutionalized residential arrangements, and by an expectation that they would not delay marriage indefinitely. Women who were perceived to have ruled out marriage entirely, however, were treated with less tolerance. Only in the late 1950s did the desire of some young women to live alone in Kampala, socializing freely, meet with occasional approval, and even this was restricted to those women with a recognizably western lifestyle: an office job, an apartment, holidays. For most women, the assertion that they could achieve a higher quality of life free from the drudgery of marriage was met with suspicion and occasional violence and repression. Legislation passed

[64] O. Arya and F. Bennett, 'Venereal disease in an elite group (university students) in East Africa', *British Journal of Venereal Disease*, 43 (1967), pp. 275–9; Arya and Bennett, 'Attitudes', pp. 160–6. Cases were more likely to have had sex in the city than controls, but the nature of relationships, rather than their location, seems to have been more significant. Taylor found a similar level of sexual experience among schoolboys in the 1950s, 43% of whom had had sex by the age of seventeen. Taylor, *Growth of the Church*, p. 281.

by the *Lukiiko* which attempted to prevent the movement to town of unmarried women without paternal permission was enforced sporadically, usually in the form of women being thrown off buses by the police. Unmarried young women were also deliberately targeted during the occasional panics about sex work in Kampala, though this usually involved little more than a few hours in a local police station. Such humiliations aside, the work of Gutkind and Southall in the early 1950s indicated that the presence of young women in town was generally tolerated by their neighbours. In part this was because the definition of pre-marital sex during the colonial era became especially imprecise in urban areas, as the proliferation of informal relationships of varying exclusivity and durability caused the distinction between an unmarried and a married state to be particularly blurred there.[65] In the countryside, women who refused to settle down to marriage, choosing instead to drift from relative to relative, and lover to lover were known as *Bakirese*, restless ones. Like *Banakyeyombekedde* they were suspected by rural wives of hoping to seduce their husbands, but did not even enjoy the status gained by farming independently and having been previously married. Moreover the *Bakirese* were considered a corrupting influence, diffusing urban attitudes and fashions on their return from their sojourns in town.[66]

Much of the previous literature on pre-marital sex has argued that state action and social disapproval targeted young women in particular.[67] Yet even male informants acknowledged the injustice of such scapegoating. 'Parents were mainly strict with girls, because they are the ones to get pregnant. A boy cannot become pregnant.' 'Parents never bothered so much if a son had a child with someone's daughter, for it would increase the clan.'[68] Interviewees all agreed that boys were responsible for starting most pre-marital affairs. 'Boys used to play around trying to tempt me into satanic acts ... The boy would try to convince me that our parents would not know.'[69] Male irrespon-

[65] Musisi, 'Colonial and missionary education', pp. 185; Autolycus, 'Spinsters', *Uganda Argus*, p. 2, 1 Apr. 1957; Southall and Gutkind, *Townsmen*, pp. 90, 167, 193–4; Anon to M. Billson, 1 Feb. 1951, Uganda 1908–54, AMSH, Women's Library, University of London, 3AMS/D/49; Musisi, 'Transformations', p. 254. Marriage in most African societies had always been a process more than an event, but the uncertain marital status which characterized many people in the later colonial period differed in nature from the classic short-term transition between being unmarried and customarily married.

[66] Obbo, 'Town', p. 187; P. Davis, 'On the sexuality of "town women" in Kampala', *Africa Today*, 47, 3/4, (2000), pp. 32–5.

[67] e.g. Davis, 'Town'; Southall and Gutkind, *Townsmen*, pp. 104–6; Obbo, *African Women*, pp. 26–8.

[68] Int. FKW, 31 Aug. 2004, Kitala, M; Int. IST, Kagezi village, 21 August 2004, Masaka, M.

[69] Int. SKKG, 25 Aug. 2004, Kabonera, Masaka District, M; Int. HGN, 10 Sept. 2004, Kiiso, F; Int. NPNK, 24 Aug. 2004, Kyanakase, F; Female FGD, Takajunge, 26 Aug. 2004; Int. JS, 26 Aug. 2004, Takajjunge, Masaka, M; Int. CNSM, 28 Aug. 2004, Butanga, M; Male FGD, Kitala, 1 Sept. 2004; Male FGD, Kisubi Kiwulwe, 4 Sept. 2004. Cf. Mair, *Native Marriage*, p. 11; Kisekka, 'Baganda', p. 153.

sibility, it seems, increased over time. According to Obbo, men born early in the twentieth century were likely to marry girls whom they impregnated, whereas 'since the 1950s, school boys or migrant laborers who made girls pregnant during vacation increasingly denied paternity.'[70]

EXTRA-MARITAL AFFAIRS, SEX WORKING AND SEXUAL CULTURE

Q Did you tell us you also suffered from gonorrhoea?
A Yes. Every one of us suffered from it. Do you expect me to deceive you? If any one of my age told you he did not suffer from gonorrhoea, he is a liar. Unless he was a Reverend Father (laughter). Yes that was it. Or maybe he was impotent. But a man who felt completely normal, who felt all his nerves alive with spasms for sex, would not deceive you that he didn't suffer from gonorrhoea.
Q Did you catch it from one of your wives or outside?
A These ones here, the barmaids, nurses, schoolteachers (laughter); so long as you had money (laughter).
Q This gonorrhoea, did you get it once or more than once?
A It was bad luck. There were times you went to a woman and, God willing, you would come back safe. Sometimes you would be trapped, you would go to a doctor, get an injection and that was all.[71]

Elders' current perception in Buganda that the young have become sexually active earlier than in the past related more to the nature of youthful sex than to its timing. Elderly informants' complaint was not so much that the age at which the young had started having sex had reduced, but that increasingly it occurred before marriage and especially that the young flaunted their affairs so brazenly.[72] Many Ganda acknowledged that sexual purity had always been difficult to maintain, but at least married Ganda had had the decency to be discreet in the conduct of their extra-marital liaisons in the past. The extreme secretiveness of such relationships—'we used to have affairs, but stealthily'—made some informants uncertain about whether they had become more common over time.[73] The furtiveness with which adulterous affairs were pursued

[70] C. Obbo, 'HIV transmission: Men are the solution', *Population and Environment*, 14, 3 (1993), p. 225.
[71] Int. JS, 26 Aug. 2004, Takajjunge, Masaka, M.
[72] K. Stewart, 'Toward a historical perspective on sexuality in Uganda: The reproductive lifeline technique for grandmothers and their daughters', *Africa Today* 47, 3/4 (2000), pp. 123–48; Int. MMA, 24 Aug. 2004, Kyanakase, F; Int. FN, 29 Aug. 2004, Butanga, F.
[73] Male FGD, Bukoto, 24 Aug. 2004; Male FGD, Kitala, 1 Sept. 2004; Male FGD, Takajjunge, 26 Aug. 2004; Int. EM, 28 Aug. 2004, Kyansi, M; Int. CNSM, 28 Aug. 2004, Butanga, M; Int. HGN, 10 Sept. 2004, Kiiso, F; Int. NPNK, 24 Aug. 2004, Kyanakase, F; Int. KJK, 31 Aug. 2004, Kitala, M.

was motivated both by fear of loss of honour and anticipation of violence. Stories of revenge against unfaithful wives and husbands, and their lovers, were reported frequently in Uganda's newspapers; a retired magistrate remembered that infidelity, drunkenness and land were the three leading causes of murder during the colonial period; and, during a period of two months in 1954, one of Peter Gutkind's research assistants witnessed five separate fights due to affairs within his Kampala suburb of 1,300 people. Ganda had just cause to be cautious.[74]

Given that interviewees agreed that affairs were immoral and dangerous, it is striking how transparent Ganda informants were about their own extra-marital history. Across this region, the elderly are permitted to discuss sex freely with their grandchildren's generation, to which my research assistants belonged, whereas sexuality was a topic of avoidance for contiguous generations. Three factors made Ganda men and women exceptionally open about their affairs, though. The first is that according to Ganda succession and inheritance laws, children conceived outside marriage are of equal status to those who are fully legitimate. It seems to have been socially accepted that the product of an affair should at some point be acknowledged, so that a number of informants were not only aware of their fathers' extra-marital children, but mentioned them without obvious bitterness.[75] The second is that one aspect of the guilt associated with affairs diminished more quickly in colonial Buganda than in many neighbouring societies, where the traditional diseases supposedly suffered by children due to their parents' infidelity were taken very seriously well into the twentieth century. Compared to informants from Buhaya and Ankole, Ganda were more likely to believe that such diseases were relatively uncommon—'they used to be there long ago and not in our generation'; that effective herbal remedies existed—'People went ahead behaving immorally, after all they knew the diseases were curable'; and to question the link between behaviour and health—'it was just a trick to keep men out of adultery.'[76] The third is that affairs after the Second World War were con-

[74] 'A European loses teeth over a woman', *Uganda Empya*, 27 Apr. 1960; 'Healer dates client's wife', *Uganda Eyogera*, 5 July 1962, p. 3; 'Wife strangles husband for adultery', *Uganda Eyogera*, 14 July 1962, p. 3; Int. JS, 26 Aug. 2004, Takajjunge, Masaka, M; Gutkind, 'Preliminary report', pp. 72, 128–30. Stories of children learning who their true father was only when their mother was on her deathbed, and of fathers disinheriting sons who bore little physical resemblance to them, were frequently told during interviews. See e.g. Male FGD, Takajjunge, 26 Aug. 2004; Int. PLGS, 31 Aug. 2004, Kitala, Busiro, M.

[75] e.g. Int. NM, 28 Aug. 2004, Lugazi, Butanga, F; Int. FN, 29 Aug. 2004, Butanga, F.

[76] Int. MGK, 26 Aug. 2004, Takajjunge, F; Int. FN, 29 Aug. 2004, Butanga, F; Int. CNSM, 28 Aug. 2004, Butanga, M; Int. JN, 29 Aug. 2004, Butanga, F. Presumably the symptoms of those illnesses associated with parental infidelity would have become less noticeable earlier in Buganda because of that region's superior colonial medical provision, which focused heavily on child health.

sidered so commonplace by interviewees that admitting to having participated in such a widespread practice was relatively easy. As one remembered: 'almost everyone did it.'[77]

Informants disagreed about the decade when extra-marital affairs became more common. As with pre-marital sex, and sexual culture more widely, the majority identified the 1960s as the time when patterns of infidelity began to change noticeably, but many older informants considered that adultery increased from the 1940s or 1950s.[78] The most common explanation for the growing incidence of infidelity was the change in patterns of socializing which enabled the sexes to mix together in new ways: 'The more fun and entertainment, the more promiscuity', as one put it. Many interviewees used the arrival of the disco in their locality as a shorthand for the hedonistic rejection of tradition associated with Milton Obote's first period of office, from 1962 to 1971. Ganda indigenous dancing styles were themselves highly erotic, so it was the fact that people danced in pairs rather than the sexualized nature of the dances themselves that gave discos such a bad name. Even so, couple dancing had existed in rural and urban Buganda since the interwar period, the rumba being displaced in popularity by the tango and calypso in the 1950s, before re-emerging in a faster form as soukous in the 1960s. Nightclubs, where married men danced with single women, were already the subject of moral concern by the early 1950s.[79] New forms of drinking also emerged in the later colonial period, again creating new opportunities for infidelity. Wives increasingly accompanied their husbands to beer-drinks, which supposedly facilitated affairs between neighbours. Modern bars where men drank, and sometimes danced, with unmarried women opened in small trading centres all over Buganda from the 1940s. Barmaids were regarded as a high-risk occupational group in the transmission of STDs long before the era of AIDS. As one informant happily remembered, 'They would seduce men to come to

[77] e.g. Int. HGN, 10 Sept. 2004, Kiiso, F; Int. NM, 28 Aug. 2004, Lugazi, Butanga, F.

[78] Int. YZ, 13 Aug. 2004, M; Int. JN, 29 Aug. 2004, Butanga, F; Int. EM, 28 Aug. 2004, Kyansi, M; Int. PLGS, 31 Aug. 2004, Kitala, Busiro, M; Int. MMA, 24 Aug. 2004, Kyanakase, F; Male FGD, Takajunge, 26 Aug. 2004.

[79] Int. JS, 26 Aug. 2004, Takajjunge, Masaka, M; Southwold, 'The Baganda', p. 167; S. Nannyonga-Tamusuza, *Baakisimba: Gender in the Music and Dance of the Baganda People of Uganda* (New York: Taylor and Francis, 2005), p. 34; Int. YZ, 13 Aug. 2004, Mbarara, M; S. Kiguli, 'Oral poetry and popular song in post-Apartheid South Africa and post-civil war Uganda: A comparative study of contemporary performance (unpublished PhD Dissertation, University of Leeds, 2004), p. 66; W. Elkan, *Migrants and Proletarians: Urban Labour in the Economic Development of Uganda* (London: Oxford University Press, 1960), p. 19; Billington, *A Tune*, p. 127; 1952 annual report of the senior community development officer, Community Development Reports, Kampala, RHO, MSS. Afr. s. 590; 'Will a man rob God?', *Uganda Herald*, 8 July 1952, p. 4; Southall and Gutkind, *Townsmen*, p. 215.

their joints . . . She would dress nicely, wear powder. Heeeei! And she would be ready for you then.'[80]

The central place of barmaids in Ganda discussions of sexual change derives from their association with three inter-related developments, which were all regarded as key to the apparent increase in extra-marital sex: urbanity, the commercialization of sex, and growing female independence. As discussed above, the growing numbers of women who were able to live unmarried in their own homes greatly expanded the range of sexual opportunity for married men. Such women were often lumped together as *malaya* or prostitutes by female informants because all independent women were regarded as equally tempting to their husbands, and by male informants because of a generalized resentment at what was perceived as an increasingly materialistic female attitude to sex. Yet on closer questioning the unhelpfulness of this stereotype was often acknowledged. Male interviewees observed that women with their own land had little need for men's money: 'they would concentrate on making good use of their hoes,' or would be as likely to give gifts to lovers as to receive them. And even women who were dependent on material support could be differentiated from sex workers: 'They would not go in for every man just because he gave her a gift or money. They had particular men they loved and accepted.' Men also, as interviews unfolded, generally acknowledged that they, not women, were responsible for the initiation of most affairs.[81]

Female materialism was most visible in town, because there opportunities for income generation sufficient for self-sufficiency were more limited than in the countryside. In most African colonial towns sex workers were the predominant source of extra-marital liaisons. This was because, until the 1940s at least, European authorities obstructed the development of the urban African family, partly due to their determination to pass the costs of the reproduction of labour onto the rural economy, and partly reflecting their concern, often shared with local chiefs, that urbanization would undermine the stability of indigenous social structures.[82] But Kampala was atypical of colonial urbanity. Most of the city was governed by Buganda's kingdom

[80] Int. HGN, 10 Sept. 2004, Kiiso, F; L. Lea Wilson, Letter to the Editor, *Uganda Herald*, 12 Aug. 1935; Beer club, 21 Nov. 1950, A. Richards papers, LSE, 7/18; Male FGD, Takajjunge, 26 Aug. 2004; Male FGD Kagezi, 25 Aug. 2004; M. Robbins and R. Pollnac, 'Drinking patterns and acculturation in rural Buganda', *American Anthropologist*, Vol. 71, No. 2. (Apr., 1969), pp. 276–285; Obbo, 'Town migration', pp. 112–15; Int. JS, 26 Aug. 2004, Takajjunge, Masaka, M.

[81] Int. ZMN, 28 Aug, 2004, Butanga, F; Int. FN, 29 Aug. 2004, Butanga, F; Int. NM, 28 Aug. 2004, Lugazi, Butanga, F; Int. JS, 26 Aug. 2004, Takajjunge, Masaka, M; Int. SKKG, 25 Aug. 2004, Kabonera, Masaka District, M; Male FGD, Takajjunge, 26 Aug. 2004; Int. NPNK, 24 Aug. 2004, Kyanakase, F; Int. HGN, 10 Sept. 2004, Kiiso, F; Male FGD, Takajjunge, 26 Aug. 2004.

[82] Cf. e.g. E. Schmidt, 'Patriarchy, Capitalism, and the Colonial State in Zimbabwe', *Signs*, 16, 4 (1991), pp. 732–56. In 1970, 60% of women in Kampala were unemployed. Shorter, *East African Societies*, p. 111.

government, which, with occasional exceptions, proved tolerant of female settlement in town. Just as important was the large proportion of Kampala's land that was owned by Ganda freeholders, whose primary concern was to maximize the number of tenants, of whatever sex, from whom they could draw rent. Kampala's sex ratio was exceptionally balanced as a result, with women and girls making up 43% of the city's population as early as 1911. By 1959, 61% of the population of Greater Kampala were women and girls, while females made up a majority of the Ganda population living in the kingdom's capital, towns, and various trading centres.[83]

Only in Kisenyi, the city's least salubrious neighbourhood, were sex workers concentrated in significant numbers. Gutkind's survey of the outer suburb of Mulago in 1954 identified only four full-time professional sex workers. Most sources suggest that this was a largely unorganized business, with the typical sex worker renting a small room where she would wait for clients, charging two or three shillings for short-time sex and, relatively rarely, ten shillings for an entire night during the 1950s. Women could expect to save thirty shillings a month, a decent income but not remarkable for Buganda. A higher rate could be charged by those women who could speak some English and possessed western clothes, and so could operate in modern bars or as street walkers in the better parts of town, often catering for European and Asian demand. Some women, especially those whose earning power was in decline, also possessed a regular lover who gave them presents, or supplemented their income from sex by selling beer, food, or charcoal.[84] Women whose main income was derived from cash for sex could also be found in bars in Buganda's towns and larger trading centres by the 1950s, but not it seems in villages during this period.[85]

It was not uncommon in contemporary accounts and interviewees' reminiscences for the presence of sex workers to be explained in terms of factors of supply: female lust, greed, or reluctance to dig; the immigration of women

[83] Obbo, 'Town migration', p. 11; Uganda Protectorate, *1911 Census Returns* (Entebbe: Government Printer, 1912); East African Statistical Department, *Uganda Census 1959* (Nairobi: Government Printer, 1961).

[84] Southall and Gutkind, *Townsmen*, pp. 79–87; Gutkind, 'Preliminary', p. 69; Int. HGN, 10 Sept. 2004, Kiiso, F; Int. TNN, 3 Aug. 2004, Kitala, F; Female FGD, Takajunge, 26 Aug. 2004; O.S.P.S. Luwaga, Letter to the Editor, 'Prostitutes in church parishes: what shall we do to save Buganda?', *Matalisi*, 25 Dec.1942, p. 2; 'Omuyindi bamukukunudde ku mukazi muddugavu', *Uganda Empya*, 26 July 1960; Davis, 'Town women', pp. 38–9. One source which does mention procurement is B. Tejani, 'Farewell Uganda', *Transition*, No. 45. (1974), pp. 64–6. He grew up in the 1950s 'above a motel famous for pimps, gamblers and whores'.

[85] Southall and Gutkind, *Townsmen*, pp. 78–9; 'Prostitutes and tax defaulters arrested', *Uganda Eyogera*, 28 June 1962, p. 2; Int. ZMN, 28 Aug, 2004, Butanga, F; Int. IST, 21 August 2004, Kagezi village, Masaka, M; Int. SKKG, 25 Aug. 2004, Kabonera, M; M. Robbins and R. Pollnac, 'Drinking patterns and acculturation in rural Buganda', *American Anthropologist*, 71, 2 (1969), p. 280.

from other societies who lacked the skills to make a living by other means; the increasing numbers of divorced or unmarried women; the development of bars.[86] But most sources tended to emphasize that sex work emerged in response to demand, that it was stimulated by the large numbers of soldiers in Kampala during the Second World War, and then sustained by the male need for short-term sexual relationships. Many Ganda men worked alone in the city, or travelled frequently on business: 'they could not stand being without sex so they would find themselves buying prostitutes,' as one informant recalled. Others simply viewed sex workers as particularly attractive. Tooro women were thought to have especially beautiful features, and Haya women to have a relatively light skin colour. But female informants felt that they could not compete even with Ganda sex workers. Liberated from physical exertion in the fields, they were 'fat and clean', their appeal enhanced by perfume, make-up, and revealing clothes, and their reputed sexual expertise. Ganda revealed considerable respect for sex workers' experience and professional competence, remembering how young men, following a visit to the city, would tempt their friends with tales of the 'tricks' and 'styles' that they had experienced. Sex work in Buganda was popular not so much because it offered the comforts of home, but because it offered guaranteed sexual excitement and novelty at a fixed price.[87]

Sex work was the subject of recurrent debate and government action throughout the colonial period, as it was associated not only with immorality and the spread of STDs, but also with Buganda's low levels of fertility, worsening marital instability, and growing female independence. Single women had been deported from the city as early as 1917, with official opposition to female autonomy being formalized in 1941 when a law passed by the *Lukiiko* defined a prostitute remarkably widely, as 'any woman who habitually gives her body indiscriminately for profit or gain or who persistently indulges in promiscuous intercourse with men even though she derives no gain or profit thereby'. In addition unmarried women under the age of

[86] Int. FN, 29 Aug. 2004, Butanga, F; D. Kawesa, 'Agriculture for girls in school. What causes prostitution?', *Matalisi*, 27 Feb. 1942, p. 5; Male FGD, Takajunge, 26 Aug. 2004; Male FGD, Kagezi, 25 Aug. 2004.

[87] Int. SKKG, 25 Aug. 2004, Kabonera, M; Male FGD, Bukoto, 24 Aug. 2004; Female FGD, Kagezi, 25 Aug. 2004; Int. IST, 21 August 2004, Kagezi village, Masaka, M; Southall and Gutkind, *Townsmen*, pp. 79–83; Int. NM, 28 Aug. 2004, Lugazi, Butanga, F; Int. NPNK, 24 Aug. 2004, Kyanakase, F; Int. EM, 28 Aug. 2004, Kyansi, M; Int. RK, 26 Aug. 2002, Takajjunge, M; Int. IST, 21 August 2004, Kagezi village, Masaka, M; Female FGD, Bukoto, 24 Aug. 2004. Some male informants emphasized that paying for sex was much cheaper than maintaining a wife or lover, and that they never had to plead for sex unlike at home. Int. KJK, 31 Aug. 2004, Kitala, M; Int. FKW, 31 Aug. 2004, Kitala, M. Cf. White, *Comforts of Home*.

twenty were forbidden from living away from home.[88] The law imposed heavy penalties on those found guilty of any breach of the regulations, but in practice prosecutions were rare—only thirty-one per annum between 1942 and 1962, the year of Uganda's independence. The main purpose of the law was to permit the harassment of sex workers and other unattached urban women. Raids seem to have grown in frequency as Ganda politics became more conservative after the deportation of the Kabaka in 1953 and respectable urban opinion became more voluble. Yet the number of sex workers was perceived to be steadily increasing. 'There are so many prostitutes in Kampala, they could stage a coup d'état,' according to one letter writer in 1965. Partly this was because attempts to clear the streets of areas such as Kisenyi simply moved sex workers into other neighbourhoods. But the main reason for the tokenistic nature of the suppression of sex work was, it seems, interference by the politically powerful. As early as the 1920s the colonial administration bemoaned the conflict of interest on the issue within Buganda's elite, and there are several recorded occasions when one branch of the royal government released sex workers who had been arrested by another. In 1957 Buganda's newspapers reported without comment an official statement which claimed that sex workers found in possession of a number of the kabaka's ministers' calling cards must have broken into their offices and stolen them. Gutkind notes that later that year a number of women charged with prostitution were discovered to be the mistresses of leading government figures.[89]

Sex work was not insignificant in Kampala. But relatively few Ganda women were professional sex workers, the largest number reportedly belonging to the Haya and Tooro ethnic groups. No doubt Ganda men figured prominently among sex workers' clients, but, according to Gutkind and Southall, in the early 1950s, paying women for short-term sex was only one extreme on the spectrum of urban sexual encounters. Some men visited sex workers very frequently. One informant remembered that 'there were men

[88] 'The law to prevent prostitution [obwamalaaya]', 1 Apr. 1941, *The Native Laws of Buganda* (Kampala, 1947), pp. 6–8. Opposition to single females in the city was far from universal by the early 1960s with even the former mayor Lwanga, responsible for repeated raids against sex workers, observing that respectable jobs needed to be created for female immigrants to the city. 'Okukwata ba malaya kiri mu mateeka', *Uganda Empya*, 15 Aug. 1960. Cf. Kyomuhendo and McIntosh, *Women*, p. 136.

[89] Uganda Protectorate, *1950 Annual Medical Report* (Entebbe: Government Printer, 1951); Anon. to M Billson, AMSH, 1 Feb. 1951, Uganda 1908–54, Women's Library, London, 3AMS/D/49; Southall and Gutkind, *Townsmen*, pp. 193–4; 'Okukwata ba malaya kiri mu mateeka', *Uganda Empya*, 15 Aug. 1960; 'Potolo Yakutte Bamalaya N'abatawa Musolo', *Uganda Empya*, 5 Mar. 1960, p. 1; Jane Musoke, Letter to the editor, *Uganda Argus*, 10 Sept. 1965; 'Who avails invitation cards to prostitutes?', *Obugagga Bwa Uganda*, 16 Jan. 1957, p. 6; P. Gutkind, *The Royal Capital of Buganda: A study of Internal Conflict and External Ambiguity* (The Hague: Mouton, 1963), pp. 79, 154–6; Gutkind, *Preliminary*, p. 128.

who had turned it into some sort of job,' while one of Southall's interviewees in the 1950s admitted that he 'might sleep with twenty of them in a month'. But more typical of male behaviour, it seems, was the search for a relatively long-term urban lover, especially where men had come to town without their wives. Women also often hoped to establish durable relationships, but few men could afford to sustain the provision of gifts and alcohol which had helped to initiate an affair. Gutkind was told that 'only by going from one man to another could "you get food"', and that 'a woman must have a lot of friends because it is very expensive to live in town.' Urban males complained that while many town women conducted simultaneous affairs, others, who tried to appear more respectable, nonetheless had several husbands, one in Kampala, another in the village, the latter relationship sustained through regular familial visits. Men deplored town women's duplicity and greed, one stating that 'when it comes to accepting money [Ganda women] do not hesitate to take it from any man, however dirty.' Yet they themselves wanted all the benefits of marriage from their urban relationships without the cost of bridewealth, and in addition often hoped to maintain the freedom to enjoy the sexual opportunities of the urban environment.[90]

Though Ganda may have regarded the city as a place of particular sexual corruption, researchers in the middle of the twentieth century were struck by how closely integrated Kampala was with its rural hinterland. Writing soon after independence Aylward Shorter observed that it had become 'increasingly difficult to make cultural distinctions between city and countryside. Ganda culture is developing more or less uniformly.' As with many African cities, urban migrants were tied to their home villages by attendance at ceremonies of naming, marriage, mourning, and inheritance, but Kampala's links to the countryside were strengthened further by the integrative nature of kingdom government, and above all by the cash-cropping wealth of the rural economy. It was not unusual for the urban poor to travel out of town daily to work on nearby farms, while wealthier migrants visited their village homes at least once a month, and usually more, partly in order to supervise their farms. A large proportion of Ganda who worked in the city chose to live in a nearby village, cycling up to twelve kilometres each way in the 1950s in order to supplement their salary with the produce of a rented plot. Other Ganda travelled much further to town to conduct business, visit relatives, or for schooling. One 1960s survey in a rural parish 120 kilometres from Kampala found that 88% of householders made visits to the city. The attitudes towards sexuality found in town infiltrated rural Buganda to a remarkable degree. Kampala's influence was felt most intensely in the peri-urban villages whose incorpora-

[90] Male FGD, Takajunge, 26 Aug. 2004; Int. SJ, 26 Aug. 2004, Takajunge, M; Southall and Gutkind, *Townsmen*, pp. 28, 66, 71–9, 88; Gutkind, 'Preliminary', pp. 62, 67–8, 71–5.

tion within the city's limits swelled Kampala's population to 330,700 in 1969, compared to 46,735 a decade earlier. But even in the early 1930s nowhere in Buganda was more than a day's journey, by foot to the local trading centre and then bus, from the capital. Small townships, comprised of a handful of shops, a butchery, and a bar or two had become the hub of rural communities by the interwar period, acting as nodes for the dispersal of city culture. 'Near the main road you never sleep', as Lucy Mair was told in one county capital. They also acted as the first and last step of the classic pattern of female urban migration in Buganda. Female life histories revealed that moving to the city was for many women more of a process than an event, beginning with a local market, progressing up the scale of settlement size, until sufficient savings had been accumulated in the trading centre, township, and town to permit a largely independent lifestyle in the city. For such women, the ideal retirement was to return to a small trading centre in Kampala's environs, their careers a metaphor for the circular links between town and country which created such long and complex sexual networks across Buganda.[91]

It is reasonable then to conceive of Buganda's sexual culture in the middle decades of the twentieth century as largely homogeneous, with the city experiencing the same forces for change as the rest of the kingdom, albeit earlier and more intensely. Attitudes towards extra-marital affairs, and sex in general, were very broad-minded in some ways. When asked to explain the frequency of infidelity in the past, one man in a focus group observed that 'it was just a natural habit', another simply stated 'poverty'. During their fieldwork in the 1950s, Gutkind heard 'endless conversations in the bars dealing with the pros and cons of having lovers', and Southwold found that 'women do not deny that Baganda women in general are adulterous; they even seem to take pride in the fact, probably in order to rile their husbands.' The proportion of cases dealt with by Buganda's local courts which related to adultery was three times higher before the Second World War compared to the period after 1940, which seems more likely to reflect a change in levels of tolerance than behaviour.[92] The local press indicated that attitudes were perhaps becoming more permissive during the era of decolonization. Papers in Buganda had

[91] Shorter, *East African Societies*, p. 113; Gutkind, 'African urban family life', p. 172; Reining and Richards, 'Report on fertility surveys', p. 359; H. Welbourn, 'Weaning among the Baganda', *African Child Health*, 9 (1963), pp. 14–24; Robbins and Pollnac, 'Drinking patterns', pp. 278–9; L. Mair, *An African People in the Twentieth Century* (London: Routledge, 1965 [1934]), p. 24; Mair, *Native Marriage*, p. 25; Southall and Gutkind, *Townsmen*, pp. 78–9, 90–1; C. Obbo, 'Dominant male ideology and female options: Three East African case studies', *Africa*, 46, 4 (1976), pp. 378–83; A. Richards, 'Kisozi village 1952' (unpublished seminar paper, n/d), A. Richards papers, LSE, 6/19.

[92] Male FGD, Kisubi Kiwulwe, 4 Sept. 2004; Gutkind, 'Preliminary', p. 21; Southwold, 'The Baganda', pp. 166–71; List of saza level cases, File 23, PPMS38/Perlman/Box 8, SOAS archive.

run stories about sexual misconduct from the interwar period, but by the 1960s the righteous moralism which characterized most of the coverage of earlier decades had been largely displaced by prurient enjoyment in the scandal of misbehaviour. Typical stories included a herbalist who took the logical step of having affairs with his female clients seeking a cure for infertility; a woman who claimed maintenance for her illegitimate child from three separate men; a man who went to use his latrine only to find his wife having sex with a neighbour; and, with rich symbolism, a man bitten by a poisonous snake while committing adultery.[93]

The Ganda press also contributed to a growing public emphasis on, and tolerance of, sexual attractiveness by printing adverts from the late 1950s which used images of scantily clad women to sell deodorant, hair removal cream, and car tyres, and, from the mid-1960s, regularly running photographs of local young women in slots such as '*The People's* beauty'.[94] Women's attempts to increase their allure and follow fashion had brought condemnation and occasional repression from at least the 1940s, with college women being forced to lengthen their hems and men cutting off their wives' 'unChristian' braids with machetes. But the growing popularity of make-up, skin lightener, wigs, and mini-skirts during the 1960s brought criticism of female indecency to a new height. Some commentators condemned modern women's lack of African authenticity. One columnist wrote in 1969 that the typical woman found in a bar, a 'red-lipped dame with buttocks and breasts well stuffed with rubber' and 'counterfeit smiles', 'must succeed in seducing you to pay a visit to her room. You discover there she is artificial all over.' Others complained that the overt display of female sensuality presented an impossible challenge to male self-control. One man interviewed about mini-skirts stated 'sometimes you feel so much involved that there and then you decide to part with her.' A police officer predicted that 'with the great increase in the use of minis, we should expect a parallel rise in the number of rape cases,' but not necessarily convictions, for a case was likely to be dismissed where 'the complainant was tantalizing the accused with her "glassy thighs".'[95]

[93] 'Healer dates client's wife', *Uganda Eyogera*, 5 Jul. 1962, p. 3; 'Naluwoza played 3 men', *Obugagga bwa Uganda*, 10 Jul. 1957, p. 8; 'Husband accompanies wife to commit adultery', *Taifa Uganda Empya*, 4 Feb. 1967, p. 10; 'Man dies committing adultery', *Taifa Uganda Empya*, 22 July 1967, p. 10.

[94] *Uganda Argus*, Jan.–Mar. 1957, *passim*; *The People*, 22 Aug. 1964, p. 4.

[95] Obbo, 'Town', p. 186; H. Stanton, 'A picture of Uganda in the 1960s. A tribute to Makerere University College and to African women' (RHO, MSS. Afr. s. 2285, n/d [*c*.1980]), Ch.5, p. 9; 'Hairstyling: bringing the past to date', *Uganda Argus*, 22 July 1971; 'Men, now is the time to act before our women take over completely', *The People*, 10 Jan. 1969, p. 7; C. Obang-Achere, *The People*, 17 Feb. 1969, p. 7; 'War on minis in Uganda?', *The People*, 14 Jan. 1969, p. 9; 'Opinions on minis: for and against', *The People*, 17 Jan. 1969. One elderly man interviewed by *The People* warned that 'the obscene behaviours of the Ugandans who are copying from the whites ... might

Interestingly both church and state were relatively quiet during this post-independence debate about sexual propriety, the Uganda People's Congress regime professing that 'Ugandans should be proud of their culture and not try to imitate foreign cultures,' but restraining its youth wing from launching a campaign against female decadence and ruling that mini-skirts were not a suitable topic for government legislation. The churches limited themselves to exhorting female adherents to wear respectable clothing, so that dresses with a low hemline were described as 'Kiwanuka' after the Catholic Archbishop.[96] To some extent this reticence was carried over from the late colonial period, when European officials and clergy withdrew from the moral debate because of a growing reluctance to criticise indigenous culture in the context of Africanization. Ganda sexuality in the 1950s had become more a topic for analysis than simple condemnation as social scientists were set the task of identifying the underpinnings of what was now termed dysfunctional rather than immoral behaviour.[97]

The East African Institute of Social Research was dominated in the 1950s by structural functionalists whose intellectual interest in Africans' ability to adapt to the stresses of modernization fitted closely with the concerns of colonial administrators. Two of the issues that particularly concerned Uganda's anthropologists were marriage and childrearing, both of which were regarded as being especially problematic in Buganda. Aidan Southall wrote in 1957 of the strain experienced by the urban family in Kampala due to endemic marital instability and the frequency with which households were headed by single women. The lack of male role models was common across urban Africa, he thought, but was especially problematic in Buganda because of the relative vagueness of its extended family relationships. Audrey Richards' concern was more with the remarkably high incidence of fostering in Ganda society, with surveys suggesting that a majority of Ganda children under the age of twelve were sent away from home to live with relatives and learn good behaviour and clanship, a practice that had become still more common due to marriage breakup, education, infertility, and the economic power of elders in

bring us a very unforgettable punishment like that one recorded in the bible where people died of water floods.' Women responded to this critique by observing that women in the countryside often exposed their breasts while working in the fields, that Ganda men wore Arab kanzus and western jeans, and that corruption came not from women's thighs but men's 'evil minds'. Maggie G.S., 'Why private parts', *The People*, 24 Jan.1969, p. 6; N. Ssabo, Letter to the editor, *The People*, 17 Jan. 1969, p. 7.

[96] 'War on minis in Uganda?', *The People*, 14 Jan. 1969, p. 9; Female FGD, Takajunge, 26 Aug. 2004.

[97] Uganda Protectorate, *Annual Medical Report, 1952* (Entebbe: Government Printer, 1953); F. Webber, CO, to General Secretary AMSH, 30 Oct. 1951, Uganda 1908–54, Women's Library, London, 3AMS/D/49; Int. HW, 31 July 2008, Bristol, F; Hastings, *Christian Marriage*.

Buganda, who held most of the kingdom's land. Parents found it difficult to refuse requests for fosterage, and often actively encouraged it, hoping that a guardian's weaker emotional tie to a child would make it easier to impose discipline. Researchers believed that the separation of a child from its parents and a husband from his wife lay at the heart of a range of social ills in Buganda: child neglect, the inadequacy of sex education, the supposed inability of many Ganda to establish durable relationships of affection. Medical researchers seeking to explain the severity of malnutrition and STD infection among children were heavily influenced by developmental psychologists such as Mary Ainsworth, who believed that removing a child from its mother early in life resulted in lasting damage to an individual's personality. The paediatrician Hebe Welbourn, in a manual on childrearing aimed at a mass Ganda audience, wrote that 'children who change homes several times... never really trust anybody and seem to make difficulties in every home they stay in for long, including their own homes when they grew up and marry.'[98]

CONCLUSION

Ganda sexuality then had been pathologized in a new way by the end of the colonial period, this time with the backing of science rather than theology, and its excesses were blamed primarily on family malfunction: the absent father, the bereft mother, and the rootless child. To some extent these problems were exaggerated. The continuing centrality of clanship meant that even where children were raised by single mothers, they rarely lost all connection to their paternal relations. Fosterage was so much a part of Ganda culture that the temporary separation of mothers and children may have been less traumatic than western researchers would have expected. Certainly many schoolchildren in the 1950s emphasized to researchers the benefits for their character formation of being sent to stay with relatives.[99] Moreover, there

[98] Southall and Gutkind, *Townsmen,* pp. 66–7; A. Richards, 'Traditional values and current political behavior', in L. Fallers, ed., *All The King's Men: Leadership and Status in Buganda on the Eve of Independence* (London, 1964), pp. 294–335; C. Potts, Memorandum on youth projects: juvenile legislation, July 1955, Community Development Reports, Kampala, RHO, MSS. Afr. s. 590; P. Robertz, 'Sharing with adolescents' (unpublished research paper, Pastoral Institute of Eastern Africa, Gaba, *c.*1969), p. 28; M. Ainsworth, *Infancy in Uganda* (Baltimore: Johns Hopkins, 1967); H. Welbourn for Uganda Council of Women, *Our Children* (Kampala, n/d *c.*1960), p. 36; H. Welbourn, 'Weaning among the Baganda', *Journal of Tropical Pediatrics*, 9, 1 (1963), p. 22. Cf. C. Summers, 'Grandfathers, grandsons, morality, and radical politics in late colonial Buganda', *The International Journal of African Historical Studies*, 38, 3 (2005), pp. 439–41.

[99] Junior secondary schoolboys, A. Richards papers, LSE, 6/26. Boys seem to have acknowledged the benefits of fosterage more than girls, perhaps because they were more indulged, and thought more in terms of long-term material opportunity. Gayaza High School, A. Richards papers, LSE, 6/27.

were indications in the 1950s and 1960s of new sources of stability within the modern Ganda family. Buganda's government began to penalize the long-term fosterage of children in order to strengthen the parent-child relationship; there were signs that some couples were adopting a more companionate style of relationship, some for moral, some for material reasons; and by the early 1960s urbanites were much more likely to live in the city with their children than they had been a decade earlier, because of rising incomes and improvements in housing and educational and medical provision within the city.[100] Ganda informants agreed with some elements in the colonial-era anthropological analysis of sexual change in their society. Many identified the increasing numbers of independent women and increasingly disobedient youth as significant factors. But fostering was considered irrelevant and even marital breakdown in itself was given little emphasis. Instead, the focus of their concern was the increase in sexual opportunity for males and females of all age groups that accompanied the new forms of socializing that emerged around the 1940s. This emphasis on sexual culture would be prominent in all three case study areas by the 1960s.

[100] Mutongole, Francis Walakira, Mawokota, 17 June 1954, A. Richards papers, LSE, 7/16; Byaruhanga, 'Divorce', p. 53; Southall and Gutkind, *Townsmen*, p. 90; Kyomuhendo and McIntosh, *Women*, p. 119; Uganda Protectorate, *The Pattern of Income, Expenditure and Consumption of African Unskilled Workers in Kampala, September 1953* (Nairobi: EAHC, 1954), pp. 1–4; Uganda Government Statistics Branch, *The Patterns of Income, Expenditure and Consumption of African Unskilled Workers in Kampala, February 1964* (Entebbe: Government Printer, 1966), pp. 1–30. The proportion of male unskilled workers who lived in the city with dependents rose from 26 to 67% between 1954 and 1964. For Ganda the rate increased from 55% to 75%. Average salaries increased 150 % over this period.

5
Prostitution in Buhaya, 1925–69

INTRODUCTION

The evolution of sexual culture in Buhaya mimicked that of Buganda in several ways. Marriage was similarly highly unstable by the middle decades of the twentieth century. A survey in the 1950s found that 22% of ever married women in their twenties were divorced or separated, and another 24% were on their second or third marriage. Extra-marital affairs seem also to have increased in frequency in Buhaya, due to diverging expectations about the ideal marital relationship, the commodification of sex, and new opportunities for social interaction. Alcohol consumption became more commercialized as spirits displaced beer as the drink of choice, and nightclubs had sprung up in small trading centres by the 1950s. Informants' memories of their young adulthood, which ranged from the late 1930s through to the 1960s, indicated that extra-marital sex had become extremely common, and was viewed with a degree of social acceptance. Typical statements were that 'every man was an adulterer', and 'what they did was normal.'[1] Divorcees and widows gained greater sexual freedom than they had historically enjoyed as legal reforms granted them new autonomy. Daughters were granted the right to inherit land while the likelihood that a widow could remain unmarried in her late husband's home increased. Informants remembered that after the Second World War the typical village possessed a number of such independent women, known as *kyegesa bazii* 'the trainers of swimmers', who conducted sexual affairs with young men. One informant, widowed while still a young woman, had romantic memories of her post-marital affairs. 'In your youth,

[1] W. Laurie and H. Trant, *East African Medical Survey, Monograph no. 2: A Health Survey in Bukoba District, Tanganyika* (Nairobi: EAHC, 1954), pp. 37–8; H. Trant, 'Not Merrion Square: Anecdotes from a woman's medical career in Africa', Rhodes House Oxford (RHO), MSS. Af.s.1872(143), p. 128; G. Hyden, *Political Development in Rural* Tanzania: *A West Lake Study* (Nairobi: East African Publishing House, 1969), p. 265; D. Muhingo to Buhaya Council Secretary, n/d [July 1961], Mwanza Provincial Archives [MPA], L5/II/B; Int. GK, 21 Aug. 2000, Nkindo, F; Int. LN, 19 Aug. 2000, Kikukwe, F.

with your beauty, with your dazzling eye, can you not fall in love with a man? We made love, but now it is over.'[2]

As in Buganda, these broad trends of growing sexual freedom and commodification concealed significant cross-currents, the most important of which was a major increase in the stability of marriage in Buhaya from the late 1950s, largely, it seems, due to a decline in infertility. Buhaya differed from Buganda in several other ways. Haya cultural antagonism to pre-marital pregnancy ensured that sex before marriage was viewed with less tolerance than among the Ganda throughout the colonial period. The anthropologist Priscella Reining found very few cases of pre-marital births during her several years of fieldwork during the early 1950s.[3] No doubt this partly resulted from the use of abortifacients, but opportunities for girls to have sex appear to have been rarer than in colonial Buganda, as parental supervision was prioritized more heavily and female schooling was relatively limited before the 1950s. A 1952 survey found that female literacy was four times higher in Buganda than Buhaya. Relatively few Haya informants who grew up in the 1940s and 1950s stated that girls had been sexually active before marriage then, in contrast to the reported situation in Buganda. Evidence of significant change in girls' sexual behaviour came with independence, and resulted in complaints about the impact of government libertarianism and respect for individual rights. The leading citizens of one rural parish protested in 1961 that '[t]here is nobody who can punish a girl who stands anyhow on the road with a man. The practice now is that this girl can sue you. Girls who get pregnant without getting married are unpunished.'[4] Relationships between young males and older women, by contrast, seem to have become more common several decades earlier. The economic diversification and administrative expansion of the later colonial period increased the ability of young men to secure wealth outside of their family's household, often drawing them into affairs rather than advancing the onset of marriage.[5]

Buhaya also differed from Buganda in that debates about sexual behaviour and attitudes were significantly more crisis-laden, moralistic, and authoritarian on the Tanganyikan side of the border, and chiefs and the colonial

[2] Native customs, Bukoba District Book, Tanzania National Archives (TNA); Judgements file (vol. II), D. Connolly papers, Rhodes House Oxford, MSS. Afr. s. 1678(2); H. Cory and M. Hartnoll, *Customary Law of the Haya Tribe, Tanganyika Territory* (London: Cass, 1971), pp. 46–57; Int. MM, 7 Sept 1999, Rubale M; Int. CM, 11 Aug. 2000, Rubya, F.

[3] A. Richards and P. Reining, 'Report on fertility surveys in Buganda and Buhaya, 1952', University of Dar es Salaam library (UDSM), Cory 373.

[4] Richards and Reining, 'Fertility surveys in Buganda and Buhaya, 1952'; Mwemage Parish School Committee to Buhaya Council Secretary, 15 July 1961, MPA, L5/II/B.

[5] Int. PEK, 7 Aug. 2000, Nkimbo Bweramutima, F; Int. GK, 14 Aug. 2000, Nkindo, F; Int. JR, 8 Aug. 2000, Rubya, F.

administration were much more likely to be the focus of popular anger. But what really set Buhaya apart, not only from Buganda but from the rest of East Africa, was that official and popular discussions about sex and marriage were dominated by the issue of sex work. As one ethnographer recorded in 1952, 'the subject of prostitution is constantly discussed by white and black in Bukoba,' Buhaya's district capital[6] The huge numbers of sex workers who migrated to and from East Africa's cities symbolized for colonial officials the corruption of Haya society, and served for Haya men as a constant source of ethnic shame. They were, moreover, repeatedly blamed from all sides for Buhaya's high levels of STDs and low fertility. This chapter will focus on the development of sex work in relation to wider changes in marriage and sexuality in Buhaya, because prostitution distinguished this society not just from the other case studies but from the rest of East Africa, and because it would play so crucial a role in the subsequent spread of HIV.

'THE MAIN EXPORTS OF BUKOBA ARE PROSTITUTES AND COFFEE, IN THAT ORDER'[7]: THE SCALE OF HAYA SEX WORK IN THE CITY

Haya women were associated with East Africa's sex trade from the First World War, but, it seems, only came to dominate it from the 1930s. Estimating the number of Haya urban prostitutes is problematic as some attempted to acquire a new ethnic identity while abroad and not all women who left Buhaya for one of the region's cities became commercial sex workers. Yet Haya do not seem to have been particularly prominent in beer brewing or market trading, two of the major alternative sources of urban income available for unskilled women during this period. Female Haya were relatively frequently employed as barmaids in the city, but this was regarded, with some justification, as so poorly paid that women had to supplement their income through short-time sex to survive. Certainly informants made no attempt to play down the scale of Haya prostitution in the past. There were 'a multitude' or 'so many I can't count'. 'If it had not been for this killer disease [AIDS] all Haya women could have gone.'[8] Various estimates of the numbers of sex workers who had left Buhaya were made during our period, which taken together reinforce the sense that prostitution among the Haya was exceptionally common. An investigation in one chiefdom in 1938 found that 3.6% of all women, including 10.5% of women in their twenties, had 'run away' to the cities, it was presumed

[6] Richards and Reining, 'Fertility surveys in Buganda and Buhaya, 1952'.

[7] E. Huxley, *The Sorcerer's Apprentice* (London: Chatto and Windus, 1948), p. 191.

[8] T. Karigata to Buhaya Council Secretary, 13 July 1961, MPA, L5/II/B; Int. YK, 19 Aug. 2000, Kikukwe, F; Int. MK, 16 Aug. 2000, Kikukwe, F; Int. LM, 12 Aug. 2000, Kanoni, F; Int. SN, 25 Aug. 1999, Katoma, M.

to become prostitutes. The East African Medical Survey reported in 1952 that 'in the little village of Gera there are thirty-five known prostitutes'. Marja-Liisa Swantz's in-depth study of thirty households in Buhaya during the 1970s recorded eight former sex workers. Occasional attempts were also made to monitor the number of prostitutes leaving Bukoba by lake steamer. At its peak in 1948 the traffic totalled 100 women per week, whereas by 1954, partly due to sustained obstruction, partly to improvements in bus transport, the weekly total had fallen to twenty. Nonetheless, the Haya were reported to constitute the largest body of sex workers in most East African towns by this time, with estimates of uncertain reliability claiming that they were the majority in Kampala in 1954, made up half of Tanganyika's sex workers in 1956, and totalled 1,000 in Nairobi alone in 1963. Given that the Haya constituted only 1% of the East African population, this was a remarkable situation.[9]

CAUSES AND CONTEXT

The origins of sex work among the Haya were discussed in Chapter 3. A combination of aesthetics, commodified sex, and growing marital discord had combined to produce the first generation of Buhaya's prostitutes. What caused Haya to engage in sex work on such a remarkable scale after the 1920s though requires consideration of a number of changes which occurred during the mid-colonial period. The best-known explanation of Haya dominance of the East African sex trade emerged from Luise White's ground-breaking work on prostitution in Nairobi. White showed how the colonial state, even while it attempted to impose patriarchal, disciplinarian control over African society, created economic niches for women to exploit. White identified two major variants of home-based, pimp-free, sex work in colonial Nairobi, which evolved out of competing strategies of wealth-creation. *Malaya* sex workers waited at home for clients to turn up, and charged a premium for providing food, conversation, and a bed for the night, as well as just sex. *Malaya* largely

[9] A. Culwick, 'The population problem in the Bukoba district', Bukoba, 1938, UDSM, EAF CORY 239; East African Medical Survey, *Annual Report, 1952* (Nairobi: EAHC, 1953); M.-L. Swantz, *Women in Development: a Creative Role Denied. The Case of Tanzania* (London: Hurst, 1985), p. 71; DC to PC, 14 Jan. 1949, Annual Report for the Bukoba District for the year 1948, TNA 215/2237; A. Southall and P. Gutkind, *Townsmen in the Making: Kampala and its Suburbs* (Kampala: East African Institute of Social Research, 1957), pp. 71–3; 'Survey of Catholic Dioceses, 1956' (Rubaga archives), pp. 495–6; Sospeter Matola Matovu to Secretary, Tanganyika African Club Nairobi Branch, 10 Jan. 1963, MPA, L5/II/B. During another local survey in 1952 the EAMS identified forty-five former prostitutes, but its report was unclear whether these forty-five were part of a sub-sample of married women over thirty, which would mean that 6.6% had been sex workers, or whether the denominator should be all 2,051 women within the surveyed community, which would mean that 2.2% had been prostitutes.

divorced themselves from their rural backgrounds in order to be free to invest their profits in urban property and small business. These sex workers helped normalize male migrant labour, while becoming some of the wealthiest Africans in the city. *Wazi-wazi*, a much larger category of sex workers, sat outside their houses, calling out their prices to potential clients, and sought to maximize the number of short-time clients they could serve in a day. Haya women, notorious for their aggression and materialism, almost exclusively adopted the *wazi-wazi*, high turnover model of sex work. Haya women needed to accumulate rapidly, according to White, because they were responsible for repaying the bridewealth that their former husbands had paid their fathers when they had got married. According to White's narrative the great depression brought about such a major decline in coffee prices that many Haya men were forced to divorce their wives in order to realize their most valuable asset. The divorcee's father then encouraged his dutiful daughter to sell her body in order to enable him in turn to clear the debt he had acquired as a result of refunding her bridewealth. *Wazi-wazi*, it was hypothesized, was sex work on behalf of elderly rural cash-crop farmers, whose power over their daughters had been strengthened by colonial capitalism. For White, *wazi-wazi* were the most professional of sex workers because they were the most loyal of daughters.[10]

White's research in the 1980s was heavily reliant on oral sources, yet none of her interviewees were Haya. No Haya sex worker of the colonial era appeared to have retired in Nairobi, reinforcing their image as target migrants, and White was unfortunately unable to conduct research within Buhaya. *The Comforts of Home*, as the title suggests, therefore tells the story of the colonial sex industry predominantly from the viewpoint of the *malaya*. The image of the Haya it depicts is derived from their competitors in the city and from missionary sources in the countryside. The argument that Haya women, having been divorced in order to save their husbands from bankruptcy, then became sex workers in order to save their fathers from ruin, was first made by the missionary academic Bengt Sundkler in 1945. The neatness of its logic, reminiscent of the best sermons, has been criticized by the Haya historian Fred Kaijage, who doubts whether financial considerations would have been the major cause of divorce even in the 1930s.[11] Falling coffee prices and debt may have encouraged a few husbands to think in terms of cashing in their

[10] L. White, *The Comforts of Home: Prostitution in Colonial Nairobi* (Chicago: University of Chicago Press, 1990). Haya so dominated the *wazi-wazi* form of sex work that it was named after them, Haya often being referred to outside Tanganyika as Waziba.

[11] B. Sundkler, 'Marriage problems in the church in Tanganyika', *International Review of Missions*, 34 (1945), pp. 253–4; F. Kaijage, 'AIDS control and the burden of history in northwestern Tanzania', *Population and Environment*, 14, 3 (1993), pp. 287–93.

wives in the early 1930s, but local administrators' annual reports indicate that Buhaya suffered less during the great depression than much of Tanganyika. In 1930, even though coffee income had fallen to a third of the previous year, the district commissioner found no hardship in Buhaya, merely a reduction in the purchase of luxuries. By the mid-1930s the reports emphasized the relative prosperity of the Haya, most of whom had responded to the initial crisis by expanding and improving their cultivation, with Buhaya's coffee production increasing by 50% between 1929 and 1934. The depression, moreover, can hardly be blamed for the consistently high numbers of Haya women who left for the cities right through to independence, given that bridewealth demands fell rapidly in the 1930s, and coffee prices recovered from 1941.[12]

None of my interviewees remembered such a lineal connection between debt, divorce, and prostitution as Sundkler proposed. Material neglect though, along with brutality and polygamy, were given as the most common reasons for a wife to leave her marriage. A woman whose husband refused to buy her clothes had long been entitled to separate on the grounds that she was being publicly dishonoured, but as the colonial period progressed, new needs emerged which had to be satisfied. After the Second World War commodities such as soap and paraffin were transformed from luxuries to necessities, while husbandly refusal to invest in children's education was mentioned frequently as the reason for women leaving their marriages in Buhaya to become sex workers.[13] Rather than blaming absolute poverty, informants attributed such neglect to husbands' excessive drinking or to their diverting family resources away from the home towards their lovers.[14] Failure to produce an heir was the only factor which informants commonly mentioned as directly causing women to be divorced and then go on to become prostitutes. Surveys supported this association. Of 140 women from one community who had left their husbands and gone to the cities in the 1930s, almost two-thirds were childless, while of fifteen former sex workers interviewed by Swantz in the 1970s, eight had become prostitutes because they were childless, and another four because they had produced no sons. The connection between infertility and sex work resulted partly from the reduced likelihood of remarriage experienced by divorcees who were childless, given the Haya fixation with

[12] Bukoba District Annual Report 1930, TNA 215/77/D; Bukoba District Annual Report 1934, TNA 215/1136; C. Smith, 'The commoditization of African agriculture and changed social relations: The case of the Haya of Tanzania' (unpublished PhD dissertation, University of Essex, 1985), p. 337.

[13] Int. VPB, 9 Aug. 2000, Busindi, F; Int. FK, 16 Aug. 2000, Kikukwe, F; Int. KM, 18 Aug. 2000, Kikuku-Kanyigo, F; Int. SG, 21 Aug. 2000, Nkindo, F; Southall and Gutkind, *Townsmen*, pp. 79–81.

[14] Int. TM, 13 Aug. 2000, Busindi, F; Int. MM, 11 Aug. 2000, Ijumbi, F; Int. EK, 7 Aug. 2000, Kanyangereko Nkimbo, F; Int. MK, 3 Sept. 1999, Rubafu, M.

securing an heir. The relative attractiveness of the city was accordingly enhanced. In addition there existed a perception in Buhaya that sex with no possibility of reproduction was a pleasurable but ultimately meaningless self-indulgence. As one informant put it, 'the parents of the husband would argue that it was justifiable for him to divorce because the wife had produced no children and so she was like a prostitute to him.' Faced with such perceptions, becoming a sex worker may have been less difficult for the childless woman.[15]

The most important factor drawing Haya women to the cities was the belief that sex work was lucrative. One informant summed up the popular stereotype of the sex worker returned from the city. 'They were rich. They used their money to buy shambas [farms], houses; they enjoyed their life with their lovers, eating well and drinking beers.' Bukoba's district commissioner estimated in 1949 that more money came into Buhaya from prostitution *per capita* than from cash crop production.[16] This wealth was displayed conspicuously, and generously redistributed. An anthropologist working in the early 1950s found that the only village women in possession of such luxuries as gold teeth, bicycles, and sewing machines were former sex workers. Women who came back from the city were remembered as celebrating their success extravagantly, buying drinks and giving presents to whoever welcomed them. But the focus of their generosity was on more durable assets within the family, investing in the education of their own children, or, more often, their nieces and nephews, setting up a relative in business, or building permanent houses for their parents or siblings. They were, as one interviewee remembered, 'like kings'.[17] In the period of decolonization several sources claimed that parents' greed caused them to encourage their daughters to abandon their marriages and seek their fortune in the city.[18] Some interviewees agreed that this had

[15] Int. MM, 12 Aug. 2000, Kanoni, F; Int. MMM, 12 Aug. 2000, Kanoni, F; A. Culwick, 'The population problem in the Bukoba district: part II', Bukoba, 1938, UDSM, EAF CORY 239, p. 15; Swantz, *Women*, p. 72; Int. MT, 24 July 1998, Igombe, F. However, the East African Medical Survey found that fertility among forty-five former sex workers was not significantly lower than among the wider population. East African Medical Survey, *Annual Report, 1952*, pp. 30–31.

[16] Int. EK, 7 Aug. 2000, Kanyangereko Nkimbo, F; Int. MM, 12 Aug. 2000, Kamachumu, F; DC to PC, 14 Jan. 1949, Annual Report for the Bukoba District for the year 1948, TNA 215/2237.

[17] P. Reining, 'The Haya: The agrarian system of a sedentary people' (unpublished PhD dissertation, University of Chicago, 1967), p. 349; H. Lapioche, 'Table d'enquête sur les moeurs et coutumes indigènes, Diocese de Bukoba', 1956, p. 34, WFA; Int. SK, 21 June 2000, Rubya, M; Int. MPM, 10 Aug. 2000, Ibare, F; Int. MK, 3 Sept. 1999, Rubafu, M; Int. KK, 15 June 2000, Bibanja, F; Int. MM, 12 Aug. 2000, Kamachumu, F; Int. SN, 25 Aug. 1999, Katoma, M; Swantz, *Women*, p. 74.

[18] S. Rwenyama to Buhaya Council Secretary, 26 June 1961, MPA, L5/II/B; D. Muhingo to Buhaya Council Secretary, n/d [July 1961], MPA, L5/II/B; Ahamad s/o Musa to Buhaya Council Secretary, 13 July 1961, MPA, L5/II/B; Swantz, *Women*, p. 75 citing an article in *Kiongozi* newspaper in 1961.

occasionally happened, but many more indicated that it was the visible signs of success enjoyed by returning sex workers that encouraged women independently to decide to become prostitutes. One of the factors that contributed to popular antagonism against sex workers was the frequency with which their visits to family ended with them returning to the city accompanied by new recruits. 'They were stealing women!', as one informant put it. But most interviewees insisted that women typically chose to leave Buhaya freely, out of 'jealousy at seeing prostitutes coming with nice clothes, buying shambas and building houses'. 'Because of this temptation some women initiated quarrels with their husbands so they could be released to go to the city.' Some newlyweds reportedly even aborted pregnancies so they could cut all ties to their marriage. A new development of the 1940s was the large number of never married women who began to join the ranks of sex workers, who previously had almost always been widows and divorcees. In some cases, daughters followed mothers, or nieces joined aunts in what had become a family business.[19]

Women may often have entered the sex trade seduced by the glamour of returning prostitutes and their tales of the city. But they were also making strategic decisions about how to live a better life, free of the economic vulnerability which marriage so often entailed. The long-term goal of Haya sex workers was not to retire in the city or return to live with their parents, but to establish themselves as independent householders within their own communities. Merely repaying their bridewealth was not enough to win the approval of their parents. The generosity of returning prostitutes was understood as compensation for the shame their career choice had brought their families. But when ex-prostitutes purchased their own land, built a house of stone and corrugated iron, and produced bananas and coffee, they were claiming entitlement to a degree of respect. One former sex worker when asked why she had gone to Arusha answered not by referring to her wooden chairs, sewing machine, or carved doors, signs of wealth which set her above most of her neighbours, but to her land, which gave her security. 'People could do nothing to prostitutes for they owned their own houses and shambas.' This was not about isolated independence, or slavishly supporting a controlling father, but the achievement of a kind of self-mastery, demonstrated by

[19] Int. AS, 27 July 1998, Bukara, M; Int. MK, 3 Sept. 1999, Rubafu, M; Int. RMR, 13 Aug. 2000, Byabusha, Busindi, M; Int. FK, 16 Aug. 2000, Kikukwe, F; Int. FR, 27 June 2000, Rubya, M; Int. VPB, 9 Aug. 2000, Busindi, F; Int. MK, 16 Aug. 2000, Kikukwe, F; Int. RK, 16 June 2000, Kanyangereko, F; Int. AM, 14 June 2000, Isikila-Irungami, F; Bukoba District Annual Report 1947, TNA 215/2154; Swantz, *Women*, p. 74.

inclusion in the affairs of the kin-group and the village as an autonomous householder.[20]

SEX WORK WITHIN BUHAYA

The significance of sex workers for the wider history of STDs and sexuality in Buhaya is that so few of them were 'lost in the cities'. By 1948 as many Haya women were coming back through Bukoba port as were setting off for the urban centres. Prostitutes were sought out by local men during their frequent visits home, and typically remained sexually active after their retirement back in the village. They tied rural Buhaya into an international network of sexual contacts, dispersing the techniques, attitudes, and pathogens they had acquired abroad throughout the Haya countryside.[21]

Haya men had had access to sex workers who operated in Bukoba town since the 1920s. These were a substantial, prosperous body of women, who occupied the bulk of the better class of urban housing until the town's commercial and administrative expansion in the decade before independence.[22] Nonetheless, the question of whether prostitutes continued their involvement in commercial sex after returning from the city to the village is much more significant, given their numbers and the rarity of rural sex work in colonial Africa. This issue is obscured by problems of definition. In 1938 the colonial administrator Arthur Culwick, charged with investigating Haya sub-fertility, wrote that while professional prostitutes operated in the villages, 'almost any Haya woman can be induced by the payment of sixpence to sleep with almost any man.' Tanganyika's government anthropologist Hans Cory, Culwick's main source of information, wrote in the same year that it was because of exceptional levels of cattle disease that, equally exceptionally, 'village prostitution developed, an otherwise unknown feature with primitives.' As Haya

[20] Swantz, *Women*, pp. 67–76, L. Stevens, 'Bananas, babies, and women who buy their graves: Matrifocal values in a patrilineal Tanzanian society', *Canadian Journal of African Studies*, 29, 3 (1995), pp. 467–75; Larsson, *Conversion*, pp. 128–9; A. Manji '"Her name is Kamundage": Rethinking women and property among the Haya of Tanzania', *Africa*, 70, 3 (2000), p. 489; Z. Bader, 'Women, private property and production in Bukoba district' (unpublished MA dissertation, University of Dar es Salaam, 1975), pp. 21, 131, 157; Kaijage, 'AIDS control', pp. 287–293; Int. MMM, 12 Aug. 2000, Kanoni, F; Int. VPB, 9 Aug. 2000, Busindi, F. Cf. J. Lonsdale, 'Kikuyu Christianities', *Journal of Religion in Africa*, 29, 2 (1999), pp. 215–25.

[21] DC to PC, 14 Jan. 1949, Annual Report for the Bukoba District for the year 1948, TNA 215/2237; Int. VPB, 9 Aug. 2000, Busindi, F.

[22] Int. RMR, 13 Aug. 2000, Byabusha, Busindi, M; Bukoba District Annual Report 1934, TNA 215/1136; G. Macgregor, 'The incidence of syphilis among antenatal women attending Kagondo and Bukoba hospitals, maternity and child welfare clinics', Mar. 1942, Bukoba District Book, TNA; Swantz, *Women*, p. 75.

could not invest in livestock, their coffee income 'had to be spent in some way'. The number of professionals was supplemented, according to Cory, 'by wives who remain with their husbands, but like to earn some pocket money in the service of Venus'. Cory, like Culwick was prone to exaggeration, but his assertion that it had become 'impossible for a man to find affection without paying for it' was not entirely unfounded.[23] A number of informants emphasized that during the colonial period sexual affairs, as in Buganda, were sustained by the transfer of gifts from men to women. But in Buhaya these gifts increasingly took the form of cash. Interviewees distinguished between affairs and sex with prostitutes, where it existed in the villages, by the nature of the relationship, not monetization. Affairs were about love not livelihood—as one informant put it, 'prostitution is commercial and promiscuity is just for pleasure'—and were, spouses excepted, theoretically exclusive.[24]

There was disagreement among interviewees about whether village prostitution existed during the colonial period.[25] It seems likely that there was a diversity of experience, partly because some communities were more successful at expelling or disciplining returned sex workers than others. More importantly though, prostitution in the city had distributed its rewards unevenly. *Wazi-wazi* was a particularly competitive form of sex work and not all Haya women possessed the confidence, beauty, or skill to secure a regular supply of clients. The most unfortunate found the work repellent, were robbed, and beaten so badly that they could not continue, or were severely infected with STDs, so that they abandoned the city before they had made

[23] A. Culwick and G. Culwick, edited by V. Berry, *The Culwick Papers 1934–1944: Population, Food and Health in Colonial Tanganika* (London: Academic Books, 1994), pp. 174–5; H. Cory, 'The Haya tribe and the incidence of venereal disease, Bukoba 1938–48', TS, UDSM, EAF CORY 104. E. Akyeampong, 'Sexuality and prostitution among the Akan of the Gold Coast *c.* 1650–1950', *Past and Present,* 156 (1997), pp. 144–73 states that a form of prostitution also existed in some colonial-era rural communities in the Gold Coast. Cf. M. Hunter, 'The materiality of everyday sex: Thinking beyond "prostitution"', *African Studies*, 61, 1 (2002), pp. 99–120 for an extended discussion of difficulties of definition arising from the 'widespread link between gifts and sex in Africa'.

[24] Int. MK, 3 Sept. 1999, Rubafu, M; Int. EK, 7 Aug. 2000, Kanyangereko Nkimbo, F; Int. PEK, 7 Aug. 2000, Nkimbo Bweramutima, F; Int. FK, 16 Aug. 2000, Kikukwe, F; Int. MM, 11 Aug. 2000, Ijumbi, F; Int. SG, 21 Aug. 2000, Nkindo, M; Int. TM, Aug. 2000, Busindi, M.

[25] Informants who stated that commercial sex work did not exist in the villages during the colonial period included: Int. YK, 19 Aug. 2000, Kikukwe, F; Int. JM 12 Aug. 2000, Kanoni, M; Int. CKM, 17 Aug. 2000, Kibanda, F. The following informants were some of those who disagreed, though several stated that it was more common for returning prostitutes to have lovers than clients: Int. MK, 3 Sept. 1999, Rubafu, M; Int. PEK, 7 Aug. 2000, Nkimbo Bweramutima, F; Int. VPB, 9 Aug. 2000, Busindi, F; Int. AK, 8 Aug. 2000, Rubya, F; Int. AMA, 15 Aug. 2000, Rwagati, F; Int. JNK, 11 Aug. 2000, Ijumbi, M; Int. SK, 21 June 2000, Rubya, M.

significant savings. Lacking the means to purchase social acceptance and unable to marry, such women were often rejected by their families, suspected by their female neighbours of trying to tempt away their husbands, and sometimes driven away from local churches, which were the main source of respectability and solace for other categories of single women in the late colonial period. These unsuccessful returnees survived by finding employment as agricultural labourers, sometimes supplementing their income through sex, at times being paid in beer, cigarettes, or food instead of cash. Those women I interviewed who had failed as prostitutes were marked by poverty, isolation, and bitterness.[26]

Even prostitutes who returned to Buhaya with enough capital to buy land appear to have adopted varying strategies within the village economy. It seems that some women sought part-time payment for sex as their farming income alone was insufficient to maintain the lifestyle to which they had become accustomed in town. But the most successful prostitutes could afford to leave sex work behind them. These women are remembered as having lived like big men, dispensing patronage, owning tractors and cattle, hiring labourers, and often maintaining lovers in both village and Bukoba town.[27] While Haya women had made their money through functional but profitable short-time sex in the city rather than offering a night of pretend domesticity, what village men wanted was to luxuriate in the exotica of urban modernity: gramophone records, perfume, mattresses, and bedsheets. A recurring trope in the dreams recorded by the impoverished revivalist village preacher Loje in the 1950s was a woman reclining voluptuously on rich material. Male informants remembered finding returned sex workers, with their skin lightener and make-up, irresistible. 'A woman is naturally beautiful and attractive, so a man felt every pain paralysed when he slept with her. What then if such a woman adds to her beauty with adornments and embroideries?' Former prostitutes' unmatchable sexual skill, meanwhile, was attributed by both male and female informants to witchcraft. Village wives felt they could not compete: 'the prostitutes knew how to treat the husband better than the wife'. Informants who had worked as prostitutes believed that men sought them out because the comforts of home in rural households were not always so great. A farmer made his wife work all day in the fields, and then was unhappy that she had rough hands,

[26] Int. AK, 8 Aug. 2000, Rubya, F; Int. FK, 16 Aug. 2000, Kikukwe, F; Int. TM, 13 Aug. 2000, Busindi, F; Int. LM, 12 Aug. 2000, Kanoni, F; Int. GK, 21 Aug. 2000, Nkindo, F; Int. CB, 13 Aug. 2000, Busindi, F.

[27] Int. TM, 13 Aug. 2000, Busindi, F; Int. SKN, 22 Aug. 2000, Maruku-Butailuka-Kasha, F; Int. AM, 24 June 2000, Kashambya, F; Int. MM, 12 Aug. 2000, Kamachumu, F. Cf. Swantz, *Women*, p. 75; Bader, 'Women', p. 156.

smelt of sweat, and was always tired. 'Whereas we were able to look after a man tenderly.'[28]

THE RESPONSE TO HAYA SEX WORK

For colonial officials, prostitution was a symptom of a wider sickness affecting Haya society. In 1947 Elspeth Huxley's investigation into the effects of the 'sorcerer's magic' of European culture and technology on East African societies took her to Bukoba. Whereas much of the region was in her opinion doomed to famine and desertification, the banana and coffee permaculture of Buhaya offered enviable food security and stable incomes. 'The Bahaya seem to have achieved, in large measure, that state towards which our own society is so painfully struggling: the enjoyment of long hours, indeed weeks, of leisure, freedom from fear and want, and the satisfaction of material needs at the expense of the minimum of effort.' The Haya appeared to the innocent observer to be a perfect advertisement for the new technocratic and welfarist developmentalism of the post-war empire. But Bukoba's district administration moved swiftly to correct this image. Huxley was warned that 'this happy state, at least in their soft tropical climate, seems to have corroded their will to work and rotted away their self-respect and morals.' The Bahaya were the victims of 'too much prosperity'.[29]

District reports had associated immorality with financial security and low labour demands as early as 1925. The farming system of the Haya evoked little admiration among their colonial rulers. Haya were regularly criticized for refusing to grow their coffee in the approved manner, neglecting to dispose of diseased berries, to prune regularly, to monocrop, or to mulch tidily. Haya showed a similar, frustrating lack of faith in colonial agronomists' prescriptions for the treatment of banana weevil, panama disease, and nematodes, believing, with some justification, that the declining productivity of their staple plantain crop was the product of colonial actions in the first place, and that the proffered cures only made matters worse. Above all, they refused to increase the area under coffee once it had reached its natural limit in the long-established villages of the eastern ridges in the mid-1930s. The large numbers of young men apparently waiting around in eastern Buhaya to inherit land from their fathers offended Europeans who wanted to see them opening up

[28] Int. SK, 21 June 2000, Rubya, M; Int. RMR, 13 Aug. 2000, Byabusha, Busindi, M; B. Sundkler, *Bara Bukoba: Church and Community in Tanzania* (London: Hurst, 1980), p. 103; Int. PKK, 18 Aug. 2000, Mshumba-Byazi, F; Int. AM, 24 June 2000, Kashambya, F; Int. YK, 19 Aug. 2000, Kikukwe, F.

[29] Huxley, *Sorcerer's*, pp. 191–3.

new coffee farms of their own. Colonial commentators as early as 1932 convinced themselves that the eastern ridges had reached their carrying capacity, and that young men were unable to marry while they waited for their inheritance. Officials were outraged that young men preferred the seductive pleasures of their village lives to the opportunity to marry and head out west to the empty, fertile lands around Lake Ikimba. This lack of pioneering spirit, yet another example of the moral weakness of the Haya, was so problematic because the stagnation of Bukoba's coffee production threatened not only the broader development of Tanganyika, but administrators' own career progression. At its peak in 1935, Buhaya produced a quarter of all the coffee in East Africa. The years that followed though saw the hopes that the Haya would drag the rest of Tanganyika out of backwardness fade, with a series of district reports bemoaning declining tax revenues and local resistance to scientific farming methods.[30] The densely cultivated villages of Buhaya, the most productive land in Tanganyika, discomforted Europeans. With their rotting mulch and humid shade, high hedges and twisting paths, they symbolized corruption and darkness, and seemed to provide a perfect environment for the nurturing of sexual affairs.[31]

Buhaya remained one of the showcase districts of colonial Tanganyika, but its wealth, literacy, and political sophistication, which so impressed outsiders, disturbed many of the British officials who actually worked there. Bukoba was seen as a 'difficult' place to govern. One district commissioner recorded that its 'complex, vociferous and mass-educated population' was interested in only two subjects, education and STDs—'they suffer from both'. The chipper tone of the memoirs of one of his successors, Tim Harris, faltered only in the chapter entitled 'Bukoba—the ultimate test'. Harris had been forewarned of 'the never-satisfied ambitions and prideful sloth of the Bahaya as a tribe', but nonetheless 'the unremitting tension in Bukoba, coupled with the volume of work and the long hours of argument . . . bred in me a near-paranoia.' Exhaustion and frustration were the lot of Bukoba administrators,

[30] Bukoba District Annual Report 1925, TNA 1733/3:46 (AB40); Tanganyika Territory, *Department of Agriculture Annual Report, 1932* (Dar es Salaam: Government Printer, 1933); G. Milne, 'Bukoba: High and low fertility on a laterised soil', *The East African Agricultural Journal*, 4 (1938), pp. 14–15; Lake Province Annual Report 1940, TNA 215/1650; Annual Report for the Bukoba District for the year 1948, TNA 215/2237; D. McMaster, 'Change of regional balance in the Bukoba district of Tanganyika', *Tanganyika Notes and Records*, 56 (1961), pp. 89–91. Banana weevils appear to have been introduced to the region in the 1930s via the colonial botanic garden in Entebbe, while the insecticide dieldrin, used on a massive scale against banana pests from the 1950s, proved not only ultimately ineffective but highly toxic.

[31] H. Cory, 'The Haya tribe and the incidence of venereal disease, Bukoba 1938–48', TS, UDSM, EAF CORY 104, p. 7.

their creative energy constantly dissipated in the adjudication of appeal court cases. The Haya were the most litigious people in Tanganyika from the mid-1920s until independence, with around one-quarter of Haya adult males involved in legal disputes in any one year. Such crippling enthusiasm for the law, rather than being taken as an indication of local support for the *Pax Britannica*, was attributed by district officers to the Haya's misuse of their wealth, education, and free time.[32]

Early histories of sexuality and law in colonial Africa often argued that European officials, frequently in alliance with indigenous authorities, used concerns about prostitution and female independence as an opportunity for the patriarchal restriction of women's autonomy.[33] This was only partly true in Buganda, and even less so in Buhaya, for while colonial commentators did write critically of the materialism and easy virtue of Haya women, it was male behaviour that was the focus of their displeasure. The older generation were condemned for marrying young women at the expense of their sons, or, worse, for corrupting unmarried girls, often believing this would cure them of gonorrhoea. Young men were regarded as particularly profligate, squandering their money on prostitutes and 'useless luxury goods' rather than saving to pay bridewealth. Europeans by contrast frequently expressed sympathy for the female predicament in Buhaya, describing prostitution as 'their only escape'. 'The men are rotten with drink and VD—too demoralised to work, as a rule . . . No wonder [women] clear out and look for easy money in the towns.'[34]

[32] Bukoba District Annual Report 1947, TNA 215/2154; T. Harris, *Donkey's Gratitude: Twenty-two Years in the Growth of a New African Nation—Tanzania* (Durham: Pentland Press, 1992), pp. 235–7, 261, 266; Bukoba District Annual Report 1923, TNA 1733/8 (AB10); Bukoba District Annual Report 1928, TNA 215/77/B; Bukoba District Annual Report 1951, TNA 215/2510; Larsson, *Conversion*, pp. 90, 105.

[33] See e.g. M. Chanock, *Law, Custom and Social Order: The Colonial Experience in Malawi and Zambia* (Cambridge: Cambridge University Press, 1985); E. Schmidt, 'Patriarchy, capitalism, and the colonial state in Zimbabwe', *Signs,* 16, 4 (1991), pp. 732–56. More recent writing though has tended to emphasize that conflict about marriage and sexuality persisted despite codification in many societies. See e.g. J. Allman and V. Tashjian, *'I Will Not Eat Stone': A Women's History of Colonial Asante* (Portsmouth NH: Heinemann, 2000); B. Shadle, *Girl Cases: Marriage and Colonialism in Gusiiland, Kenya, 1890–1970* (Portsmouth NH: Heinemann, 2006); R. Jean-Baptiste, '"These laws should be made by us": Customary marriage law, codification and political authority in twentieth-century colonial Gabon', *The Journal of African History,* 49, 2 (2008), pp. 217–40.

[34] A. Culwick, 'The population problem in the Bukoba district', Bukoba, 1938, UDSM, EAF CORY 239, pp. 32–3; H. Cory, 'The Haya tribe and the incidence of venereal disease, Bukoba 1938–48', TS, UDSM, EAF CORY 104, pp. 3–6; G. Macgregor, 'The incidence of syphilis among antenatal women attending Kagondo and Bukoba hospitals, maternity and child welfare clinics', Mar. 1942, Bukoba District Book; EAMS, *Annual Report, 1952*, pp. 68–9; Huxley, *Sorcerer's*, pp. 192–3. The belief that sex with a virgin would cure STDs reappeared in the early years of the AIDS epidemic.

Hans Cory explained the dissipation of Haya males in classic terms, their cultural integrity having been lost with their twin roles of herdsman and warrior. 'Because of the pacification of the country by the Europeans and the advent of rinderpest the men lost the purpose of their life and with it the concrete basis of their tribal customs and institutions.' Arthur Culwick agreed that the 'breaking up of Bantu society' lay at the heart of the crisis of masculinity and morality in Buhaya, but viewed its collapse as the consequence of the very nature of colonial rule. Tribal discipline had been undermined by European libertarianism and the atomizing and degrading economic independence provided by cash cropping. Indirect rule had permitted the local kings, the Bakama, with their 'passive resistance and courteous obstruction', to blunt European guidance, causing Haya to laugh 'at our administration as effete and incapable of even making the most highly paid native official do any work'. The result was 'the complete breakdown of sexual morality in the tribe. The Bahaya could hardly achieve a greater degree of promiscuity if they tried.' Haya women, regarded 'as an agricultural machine and a domestic drudge' by their 'drunken, lazy and generally dissolute' husbands, had understandably chosen a life of prostitution. For Culwick, these women symbolized the corrupting, deracinating nature of colonial capitalism: they 'sell themselves in Bukoba during the coffee season and then migrate to Mwanza or Uganda for the cotton season'. The absence of restraint, and the prevalence of STDs which resulted, had caused 'a much greater degree of neurosis than I have seen in any other tribe' and lay behind Bukoba's notorious difficulty as an administrative posting. Freedom from compulsion had made Haya men not only bad husbands but also unruly subjects. Culwick's solution was to force the Haya to control sexual misbehaviour within their own communities. He was 'unable to see that any able-bodied man has any right whatsoever to fritter away his life in an orgy of drink and women', and predicted that coercion would not only improve public health and morality, but that 'beneficial psychological changes would follow which would make the tribe much easier to deal with'.[35]

Culwick, seeing himself as an ideas man, left the details of the programme of compulsion to be worked out by Cory, who in late 1938 provided a remarkable set of proposals based on the establishment of highly intrusive village-level societies or *viama*. These would act as channels of moral propaganda, agents for the organization of STD testing and treatment, and sources of improving entertainment. Primarily though they would 'separate the healthy

[35] H. Cory, 'The Haya tribe and the incidence of venereal disease, Bukoba 1938–48', TS, UDSM, EAF CORY 104, p. 1; Culwick, Culwick and Berry, *Population*, pp. 124, 174–7, 228–9; A. Culwick, 'The population problem in the Bukoba district', Bukoba, 1938, UDSM, EAF CORY 239, pp. 29–35, 41, 66.

from the sick', with membership dependent on a negative STD test. Members would wear a badge, inform on fellow villagers who were infected with STDs, and agree never to pay nor receive money for sex. Cory's vision was one of gradualist moral reform, so several concessions were made to limit the damage caused by inevitable lapses. Female members, for example, would be advised to ensure 'that after marriage they will select their lovers from the membership of the [v]iama'. The real target of the campaign would be 'the worst offenders, the prostitute and the men of similar character. These mobile incubators of bacilli have to be rendered innocuous as soon as possible.' Cory anticipated that as a result of isolation and harassment 'a lot of the village beauties would emigrate', so he planned that quarantine stations would be set up at Bukoba port and the Uganda border where all female travellers would be forced to accept examination and treatment for STDs.[36]

Cory and Culwick's proposals came to nothing in the short term. Culwick's critique of indirect rule and cash cropping was hardly likely to win the approval of central government, while Cory's programme required the energetic moral leadership of Bakama and local chiefs across Buhaya. Yet, as one informant remembered, 'the chiefs themselves were notorious adulterers.'[37] Local communities, frustrated at the inaction of both colonial and chiefly governments, now took the lead in trying to deal with the problem of prostitution. Women were expelled from some villages where they were blamed for infecting a man who had paid them for sex with an STD, which he then passed on to his wife. In other cases, parents who were unable or unwilling to recall their daughters from the cities were boycotted. And throughout Buhaya chiefs came under increasing pressure to prevent women from leaving the district. On one occasion a Mukama who had protected a woman's freedom of movement against the wishes of her father had to seek colonial protection, chased from his kingdom by a mob of angry subjects.[38] In 1946 Buhaya's chiefly council passed new rules forbidding women suspected of being prostitutes from boarding the lake steamer. The district commissioner, facing accusations that colonial obstruction would be further proof of a British plot to reduce Haya numbers, approved the rules, only for them to be overturned by the central government on the grounds that they interfered with the liberty of the individual.[39] Accordingly local government endeavoured to undermine prostitution within Buhaya. A dual strategy emerged which attempted to

[36] H. Cory, 'The Haya tribe and the incidence of venereal disease, Bukoba 1938–48', TS, UDSM, EAF CORY 104, pp. 9–19.

[37] Int. RMR, 13 Aug. 2000, Byabusha, Busindi, M.

[38] Int. AK, 8 Aug. 2000, Rubya, F; Int. FK, 16 Aug. 2000, Kikukwe, F; Int. YK, 19 Aug. 2000, Kikukwe, F; Harris, *Donkey's*, pp. 261–5. Cf. Hyden, *Political*, p. 110.

[39] Harris, *Donkey's*, pp. 261–5; Huxley, *Sorcerer's*, p. 192.

both reduce the attractiveness of sex work, and offer 'respectable women . . . a glimpse of progress to better things for themselves without resorting to the usual course of emancipation through prostitution'. So rules were passed against prostitutes operating in the trading centres and buying land in the villages, but daughters were allowed to inherit part of their fathers' estates, and substantial funds were voted for female education and women's clubs.[40]

As the 1950s progressed the colonial administration increasingly focused on the consequences rather than the causes of immorality, targeting its energy on mass, compulsory treatment for STDs. Buhaya's chiefs meanwhile spent a number of years debating Uganda's repressive 1941 legislation against local prostitution. Ignoring all warnings that the Uganda system had reduced merely the visibility not the prevalence of sex work, Buhaya's council drafted near-identical regulations in 1958, which by 1961 were found to be 'quite useless'.[41] By this point political leadership within Haya society had shifted from Bakama to nationalists, whose primary concern was Buhaya's place in the emerging Tanganyikan nation and the ever more integrated East African region. As Derek Peterson has argued, prostitution had been regarded as something of an ethnic embarrassment by conservative patriots since at least the 1940s.[42] In 1950 the Haya Union revived the issue of female emigration, and set up its own checkpoint at Bukoba port, turning away women who could not prove that they were travelling on legitimate business and had chiefly, husbandly, or parental approval. The district administration turned a blind eye, only restoring freedom of movement in 1951, after several Haya women had sued the Union for obstruction and assault, though popular belief held that the blockade crumbled when a group of prostitutes chartered a plane to take them to Nairobi. Popular disgust with Haya sex workers was often tinged with admiration of their flair.[43]

[40] Annual Report for the Bukoba District for the year 1953, TNA 215/2700; Minutes of Buhaya Council, 3–4 Dec. 1956, MPA, L5 II B; Swantz, *Women*, p. 61; Bukoba District Annual Report 1946, TNA 215/2070; Bukoba District Annual Report 1944, TNA 215/1898.

[41] DC to PC, 10 Apr. 1951, in Bukoba: Official Correspondence relating to constitutional matters, politics and land, including notes and memoranda by Hans Cory, 1950–8, UDSM, EAF Cory 21; Minutes of Buhaya Council, 3–4 Dec. 1956, MPA, L5 II B; Locgov, Dar es Salaam, to Buhaya Native Council, 10 Sept. 1958, MPA, L5 II B; Political Bukoba to Provincer Bukoba, 6 May 1961, MPA, L5 II B.

[42] D. Peterson, 'Prostitution and patriotism in Northwestern Tanganyika' (unpublished seminar paper, African History Group, Cambridge, 30 October 2007).

[43] Peterson, 'Prostitution'; Swantz, *Women*, p. 77; H. Trant, 'Not Merrion Square: Anecdotes from a woman's medical career in Africa', RHO, MSS.Af.s.1872(143), p. 128. An example of the contempt with which many Haya viewed sex workers was the belief that they were the source of a new STD known as *kauzi*, named after its thread-like discharge. Local doctors consider *kauzi* to be advanced penicillin-resistant gonorrhoea, but it is popularly thought to be a canine disease, the result of Europeans paying Haya prostitutes to have sex with their dogs. Pers. comm. Y. Swai.

Male migrants in the cities then unsuccessfully sought to restore their ethnic good name by attempting to register and repatriate all Haya sex workers, until approaching independence offered hope that Bukoba's executive authority, freed from chiefly inertia and colonial weakness, could be projected into East Africa's urban slums.[44] Haya men in the city were shamed by the behaviour of their female compatriots. Men from other ethnic groups thanked Haya men for providing them with such sensual bedfellows, greeted them as their in-laws, and mocked their inability to control their womenfolk.[45] In May 1961, coinciding with Tanganyika's achievement of self-government, the Buhaya Council distributed a survey entitled 'How to stop prostitution' throughout the district and among the Haya diaspora, signalling its new attentiveness to popular concerns. The seventy or so responses blamed prostitution for a host of Buhaya's ills: growing marital instability, declining fertility, high levels of STDs, underdevelopment, weakening religious fervour, theft, and violence. But above all respondents emphasized the 'shame and disgrace' that prostitutes 'who . . . sell themselves like oranges in the market' brought to their 'nation' of Buhaya. Some writers displayed a bucolic antagonism to the corrupting influence of town life, but others argued that Haya men were deterred from conquering the city by the derision they knew they would encounter. Sex work prevented Buhaya from reaping the rewards of its educational advantages.[46] Haya males were outraged by prostitutes' abuse of their ethnic identity. Nairobi's most famous prostitute had not only written in stone that Buhaya was the home of prostitution by naming her residence in Kenya's capital Bukoba House, but, with a number of her colleagues, she had publicly declared that they were Baziba from Kiziba, not Haya, a deliberate insult aimed at the male-dominated Haya Union.[47] This rejection of an amalgamated ethnicity further threatened the prominence that the Haya, as Tanganyika's third-largest grouping, claimed within independent Tanganyika. Haya patriotism, evolving rapidly in response to nationalist politics and the collapse of royal authority, sought an alliance with the emerging bureaucratic state in order to eradicate prostitution. Many Haya expressed confidence that

[44] 1952 Annual Report of the Senior Community Development Officer, Community Development Reports, Kampala, RHO, MSS. Afr. s. 590.

[45] Int. SN, 25 Aug. 1999, Katoma, M; Sospeter Matola Matovu to Secretary, Tanganyika African Club Nairobi Branch, 10 Jan. 1963, MPA, L5/II/B.

[46] S. Rwenyama to Buhaya Council Secretary, 26 June 1961, MPA, L5/II/B; Haya students of Saint Andrew's Teacher Training College, Korogwe to Buhaya Council Secretary, 6 July 1961, MPA, L5/II/B; E. Muhigi to Buhaya Council Secretary, 12 July 1961, MPA, L5/II/B; T. Karigata to Buhaya Council Secretary, 13 July 1961, MPA, L5/II/B; Y. Sulemani to Buhaya Council Secretary, 7 July 1961, MPA, L5/II/B.

[47] Sospeter Matola Matovu to Secretary, Tanganyika African Club Nairobi Branch, 10 Jan. 1963, MPA, L5/II/B.

Buhaya could, and must, be saved from its degradation by the new national government. Independence, they argued, brought empowerment, but also serious responsibility. 'Tanganyika and all the citizens have hated prostitution for a long time, but the colonial government was deaf to the cries of the people . . . Now we, from the coast to the hinterland, rule, so we have the powers to stop prostitution.' Sex work 'spoils and disparages our independent and holy nation of Tanganyika'. National pride dictated that Tanganyikans 'imitate the civilised countries like UK where such acts of disgrace are not visible'.[48]

The growing popular reaction against the exploitation and brutality of royal rule meant that Haya campaigners for moral reform, unlike those in Buganda, tended not to glorify a distant, purer past, before cultural integrity was contaminated by western influence. Informants in Buhaya were much more likely to complain of chiefs' sexual acquisitiveness than those in Ankole and Buganda. For several respondents to the 1961 survey, 'customs are the source of prostitution—many children are brought up to copy the bad behaviour of their parents.'[49] The fathers of sex workers in particular were the subject of sustained criticism. Their greed for high bridewealth forced the young to marry for money not love, their inattentiveness ensured that Buhaya's bars and dance clubs were full of young girls, their profligacy forced their divorcees to repay their own bridewealth through sex, and their shamelessness caused them to accept with joy the money, clothes, and cars earned through their daughters' dishonest sweat.[50] The responses to the survey, even though they were almost entirely authored by men, were surprisingly even-handed in their criticisms. One asserted that 'the root cause of prostitution is

[48] Mwemage Parish School Committee to Buhaya Council Secretary, 15 July 1961, MPA, L5/II/B; Ahamad s/o Musa to Buhaya Council Secretary, 13 July 1961, MPA, L5/II/B; David Sekabembe to Buhaya Council Secretary, 9 July 1961, MPA, L5/II/B; A. Salim to Buhaya Council Secretary, 4 July 1961, MPA, L5/II/B; Sospeter Matola Matovu to Secretary, Tanganyika African Club Nairobi Branch, 10 Jan. 1963, MPA, L5/II/B; Fr. D. Kashagaki to Buhaya Council Secretary, 12 July 1961, MPA, L5/II/B. Kashagaki though did have some doubts whether the new era of party politics could bring moral uplift, noting that prostitution caused 'quarrelling, hatred and even deaths because sex workers . . . have to argue and compete just like politicians do for votes'.

[49] e.g. Int. RMR, 13 Aug. 2000, Byabusha, Busindi, M; D. Muhingo to Buhaya Council Secretary, n/d [July 1961], MPA, L5/II/B; E. Mutoka to Buhaya Council Secretary, 12 July 1961, MPA, L5/II/B; Fr. D. Kashagaki to Buhaya Council Secretary, 12 July 1961, MPA, L5/II/B. But see Mwemage Parish School Committee to Buhaya Council Secretary, 15 July 1961, MPA, L5/II/B.

[50] D. Muhingo to Buhaya Council Secretary, n/d [July 1961], MPA, L5/II/B; David Sekabembe to Buhaya Council Secretary, 9 July 1961, MPA, L5/II/B; Y. Lutabanzibwa and M. Kamondo to Buhaya Council Secretary, n/d [July 1961], MPA, L5/II/B; S. Rwenyama to Buhaya Council Secretary, 26 June 1961, MPA, L5/II/B; Fr D. Kashagaki to Buhaya Council Secretary, 12 July 1961, MPA, L5/II/B; Ahamad s/o Musa to Buhaya Council Secretary, 13 July 1961, MPA, L5/II/B; Haya students of Saint Andrew's Teacher Training College, Korogwe to Buhaya Council Secretary, 6 July 1961, MPA, L5/II/B.

men mistreating their wives; treating them like strangers in their own homes ... hiding the amount of salaries they earn, or selling harvests that they worked hard together to plant ... and spending the whole night in night clubs.' The wife's 'heart breaks and she starts thinking about running away'. Another asserted that prostitution would only end if their clients were heavily penalized: 'Then to whom would sex workers sell their bodies? Maybe dogs.' Others made pragmatic suggestions about how to reduce the attractiveness of sex work, such as ensuring that couples were better prepared for marriage and enhancing career opportunities for women.[51]

Nonetheless, even though respondents accepted that male behaviour must also be monitored and forced to change, their prescriptions focused on the need to regulate the movement and actions of prostitutes, the 'disseminators of disease' and 'the biggest enemy of Buhaya'.[52] The idea of stopping Haya women from leaving for the cities was revived yet again, but new optimism was engendered by the bureaucratic power of the Tanganyikan nation. Women on the move would have to carry a passport, licence, or marriage certificate so that their identities and destinations could be approved.[53] Respondents also wanted to see prostitutes forcibly returned from the cities, partly because of the belief that sex workers' success attracted others to follow them, but primarily to end Haya ethnic shame. Again the responses rang with confidence in the executive capacity of free government. Even Haya women who pretended to belong to local ethnic groups could be hunted down by plain-clothes investigators and extradited from the cities.[54] Once returned to

[51] D. Muhingo to Buhaya Council Secretary, n/d [July 1961], MPA, L5/II/B; Mwemage Parish School Committee to Buhaya Council Secretary, 15 July 1961, MPA, L5/II/B; Fr. D. Kashagaki to Buhaya Council Secretary, 12 July 1961, MPA, L5/II/B; S. Rwenyama to Buhaya Council Secretary, 26 June 1961, MPA, L5/II/B; David Sekabembe to Buhaya Council Secretary, 9 July 1961, MPA, L5/II/B; Bushasha Village Council to Buhaya Council Secretary, 11 July 1961, MPA, L5/II/B; Ahamad s/o Musa to Buhaya Council Secretary, 13 July 1961, MPA, L5/II/B; Y. Lutabanzibwa and M. Kamondo to Buhaya Council Secretary, n/d [July 1961], MPA, L5/II/B; Haya students of Saint Andrew's Teacher Training College, Korogwe to Buhaya Council Secretary, 6 July 1961, MPA, L5/II/B.

[52] Haya students of Saint Andrew's Teacher Training College, Korogwe to Buhaya Council Secretary, 6 July 1961, MPA, L5/II/B; E. Muhigi to Buhaya Council Secretary, 12 July 1961, MPA, L5/II/B. Cf. Peterson, 'Prostitution'.

[53] T. Karigata to Buhaya Council Secretary, 13 July 1961, MPA, L5/II/B; Mwemage Parish School Committee to Buhaya Council Secretary, 15 July 1961, MPA, L5/II/B; Bushasha Village Council to Buhaya Council Secretary, 11 July 1961, MPA, L5/II/B.

[54] Mwemage Parish School Committee to Buhaya Council Secretary, 15 July 1961, MPA, L5/II/B; T. Karigata to Buhaya Council Secretary, 13 July 1961, MPA, L5/II/B; David Sekabembe to Buhaya Council Secretary, 9 July 1961, MPA, L5/II/B; Y. Sulemani to Buhaya Council Secretary, 7 July 1961, MPA, L5/II/B;. Cf. Sospeter Matola Matovu to Secretary, Tanganyika African Club Nairobi Branch, 10 Jan. 1963, MPA, L5/II/B.

their homeland, many respondents recommended that ex-prostitutes should be forced to rejoin their husbands, or to accept whoever would be prepared to marry them. Those who refused to accept marital discipline would be incarcerated in a designated prostitutes' prison, where the performance of public works would cure their selfishness.[55]

The curative potential of honest labour recurred as a theme even in those responses which favoured prostitutes being reabsorbed into society, rather than institutionalized. Male Haya wanted prostitutes to be producers not parasites, blaming them for the food shortages which were in fact largely due to declining yields. 'Prostitution brings about hunger in the country because prostitutes like feasting on other people's sweat.' Sex workers 'visit their parents when there is food then leave when it is finished', and men 'give prostitutes money at the expense of their wives and children'. Many writers mused on the TANU slogan *Uhuru na Kazi*, observing that 'Freedom and Work does not mean Freedom and Idleness.' Anxious husbands complained that prostitutes, 'the leaders of laziness', infected previously industrious wives with their indolent example. Many societies in this region viewed unmarried women as a burden on their families, but in Buhaya, with its densely settled villages, unproductive females were viewed with particular hostility. 'The hoe is the source of good livelihood here in Buhaya. Eating our food without cultivating is like sucking our blood.' In language reminiscent of colonial agronomists in the 1930s, prostitutes were told to go and dig on the infertile *rweya* grassland surrounding the villages or settle the empty lands to the west.[56]

This utopian vision of reformed sex workers building the nation was not shared by all respondents. Some believed that rigorous border control could end Haya prostitution abroad but feared that eradicating it within Buhaya itself 'is maybe just impossible'. Again the answer lay in regulation, to physically contain illicit sex so that it could be effectively monitored. Sex workers within Buhaya should be licenced, so that their STD status could be regularly checked, they could be forced to operate within designated zones, and above all so that clients would be deterred from using them. 'A licence costing one hundred shillings per month would push the cost of a visit to fifteen or thirty shillings for a night, which would be too expensive for most men.' The most complex proposal, from a teacher named Karigata, recommended that two

[55] Y. Lutabanzibwa and M. Kamondo to Buhaya Council Secretary, n/d [July 1961], MPA, L5/II/B; Fr. D. Kashagaki to Buhaya Council Secretary, 12 July 1961, MPA, L5/II/B.

[56] Bushasha Village Council to Buhaya Council Secretary, 11 July 1961, MPA, L5/II/B; Ayubu Saidi to Buhaya Council Secretary, 10 July 1961, MPA, L5/II/B; David Sekabembe to Buhaya Council Secretary, 9 July 1961, MPA, L5/II/B; Y. Sulemani to Buhaya Council Secretary, 7 July 1961, MPA, L5/II/B; Haya students of Saint Andrew's Teacher Training College, Korogwe to Buhaya Council Secretary, 6 July 1961, MPA, L5/II/B. Cf. Stevens, 'Bananas', p. 475.

forms of prostitution be permitted in Buhaya. 'Village girls' should be registered and regularly treated for STDs, and only allowed to operate from their own homes. 'Town girls' in Bukoba and the larger trading centres would be accommodated in government brothels and pay income tax and a higher licence fee. Karigata's proposals, like Cory's a generation before, were all about sharpening the blurred edges of Haya sexuality. Commercial sex would be physically separated from neighbourly, social sex in both town and village, and part-time prostitutes would be forced to accept the responsibilities of full-time professionalism or be driven away.[57]

Buhaya's citizens in 1961 seem to have over-estimated the bureaucratic capacity and unity of purpose of the emergent independent state. There is no record of the Buhaya Council's Sub-committee for the Prevention of Prostitution acting on any of the recommendations it sought. In 1962 Edward Barongo, the highest ranking Haya official within the ruling party, gave a speech in Bukoba where he complained that his audience was almost entirely male. According to Barongo, Bukoba's women were all prostitutes who preferred private business in bars to debating public concerns, and wore barbarous *cha cha cha* clothes 'that dirty the nation'. Two days later, in response to Barongo's call, prostitutes shopping in Bukoba's markets were verbally criticized for dressing indecently, prompting one to strip naked. Bukoba's member of parliament then intervened, defending the right of prostitutes to dress as they pleased. Then in January 1963 several Haya sex workers from Nairobi informed a Kenyan national newspaper that the Tanganyika African Club no longer represented their interests, and instead they had appointed one Amnazo Juma as their 'chief of general staff', and indeed 'queen of the women of Bukoba'. In response a male migrant wrote directly to TANU complaining that the growing profile of Haya prostitutes abroad was 'a source of embarrassment for our holy nation of Tanganyika'. TANU merely passed the issue on to the semi-official National Council of Tanganyika Women. Prostitution next resurfaces in the historical record only in the wake of the Arusha Declaration which heralded not only villagization, but also a much more intensely interventionist and bureaucratic form of government. In Missenyi, an area already dominated by the cross-border smuggling that would shape the early development of the HIV epidemic in Buhaya and Buganda, medical officers in 1967 reported that STDs had 'become rampant . . . due to an increase in prostitution'. The response of the local administration was perhaps indicative of the continuing difficulty of defining the sex worker, as petty urbanization reshaped rural economies and

[57] T. Karigata to Buhaya Council Secretary, 13 July 1961, MPA, L5/II/B; David Sekabembe to Buhaya Council Secretary, 9 July 1961, MPA, L5/II/B; A. Salim to Buhaya Council Secretary, 4 July 1961, MPA, L5/II/B.

patterns of socializing. All women working in bars and hotels across the area were to be sent in for medical certification twice a month, while women in 'trading centres and minor settlements' without formal employment were to be arrested and 'chased back to their homes'. Two months later the local administrator was forced to warn bar and hotel owners that their businesses faced closure, as their failure to ensure their staff were medically examined was 'not a way of fulfilling our politics of *ujamaa* [familyhood] and self-independence'. Controlling sex work had proven impossible for colonial administrators and kings, and then for local patriots energized by the victory of nationalism. Whether Missenyi's Sublocation Executive Officer could do better, supported by the disciplinary power that gave the moralizing ideology of *ujamaa* its edge, is unknown, for the local archival trail ran cold after 1967. The experience of the 1970s though would suggest that any success must have been short-lived.[58]

CONCLUSION

The pattern of sexual behaviour which would facilitate the rapid rural diffusion of HIV across Buhaya in the late 1970s was already well established by the 1960s. Extra-marital affairs had long been common, and pre- and post-marital sex had increased significantly in frequency in the later colonial period. But what made Buhaya distinct was the highly commercialized nature of sex there. A remarkably large number of women left Buhaya for the cities, where, as Luise White's classic study has shown, they dominated short-time prostitution. Viewing sex work from the point of origin and return, rather than from the city itself, however, has added several strands to the story of Haya prostitution. Haya women may often have gone to urban areas in order to enable their fathers to repay their bridewealth, but they stayed in order to earn enough money to purchase social acceptance and autonomy. Not all women succeeded in this goal, however, and the sad fate of the failed prostitute should temper any tendency to glamorize the East African sex industry. Yet those prostitutes who returned to Buhaya 'with a bicycle, a sewing machine, and enough money to buy a small farm' undoubtedly were perceived as alluring objects of desire because of the luxurious urbanity with which

[58] E. Barongo, Deputy General Secretary TANU to Shell Muhanna MP, 18 Jan. 1962, MPA, L5/II/B; Sospeter Matola Matovu to Secretary, Tanganyika African Club Nairobi Branch, 10 Jan. 1963, MPA, L5/II/B; Abdu Semanda, Deputy Area Secretary TANU, Bukoba to the Secretary General, National Council of Tanganyika Women, 18 Jan. 1963, MPA, L5/II/B; Hyden, *Political*, p. 136; Divisional Executive Officer to All Assistant Divisional Officers and All Village Executive Officers, Missenyi, 2 Mar. 1967, MPA, F37/54; Sublocation Executive Officer to All Bar and Hotel Owners, Minziro-Missenyi, 12 Apr. 1967, MPA, M1/188.

they tempted local men.[59] Haya prostitutes may have been *wazi-wazi* in the city but they were more like *malaya* in the countryside. Haya women may not have continued as full-time pure prostitutes when they returned from the city to the village, but they helped ensure that exchanging money for sex became one of the characteristics of rural life in Buhaya. Meanwhile, fully commercial sex was available from the 1920s in Bukoba town and in large townships like Muleba, Kamachumu, and Kyaka a couple of decades later. By the 1960s even small trading centres seem to have supported bars and hotels where barmaids and waitresses offered paid sex.

Haya society was highly mobile and intensely social. Haya found spouses outside their home villages, women frequently visited relatives, while males commonly possessed a second occupation in addition to farming, which required them to commute on a daily or weekly basis. Bukoba town, which had a population of 8,141 by 1967, 43% of whom were female, was the hub of the district's commercial and social economy. Securing contracts and trading depended on a wide circle of acquaintance, maintained by frequent socializing. An economy based on banana and coffee permaculture created village settlements of exceptional population density, often extending over two square miles, and allowed for extensive opportunities for leisure and non-agricultural work. This was a society that was very different from much of colonial Tanganyika. In Buhaya social networks and behavioural norms were shaped by neighbours and acquaintances more than kin groups, due to historic low fertility, while the agricultural system relied on careful, constant, low-level nurturing, in contrast to the intense, sporadic nature of arable cultivation. These social characteristics created a rich, complex culture, but could also be interpreted as providing ideal conditions in which individuals could pursue multiple sexual contacts. Certainly colonial officials tended to see only unusual potential for idleness and immorality. The East African Medical Survey, for example, finished its analysis of the causation of STDs in Buhaya by discussing 'one more disease, namely prosperity'. This provoked the anthropologist Priscilla Reining to comment how curious it was:

> that, in a world where underdevelopment was already becoming a keyword, a people whose average income was no more than £30 a year were thought to be 'too wealthy' by the Europeans who lived among them. The people, whose system of cultivation was such that there were no 'hunger months', were somehow downgraded because 'it makes their life too easy', as if poor nutrition were a goal to be achieved rather than a state to be avoided.

[59] Trant, 'Not Merrion Square', p. 128.

The problem for colonial administrators was that they were trying to control a rural society which had a semi-urban way of life.[60]

By the 1950s the animosity felt towards the Haya by colonial officials was fully reciprocated, and the attempts of the Bakama to regulate their subjects' behaviour foundered as populist antagonism to royal domination took on a more organized form.[61] Nationalist politics heightened male Haya's sense of shame at the notoriety which prostitution had earned their ethnic group, their desire for national leadership reinvigorating the drive for moral uplift in their homeland. The Haya world was transformed in the 1960s, but Haya patriots' prescriptions for the prostitution problem had much in common with colonial reformers like Hans Cory and Arthur Culwick. The determination to sharpen the distinction between affairs and prostitution and to control sexual behaviour through regulation and intrusive supervision survived independence intact, but Haya males appropriated colonial criticisms of endemic laziness and refusal to settle new land that had been targeted at men and redirected them at prostitutes. Letters written by Haya men in the early 1960s frequently referred to the TANU slogans 'Freedom and Work' and 'Freedom and Justice' which promised that independence would bring true liberty, but in their vision of the good society, freedom belonged only to the righteous. Incarceration, forced labour, forced marriage, licensing, and registration—these restrictions on the rights of citizenship would cure Buhaya's sickness, if the bureaucratic power of the new state lived up to popular expectations.

The various attempts to eradicate prostitution within Buhaya over this period appear to have been entirely unsuccessful, but the export of Haya sex workers to the region's cities does seem to have slowed down from the 1950s. The repeated obstruction of female emigration may have played a part in this, though the blockade of the port was never sustained for long and road transport was more difficult to control. Both documentary and oral sources considered that allowing women to inherit land, expanding girls' education, and improving female opportunities to secure a legitimate income did provide alternatives to sex work for some women. In addition husbandly behaviour

[60] Tanzania, *1967 Population Census: Vol. II, Statistics for Urban Areas* (Dar es Salaam: Government Printer, 1970), pp. 2–13; Hyden, *Political*, pp. 264, 271; Laurie and Trant, *East African Medical Survey*, p. 140; Reining, 'A sedentary people', pp. iv, 75–8, 131–6, 315–20. Reining observed that 'the Haya display a division of labour, relatively reliable productivity per cropping unit, individual tenure of land and an emerging emphasis on the small domestic group which are urban-like. These social characteristics suggest that for the Haya, and inferentially, other Lacustrine Bantu, the urban:rural dichotomy is inadequate and should be enlarged to comprehend true urban life . . . high density rural societies, of which Haya is one example, and low density rural societies.'

[61] Reining, 'A sedentary people', p. 320; Harris, *Donkey's*, p. 266; Annual Report for the Bukoba District for the year 1957, TNA 215/3449; Hyden, *Political*, pp. 113–19, 130.

supposedly improved towards the end of the colonial period, in some cases in recognition of the frequency with which unhappy wives escaped to the city, more broadly because high coffee prices enabled greater generosity at home, and, for a growing number of men, because of the impact of the East African Revival on conceptions of marriage.[62] Certainly marriage does seem to have become more stable over time, surveys indicating that the proportion of women who were on their second or third marriage declined between the early 1950s and early 1970s from 35 to 20%, while the proportion of women who were currently divorced also fell from 15% to 11.5%.[63] The final element in this limited reform of sexual behaviour was the decline in socially legitimate extra-marital sex. Paternal or fraternal demands to sleep with a man's wife were increasingly seen as unChristian and backward, while *bisisi*, regarded by local churches as 'the great door to immorality and the disorganization of the family', gradually reduced in frequency, as fertility and child survival rates improved, belief in vengeful spirits declined, and *bisisi* children's rights of inheritance were ruled invalid by the Buhaya Council.[64] The sexual history of the Haya is not one of ever increasing decadence, but of gains and losses in an ever-evolving contest between growing freedom and heightened restriction, and between marital conflict and reconciliation. If the period of independence brought Haya new hedonism in some contexts and growing restraint in others, the 1970s, a decade of economic collapse and war, entailed rapid change in only one direction.

[62] Bukoba District Annual Report 1953, TNA 215/2700; Survey of Catholic Dioceses, 1956 (Rubaga archives), p. 496; P. Reining, 'Village organisation in Buhaya' (unpublished conference paper, EAISR conference, June 1952), p. 50; S. Samson to Buhaya Council Secretary, 26 June 1961, MPA, L5/II/B; Int. MM, 7 Sept. 1999, Rubale, M; Int. AM, 14 June 2000, Isikila-Irungami, F; Sundkler, *Bara*, pp. 117–23, 133. Haya though still dominated prostitution in many East African cities through to the 1980s. F. Kaijage, 'AIDS control and the burden of history in northwestern Tanzania', *Population and Environment*, 14, 3 (1999), pp. 279–300; W. Nkya et al., 'The role of self-proclaimed prostitutes in STD transmission in Tanzania', in Tanzania Public Health Association, 'Epidemiology and control of communicable diseases in Tanzania. Proceedings of the 8th Annual Scientific Conference, Dar es Salaam, 14–17 November 1989 (Dar es Salaam, 1991), pp. 12–40.

[63] Richards and Reining, 'Fertility surveys in Buganda and Buhaya, 1952'; Laurie and Trant, *East African Medical Survey*, p. 37; R. Henin, *National Demographic Survey of Tanzania, 1973: Volume II, Data for Socioeconomic Groups* (Dar es Salaam: Tanzania Bureau of Statistics, 1973), pp. 78, 32.

[64] Larsson, *Conversion*, p. 116; Int. AMR, 26 July 1998, Kenyana-Kilimilile, F; Richards and Reining, 'Fertility surveys in Buganda and Buhaya, 1952'. For an extended discussion of legitimate extra-marital sex and *bisisi* see Chapter 1.

6

Ankole: Marriage and the Ethnicity of Sex, 1925–69

INTRODUCTION

Chapter 1 detailed some of the practices and attitudes which meant that in Ankole marriage was more stable and, among the agriculturalist majority at least, sexuality more constrained than in the other two case study areas. This chapter will focus on the reasons why divorce and illicit extra- and post-marital sex remained relatively rare among the Nkole, in sharp contrast to Buganda and Buhaya, and also why this district, until the period of independence, remained largely immune to the forces which encouraged a rapid increase in the frequency of pre-marital sex among the Ganda during the colonial period. It will show that labour migration, the dominant form of economic activity in this society, did bring about some changes in sexual behaviour, and more importantly integrated Ankole intimately with the Ganda. But economic migration appears to have had a much less destabilizing impact on marriage and systems of sexual control than did cash crop farming. Given the role frequently ascribed to labour migrants as the bearers of STDs to the African countryside over the past century, this is perhaps the most significant aspect of Ankole's story during this period.[1]

PREMARITAL SEX

Q. If a girl was found not to be a virgin at marriage, what would happen?

A. The husband's family would put a hole in a barkcloth and they would use it to wrap up a cent (a ring-shaped coin) and give this to the girl's aunt. If the aunt

[1] Cf. F. Sanderson, 'The development of labour migration from Nyasaland, 1891–1914', *Journal of African History*, 2, 2 (1961), pp. 259–271; I. Schapera, *Migrant Labour and Tribal Life: A Study of Conditions in the Bechuanaland Protectorate* (London: Cambridge University Press, 1947); K. Jochelson, *The Colour of Disease: syphilis and racism in South Africa, 1880–1950* (London: Palgrave Macmillan, 2001); M. Belsey, 'The epidemiology of infertility: a review with particular reference to sub-Saharan Africa', *Bulletin of the World Health Organization*, 54 (1976), p. 336.

> saw the hole and the coin instead of blood, she would beat the girl's mother with that cloth.[2]

The language used by informants from Ankole when discussing sex before marriage in the 1940s, 1950s, and 1960s differed strikingly from that employed by Ganda. People in Ankole talked about pre-marital sex during these decades in terms of fear, scorn, and shame. Some interviewees remembered being terrified of STDs, or of sex in general. As a girl, one informant told her grandmother that she had just started to menstruate. 'She said something has cut you. If you go to those people with a different genitalia from you, it will cut you again. So make sure you run away from the penis. Because even merely seeing it will lead to a heavy flow. We were taught that the penis was a very bad thing. So we would avoid it.' Other interviewees recalled that 'a girl who was promiscuous would be called everybody's wheelbarrow', and songs would be sung at village weddings mocking her and her parents. Boys too who slept around would be condemned as *malaya* or prostitutes.[3] An even greater deterrent than the horror of public humiliation were the stories girls were told about relatives or neighbours who had been ritually killed for falling pregnant before marriage. 'We grew up hearing about my aunt who was buried alive for this so no-one dared to get involved with the boys.' Such extreme penalties were outlawed by the time interviewees were growing up, but girls who fell pregnant were still treated harshly in both pastoralist and cultivating communities, typically with a long or even permanent exile. In the late 1960s the anthropologist Yitzchak Elam witnessed 'a red-eyed father chas[ing] his pregnant daughter away from the camp with an upraised spear'. The unmarried mother continued to be regarded as ritually dangerous, being kept away from people's gardens and livestock lest their abuse of their fecundity caused crops to wither and cows to cease milking. Marriage offered the only chance of redemption, but if the new husband was polygamous and neglected to perform elaborate preventive rituals, his contamination would burn the skin of his senior wives when he next had sex with them.[4]

Individual informants' testimonies about local sexual norms and their own personal sexual experiences should always be viewed with caution. But when the same answers are provided in a succession of different interviews,

[2] Kiyungi Focus Group Discussion (FGD) Female, 21 Aug. 2004.

[3] Male FGD Ruti, 19 Aug. 2004; Female FGD Ruti, 19 Aug. 2004; Bumbire (Bushenyi) FGD Female, 2004.

[4] Kiyungu Shema FGD Male, 21 Aug. 2004; Kiyungi FGD Female, 21 Aug. 2004; Y. Elam, *The Social and Sexual Roles of Hima Women: A Study of Nomadic Cattle Breeders in Nyabushozi County, Ankole, Uganda* (Manchester: Manchester University Press, 1973), p. 55; Bumbire (Bushenyi) FGD Female, 2004; Death of Spouses, D. Stenning Papers, Cambridge University, ADD 7916, B9; Kyenjenyi female FGD, 22 Aug. 2004.

then the burden of proof shifts, and in the case of this study, the question to be asked is why would more than a hundred elderly people from a dozen or so villages across Ankole transmit a largely consistent body of material about sexual attitudes and behaviour in the past which is distinctly different from the oral information repeated again and again by a similar number of people scattered across Buganda. Either norms and practices in each society did indeed differ fundamentally in the 1940s, 1950s, and 1960s, or the way in which Nkole talk about sex today is radically different from how it is discussed in Buganda. Given that the two societies are much more integrated in the present day than they were in the middle of the twentieth century, the former seems more likely.

Most informants in Ankole acknowledged that sex before marriage occurred during the period of their youth, but insisted that it was rare, for females at least. When one group of women who came to maturity around the 1950s were asked if they knew many girls who had pre-marital sex when they were young, they responded 'in Kakyuki there was one. And another even in Nyarubaare.' This was an individual not societal phenomenon. Some young women 'were too lustful', others drank too much at weddings, so that they were found asleep by fellow guests and raped. But village society discouraged the young from mixing. 'Boys in the village feared us girls, and we feared them . . . We would not meet, we did not know each other.' 'If a boy found a girl on the path, she would put her face down and walk fast.' Even at dances 'your aunt would be behind you so if you made the mistake of looking up she would roughly push your head down. A girl's eyes were supposed to be on the ground always.'[5] Many unmarried males did continue to have sexual access to their relatives' wives well into the post-independence era, especially among Hima pastoralists. But young men appear to have been less likely to engage unrelated married women in affairs than their counterparts in Buganda and Buhaya, because their access to cash was more limited and Ankole's sexually conservative culture caused its women to value discretion particularly highly. 'Married men maintain confidentiality', as one elder observed, 'whereas young boys want to show off.'[6]

In marked contrast to Buganda, no female informants and few male informants admitted to having had sex before marriage. Even among men from Mbarara town, who certainly regarded themselves as sexually

[5] Bumbire (Bushenyi) FGD Female, 2004; Kyenjenyi female FGD, 22 Aug. 2004. Musa Mushanga, however, indicates that informants may have exaggerated pre-marital chastity a little. M. Mushanga, 'The Nkole of South-Western Uganda', in A. Molnos (ed.), *Cultural Source Materials for Population Planning in East Africa III* (Nairobi, University of Nairobi, 1973), pp. 181–3.

[6] Elam, *Social*, p. 166; Kiyungu Shema FGD Male, 21 Aug. 2004; Male FGD Nyamitanga, 19 Aug. 2004; Int. YZ, 13 Aug. 2004, M; Int. RNT, 9 Aug. 2004, Mbarara, M.

sophisticated, half claimed to have married as virgins.[7] The sexual restraint of the young lasted further into the twentieth century in Ankole than in the other societies, partly because of its economic peripheralization, and the limited petty urbanization that resulted, partly because education developed relatively slowly there. Ankole was the least urbanized society in southern Uganda in the 1950s. The population of its district capital, Mbarara, at 2,724, was only 20% larger in 1959 than it had been in 1911. Meanwhile by 1969 only 14% of females aged fifteen and over had ever been to school, compared to 40% in Buganda and 36% in Buhaya by 1973. Nonetheless missionaries complained of Mbarara's corrupting influence on the local youth from as early as the 1930s, and girls made up a large minority of Ankole's limited school population from the 1940s. Informants remembered that 'we no longer feared each other, as we used to sit together.'[8] By the early 1960s boyfriend-girlfriend relationships were beginning to develop, the young started to go to dance clubs, and stories appeared in Ankole's newspapers complaining of girls coming back from school pregnant or drinking in town bars. But independent unmarried women were still very uncommon in Ankole, and the most dramatic changes in youthful sexual culture would wait until the 1970s, 'the decade of the striptease' as one informant described it.[9]

EXTRA-MARITAL SEX

Ankole's sexual conservatism ensured that socially legitimate extra-marital sex remained relatively common well into the second half of the twentieth century, especially among Hima pastoralists. The demographer James Ntozi found in the early 1980s that 85% of Hima men claimed to have had permitted sex with their sisters-in-law, compared to 41% of cultivators and 46% of

[7] Cf. e.g. Male FGD Nyamitanga, 19 Aug. 2004; Kiyungu Shema FGD Male, 21 Aug. 2004; Kyenjenyi female FGD, 22 Aug. 2004.

[8] Uganda Protectorate, *Uganda Census 1959: African Population* (Entebbe: Ministry of Economic Affairs, 1960), p. 85; Uganda Protectorate, *1911 Census Returns* (Entebbe: Government Printer, 1912); Republic of Uganda, *Report on the 1969 Population Census: Vol. III Additional Tables* (Entebbe: Statistics Division, 1973), pp. 72, 81; R. Henin, *National Demographic Survey of Tanzania, 1973: Volume II, Data for Socioeconomic Groups* (Dar es Salaam: Tanzania Bureau of Statistics, 1973), p. 21; O. Beaudoin to E. Michaud, 26 Mar. 1933, Mbarara in E. Michaud, 'Enquêtes sur les conditions morales dans le vicariat de l'Uganda, 1933', Rubaga archives, 904.1; A. Kagume, 'Church and society in Ankole, Uganda: an analysis of the impact of evangelical African Christianity on ethnic and gender relations in Ankole, 1901–1961' (unpublished PhD dissertation, University of Bristol, 1993), p. 262; Kyenjenyi female FGD, 22 Aug. 2004.

[9] Int. RNT, 9 Aug. 2004, Mbarara, M; Imelda Batwangiraki, 'Murekye Kugabura Okwega Kw'abaishiki', *Ageteraine*, 1 Apr. 1960; N. Ndyanga, 'Baishiki mwegarukyemu mwahangara', *Ageteraine*, 5 Nov. 1960; Elam, *Social*, p. 87; Kagume, 'Church', p. 272; Kyenjenyi female FGD, 22 Aug. 2004.

mixed farmers.[10] The anthropologists Oberg and Elam both regarded sexual openness as a strategic necessity for Hima nomadic pastoralists, whose individual survival and prosperity depended on the strength of their familial bonds and the breadth of their herding alliances. These ties of fraternity and friendship were sustained by a man's willingness to share his wife with guests and fellow members of the kraal. During the Hima wedding ceremony wives were warned that they must welcome the sexual demands of their in-laws, and a wife who undermined her husband's system of sexual insurance might be beaten, ostracized, or divorced. These legitimized liaisons were believed by contemporary observers to have resulted in exceptionally wide sexual networks within Hima society.[11] Among cultivators, by contrast, wife-sharing was not only less common, but the range of male beneficiaries was much narrower. Only brothers-in-law could claim a socially recognized right to sex, though fathers-in-law who had paid bridewealth on behalf of their sons might demand it. Informants stated that cultivators may have regarded this practice as morally wrong, but they tolerated it, if conducted discreetly, because it helped contain the dangerous lustfulness of unmarried males, reduced the risk of a wife going astray while her husband was working abroad, and increased the chance that the wife of an infertile man would fall pregnant.[12]

Informants disagreed about the dating of the decline in wife-sharing. Some suggested the 1950s, others the 1980s. It seems likely that its disappearance was gradual and uneven. In one group discussion a woman born in the early 1920s revealed that she had once agreed to her husband's request to show his younger brother how to have sex so that he would not embarrass himself when attempting to consummate his upcoming wedding. Two neighbours, a decade or so younger, mentioned that they had also come under pressure to sleep with their brothers-in-law, but had had sufficient confidence to evade their demands. 'I would find excuses every time he came. The last time I told him I was in my periods.'[13] Other women argued more explicitly that growing female resistance to the claims of patriarchy reduced the frequency of legitimate extra-marital sex, though the specific role of religion, education, and the increasing awareness of STDs were also emphasized by interviewees who explained the demise of this practice in terms of their

[10] J. Ntozi, *The Role of Men in Determining Fertility among the Banyankore of Southwestern Uganda* (Kampala: Marianum Press, 1993), pp. 74–5.

[11] K. Oberg, 'Kinship organization of the Banyankole', *Africa*, 11, 2 (1938), pp. 146–52; K. Oberg, 'Analysis of the Bahima marriage ceremony', *Africa*, 19, 2 (1949), p. 114; Elam, *Social*, pp. 124–5, 160; Female FGD Ruti, 19 Aug. 2004; Int. EM, 27 Sept. 2001, Kampala, M.

[12] Oberg, 'Kinship', p. 142; Female FGD Nyamitanga, 19 Aug. 2004; Male FGD Nyamitanga, 19 Aug. 2004; Kyenjenyi female FGD, 22 Aug. 2004; Kyangyenyi/Kiyungu Male FGD, 22 Aug. 2004; Kiyungu Shema FGD Male, 21 Aug. 2004.

[13] Kiyungu Shema FGD Male, 21 Aug. 2004; Male FGD Ruti, 19 Aug. 2004; Kyenjenyi female FGD, 22 Aug. 2004; Bumbire (Bushenyi) FGD Female, 2004.

society's enlightenment. A number of informants emphasized that they rejected wife-sharing 'because we were learned' or had converted to Christianity, especially to the Balokole revivalist movement. These factors altered many individuals' perceptions, but it should be noted that only 1.6% of Ankole's population were Balokole in the late 1950s, and of these a large proportion were women of advancing years. Moreover, Ntozi found that experience of wife-sharing was more common among men with secondary and tertiary education than the uneducated, presumably because schooling tended to delay male marriage. It seems likely that the decline in labour migration from the 1950s and a growing sense of marriage as a personal, companionate relationship, which elders regarded as a symptom of selfishness and pride, were just as significant. It appears that men became less willing, and had less need, to relinquish their exclusive sexual rights over their wives.[14]

When informants discussed illegitimate adulterous affairs in the middle decades of the twentieth century the theme that recurred more than any other was the ritual danger associated with such behaviour. Interviewees mentioned a remarkable range of negative consequences arising from adultery, from miscarriage to the sickness, disfigurement, sterility, or death of perpetrators, their spouses, or their children. Even salt would lose its taste. The risks of adultery were greatest when the marital relationship was under most strain, during a husband's absence, or when spousal support was most needed, during pregnancy and breastfeeding. While Ganda appear to have lost respect for such prohibitions by the early colonial period if not earlier, as late as 1968 a third of all Nkole surveyed still believed in them. Male informants acknowledged that the primary purpose of such proscriptions was to maintain female fidelity. 'They constrained the women. But today they are educated. Even if you lied to them like that, they cannot keep still.'[15] Compared to Ganda and Haya, moreover, Nkole were much more likely to emphasize the violence that could

[14] Female FGD Nyamitanga, 19 Aug. 2004; Male FGD Ruti, 19 Aug. 2004; Female FGD Ruti, 19 Aug. 2004; Int. JH, 10 Aug. 2004, F; Kiyungu Shema FGD Male, 21 Aug. 2004; P. Nicolet, 'Table d'enquête sur les moeurs et coutumes indigènes, Vicariat Apostolique de Rwenzori: Tribu des Hamites Abahima et Bantu Abairu de l'Ankole', 1951, p. 48, WFA; D. Stenning, 'Preliminary observations on the Balokole movement particularly among Bahima in Ankole district', (EAISR conference paper, 1958, ASC, Cambridge); Elam, *Social*, pp. 166, 177, 202, 213–5; D. Stenning, 'Persistence of cult elements in an East African population', British Psychological Society Annual Conference, Cambridge, April 1959, D. Stenning Papers, Cambridge University, ADD 7916, B6; Ntozi, 'Role', p. 75; Kiyungi FGD Female, 21 Aug. 2004.

[15] Kiyungi FGD Female, 21 Aug. 2004; Kyenjenyi female FGD, 22 Aug. 2004; Kiyungu Shema FGD Male, 21 Aug. 2004; Bumbire (Bushenyi) FGD Female, 2004; Oberg, 'Analysis', p. 114; Ntozi, 'Role', p. 70; R. Cook, 'Child health in Ankole, Uganda: A programme of immunization and health education and its evaluation' (unpublished DMed dissertation, University of Oxford, n/d [*c*.1968]), p. 106; Male FGD Nyamitanga, 19 Aug. 2004.

result from affairs. An adulterer 'would be speared and killed, and if he was not of the husband's clan, they would attack his family'. 'At that time, there were no laws' to stop such vendettas.[16]

Missionaries appreciated the effect of this culture of fear on marital behaviour. In the 1930s one wrote that 'generally speaking . . . the moral condition of Ankole remains relatively good.' Twenty years later another observed that 'fidelity on the whole is the rule rather than the exception.' Some, especially male, informants agreed that affairs in the past were 'uncommon', 'minimal', or 'non-existent', often noting that children conceived outside of marriage in Ankole, unlike Buganda, could not legally be claimed by their genitor and 'would bring chaos'.[17] None of the informants from Ankole admitted to having had extra-marital affairs, but a number of women suggested that infidelity was more common in the past than some sources indicated. It was, they argued, 'normal' male behaviour. 'Can you stop a man?', they asked. Women claimed that by contrast wives used to fear and respect their husbands, and viewed divorce, the penalty for female adultery, with horror.[18] Still some female informants acknowledged that women in the past did secretly engage in affairs to avenge their husbands' infidelities, or because labour migration had left them alone and unsupported for so long. The abortion of an ill-timed pregnancy was, according to some sources, not uncommon in colonial Ankole, due to the frequency and duration of male absences. Missionaries had hoped that cash cropping would involve fewer moral hazards than labour migration, but in fact the sudden wealth associated with the rapid expansion of coffee brought new problems. Informants remember the celebrations associated with the first coffee sales of the 1960s as times of exceptional sexual freedom.[19]

Even where female informants were prepared to admit that married women also had affairs in the past, they still maintained that men tended to be more adulterous. The corollary of this proposition was that some women

[16] Male FGD Nyamitanga, 19 Aug. 2004; Kyangyenyi/Kiyungu Male Focus Group Discussion, 22 Aug. 2004.

[17] O. Beaudoin to E. Michaud, 26 Mar. 1933, Mbarara in E. Michaud, 'Enquêtes sur les conditions morales dans le vicariat de l'Uganda, 1933', Rubaga archives, 904.1; Survey of Catholic Dioceses, 1956 (Rubaga archives), p. 287; Kyangyenyi/Kiyungu Male FGD, 22 Aug. 2004; Kiyungu Shema FGD Male, 21 Aug. 2004; Male FGD Nyamitanga, 19 Aug. 2004; Bumbire (Bushenyi) FGD Female, 2004.

[18] Female FGD Ruti, 19 Aug. 2004; Kiyungi FGD Female, 21 Aug. 2004; Female FGD Nyamitanga, 19 Aug. 2004; Kyenjenyi female FGD, 22 Aug. 2004.

[19] Bumbire (Bushenyi) FGD Female, 2004; Oberg, 'Kinship', pp. 152–3; O. Beaudoin to E. Michaud, 26 Mar. 1933, Mbarara in E. Michaud, 'Enquêtes sur les conditions morales dans le vicariat de l'Uganda, 1933', Rubaga archives, 904.1; C. Byaruhanga, 'Divorce in Uganda sociologically viewed' (unpublished thesis ad lauream, Pontifical Gregorian University, 1954), p. 90; Int. RNT, 9 Aug. 2004, Mbarara, M.

in Ankole must have had a large number of sexual contacts. Prostitution was relatively rare in Ankole before independence, with a small number of sex workers, mostly from Tooro and Buganda, operating in Mbarara and the large, regular cattle markets that provided Hima with the bulk of their income. According to informants from rural areas the expansion of the graded road network in the late 1960s brought small numbers of sex workers to the larger trading centres, first serving the construction workers, then staying to cater for both passing truck drivers, who paid them in cash, and local men who offered only 'vaseline, tobacco, or a bottle of local brew'.[20] More common were the women who owned or worked in bars, and offered sex as a means of supplementing their income. Drinking patterns were reported as having changed by the 1930s as beer made from bananas, as in Buganda, rather than from millet, traditionally drunk communally, began to be sold in shops in the various county capitals. By the late 1950s modern bars had become relatively common in Mbarara, with customers 'also wanting a taste of the very attractive girls before they went home'. Couple dancing had come into Ankole from Buganda by this time. One interviewee reminisced that 'when men danced with women and held them tight, they would feel attracted to each other. So they went to a lodge and after he would give her a piece of soap.' Informants remembered though that a woman who worked in a bar 'would never allow anyone to call her a prostitute. So she would not be paid for sex.' However, 'they would be given a small token like perfume . . . There was nothing for nothing.'[21]

DIVORCE AND POST-MARITAL SEX

Marriage in Ankole appears to have been much more stable than in Buganda and Buhaya. Surveys in the 1950s and 1960s found that only 6% of cultivators' marriages had ended in divorce, and that a Hima community of 1,004 people contained only eleven divorcees.[22] Most informants agreed that divorce

[20] Kiyungi FGD Female, 21 Aug. 2004; Male FGD Ruti, 19 Aug. 2004; Female FGD Ruti, 19 Aug. 2004; W. Bazley, 'Reminiscences as a district officer in Uganda, 1951–1953, 1958–1960', RHO MSS Afr. s. 924, p. 90; Female FGD Nyamitanga, 19 Aug. 2004; Kyenjenyi female focus group discussion, 22 Aug. 2004; Kiyungu Shema FGD Male, 21 Aug. 2004; Male FGD Nyamitanga, 19 Aug. 2004. No informant reported having engaged in same-sex relationships.

[21] Female FGD Nyamitanga, 19 Aug. 2004; Male FGD Ruti, 19 Aug. 2004; O. Beaudoin to E. Michaud, 26 Mar. 1933, Mbarara in E. Michaud, 'Enquêtes sur les conditions morales dans le vicariat de l'Uganda, 1933', Rubaga archives, 904.1; Kiyungi FGD Female, 21 Aug. 2004; P. van Thiel, *Multi-tribal Music of Ankole: an Ethnomusicological Study Including a Glossary of Musical Terms* (Tervuren: Musée royal de l'Afrique, 1977), pp. 183, 198–200.

[22] 'Families and land parcels', D. Stenning Papers, Cambridge University, ADD 7916, D7; Elam, *Social*, pp. 150–1. Divorce here refers to the socially recognized termination of a marriage.

was rare before the 1970s, except in cases of impotence and female sterility. The extreme pro-natalism of Ankole culture was once again evident in interviewees' explanations for marital breakdown in such situations. In contrast to Buganda, women here justified separation from an impotent husband more in terms of their wasted fertility than sexual dissatisfaction. 'If you could not get pregnant then why would you be married in the first place? You would leave him alone.' Barrenness was not a universally recognized reason for divorce, as men were expected simply to marry an additional wife. But infertile women often left their marriages, driven away by the taunts of their co-wives and the neglect of their husbands. Sterility was popularly believed to be both contagious and a sign of moral failing. An infertile wife could not be a good wife: 'How can you be well mannered without giving birth? To husbands that was the worst behaviour.'[23]

Compared to Buganda, marriage in Ankole during this period was little affected by legal and economic changes. Because divorce here was relatively rare, and bridewealth in Christian marriages was no higher than with customary unions, Nkole were less concerned by the commitment involved in marriage under the Ordinance. Surveys showed that in the 1950s Ankole's Anglicans were 68% more likely to have married in church than their Ganda brethren, while by the 1960s the Catholic marriage rate was 233% higher in Ankole than Buganda. Converts in Ankole appear to have accepted the Christian model of marriage more wholeheartedly than in Buganda, where only 52% of male converts remained monogamous in the late 1950s, compared to 83% in Ankole. There is some evidence that husbandly behaviour was modified relatively significantly following conversion in Ankole, and that the popularity of church women's groups in the district helped many wives mediate some of the tensions of modern married life. Certainly Christian marriage in Ankole appears to have been very stable, with one study showing that the ratio of marriages to separations within the Anglican church in 1938 was 26.2:1 in Ankole and 3.4:1 in Buganda.[24] Bridewealth meanwhile remained not only universal and extremely high by regional standards, but fully refundable in case of divorce. Marriage payments moreover were relatively unmonetized until the period of independence. Derrick Stenning's study of a cultivating community found that no bridewealth had been paid in cash until

[23] Bumbire (Bushenyi) FGD Female, 2004; Kyenjenyi Female FGD, 22 Aug. 2004; J. Ntozi and J. Kabera, 'Marriage patterns in Ankole, South-Western Uganda' (African Demography Working Papers no. 16, University of Pennsylvania, August 1988), p. 21.

[24] J. Taylor, 'Analysis of parishes', CMSA, Acc. 265 Z5; A. Hastings, *Christian Marriage in Africa, Being a Report Comissioned by the Archbishops of Cape Town, Central Africa, Kenya, Tanzania, and Uganda* (London: SPCK, 1973), pp. 141–3; 'Families and land parcels', D. Stenning Papers, Cambridge University, ADD 7916, D7; Kagume, 'Church', pp. 255–8, 271; 'Women's clubs', *Taifa Empya*, 15 Oct. 1970; Bumbire (Bushenyi) FGD Female, 2004; Int. RNT, 9 Aug. 2004, Mbarara, M.

the 1950s. This combination of factors ensured kingroup interest in resolving marital disputes and discouraging divorce.[25] The final element in Ankole's marital stability was that, in contrast to Buganda, children invariably continued to remain with the father when a relationship broke up. Informants emphasized this as the key reason why so many women endured an unhappy marriage. A husband might 'put out your eyes, kick in your teeth, but you don't go anywhere. You remain for your children.' 'Those days a women who had a drunkard of a husband would be beaten everyday like a drum. And she would stay around or else it would be the children to suffer.'[26]

Marriages in Ankole did nonetheless end through death or separation, but the sexual freedom of widows and divorcees was often carefully controlled right into the 1980s. Widow inheritance seems to have been the most frequent response to the death of a male relative, unless the woman had not yet borne children, with the wife being taken by a brother, stepson, or occasionally her father-in-law immediately after the funeral. Informants in Ankole were much more likely than those in Buganda and Buhaya to assert that a wife was possessed by the clan which had paid bridewealth for her. 'She would not be let out.' 'They do not like their wife to go outside . . . If you're married, you're married.' The insistence that 'a wife belongs to the family' was influenced by the exceptional importance ascribed to maximizing the size of the lineage. Only apparently sterile women or widows nearing or past menopause were exempt from the expectation of remarriage. Elderly Nkole men claimed that widow inheritance survived because it was 'very healthy. It was a way of ensuring this woman would not misbehave.' In fact though as independence approached widows were allowed to veto suggestions that they should accept a new husband from among their in-laws. The frequency with which widows were inherited after the 1950s was a reflection less of direct patriarchal control than the absence of the alternative routes to security that existed in Buganda.[27] Divorcees it seems also frequently remarried quickly, in the cultivating community at least. Usually they could only be married polygamously, with the discounted bridewealth gained from the new suitor being used to help reimburse the estranged husband. The frequency of female remarriage

[25] 'Families and land parcels', D. Stenning Papers, Cambridge University, ADD 7916, D7; Int. RNT, 9 Aug. 2004, Mbarara, M; Kiyungi FGD Female, 21 Aug. 2004. Cf. L. Fallers, 'Some determinants of marriage stability in Busoga', *Africa*, 27, 2 (1957), pp. 214–21.

[26] Kiyungi FGD Female, 21 Aug. 2004; Male FGD Nyamitanga, 19 Aug. 2004; Int. YZ, 13 Aug. 2004, Mbarara, M.

[27] Male FGD Nyamitanga, 19 Aug. 2004; Int. YZ, 13 Aug. 2004, Mbarara, M; Int. RNT, 9 Aug. 2004, Mbarara, M; P. Nicolet, 'Table d'enquête sur les moeurs et coutumes indigènes, Vicariat Apostolique de Rwenzori: Tribu des Hamites Abahima et Bantu Abairu de l'Ankole', 1951, p. 36, WFA.

depended to a large extent on the woman's natal family's reluctance to be responsible for her upkeep and good behaviour. These various forces ensured that female autonomy was uncommon in Ankole right through to the 1970s. A large-scale rural survey in 1968 found not one female-headed household in its Ankole sample, in sharp contrast to the situation found in Buganda.[28]

CROSS-ETHNIC SEX

The story told of sexual change in Ankole so far has emphasized conservatism and restraint until the 1950s and then gradually increasing openness due to expanding communications, education, and cash crop farming. One of the most striking aspects of this widening of sexual networks was the growing willingness to seek sexual partners across ethnic or sub-ethnic lines. Compared to the other societies examined for this study Ankole historically had had a relatively closed sexual culture. Nkore and the principalities to the west had imported few slaves in pre-colonial times, and there is little indication of significant economic immigration before the colonial takeover, unlike Buganda in particular. Moreover, Ankole's Hima pastoralists maintained norms of sexual exclusivity longer than the ruling elites in some of the region's other cattle kingdoms. Pastoralists began to marry into wealthy agricultural lineages in Bunyoro during the nineteenth century, if not before, while some of Buhaya's kings took wives from cultivating clans in the early twentieth century. The cultural ideals of separateness and superiority seem to have survived the European takeover largely intact in Ankole, and indeed pastoralists were able to reify their ideal of sexual isolationism into the later decades of colonial rule, due to the exceptional wealth of their livestock economy, and the political hegemony they were granted in the 1890s when the British granted Hima-dominated Nkore suzerainty over the mainly agricultural lands to the west. In the early twentieth century Hima associated Ankole's cultivators with uncleanliness, ugliness, and stupidity, and supposedly would not consider marrying into agriculturalist clans. Inevitably though there were exceptions to this rule. In the pre-colonial era there were isolated cases of intermarriage with cultivators in Nkore, and, according to Edward Steinhart,

[28] Kyangyenyi/Kiyungu Male Focus Group Discussion, 22 Aug. 2004; Kiyungu Shema FGD Male, 21 Aug. 2004; Ntozi and Kabera, 'Marriage patterns', pp. 22–8; Ministry of Planning and Economic Development, *Rural Food Consumption Survey, 1968, in Ankole, Busoga, Masaka and West Nile* (Entebbe: Government Printer, 1970), p. 33; 'Death of spouses' and 'Hima marriage', D. Stenning Papers, Cambridge University, ADD 7916, B9, C2, C6A. Three percent of the Hima community studied by Elam were widows and divorcees but these lived, usually unhappily, with agnates. Elam, *Social*, p. 37. Even the kings of Ankole, it seems, were prepared to accept as wives previously married women. Nyamitanga mission diary, enclosure, 30 Sept. 1945, WFA.

destitute male cultivators who sought employment as servants sometimes gained sexual access to the wives of their Hima patrons. Agriculturalist female slaves moreover would be expected to provide sexual services to their masters and their relatives, and would gain some of the rights of a wife if they became pregnant. Such patterns of behaviour seem to have continued throughout the colonial period, despite Hima rhetorical emphasis on the maintenance of social distance.[29]

Still, the sexual separation of pastoralists and cultivators, never absolute, weakened significantly in the last years of colonial rule. By the 1930s the foundations of Hima pre-eminence were beginning to disintegrate. British officials' admiration of the Hima diminished as early excitement about their supposed Hamitic origins dissipated due to Uganda-wide concerns about the exploitation of African peasants, and local frustration at stockowners' insistence that their cattle should be a source of status, aesthetic pleasure, and food security more than profit and government revenue. Agriculturalists meanwhile found that conversion to Christianity led to education, wealth, and power. By the 1940s Ankole's elite secondary schools, established for the sons of Hima chiefs, contained as many agriculturalist as pastoralist children, with the former being maintained by government scholarships or community support. Ankole's labour migrants invested their wealth in livestock as well as schooling, the two measurable markers of their inferiority, so that cultivators owned three-fifths of the district's cattle by 1947. Whereas in 1907 none of Ankole's ten county chiefs, and only eight of seventy-four sub-county chiefs, were agriculturalists, by 1942, as academic achievement became the key to administrative appointment, they held a fifth of the county chiefships and 62% of the sub-counties. The post-war imperial commitment to representative local government, moreover, saw cultivators take the prime ministership in 1948 and form a majority on the kingdom's ruling council in 1952.[30] One

[29] E. Steinhart, 'Slavery and other forms of social oppression in Ankole, 1890–1940', in H. Médard and S. Doyle (eds.), *Slavery in the Great Lakes Region of East Africa* (Oxford: James Currey, 2007), pp. 191, 194–200; H. Johnston, *The Uganda Protectorate* (London: Hutchinson and Co., 1902), pp. 568–72; G. Hyden, *Political Development in Rural Tanzania: A West Lake Study* (Nairobi: East African Publishing House, 1969), p. 113; M. Doornbos, 'Ethnicity, Christianity, and the development of social stratification in colonial Ankole, Uganda', *The International Journal of African Historical Studies*, 9, 4 (1976), pp. 556–67; Oberg, 'Analysis', pp. 107, 116; Kiyungu Shema FGD Male, 21 Aug. 2004; Int. YZ, 13 Aug. 2004, Mbrara, M. By the 1950s political tension between the former pastoralist elite and the agriculturalist majority empowered by democratization had become intense in Ankole and Buhaya, where the nobility were told by populist leaders '"Everything is at an end between us. When you die none of us will be there to assist at the burial."' Buganda was almost unique in this region for the absence of radical disenchantment with monarchy in the late colonial period. B. Sundkler, *Bara Bukoba: Church and Community in Tanzania* (London: Hurst, 1980), p. 183.

[30] Kagume, 'Church', pp. 38, 71, 85–92, 120–9, 180–5; S. Karugire, *A History of the Kingdom of Nkore in Western Uganda to 1896* (London: Clarendon, 1971), p. 41; Doornbos, 'Ethnicity', pp. 566–70; Notes on meeting with Lord Hailey re Ankole, 31 Aug. 1947, NA, CO/1018/82.

of the consequences of this political revolution was that marriage between cultivators and pastoralists became more common. Partly this was a response to the shift in wealth which had occurred, with women from poor Hima families seizing the prosperity that was offered by the socially ambitious new commoner elite. But it also reflected a change of perspective among many Hima, especially those who had been most exposed to education and Christianity. Mission educators forced all pupils to cultivate in the school gardens and to eat the crops they produced, despite Hima repugnance for such degrading practices. The Balokole revival further narrowed the cultural gap by encouraging Hima adherents to abandon food taboos, to confront the deadly sin of pride, and to sedentarize near their local church, as nomadism was thought to encourage idleness and immorality.[31]

The sexual barriers between pastoralists and agriculturalists were beginning to come down by the late colonial period, but the changes detailed above would not in themselves have integrated the cultivating majority into the higher-risk relationship culture of the Hima. By definition, both Balokole and Hima women who married into the agricultural elite were essentially removed from the wife-sharing relationships that held pastoralist society together. It is possible that cultivators' growing political and economic power altered Hima attitudes towards what was sexually possible more generally, and encouraged an increase in sexual affairs between members of the two communities. It seems likely though that it was labour migration that played the larger role in integrating Ankole's agriculturalists into wider sexual networks.

According to oral informants, when labour migrants first left Ankole to go to work for Buganda's cotton and coffee farmers they feared Ganda women, who had a reputation for drunkenness, promiscuity, and shockingly deviant behaviour. This fear of the sexually unknown was not uncommon in East Africa, often serving to bolster group solidarity. Members of some societies supposedly would not countenance relationships with foreigners who, for example, had not been circumcised. Other ethnic groups were less specific, with Haya informants regarding any marriage with outsiders, almost invariably regarded as inferiors, as shameful. 'It would be as if the person was dead.'[32] But over time it seems that affairs between Nkole men and Ganda women became common. The geographical context in which these sexual

[31] G. Kyomuhendo and M. McIntosh, *Women, Work and Domestic Virtue in Uganda, 1900–2003* (Oxford: James Currey, 2006), p. 55; Kagume, 'Church', pp. 103, 110, 130, 156–67.

[32] Male FGD Ruti, 19 Aug. 2004; N. Nelson, '"Selling her kiosk": Kikuyu notions of sexuality and sex for sale in Mathare Calley, Kenya', in P. Caplan (ed.), *The Cultural Construction of Sexuality* (London: Tavistock, 1987), pp. 219–20; Int. EB, 1 Sept. 1999, Bukoba, M; Int. SN, 25 Aug. 1999, Katoma, M; Int. PKK, 18 Aug. 2000, Mshumba-Byazi, F. In fact though some Haya men specifically sought out wives from ethnic groups with a reputation for high fertility.

interlinkages developed was unusual in this region. Usually in Africa European officials and indigenous authorities alike focused their moral displeasure on colonial towns, deplored for their detribalizing squalor, which corroded the ethnic distinctions and moral purity of the countryside. But in Uganda the destination of choice for most labour migrants was not Kampala or Jinja, nor even the sugar and tea plantations surrounding those towns, but the cash crop farms of tens of thousands of individual Ganda households. This is yet another example of the rural character of so much of these societies' sexual networking practices.

At first, male Ganda regarded the presence of these migrant labourers, often referred to as 'God's blessing', with approval, as the prestige of a Ganda householder was enhanced by being liberated from manual work and by being able to assume the role of patron to these seasonal clients. The Ganda sense of ethnic superiority was naturally enhanced by the poverty and apparent backwardness of their workers. According to one informant, 'they used to have diseases that caused them sores . . . They also were careless about washing their faces. So all this made people despise them and isolate them.' But Ganda men were frequently taken away by business interests or social engagements, so that it often fell to their wives to manage these foreigners who offered their sweat in exchange for money. As immigrants returned to the same families year after year, adopted Ganda standards of hygiene, learnt to speak Luganda, and relieved local women of much of their work, the mistress-servant relationship often became something more intimate. Ganda informants remembered that '[w]hen those men started becoming clean and cured of the diseases, sometimes they would have affairs with the wives of their employers. They would even impregnate those women but it was kept as a secret even when the husbands discovered it. It would be a shame if the whole village knew of it.' Typically Ganda men suggested that such incidents arose where a wife was neglected. One informant revealed that a relative had an affair with her labourer 'because her husband ignored her. I think whenever he came back home drunk, he would just sleep. So this porter did the needful.' Or 'if say a man had four wives. By the time it comes to the last wife's turn, it would be too much for her already. So she would decide to go in for the porters.'[33]

But some Ganda men acknowledged that migrant labourers from Ankole as well as those from Rwanda, Burundi, and Buhaya, were more attractive than they first appeared. 'The shamba boys had their own system of doing it. They used to do *kakyabali* [a technique of foreplay used to the south and west

[33] Int. CSNM, M, 28 Aug. 2004, Butanga, M; Male FGD, Kitala, 1 Sept. 2004; A. Richards, 'The assimilation of the immigrants', in A. Richards (ed.), *Economic Development and Tribal Change: A Study of Immigrant Labour in Buganda* (Cambridge: Heffer, 1952), pp. 161–6; G. Mut. 7, Kyagwe, M. Musaale, 1951, A. Richards papers, LSE, 7/19.

of Buganda] . . . and the women would really enjoy... And she would tell other women about it.' When one group of female Ganda were asked what women used to do if they were not sexually satisfied by their husbands, their answer was 'If you had your *bakayanda* [labourers] at home, they would handle this very well', and then sang *Bwogoba Kayanda anga nange ngenda* [If you chase Kayanda I will leave with him].

Now my friends told me that Kayanda had a child with my wife...

I told him, Kayanda, leave my home, leave my wife, leave my son.

He told me: Master, you can't take my child, except if you want to die. I will go with my child . . .

My wife said: If you dare send Kayanda out of this home, I will follow him ... Kayanda is better than the undisciplined Baganda. Kayanda is better than seventy men put together. Kayanda does the *kakyabali* best.[34]

Interviews in Ankole and Buganda jokingly referred to the acceleration in sexual exchange after the Second World War as a form of globalization, with Ganda men begrudgingly learning *kakyabali*, and Nkole women imitating the use of beads, erotic language, and kissing that had made female Ganda the object of both lust and mistrust across the region. Ankole informants remembered that as patterns of migration became well established and sexual openness increased, men often maintained two households, with wives in both Ankole and Buganda, each usually ignorant of the existence of the other. Interestingly though, sources from Buganda indicate that marriage between Ganda and immigrants was rare. Oral interviewees in Buganda generally viewed intermarriage with disquiet. A typical comment was that it diluted Ganda culture, undermined traditional childrearing, encouraged divorce, and typified the arrogance of the young, thinking that love could overcome ethnic difference.[35] In the 1950s Audrey Richards recorded similar concerns in her fieldnotes. Most foreigners were too culturally different or too poor to regard as appropriate marriage partners. Men might consider marrying foreigners, but baulked at the thought of allowing their sisters and daughters to marry out. Similarly foreigners also appeared to lack enthusiasm for marrying their hosts. The immigrants she spoke to often questioned the fidelity and fertility of Ganda women and feared the notorious litigiousness and greed of their menfolk. Those migrants who admitted to having married a

[34] Male FGD, Kisubi Kiwulwe, 4 Sept. 2004; Female FGD, Takajunge, 26 Aug. 2004. Kayanda is a personal name common to the societies of the southern interlacustrine region often used as a synonym for labourer.

[35] e.g. Male FGD Namitanga, 19 Aug. 2004; Male FGD Ruti, 19 Aug. 2004; Int. IST, 21 Aug. 2004, Kagezi village, Masaka, M; Male FGD, Kitala, 1 Sept. 2004; Kiyungu Shema FGD Male, 21 Aug. 2004; Int. PLGS, 31 Aug. 2004, Kitala, Busiro, M.

Ganda woman emphasized the atypicality of their wives. 'Mine is a good one. She doesn't like beer. She stays at home.'[36]

Data from church records seem at first to back up this thesis that intermarriage was rare. The Roman Catholic parish of Kisubi, located between Kampala and Entebbe in Buganda, was chosen for this study partly because it was reputed to belong to a part of Buganda where immigration was relatively limited. In order to investigate the prevalence of inter-ethnic relationships in this area, the details of tens of thousands of baptisms and marriages during the colonial period were entered into a database. Then those individuals within the dataset who had unmistakably non-Ganda names were identified. This process revealed that between 1900 and 1962, of the approximately one thousand marriages registered by the parish, about 5% were between non-Ganda, and only 2% were mixed, with a Ganda spouse marrying a non-Ganda. These data appear to confirm the story told by Ganda both today and in the 1950s. However, the ethnic profile of the baptism register is very different from that which recorded marriage. Overall 21.4% of parents were non-Ganda. Partly the disparity between the frequency with which non-Ganda appeared in the marriage and baptism registers was due to immigrants marrying in their homelands and bringing their spouses with them to Buganda, where they settled and had children. But it was also because Ganda were much more willing to have children with immigrants than to formally marry them in church. Of non-Ganda men who brought children for baptism in Kisubi during the colonial period, 47% cohabited with a Ganda woman. Meanwhile, 37% of non-Ganda women who appeared in the baptism register as mothers, had a Ganda man as their partner. These results question two of the assumptions about inter-ethnic relationships made by Audrey Richards' team of researchers in the 1950s: that they were a generally novel phenomenon, and that the Ganda involved in them belonged to the group of restless, independence-loving women who preferred temporary, informal unions to permanent, official marriage. In fact immigrants were more likely to be in a relationship with a Ganda than with a fellow foreigner in each of the first four decades of the twentieth century. Moreover, proportionally the Kisubi data show that almost as many Ganda men as women had children with immigrants, and that cross-ethnic relationships were so common that they could not be described as restricted to the margins of Ganda society. That is not to say that they were well regarded. The infrequency with which couples of mixed ethnicity married in church was no doubt partly the result of family disapproval and the costs involved, but may also have reflected scepticism about the durability of cross-cultural relationships. Certainly the Catholic Church was

[36] Busiro, Musisi (Musigiri Semeoni Kayanda), 17 Nov. 1950, and Buganda attitudes, Sesiriba, Busiro A. Richards papers, LSE, 7/16.

reluctant to marry couples from different ethnic backgrounds because of such unions' reputation for rapid dissolution. Nonetheless, even if church weddings between Ganda and immigrants were rare, sex and less formal relationships were not.[37]

CONCLUSION

Compared to Buganda and Buhaya, the story of sex and marriage in Ankole before the 1970s is one of stability and restraint. Pre- and post-marital sex remained heavily regulated, and extra-marital affairs were associated with danger and dishonour. By the 1950s mixed schooling and growing prosperity led to new kinds of social encounters, and the 1960s brought a major expansion of the road network and a slow spread of modern bars and dance clubs. The most significant changes though were associated with Ankole's links with its more cosmopolitan neighbour, Buganda. Prostitution, couple dancing, new sexual styles, and new STDs were all thought to have come from there, often brought by returning migrants, who had frequently performed more than just agricultural labour for their hosts. Buganda was in some ways the region's sexual interchange. News of the beauty and exotic skills of Kampala's Haya and Tooro sex workers spread rapidly amongst Ganda men during the colonial period. The particular abilities of Ganda women as lovers drew in men from across the region. Male informants remembered that 'on setting foot here, the first thing Kenyans would ask was for us to get them Baganda women.' Ganda women meanwhile encouraged their friends to discover the pleasures of *kakyabali*. 'That is why Baganda like men from western Uganda', explained Ankole interviewees. This was where the growing openness and homogenization of sexual culture across the region began, a process that would intensify during the 1970s, as will be discussed in Chapter 9.[38]

[37] Richards, 'Assimilation', p. 178; Nabanga, Busiro, 1951, A. Richards papers, LSE, 6/18; Int. SJ, 26 Aug. 2004, Takajunge, M. It was not possible to identify people from Ankole with absolute certainty in the parish registers as many of their names are shared with neighbouring ethnic groups. Ganda naming patterns are unusually distinctive.

[38] Male FGD, Kitala, 1 Sept. 2004; Male FGD Nyamitanga, 19 Aug. 2004. Cf. F. Bennett, 'Gonorrhoea: a rural pattern of transmission', *East African Medical Journal*, 41, 4 (1964), pp. 163–7.

7

Fertility in Ankole, Buganda, and Buhaya, 1925–69

INTRODUCTION

The previous three chapters have argued that sexual culture in Ankole, Buganda, and Buhaya varied markedly until the mid-twentieth century, but tended to become more homogeneous in the era of decolonization. The story of fertility change in modern Africa by contrast is one of evolving extreme diversity. In some states, such as Zimbabwe, birth rates rose steeply from the 1940s, if not earlier, until around 1980, and then halved in less than a generation. For most countries fertility rates seem to have risen somewhat later and have as yet shown little sign of a marked reduction. In a few cases, such as Chad, recorded birth rates have barely changed over at least the past sixty years. It is natural to direct attention to the most dramatic aspect of this story, the radical shift from sustained expansion to sudden limitation, but the divergence that existed between and within African countries is equally significant. In the 1950s Rwanda's total fertility rate (TFR) was almost twice as high as Gabon's, while within Uganda district-level TFRs ranged between 3.2 and 7.0 live births per woman. Similar diversity could be found in the first decade of the twenty-first century, with the unevenness of fertility decline meaning that Angola's TFR was more than double that of Botswana, and within Uganda women in Kibaale district had twice as many live births as women in Kampala.[1]

Given such wide variation in demographic experience, it is unsurprising that the causes of fertility change in modern Africa have been the subject of intense academic debate. Two broad approaches have been adopted in the attempt to explain the increase in birth rates which was observed in much of Africa during the middle decades of the twentieth century. The first focuses on the release of the physical limitations on reproduction imposed by diet

[1] UN Fertility Data, http://data.un.org/Data.aspx?d=PopDiv&f=variableID%3a54, accessed 15 Nov. 2010; Uganda Protectorate, *Uganda Census 1959: African Population* (Entebbe: Ministry of Economic Affairs, 1960); Uganda Bureau of Statistics, *The 2002 Uganda Population and Housing Census, Population Dynamics* (Kampala: UBOS, 2006), pp. 26–30.

and disease, with scholars such as John Iliffe, Anne Retel-Laurentin, and Anatole Romaniuk arguing that fertility rose primarily in response to improvements in nutrition, the medicalization of childbirth, and, above all, the antibiotic treatment of STD-related sterility.[2] The second is more concerned with the social context of fertility change. Scholars, such as Jack Caldwell, have emphasized that Christianity, education, and urbanization helped to reduce birth intervals by breaking down traditions of prolonged breastfeeding and post-partum sexual abstinence, whereas neo-Marxists, such as Dennis Cordell and Joel Gregory, have claimed that colonial taxation pushed young men into labour migration, enabling them to marry earlier, and caused parents to produce more children to help meet the labour demands associated with cash cropping.[3]

The attempt to construct a theory of fertility change that holds true across Africa's thousands of societies is an intellectual task of huge ambition, given the diversity of reproductive experience over time and space, the uneven impact of the western concept of the family within indigenous cultures, and the need to identify which of the many proximate determinants of fertility were significant at any particular moment before investigating how they were affected by background social change.[4] This chapter will attempt to make some contribution to this endeavour, but makes no claim to have developed an interpretation of continent-wide application. It is, however, based on sources of unusual richness by contemporary standards, even if they seem entirely inadequate compared to modern-day censuses, Demographic and Health Surveys, or Knowledge, Attitudes and Practice Surveys. Uganda collected more demographic information on its population than perhaps any other African colony between the wars. Its 1931 census not only counted each person individually, but also identified their sex, marital status, and age group. Uganda's system of vital registration also required its population to record live births, still-births, and deaths in infancy and at older ages, though

[2] J. Iliffe, *Africans: the History of a Continent* (Cambridge: Cambridge University Press, 1995), p. 240; A. Retel-Laurentin, 'Sub-Fertility in Black Africa: The case of the Nzakara in Central African Republic', in B. Adadevoh (ed.), *Subfertility and Infertility in Africa* (Ibadan: Caxton Press, 1974); A. Romaniuk, 'Increase in natural fertility during the early stages of modernization: Evidence from an African case study, Zaire', *Population Studies*, 34 (1980), pp. 293–310.

[3] J. Caldwell, 'The social repercussions of colonial rule: demographic aspects', in A. Adu Boahen (ed.), *UNESCO General History of Africa, VII* (London: Heinemann, 1985), pp. 458–80; D. Cordell and J. Gregory, *African Population and Capitalism: Historical Perspectives* (London: Westview, 1987); G. Kitching, 'Proto-industrialisation and demographic change: a thesis and some possible African implications', *Journal of African History*, 24, 2 (1983), pp. 229–30.

[4] Cf. M. Lockwood, *Fertility and Household Labour in Tanzania: Demography, Economy, and Society in Rufiji District, c.1870–1986* (Oxford: Oxford University Press, 1998). Proximate determinants of fertility are factors which directly influence fertility levels such as contraceptive prevalence or the proportion of adults in a relationship.

compliance was far from universal. Information, albeit of imperfect quality, therefore exists about two of the key determinants of fertility, the proportion of adults in union and the level of pregnancy loss, at an exceptionally early date, but estimates of other determinants of fertility, such as the age at first marriage, only became available through conventional sources with the 1948 censuses. The greatest problem in African historical demography is in locating consistent and comparable data sources. Most of Uganda's 1980 census results, for example, were lost due to the unrest affecting the country in that year. Tanganyika's censuses were extremely basic before 1967, and even though Buhaya's chiefs did register some vital events, they did not record still-births.

Additional sources of data relating to fertility change are required in order to build on the demographic foundations provided by government censuses and vital registration. This chapter will utilize four alternative types of information. Parish baptism and marriage registers permit shifts in age at first marriage and birth intervals to be traced between 1925 and 1969.[5] For the same years in Buganda hospital maternity records documented patients' parities and their experiences of pregnancy loss and stillbirth. Finally, both a series of small-scale demographic surveys from the 1930s to the early 1970s and oral interviews with elderly men and women provide information on factors such as the take-up of contraception and the changing duration of breastfeeding and post-partum abstinence, as well as the motivations underlying such developments. These sources need to be used with caution. The quality of data recording can be questioned, as can the accuracy of informants' recall. The most significant concerns relate to the representativeness of the individuals who gave birth in a clinic, participated in church sacraments or lived in an area deemed suitable for an intensive survey. It is to be expected, for example, that people whose life events were recorded in church and hospital registers would have experienced fertility change in advance of the wider population. They were predominantly Christianized, probably possessed at least basic literacy, resided in or near an urban centre, and were likely to have been exposed to medical advice on supplementary feeding and birth spacing. Nonetheless, these sources generally corroborate the trends identifiable in the censuses, and, used in combination and with caution, provide a richly textured narrative of reproductive change.

The story told by these sources does not fit comfortably with existing explanations of the transition to higher fertility, all of which associate this development with particular aspects of modernization. Ankole's transition to high fertility occurred decades in advance of that of Buganda and Buhaya,

[5] Unfortunately in Bukoba I was only permitted to access the baptism registers that dated from the colonial period, due to the sensitivity of the information they contained.

yet colonial Ankole was a much poorer society, with a distinctly inferior level of medical and educational provision, and a far lower rate of conversion to Christianity. It also suffered the recurrent absence of much of its adult male population to labour migration. What has made the apparent exceptionalism of this region comprehensible in the past was the much higher level of reported STD prevalence in Buganda and Buhaya. This chapter will investigate whether this is an entirely adequate explanation. Because a unique combination of factors shaped fertility patterns in each case study area, the chapter will examine the three societies separately, before identifying key similarities and differences in the concluding section.

Ankole

By 1924 the early colonial fear that Ankole was experiencing population decline due to high levels of syphilis had been erased by the sustained increase in the number of births registered each year by the district's chiefs. Officials from time to time doubted the accuracy of the annual compilation of births, deaths, and still-births, but their utility as an indicator of broad trends was generally accepted, especially in the 1930s when the reduction in reported death rates could be used as evidence of the impact of various health interventions. This cautious confidence in the system of vital registration collapsed in 1948 when the results of Uganda's first proper census were released. The national crude birth rate (CBR) recorded by the vital registration system was 60% lower than that calculated from the census returns. All the vital rates recorded by chiefs throughout Uganda were affected by endemic under-reporting, but a closer examination of each district's figures suggests that some areas were more consistent than others. Ankole's reported rates, for example, were much more erratic than those of Buganda, perhaps reflecting the more bureaucratic nature of chiefship in the latter society. Ankole's reported CBR of 1930, 38.5 per 1,000, was reasonably plausible, whereas the 1935 rate, 21.8, was not. Nothing in the medical records, moreover, could explain why Ankole's still-birth rate in the 1920s was almost four times as high as in the 1930s, nor why the rate should have dropped from 17.8% of all births in 1929 to 4.4% in 1930 (see Figures 7.1 and 7.2).[6]

Vital registration then proves to be of limited value in helping to trace and explain fertility change during the mid-colonial period, in the case of Ankole at least. Uganda's censuses before 1948 though were superior to the norm for

[6] Uganda Protectorate, Annual Medical Reports 1912–49, NA, CO/685; C. Martin, 'Some estimates of the general age distribution, fertility and rate of natural increase of the African population of British East Africa', *Population Studies*, 7, 2 (1953), pp. 188–9. The sharp fall in the vital registration crude birth rate between 1947 and 1948 was due to the incremental underestimation of the total population between the 1931 and 1948 censuses.

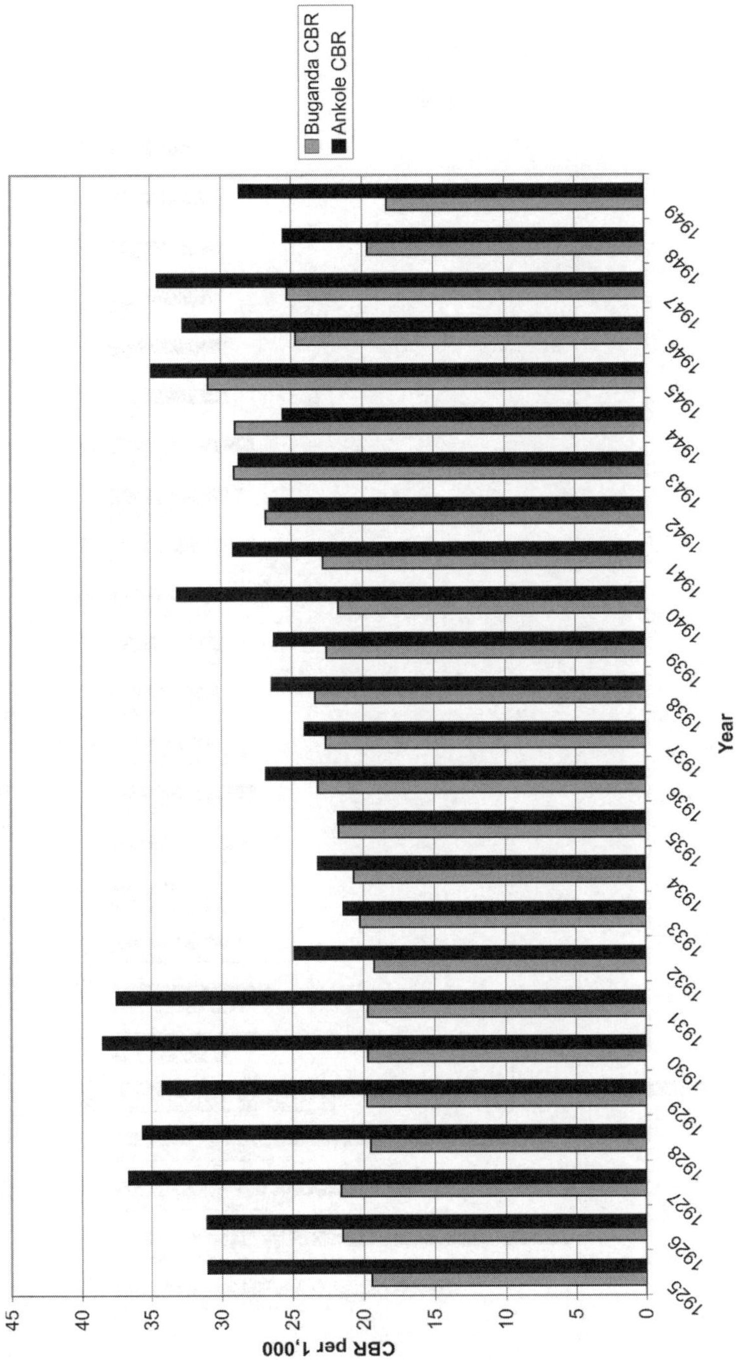

Figure 7.1 Crude birth rate per 1,000 in Ankole and Buganda 1925–49, from vital registration records

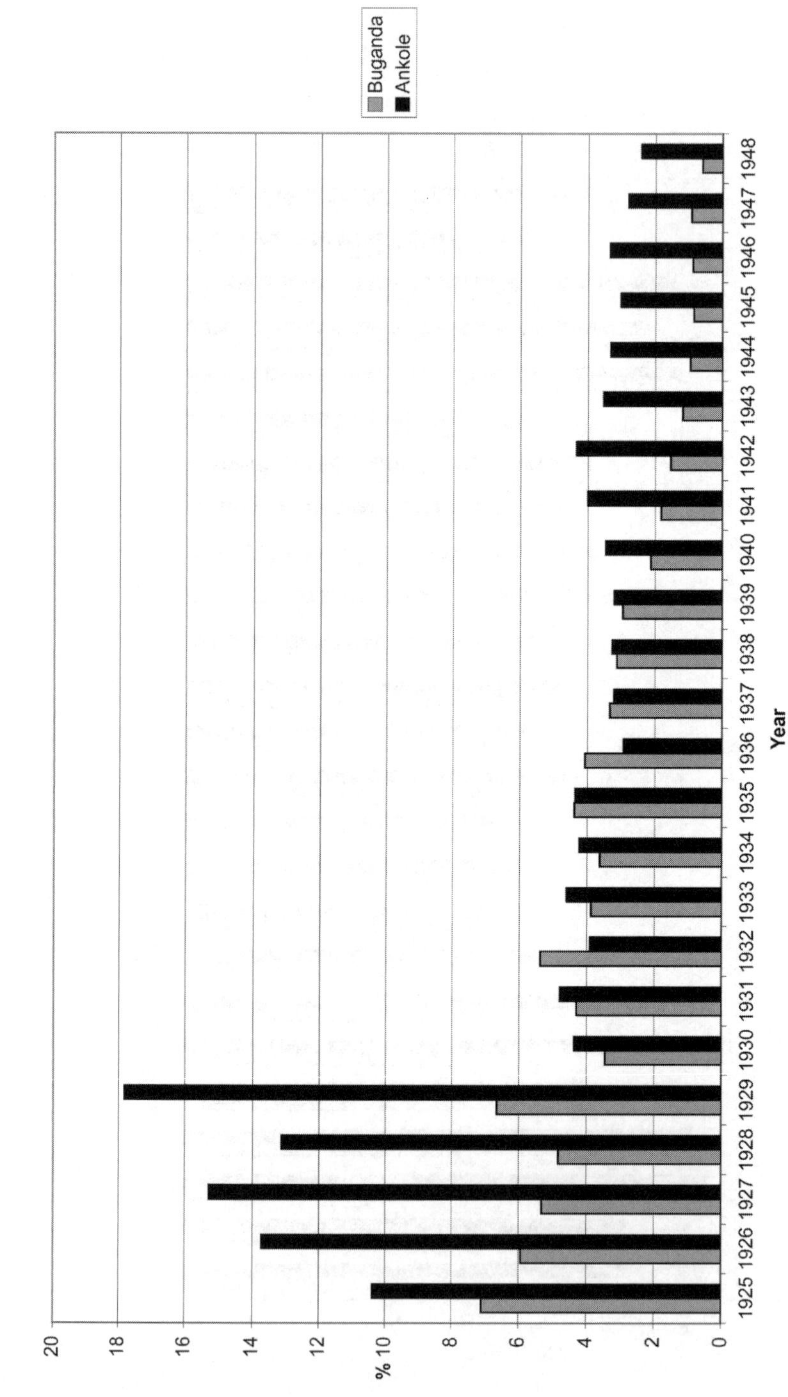

Figure 7.2 Stillbirths as a percentage of all registered births in Ankole and Buganda 1925–48

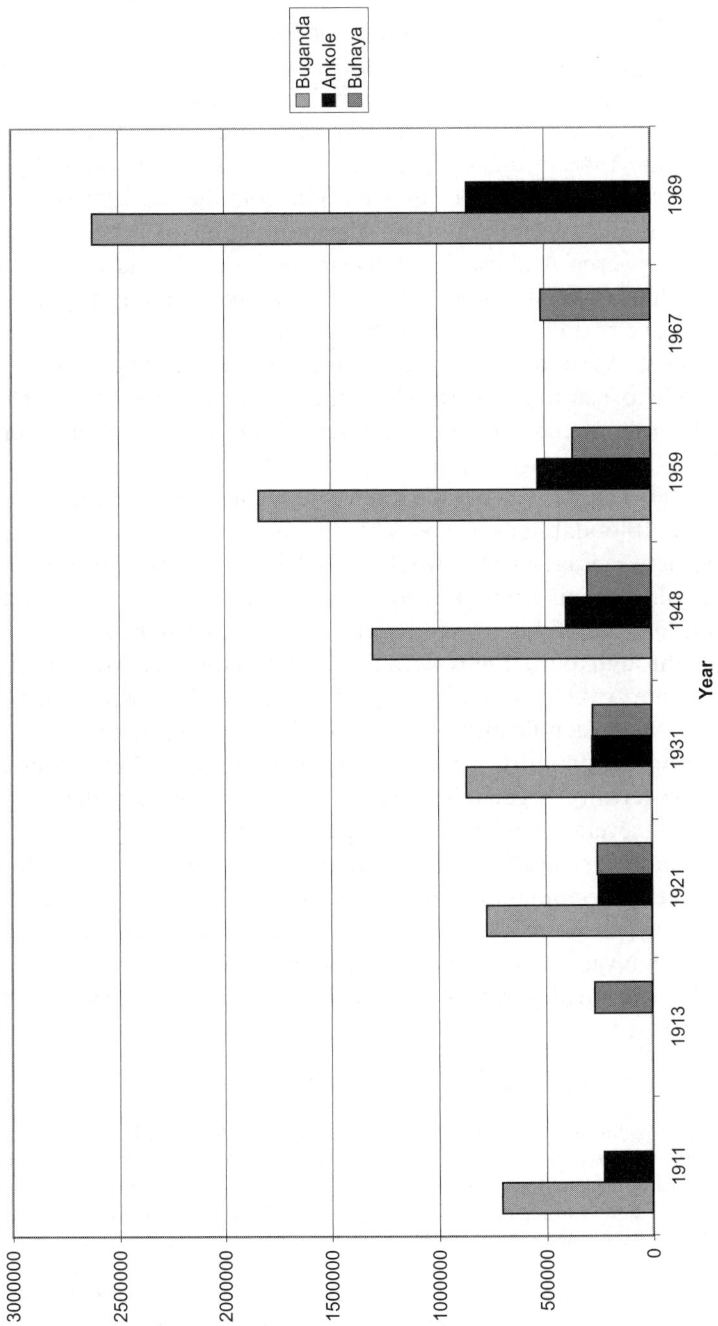

Figure 7.3 Population totals for Ankole, Buganda and Buhaya according to census data

inter-war Africa, in that they did at least attempt to count the entire population. But as the method of enumeration was for each sub-parish headman to gather his villagers together to be recorded, there existed great potential for omission, both deliberate and unintentional. It is likely that the district totals for the censuses of 1911, 1921, and 1931 were underestimates, which helps explain why the 1948 results caused such consternation in colonial government circles (see Figure 7.3). The information from the pre-1948 censuses on the age profile and marital status of the population of Ankole is of real significance, however. A marked increase in the ratio of children to adults in a society such as colonial Ankole tends to be associated with rapid population growth, due to an increase in birth rates or child survival, or a combination of the two.[7] As so many male labour migrants left Ankole for Buganda it seems sensible to examine only the changing age structure of the female population, which shows that whereas there were almost twice as many women as girls under fifteen in Ankole in 1911, by 1969 their numbers had equalized (see Table 7.1). The various census reports used slightly different ages as the marker of adulthood, but as it is possible that in a largely illiterate culture the distinction between age-groups would have been socio-biological as well as chronological, it seems safest not to adjust the raw data. The district level figures indicate that children made up an ever increasing proportion of the population through to the 1960s, with the fastest change occurring after 1959, but results from Ankole's counties suggest that rates of growth varied across the society. Most significantly, the Nyabushozi census data suggest that Ankole's pastoralist minority, like several other African communities with a history of low fertility, began to experience relatively rapid population growth only after 1948, several decades after the agriculturalist majority. Unfortunately most of Uganda's censuses failed to distinguish between Ankole's cultivating and cattle-keeping populations, but it is possible to compare the age profiles of counties which were predominantly agricultural, such as Igara and Mitooma, with Nyabushozi, Ankole's pastoralist heartland. Table 7.1 suggests that Ankole's sustained growth was the result of successive, localized periods of rapid increase.[8]

[7] Cf. B. Fetter, 'Decoding and interpreting African census data: Vital evidence from an unsavory witness', *Cahiers d'études africaines*, 27, 105/106 (1987), pp. 83–105. Evidence supporting the alternative causative explanation of a more youthful population, a sustained increase in adult mortality or migration, is difficult to find for this period with the exception of Nyabushozi from 1921 to 1931, where the number of children rose by 9% while that of adults fell by 21%.

[8] Uganda Protectorate, 'Sample census 1948' (I am grateful to Sarah Walters for sharing this unpublished document with me). In the late 1950s Derrick Stenning calculated that among the Hima community he surveyed in Nyabushozi, only 30.4% of the female population was aged under 15. It is possible that Nyabushozi's population became so much younger in the 1950s primarily because of the immigration of non-pastoralist families.

Table 7.1 Girls as a percentage of the female population in Ankole

Age group	Census date	Ankole	Igara	Mitooma	Nyabushozi
Under 15	1911	37.4	42.7	26.7	26.5
Under 15	1921	39.2	43.4	38.2	33.7
Under 15	1931	43.5	50.8	36.5	No data
Under 16	1948	44.3	49.3	42.0	32.9
Under 16	1959	46.9	50.0	45.6	39.7
Under 15	1969	49.8	No data	No data	No data

The 1948 census indicated that Ankole's pattern of fertility change was shaped by generational as well as geographical factors. The most surprising finding of the 1948 sample census in Ankole was the remarkably high level of childlessness among women aged over forty-five. Of Nkole women who had passed the age of childbearing, 39% had never given birth, by far the highest rate in Uganda, and more than double the national average. Yet women who had given birth at least once had relatively high fertility. Sixty-three percent had had five or more babies, and their average completed family size was 5.77.[9] By contrast, only 24.2% of Nkole women aged thirteen to forty-five had had no children, and it is reasonable to assume that some of these women were not yet married rather than sterile.[10] Ankole had Uganda's third-lowest level of childlessness among women of reproductive age, a dramatic transformation in the likelihood of motherhood in this society, which, more than anything else, would have accounted for Ankole's shift towards extremely high fertility during the colonial period. Appreciating the significance of this change is much easier than explaining it, but it seems likely that early colonial pressure to bolster marriage and reshape sexual norms played a major role, with improvements in reproductive health perhaps playing a secondary role in this pre-penicillin era.

One factor that would have contributed to the decline in the rate of childlessness would have been the reduction in the proportion of Nkole women

[9] Uganda Protectorate, 'Sample census 1948'. The average completed family size is an underestimate as the census report grouped together all women with ten or more births. My calculation assumed they had no more than ten. Gorju had commented on the frequency of sterility in Ankole before 1920. J. Gorju, *Entre le Victoria, l'Albert et l'Edouard* (Rennes, 1920, translated by Ralph Butler, 1957, A. Richards papers, LSE archive), pp. 15–16.

[10] It is likely that some women may have stated that they were childless whereas in fact they had had a child which died soon after birth, and that this would have been a more significant factor among the older women.

[11] Uganda Protectorate, *1911 Census Returns* (Entebbe: Government Printer, 1912); Uganda Protectorate, *1921 Census Returns* (Entebbe: Government Printer, 1922); Uganda Protectorate, *1931 Census Returns* (Entebbe: Government Printer, 1932); B. Sheku, 'Pathological determinants of *sterility* in rural Uganda' (unpublished PhD dissertation, University of Pennsylvania, 1987), p. 27.

who were unmarried in the early colonial period. In 1911 and 1921 16% of Nkole women had never married, compared to the Ugandan average of 11%. By 1931 only 8% of women in Ankole had not married, while the Ugandan average had increased to 13%. This trend towards near universal marriage in Ankole was sustained through to the 1970s, with a large-scale demographic survey in 1972 reporting an almost identical proportion of women who had never married, 9%. Ninety-seven percent of women aged over thirty had been married, an exceptionally high rate.[11] Not only did almost all Nkole women marry after the First World War, they tended to stay married. In many societies in Africa which suffered high levels of childlessness, Buganda and Buhaya among them, failure to quickly conceive often led to rapid divorce, helping to create a vicious circle of marital instability and infertility.[12] The case of Ankole demonstrates that such a response was not automatic. Ankole's pre-existing cultural opposition to separation appears to have been reinforced during the colonial period. Most informants stated that when divorce did occur, remarriage was common. This was also true for widows, unless they were near the end of their reproductive lives. A recurring theme in interviews in Ankole was opposition to the reproductive potential of young women being wasted.[13] The 1972 survey found that 82% of women aged between fifteen and forty-five were currently married. Childlessness had not disappeared from the female experience in Ankole but it had increasingly become a temporary phenomenon, associated with delayed marriage. Only 13% of women aged over forty-five had never borne a child, a third of the level found in the 1948 sample census. By contrast the proportion of women of reproductive age who were still childless was now 31%, the great majority of whom were aged under twenty-five. An increase in marriage age due to schooling and, to a lesser extent, employment seems to have caused many Nkole women to start their reproductive lives relatively late by the early 1970s.[14]

Ankole's marriage rate was relatively low before 1931, but was certainly not low enough to account for the extremely high levels of childlessness among older women recorded in 1948. It seems likely therefore that disease-related primary sterility must have been extremely common in the early colonial period. Few data on disease prevalence and incidence are available from colonial Ankole, but none of the evidence which exists indicates that trypanosomiasis, schistosomiasis, or malaria, some of the most important pathological causes of infertility in Africa, were particularly significant in this

[12] E. Boserup, 'Economic and demographic interrelationships in sub-Saharan Africa', *Population and Development Review,* 11, 3 (1985), pp. 383–97; O. Kokole, 'The politics of fertility in Africa', *Population and Development Review,* 20 (1994), pp. 73–88.

[13] Kyenjenyi Focus Group Discussion (FGD) Female, 22 Aug. 2004; Male FGD Namitanga, 19 Aug. 2004; Kiyungi FGD Female, 21 Aug. 2004.

[14] Sheku, 'Sterility', pp. 27–51.

district, although tuberculosis was reported to be very common. This leaves STDs as the most likely alternative explanation for this district's primary infertility. No reliable data on prevalence levels exist before 1948. Ankole's population was described as highly syphilized by early colonial observers, but the tendency to over-diagnose syphilis in this period has been well documented. The sources give no indication before the Second World War of the frequency of infection with gonorrhoea and chlamydia, much more serious causes of sterility, so it is possible that their prevalence fell dramatically after the First World War. But as is also the case with tuberculosis, no medical intervention that existed in Uganda before 1948 is likely to have brought about such a major fall in infection rates. The possibility exists that sexual behavioural change on a large scale occurred in the early decades of the twentieth century in Ankole, reducing STD-related sterility dramatically, but the evidence for such a radical change is relatively slim. The moralistic Balokole movement was prominent in Ankole, but only affected less than 2% of the population before the 1950s. However, mainstream Christianity, which spread rapidly from the 1930s, does seem to have been more associated with heightened sexual probity in Ankole than in Buganda, for example (see Chapter 6). Certainly missionary opposition to under-age marriage may have reduced the number of women who became sterile as a result of being exposed to sexual contact before they were physically mature. It may be, moreover, that the increase in the proportion of the adult population which was married after 1921 was part of a broader shift in sexual morality generated by chiefly pressure and ethnic rivalry.[15]

The decline in the level of primary sterility was only one of several factors which together resulted in Ankole having some of the highest fertility rates in Africa between 1959 and 1969. Family reconstitution offers additional insights into the causes of fertility increase in this society. The results of the reconstruction of family relationships using the baptism and marriage registers of the large Catholic parish of Nyamitanga, whose headquarters lay on the outskirts of the district capital of Mbarara, show that birth spacing changed significantly during this period. The average gap between each birth lengthened until it peaked in the early 1930s at 32.3 months, before falling steadily to around 28.6 months in the late 1950s, a level at which it remained

[15] Uganda Protectorate, *1957 Annual Medical Report* (Entebbe: Government Printer, 1958); Frazer Committee meeting with the Ankole district team, 20 Sept. 1955, Wellcome Archive, PP/CDW E.3/2; Lambkin, Mission to the Uganda Protectorate on the prevalence of venereal diseases. Summary of evidence, Dec. 1907, NA, CO/536/15; Annual medical report 1918, NA, CO/536/95; Kyangyenyi/Kiyungu Male FGD, 22 Aug. 2004; Int. ML, 12 Aug. 2004, Mbarara, F; C. Costello, 'Maternal and child health in rural Uganda: the role of nutrition' (unpublished PhD dissertation, University of Pennsylvania, 1986), p. 291.

until the end of the 1960s. This was a major change, but it was not an exceptional decline in birth spacing, by modern Africa standards. Comparing the reconstitution results from Buganda and Ankole, it seems clear that after 1930 Ganda women had shorter birth intervals than women in Nyamitanga, no doubt in part because of reduced coital frequency in Ankole due to labour migration. Yet we know that Nkole women had much higher fertility during this period. The reconstitutions help to resolve this apparent problem. They show that the average number of children baptized per family in Nyamitanga exceeded that in the Buganda and Buhaya parishes by 42%, with the biggest increase occurring between 1910 and 1924 (see Figure 7.7).[16] Moreover, the proportion of women in each parish who had baptized five or more children was, at 15.2%, 2.3 times higher in Ankole than Buganda and Buhaya (see Figure 7.8). The possibility must be acknowledged that variations in data quality across these three parishes may have artificially generated these differences in birth spacing. For example, the higher frequency with which parishioners in Nyamitanga married in their local church could be interpreted as a marker of greater population stability compared to Bukoba and Kisubi, or of greater religious devotion, which could indicate that Nkole were more likely to seek baptism for their children more urgently than elsewhere. But in fact Ankole was one of East Africa's great labour exporting regions during the colonial period. Moreover, while the average delay between birth and baptism differed significantly across the three parishes, a factor which, given the high levels of infant mortality in these societies, might have been of great importance, it was actually highest in Nyamitanga, at 363 days, compared to 254

[16] Birth intervals of less than nine and more than sixty months were excluded, as were those where one of the children's dates of birth did not specify at least the month in which the birth occurred. The interval between marriage and birth, and the last open-ended interval, were excluded from these calculations. There was no attempt to refine this sample to exclude poor recorders because no records exist relating to, for example, attendance at festivals or tithe payment. The birth interval calculations were based on 11,284 individuals. These figures tally well with the average birth interval of 30.5 months which was recorded in 1972 by the Ankole Demographic Research Project. The 1972 figure was calculated from reproductive histories obtained from a large sample of women aged between fifteen and forty-nine. Some of the birth intervals included in this average figure therefore would have dated from the late 1930s. Costello, 'Maternal', p. 161. The 1972 total is likely to have been inflated due to informants' forgetting some pregnancies which did not result in a living child. Equally the parish reconstitution data would have exaggerated true birth intervals, while the total number of children baptized grossly underestimated true fertility levels. As noted above, many babies would have died before being baptized, given the size of these parishes; couples often would have been lost to observation in the middle of their reproductive lives due to permanent or temporary migration or the creation of daughter parishes; and, given the inaccuracy of missionary recording of personal names, reconstitution was far from complete. Many of these problems, it should be noted, were common in historic European parishes as well.

days in Bukoba and 182 in Kisubi. The delay increased steadily in all three parishes over time, yet there was no obvious correlation between this worsening, uneven problem of delayed baptism and birth spacing trends. Overall, it does not seem that the inconsistencies within the parish registers undermined the reliability of the results of the reconstitution in any obvious way. In the absence of age-specific marital fertility rates, it cannot be demonstrated beyond reasonable doubt that, as an explanation of Nkole women's high fertility, the longevity of their reproductive lives within marriage was more important than the rapidity with which they gave birth. But it can certainly be suggested that lower levels of divorce and secondary sterility contributed greatly to Ankole's higher fertility compared to Buganda and Buhaya.

On balance, it seems that the apparent lengthiness of Nkole women's reproductive lives was not due to women entering marriage at an exceptionally young age. Neo-Marxist models of demographic growth in colonial Africa hypothesize that women reproduced for longer periods of their lives because of economic pressures which encouraged earlier marriage than had historically been the norm. In Ankole, however, the parish registers indicate that average marriage age for men and, more importantly, for women rose gradually from the 1920s until the 1950s and then stabilized. On average, before 1970 Catholic men married, supposedly for the first time, at 23.7 years of age, women at 21. While Nkole men married about nine months earlier than Ganda and Haya males, Catholic brides in Ankole were around nine and twenty-one months older than their counterparts in Buganda and Buhaya (see Figures 7.5 and 7.6). The recorded age at marriage in church though should be assumed to be higher than the norm in African societies in this period. Parish weddings were unlikely to be representative of marriage more generally. Many who underwent a Christian ceremony did so as a marker of status or aspiration, and are likely to have had their marriages delayed by prolonged education or paid employment. Moreover, it would be optimistic to believe that church authorities were always aware of situations where a couple sought a Catholic wedding simply to add a spiritual blessing to a pre-existing union. Other sources indicate that Christian weddings did indeed occur later than the societal norm. James Ntozi calculated the female singulate mean age at marriage (SMAM) from the 1969 census data to be 18.1 years in Ankole, while a rural survey in 1972 reported that women had on average first married at 16.7 years of age. The value of the parish data then is primarily longitudinal and comparative. The church records indicate that marriage age rose rather than fell over time, and that women married later in Ankole than in the other case study areas. Therefore the seemingly greater longevity of Nkole women's reproductive lives cannot be explained by their having started earlier than their neighbours, but from their having been able to have children over a longer period once they started. Marital stability and sustained reproductive health were key.[17] A survey conducted by Derrick Stenning in the late 1950s helps to explain why labour migration appears to have had only a marginal impact on average male marriage age. The men who had worked as migrant labourers comprised three distinct groups. A third of the men were the poorest in the community who had had to rely purely on labour migration to raise bridewealth, making up to six annual trips to Buganda to secure the funds needed. Such men might never have acquired the resources to marry before the introduction of a cash economy, so labour migration in this case was perhaps significant more for increasing the proportion of Nkole men who ever married, rather than for reducing the average marriage age. Another third had worked as migrant labourers for several years to supplement the livestock they had set aside for bridewealth, and it is likely that this did enable them to marry earlier than they otherwise would have done. The third group were men who possessed sufficient personal wealth to secure a wife but who delayed getting married while they worked away earning money to satisfy other material needs.[18]

It seems then that it is the information on birth intervals rather than marriage age which is the most valuable product of the Nyamitanga reconstitution. It is likely that birth spacing began to shorten because of the cumulative effect of a number of factors during the interwar period rather than one particular trigger in the late 1930s, the point at which average intervals began

[17] J. Ntozi and J. Kabera, 'Marriage patterns in Ankole, South-Western Uganda' (African Demography Working Papers no. 16, University of Pennsylvania, August 1988), p. 11; Sheku, 'Sterility', p. 27.

[18] D4 Background Information, D10 Marriage, D12 Migrant Labour, D. Stenning papers, Cambridge University Library.

[19] Source: Bukoba, Kisubi, and Nyamitanga Catholic parish baptism registers. The graphs display only those five-year periods with more then fifty birth intervals. No data were available for Bukoba after independence.

[20] Only five-year periods when twenty-five or more marriages occurred are included. Marriage ages below twelve and above forty-five are excluded, because it is unlikely that individuals would marry for the first time at such ages, and that they would be fertile. Marriage ages were taken from the baptism rather than the marriage registers from these parishes, partly because the former were more likely to identify individuals who should be excluded from the calculations because they were widowed or were seeking a religious blessing for a pre-existing customary marriage. Moreover, individuals were unlikely to state their true ages when marrying if they were very young. Thus only 3.1% of brides in the Kisubi marriage register stated their age at less than sixteen, none less than fourteen. None of the 1,051 husbands in this marriage register were younger than sixteen, only eight younger than 18. But the marriage dates recorded in the notes column of the baptism register indicated that 10.8% of brides and 4.6% of husbands were younger than sixteen. In May 1937 a woman named Namayanja married at Kisubi, her age being recorded as fifteen in the marriage register. Yet by linking the personal details recorded in the marriage and baptism registers we find that she was in fact just over thirteen years old. In March 1925 a woman named Namutebi claimed to be twenty-three when getting married. She was in fact twelve years and three months old.

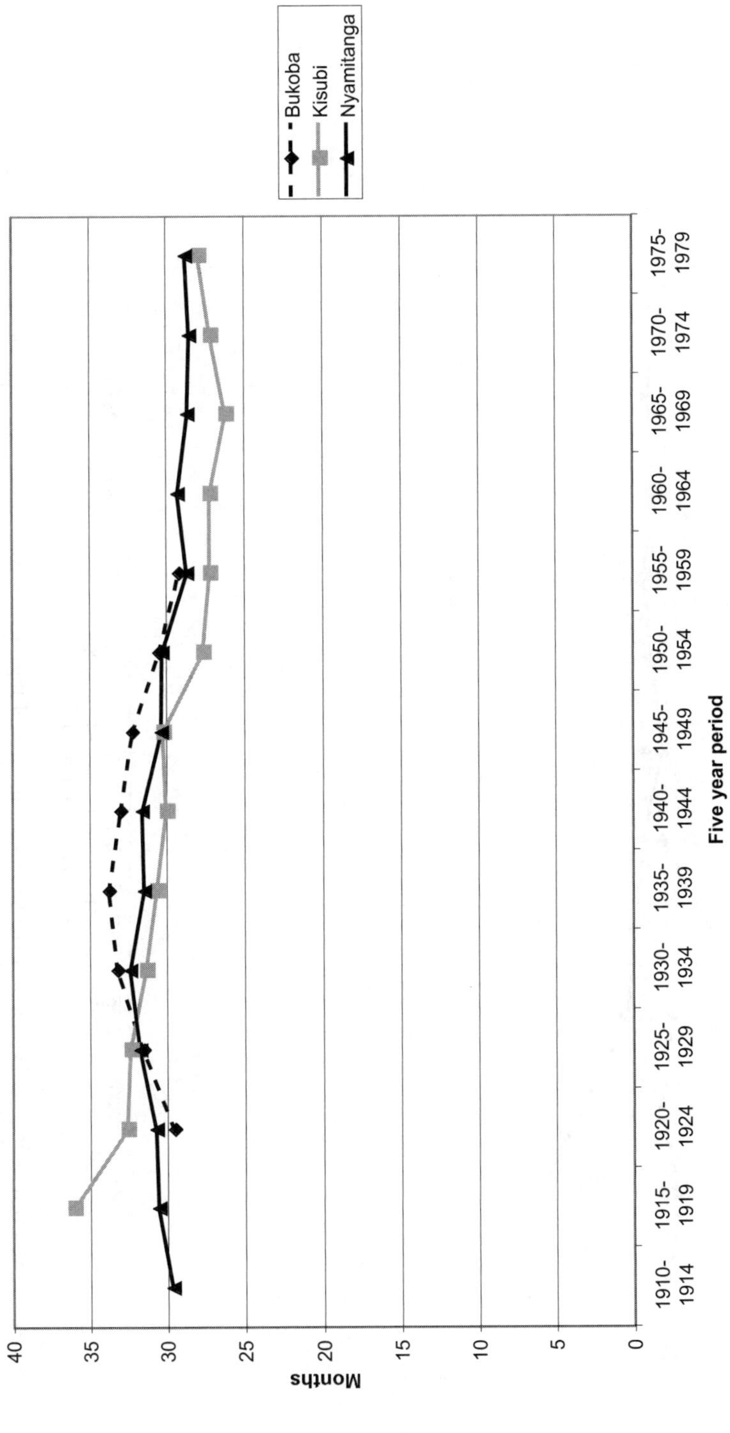

Figure 7.4 Average birth intervals in months for the Catholic parishes of Bukoba (Buhaya), Kisubi (Buganda), and Nyamitanga (Ankole)[19]

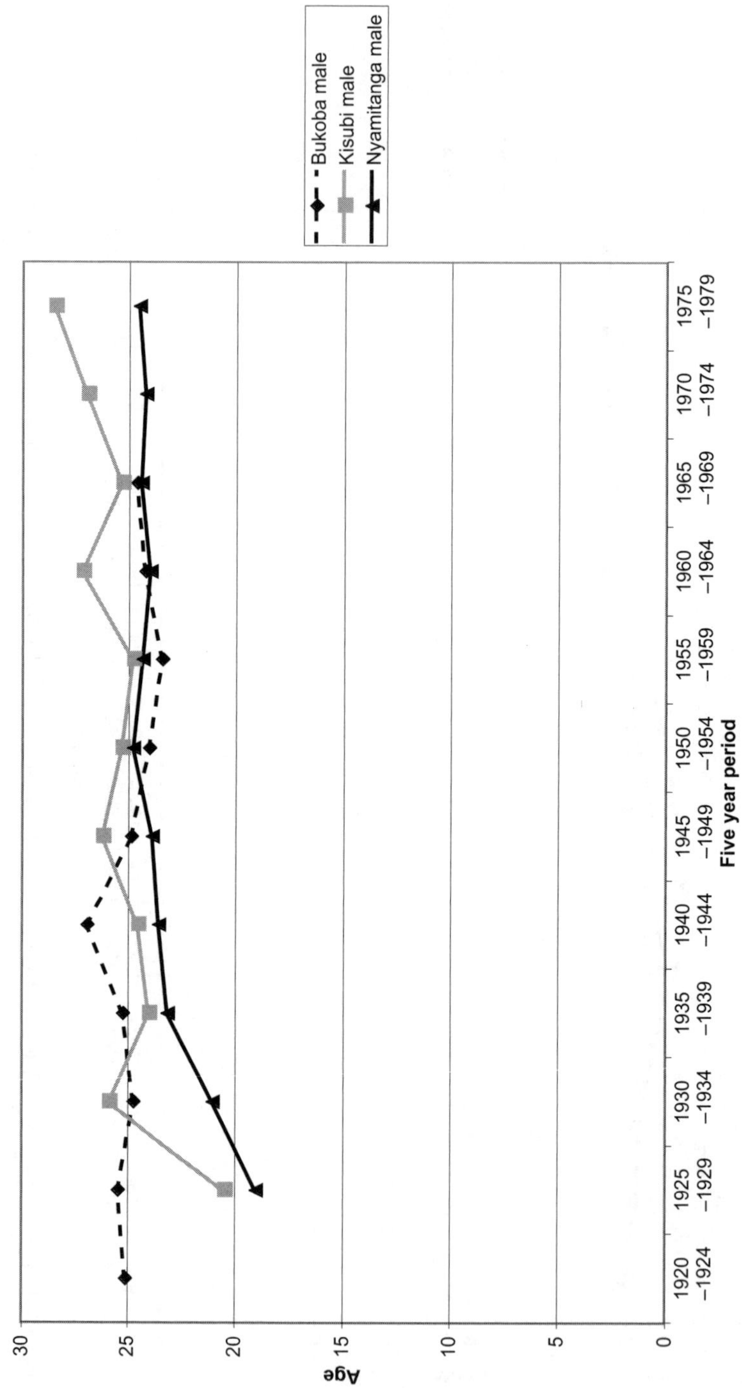

Figure 7.5 Mean age at first marriage for males in the Catholic parishes of Bukoba (Buhaya), Kisubi (Buganda) and Nyamitanga (Ankole)

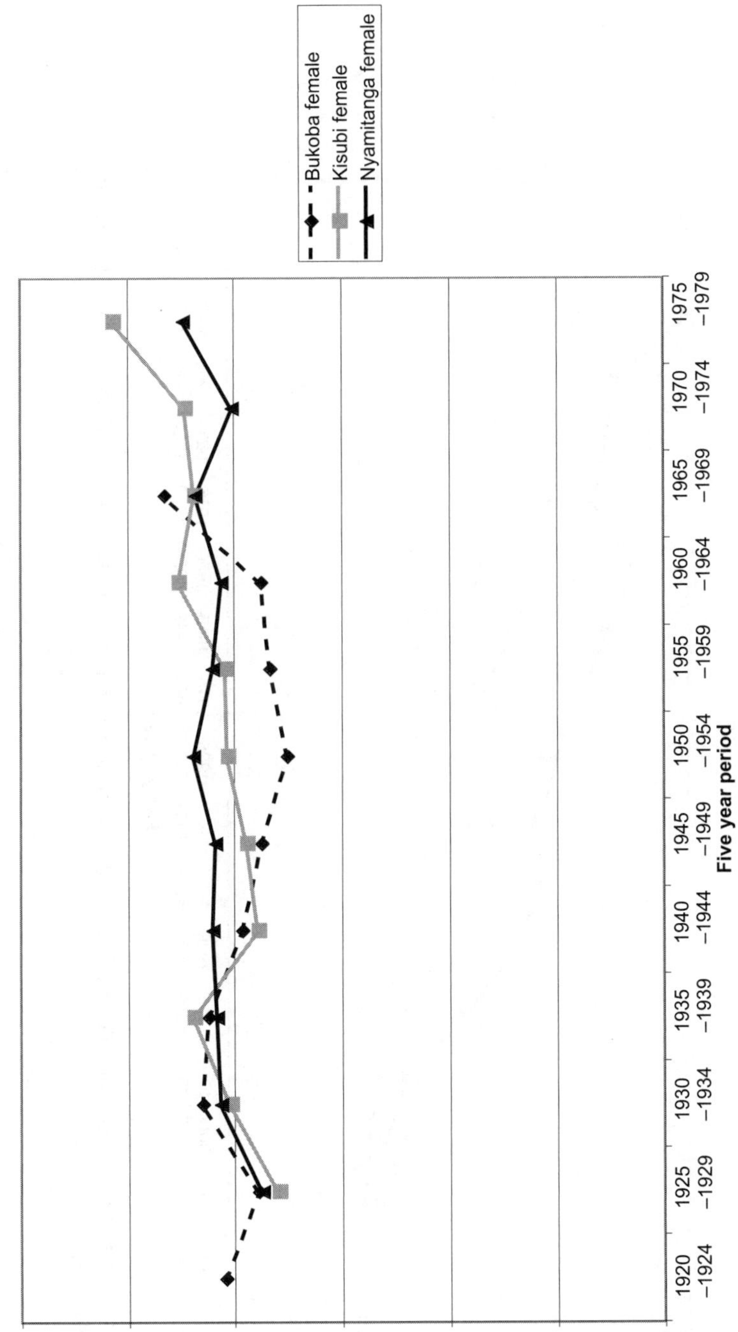

Figure 7.6 Mean age at first marriage for females in the Catholic parishes of Bukoba (Buhaya), Kisubi (Buganda) and Nyamitanga (Ankole)[20]

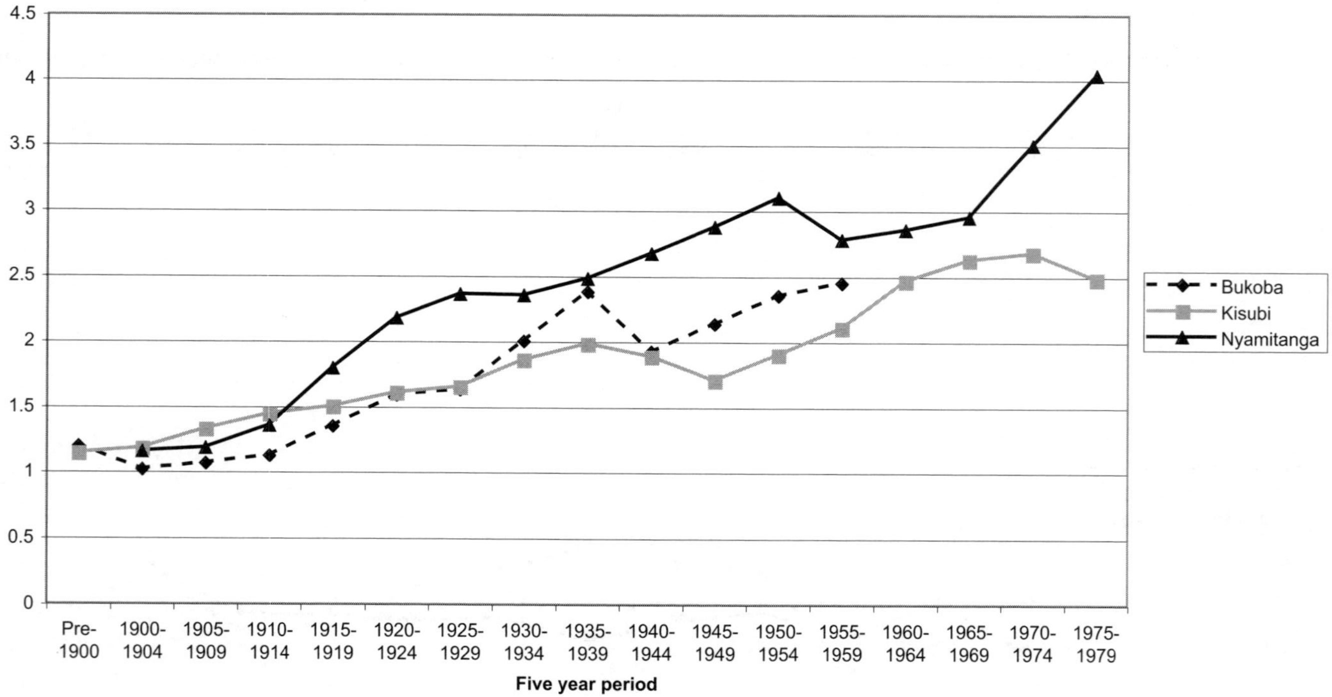

Figure 7.7 Mean number of children ever baptized per woman in the Catholic parishes of Bukoba (Buhaya), Kisubi (Buganda), and Nyamitanga (Ankole)[21]

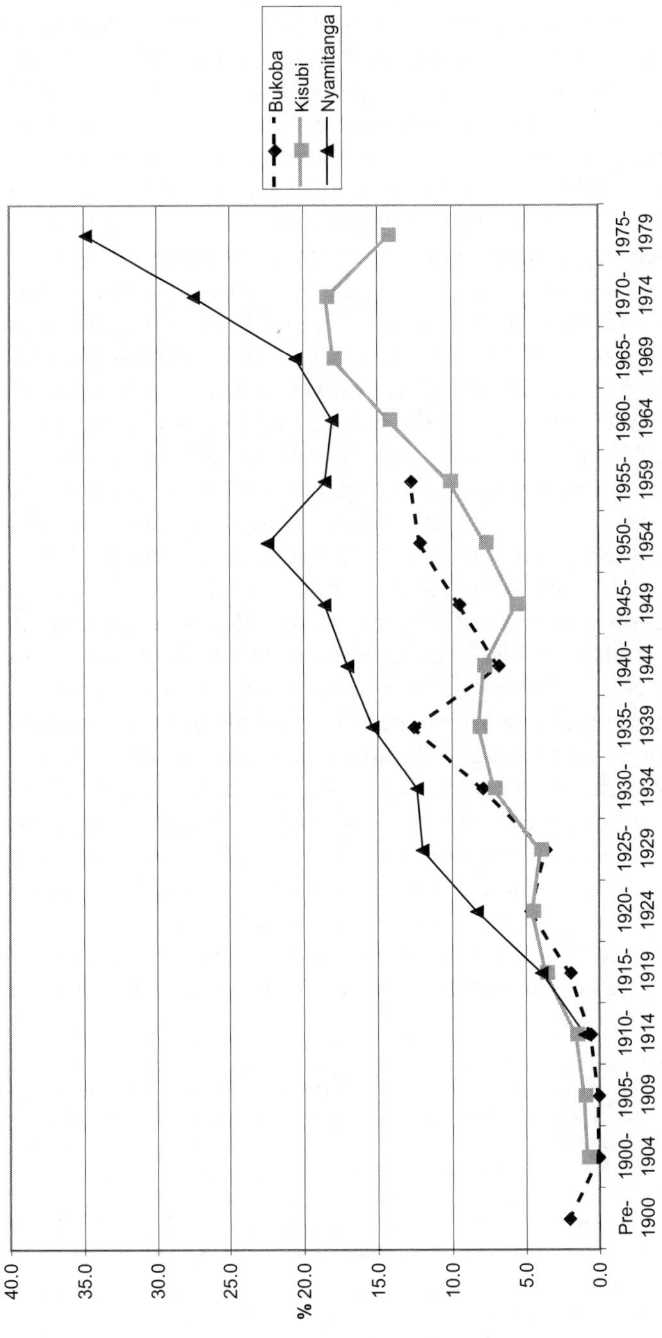

Figure 7.8 Percentage of mothers with five or more baptized children in the Catholic parishes of Bukoba (Buhaya), Kisubi (Buganda), and Nyamitanga (Ankole)

to fall. An examination of birth intervals by parity provides some evidence that in Ankole there was a cohort effect at play, for birth intervals began to decline among women having their second baby in the early 1930s, for para 3 and 4 women in the late 1930s, and for para 5 and 6 women between 1945 and 1949.[22] If this is true, then it suggests that women born in the second decade of the twentieth century came to maturity with a body of experiences which encouraged or enabled them to space their births more closely together. Almost all the parents in the Nyamitanga dataset were Catholics, and so would have been exposed to clerical criticism of prolonged breastfeeding and post-partum sexual abstinence, which many missionaries believed were used as justifications for male adultery and polygamy. It was also commonplace for such practices to be regarded as unmodern by women who had gone to school in colonial Africa, but formal education was the exception rather than the rule for Ankole females during the colonial period. According to the 1959 census only 5.4% of women who were born between 1914 and 1943 had had any schooling, hardly enough to change district-level behaviour noticeably. Male education rates were much higher, though not nearly so high as in Buganda and Buhaya, and it is possible that some husbands may have encouraged their uneducated wives to abandon traditional spacing practices. Colonial and missionary healthcare moreover affected a still larger proportion of the population. All Catholic mission stations in Ankole possessed a dispensary after the First World War, and Church Missionary Society medical activity operated at a smaller scale but provided higher quality healthcare, while the colonial state opened a number of dispensaries between the wars to supplement Mbarara's district hospital. Famine policy too was a universal benefit, with no famine mortality being recorded in Ankole during this period, though widespread hunger was experienced in 1943. The 1948 census found that the experience of child loss had declined substantially among women born after 1903. Subsequent censuses showed that infant mortality continued to fall rapidly into the 1970s. Growing confidence in the likelihood of child survival may have permitted Nkole women from the 1930s to pay less heed to

[21] These data will underestimate the true family size in these parishes. Not all baptized children had a legible date of birth, it is likely that some parents' names were misspelt, many families would have had some children baptized outside the parish due to migration, and few babies who died soon after birth would have been baptized. Therefore family reconstitution here would have been incomplete. It is important again to note that many of these problems are universal and also affected European reconstitutions. The purpose of this graph is primarily comparative. All three parishes are of similar age and grew more or less at a similar rate. The low family sizes of the early period would partly reflect the Christianizing nature of these communities, so that not all children in a family would necessarily have been baptized.

[22] Due to the inevitable incompleteness of the family reconstitution, it should not be assumed that all parities are entirely accurate. This though should not affect the broad argument made here.

traditions supporting prolonged breastfeeding and abstinence.[23] Another possible cause of the reduced length of breastfeeding was the improving health and nutritional status of Nkole women. It was striking how many elderly informants reported that they had fallen pregnant on several occasions before they had realized that their post-partum amenorrhoea had ended. Such women wanted to breastfeed their babies for at least twelve months and space their pregnancies further apart, but found that lactation did not have the spacing effect that their elders had promised. Instead they found they were pregnant five or six months after their previous delivery, so that they were forced to wean their babies prematurely. Whatever the reason, by the mid-twentieth century on average women resumed having sex less than a month after giving birth, while by the end of our period only 8% of women breastfed for two years or more, the cultural norm.[24]

It is probable that it was only from the 1950s that improvements in reproductive healthcare contributed significantly to Nkole women's shortening birth intervals and increasing average parity. The district's first maternity hospital closed in 1921 due to lack of interest, and births in non-specialist medical units were a rarity for decades thereafter. Increased investment in maternity services and health education saw institutional births rise by 36% in 1951, but as late as 1958 there were more than three times as many maternity beds per woman in Buganda as Ankole. It was not until 1970 that medicalized delivery became anything like the norm in Ankole. Various reports from this period emphasize the unusual strength of local antagonism towards biomedical maternity services. Proverbs described childbirth as a battle which provided women with an opportunity to demonstrate their bravery. Elders identified the desire of pregnant women for medical assistance as a sign of weakness, although in fact many younger women avoided the maternity ward because

[23] Uganda, *1959 Census*; Uganda Protectorate, Annual Medical Reports, 1926–1949, NA, CO/685; Uganda, 1948 Sample Census. Cf. S. Walters, 'Fertility, mortality and marriage in northwest Tanzania, 1920–1970: A demographic study using parish registers' (unpublished PhD dissertation, University of Cambridge, 2008), p. 275. In the mid-1950s Derrick Stenning interviewed thirty-seven women aged between twenty and sixty about their reproductive histories. Only 7.5% of pregnancies had ended in miscarriage or stillbirth while 23.5% of children had died. This was a small sample but suggests that women here could have contemplated shortening their birth intervals. 'Age and sex composition by parcels', Stenning papers, D7, CUL.

[24] Female FGD Ruti, 19 Aug. 2004; Kyenjenyi FGD Female, 22 Aug. 2004; Bumbire (Bushenyi) FGD Female, 2004; Y. Elam, *The Social and Sexual Roles of Hima Women: A Study of Nomadic Cattle Breeders in Nyabushozi County, Ankole, Uganda* (Manchester: Manchester University Press, 1973), pp. 147, 150–2, 174, 186–7; M. Mushanga, 'The Nkole of South-Western Uganda', in A. Molnos (ed.), *Cultural Source Materials for Population Planning in East Africa III* (Nairobi, University of Nairobi, 1973), p. 178; J. Ntozi, *The Role of Men in Determining Fertility among the Banyankore of Southwestern Uganda* (Kampala: Marianum Press, 1993), pp. 67, 71; Costello, 'Maternal', p. 234. Cf. C. Varkevisser, 'The Sukuma of northern Tanzania', in Molnos, *Cultural III*, p. 236.

they associated it with excessive pain and danger. Midwives' insistence that women wait until they were fully dilated before pushing was regarded as unnecessarily prolonging the agony of childbirth, while exaggerated rumours about the frequency of caesarean section kept many women away from the clinic. In consequence, although one-third of Nkole women gave birth in the clinic in the late 1960s, emergency cases made up an exceptionally high proportion of maternity admissions, so that this district had Uganda's highest institutional rates of stillbirth and maternal and neo-natal mortality. Female interviewees spoke with distaste of the atmosphere of 'chaos' in maternity wards in the 1960s due to the unplanned arrival of women suffering from disproportion, ruptured uterus, and post-partum haemorrhage. Nonetheless, the expansion of maternity services after the Second World War did reduce maternal death and pregnancy loss. In one focus group alone, five out of seven women had required medical intervention to resolve potentially life-threatening complications associated with childbirth. Minor surgical intervention helped women who had suffered habitual abortions due to cervical incompetence. Ante-natal clinics tested and treated pregnant women for syphilis and identified those who required assisted delivery due to problems such as malpresentation, thus reducing levels of miscarriage and stillbirth. They also supplied women who were determined to deliver at home with drugs that would reduce the risk of severe haemorrhage, and, through sustained health education, ensured that it became common by the 1960s for traditional birth attendants to observe basic hygiene during delivery and use a new razor blade when cutting the umbilical cord, thus reducing levels of tetanus. The impact of these improvements in the provision of medical care and advice was reinforced by a dramatic increase in levels of female schooling, with a rural survey in the 1960s finding that educated women suffered 71% fewer stillbirths and neo-natal deaths than the uneducated.[25]

Criticism from medical staff also helped to reduce the number of women who used powerful oxytocic herbal medicines during delivery, with the aim of strengthening contractions and so shortening childbirth. Such herbal medicines were particularly dangerous in cases of malpresentation, where the

[25] Western Province Annual Report, 1922, ESA, A46/1094; Uganda Protectorate, *1951 Annual Medical Report* (Entebbe: Government Printer, 1952); E. Grech, J. Galea and R. Trussell, 'Maternal mortality in Uganda', *International Journal of Gynaecology and Obstetrics*, 7, 6 (1969), p. 263; Kiyungi FGD Female, 21 Aug. 2004; Kyenjenyi FGD Female, 22 Aug. 2004; Female FGD Ruti, 2004; Monica Byrne papers, RHO, MSS.Afr.s.1872 (23); R. Cook, 'Child health in Ankole, Uganda: A programme of immunization and health education and its evaluation' (unpublished DMed dissertation, University of Oxford, n/d [*c*.1968]), p. 88; K. Masters and J. Iraka, 'The influence of custom and tradition on maternity care in Ankole district', *East African Medical Journal*, 47, 11 (1970), p. 553. Of course some of the women treated for syphilis may have been misdiagnosed, given the inaccuracy of colonial era tests.

baby's head was too large to fit through the mother's pelvis, or when they were administered before the mother's cervix was sufficiently dilated. Researchers in 1968 found that among women admitted to Mbarara Hospital's maternity ward, the incidence of stillbirth, neo-natal death, maternal death, and ruptured uterus was almost four times higher among women who used oxytocic medicines compared to those who did not. To a large extent this was because such medications were particularly likely to be given by birth attendants when a delivery was not progressing normally. Patients who had used oxytocic medication were four times more likely than non-users to suffer from problems of disproportion and malpresentation. The hospital data then, being drawn from a sample of oxytocic users who ended up requiring emergency intervention, would tend to exaggerate the risk of taking herbal medication during delivery. But in fact the 1968 study also surveyed women who had had no assistance from maternity services about their use of medicinal herbs and experience of stillbirths and neonatal deaths, and this found that oxytocics were still associated with a 59% increase in the risk of perinatal death.[26]

Ankole's high fertility has been discussed as a product of various changes, but it was also the result of a particularly resilient pro-natalism.[27] Many elderly informants when asked whether they had an ideal number of children they had wished to produce stated that a woman should keep producing for as long as she was physically able. One women when asked how many full-term births she had had replied 'five only'. Another was named Mpirirwe because her mother was considered to have taken such a long time—three years—to fall pregnant. When asked how many children would be considered to be a lot, male informants responded fifteen or twenty. It is striking how many aspects of Ankole's reproductive culture, such as the remarkably high number of occasions when a couple were expected to have ritual sex, and the

[26] Int. BK, 12 Aug. 2004, Mbarara, F; Masters and Iraka, 'The influence', pp. 550–6. This study found that 36% of women used oxytocics, that their use reduced with educational attainment, that among women admitted to hospital 34.2% of oxytocics users' pregnancies ended with uterine rupture or the death of mother or baby, and that 28.8% of oxytocics users were affected by disproportion or malpresentation.

[27] Hima culture was much less pro-natalist than the agriculturalist majority, due to the pressure to maximize the size of cattle herds. Fertility increase among the Hima was it seems partly due to the effect of antibiotic treatment on the high levels of recorded STDs within pastoralist society, but was also due to the Balokole Revival, which had a disproportionate impact among the Hima, reducing STD transmission caused by wife-sharing, limiting spousal separation through sedentarization (driven by a desire to maintain close contact with the church), and discouraging women from returning to their parents' homes after each delivery, which had ensured long periods of post-partum abstinence, but was now regarded as a dangerous challenge to husbands' fidelity. Cf. K. Oberg, 'Kinship organization of the Banyankole', *Africa*, 11, 2 (1938), p. 136; J. Ntozi et al., 'The value of children as a major influence on fertility in Uganda: A case study of Ankole', *Fertility Determinants Research Notes*, 23 (1988), pp. 20–7.

association of barrenness with moral failure and spiritual danger, survived largely unchanged through colonialism and decolonization. Ankole, moreover, seems to offer much clearer support than Buganda or Buhaya for the neo-Marxist thesis that the development of a modern economy supported pro-natalism. Informants claimed that polygamy remained relatively common in Ankole because men came to appreciate the labour value of children more once their agricultural work brought a cash return. 'You see, many children meant more workers on the farm.' According to one interviewee, one of her neighbours 'even dressed his children in a uniform. When they turned ten they would be given a hoe and a uniform and put to dig. They would be like labourers to him.'[28]

Buhaya

In many ways Bukoba in the mid-1920s was a model district, with which much of the rest of Tanganyika was compared unfavourably by Britain's colonial administration. Buhaya's authoritarian yet relatively respected and effective chiefs fitted well with indirect rule's ideal of the traditional ruler. Its tens of thousands of coffee farmers were an advertisement for colonial capitalism, their efforts proving crucial in Tanganyika's attempt to wean itself off metropolitan subsidy. In their appetite for schooling, the Haya again seemed to demonstrate a pleasing commitment to the imperial vision of progress.[29] But the Haya village, for all its ordered prosperity, jarred with European observers. In contrast to the dominant image of Africa, within Haya society children were remarkable for their scarcity rather than their ubiquity. Officials, convinced that the Haya population was falling or at best stagnating, and worried about declining tax revenues, fixated on the low fertility of the Haya people. By associating low birth rates with high reported rates of STD infection, both missionaries and administrators over the decades that followed

[28] Kiyungu Shema FGD Male, 21 Aug. 2004; Kyenjenyi FGD Female, 22 Aug. 2004; Male FGD Namitanga, 19 Aug. 2004; Kiyungi FGD Female, 21 Aug. 2004; Ntozi, *Role of Men*, p. 71; Male FGD Ruti, 19 Aug. 2004; Female FGD Nyamitanga, 19 Aug. 2004.

[29] This popularity proved ephemeral. Within a decade, colonial officials bemoaned Buhaya's chiefs' corruption, incompetence, and inability to contain populist agitators; the stagnation of coffee exports prompted ever more aggressive colonial criticism and intervention; and one of the most prominent African allies of the colonial state, Felix Lwamgira from Kiziba, began to question whether colonial-style education was in fact the best route to modernization. Cf. R. Austen, *Northwest Tanzania under German and British Rule: Colonial Policy and Tribal Politics, 1889–1939* (New Haven: Yale University Press, 1968), p. 135; K. Curtis, 'Capitalism fettered: state, merchant & peasant in northwestern Tanzania, 1917–1960', (unpublished PhD thesis, University of Wisconsin-Madison, 1989), pp. 282–95; J. Iliffe, *A Modern History of Tanganyika* (Cambridge: Cambridge University Press, 1979), pp. 281–6, 348.

repeatedly discussed Haya sub-fecundity as a symptom of a moral crisis within this society, a discourse that would be sustained by Haya themselves into the era of independence.[30]

Concerns about Buhaya's demographic situation came to a head in the late 1930s, as the last areas of farmland that could be easily turned over to coffee cultivation came to maturity and as tax receipts steadily declined. Inspired by the East African Revival, Protestant missionaries used cataclysmic language when discussing sub-fertility. In 1938 one missionary doctor preached that 'venereal disease has become rampant. We try to heal but it does not seem to help. The Haya are a dying people. Your country will be eaten up by another people. Hayaland stands at the door of death.'[31] In the same year the colonial administrator Arthur Culwick and his wife Geraldine, both regarded as specialists in the field of demography, were despatched to Buhaya to propose solutions to what was regarded as a demographic crisis. The Culwicks' report shared the missionaries' millenarian doom. 'The Bahaya are threatened with extinction as the result of venereal disease', they warned.[32] When the 1948 census showed that Buhaya was one of the few areas in East Africa whose population had failed to increase since 1931, its district commissioner believed that this confirmed 'the trend foretold by Culwick . . . the population is rapidly disappearing due to VD, prostitution and the general break-up of family life.'[33]

In response to these repeated warnings of imminent demographic collapse, Tanganyika's government requested that the newly established East African Medical Survey (EAMS) select Buhaya as one of its survey sites. The EAMS obliged, keen to understand why the Haya had not responded appropriately to the opportunities offered by colonial development.

> Here we have a productive area with a high rainfall, much money from cash crops, with available all the advantages of civilization, e.g. good educational facilities, first-class medical care and attention with a good general hospital, and readily available expert advice on agricultural, veterinary and other matters, with a central thoroughly efficient administration in command. And yet the tribe is dying.

[30] e.g. Bukoba District Annual Report 1926 TNA (Tanzania National Archives, Dar es Salaam) 215/77/A; B. Sundkler, *Bara Bukoba: Church and Community in Tanzania* (London: Hurst, 1980).

[31] B. Larsson, *Conversion to Greater Freedom? Women, Church and Social Change in North-Western Tanzania under Colonial Rule* (Uppsala: University of Uppsala, 1991), pp. 107–8.

[32] A. Culwick, 'The population problem in the Bukoba district' (Bukoba, 1938, UDSM, EAF CORY 239), pp. 7–9.

[33] Bukoba District Annual Report 1948, TNA 215/2237.

The explanation, once again, was idleness and immorality. While the survey's 1953 annual report noted that there was no correlation between the results of STD tests and fertility levels, blaming high levels of divorce for Haya sub-fertility, the final EAMS report in 1954 returned to familiar ground. 'Extra-marital intercourse' and consequent infection with gonorrhoea were hypothesized to be the primary causes of the low reproduction rate. Only when the Haya were shown 'the evil of their ways' might their demographic problems be resolved.[34]

These repeated assertions that Bukoba district's low fertility was due to STDs were internalized by Haya themselves. The EAMS found that the likelihood that a woman would claim that she was infected with an STD was correlated not with a positive serological test, but with a history of miscarriage, stillbirth, and infant mortality. Haya women had come to associate reproductive misfortune with sexual misconduct, often wrongly. As late as 1961 Haya commentators continued to state baldly that 'production of children has gone down in Buhaya because of VD.'[35]

The dominance of STDs in the analysis of Haya population history survived unchallenged until 1967 when Priscilla Reining completed a doctoral thesis based on her anthropological fieldwork from the early 1950s. Reining had assisted the EAMS during their investigations, and believed that the nature of Buhaya's demographic situation had been consistently misrepresented. As she observed, there was no evidence of population decline in Buhaya after the mid-1920s, and the relationship between syphilis infection and low fertility was not statistically significant. Reining found it peculiar that the Haya should have been condemned locally for failing to increase rapidly in numbers at a time when global concerns were beginning to focus on the problems arising from accelerating demographic growth in the developing world. Whereas colonial officials had described the Haya population as stagnant or on the brink of collapse, viewed Bukoba's farmers as frustratingly idle, and bemoaned the reluctance of the youth to colonize the interior of the district, Reining admired the stability of Buhaya's demographic system, the labour efficiency of Haya agriculture, and the entrepreneurialism and craftsmanship of young Haya men, asking why pioneering settlers should be

[34] East African Medical Survey, *Annual Report, 1952* (Nairobi: EAHC, 1953), pp. 23–32; East African Medical Survey, *Annual Report, 1953* (Nairobi: EAHC, 1954), pp. 12–13; W. Laurie and H. Trant, *East African Medical Survey, Monograph no. 2, A Health Survey in Bukoba District, Tanganyika* (Nairobi: EAHC, 1954), pp. 1–4, 138–40.

[35] P. Reining, 'The Haya: the agrarian system of a sedentary people' (unpublished PhD dissertation, University of Chicago, 1967), pp. 87–8; Haya students of Saint Andrew's Teacher Training College, Korogwe to the Secretary of the Council of Buhaya, 6 July 1961, Mwanza Provincial Archives (MPA), L5/II/B; S. Samson to the Secretary of the Council of Buhaya, 26 June 1961, MPA, L5/II/B.

admired more than traders and artisans. Reining never explicitly stated that the Haya deliberately limited their family size to avert a crisis of landlessness in Bukoba's densely settled villages. But this was implied in her description of the broad harmony between the size of farm and family as a 'desirable status quo', and by her suggestion that Buhaya possessed a mature demographic regime characterized by low fertility and mortality which had evolved in a context of limited usable land.[36]

Reining's dissertation was an essential corrective to earlier studies' moralistic overemphasis on STDs, and especially syphilis, but the delay between her research and submission was unfortunate. In the intervening fifteen years the Haya had experienced a dramatic increase in fertility rates, which had prompted the mass migration of young families away from the established coffee and banana areas of the Lake Victoria littoral to the drier, emptier lands to the west. Evidently Bukoba's demographic system was neither mature nor stable, and the Haya were not so fundamentally opposed to opening new land as generations of agricultural officers had complained. The number of Haya in Bukoba district, which had remained static for decades, increased by 20% between the 1948 and 1957 censuses. From 1957 to 1967 Buhaya's population then grew at an average of 3.8% per annum, one of the fastest rates in Tanzania. Around a quarter of this demographic expansion was due to immigration, but natural increase, at 2.8% per annum, was the primary agent of change. The TFR had been estimated in 1952 at three children, albeit from a large survey associated with the EAMS, whereas the more reliable 1967 census reported a TFR of 7.2. A sense of the suddenness of this change can be gained from a comparison of the 1967 TFR, which was a measure of current fertility patterns among women of reproductive age, with the 1967 figure for completed family size, four, which was obtained from women aged fifty and above. It seems that Haya fertility had risen very rapidly since the early 1950s. As a consequence of this and declining infant mortality, the percentage of children in Buhaya's population increased enormously, from 32.9% in 1948 to 47.3% in 1967.[37]

[36] Reining, 'Agrarian system', pp. iii, 87, 95, 115, 225–6, 304, 315–9; P. Reining, 'The Haya of north-western Tanzania', in Molnos, *Cultural III*, pp. 204–5.

[37] East Africa High Commission, *African Population of Tanganyika Territory: Geographical and Tribal Studies* (Nairobi: East African Statistical Department, 1950); East Africa High Commission, *Tanganyika African Population Census 1957: Analysis by Sex and Age for Province, District, and Territorial Census Areas* (East African Statistical Department, 1958); R. Henin and B. Egero, '1967 population census of Tanzania: a demographic analysis' (BRALUP Research Notes 19, UDSM, 1972); I. Sembajwe, 'Impact of urbanization on fertility and child mortality. The case studies of Tanzania and Uganda' (unpublished MA dissertation, UDSM, 1973), pp. 30–7.

Few societies in recorded history have ever experienced such a rapid increase in their fertility rates. Before the reasons for this transformation are examined though, it is necessary first to explain why Haya birth rates remained so low, for so long. Two factors can be immediately ruled out. Very few Haya women failed to marry during the colonial period, and few married late. Only one woman out of 2,079 surveyed by the EAMS in 1954 had not yet married by the age of thirty. The Catholic parish registers meanwhile show that the average age at which women married in colonial Bukoba was 19.2, almost a year younger than women in Kisubi in Buganda, and more than a year and a half younger than in Nyamitanga, Ankole. Other sources suggest, moreover, that Catholic weddings in Buhaya occurred at a later age than customary marriages. In the villages sampled by the EAMS in 1951 the average age at first pregnancy was 19.1 years, with only 0.2% of women reportedly having fallen pregnant before marriage. Women aged over forty who were interviewed by the 1973 National Demographic Survey (NDS) reported a mean marriage age of 16.5. In addition to the factors discussed above, evidence from Buhaya provides one additional explanation for the discrepancy between the age at which women married in and out of church. According to the NDS 32% of older women had married between the ages of eight and fourteen, whereas only 11.2% of Catholic brides married before fifteen, and almost all of these were fourteen. The church's policy on child brides, even if it was not consistently applied, seems to have had some deterrent effect.[38]

Haya women then were universally exposed to the possibility of conception from a relatively early age. Yet, on average, they had an extremely low number of live births over their lifetimes. One contributory factor was that the pace of reproduction was slower in Buhaya than in both Ankole and Buganda. Bukoba parish records indicate that the average birth interval during the colonial period was 31.5 months, more than one and a half months longer than in Nyamitanga and Kisubi. Average intervals, moreover, peaked higher and later than in the other two societies, reaching 33.7 months in the

[38] East African Medical Survey, *Annual Report, 1954* (Nairobi: EAHC, 1955), p. 37; East African Medical Survey, *Annual Report, 1951* (Nairobi: EAHC, 1952), p. 65; R. Henin, *National Demographic Survey of Tanzania, 1973: Volume II, Data for Socioeconomic Groups* (Dar es Salaam: Tanzania Bureau of Statistics, 1973), p. 32. While this 1973 survey is believed to have suffered from significant methodological problems (pers. comm. Sarah Walters), it was superior to censuses of that era in terms of the local scale at which data were presented, and the range of questions asked about marriage and fertility. H. Lapioche, 'Table d'enquête sur les moeurs et coutumes indigènes, Diocese de Bukoba', 1956, pp. 62–3, WFA. Bukoba parish did not create a separate marriage register until after independence, so marriage details during the colonial period were added into the baptism register. This meant that clergy did not have to formally record brides' ages, making it easier to turn a blind eye to under-age weddings, although it is likely girls would not have given their true ages in any case. Around 14% of all marriages took place in church in the 1950s.

late 1930s.[39] Birthspacing was a topic of greater importance for my informants in Buhaya than elsewhere, with Haya women repeatedly stressing the dangers associated with falling pregnant too quickly after a previous delivery. Female informants were unusually concerned about the physical strain placed on their bodies by pregnancy, childbirth, and breastfeeding. But even more emphasis was placed on the threat posed to the suckling child by its mother conceiving again, a situation referred to in Buhaya as 'child-strangling'. The early cessation of breastfeeding by pregnant mothers was regarded with great anxiety during the colonial period, being blamed for causing infant malnutrition. A few informants reported that such ill-timed pregnancies might be aborted, others employed prolonged abstinence to ensure long birth intervals, but much more common was the use of herbal medicines that were believed at the time to have a contraceptive effect. Interviewees gradually lost faith in the value of such medicines after independence, having seen birth intervals fall so rapidly over their lifetimes, but the frequency with which they were used in the past is certainly indicative of Haya intentions. Haya women retained faith for longer in the contraceptive effect of prolonged lactation. Elderly informants reported that the Haya ideal was to breastfeed for three years, though in practice none had lasted more than thirty months. Still, the minimum reported length of breastfeeding was nine months, and a year and a half was the most common period cited. Perhaps more importantly, Haya women knew that breastfeeding had the greatest negative impact on fecundity when it was babies' exclusive source of nutrition. It was striking how many women claimed that they had only started to wean their children at the age of eight, ten or twelve months, very late by comparative standards.[40]

Buhaya's relatively long birth intervals must have contributed to the district's low fertility, but other factors were also important. One informant who reported that she had produced a baby every two and a half years ended up with nine live births.[41] Her birthspacing was typical, but her overall reproductive experience was not, for Haya interviewees were characterized above all by their sub-fertility. Answers to the question: 'How many live births were

[39] So few families had large numbers of children that any cohort effect in changing birth intervals is impossible to identify with confidence.

[40] e.g. Int. VPB, 9 Aug. 2000, Busindi, F; Int. AM, 14 June 2000, Isikila-Irungami, F; Int. KK, 15 June 2000, Bibanja, F; Int. VM, 16 June 2000, Kanyangereko, F, 4; Int. EK, 7 Aug. 2000, Kanyangereko Nkimbo, F; Int. YK, 19 Aug. 2000, Kikukwe, F; Int. PB, 22 Aug. 2000, Maruku, F; Int. PKK, 18 Aug. 2000, Mshumba-Byazi, F; Int. LN, 19 Aug. 2000, Kikukwe, F; Int. FK, 16 Aug. 2000, Kikukwe, F; Int. MK, Kikuku, 16 Aug. 2000, F. Cf. C. Bledsoe, *Contingent Lives: Fertility, Time, and Aging in West Africa* (Chicago: University of Chicago Press, 2002). Some women did breastfeed when pregnant, taking medicinal herbs which supposedly minimized the danger to themselves and their babies, but this was reported to be uncommon. It is possible that delayed weaning may have contributed to morbidity among older infants.

considered to be many in the past?', were particularly revealing. Five was thought by most to be 'impossible'. Four was described as 'extraordinary' or 'the maximum, and the woman would have to be a witch'. Someone with two children 'was a man, a boss'. 'He would be so proud.' A number of informants' names reflected this struggle to have children. One, an only child like so many others, was called Mukamutachumwa, indicating that she would be both son and daughter to her parents.[42] Only a handful of female informants had more than three children. Many more were childless. It was perhaps the ubiquity of infertility—some informants believed that the childless had been the majority in the villages of their youth—as well as the disastrous consequences of heirlessness that made the Haya unusual in Africa in their ready acceptance of the possibility of male sterility. In these densely settled communities it would have been impossible to be unaware of cases of men fruitlessly marrying woman after woman, or of women conceiving after leaving childless marriages. Of course the latter situation had been rationalized through the *bisisi* custom (see Chapter 1) as a revival of a dormant pregnancy from the previous marriage. But as Haya went to the clinic with ever increasing frequency, knowledge of the reproductive process became more accurate. Informants came to acknowledge that 'diseases could kill men's seeds' and that *bisisi* was in essence a means, biologically fraudulent but socially useful, by which childless men could secure an heir.[43]

Some informants considered infertility to have been the most serious medical problem in colonial Buhaya. Tragic everywhere, childlessness was unusually destructive here because until the late colonial period the lack of a male heir resulted in the loss of the family farm to a landlord or the Mukama. As a result, according to one informant, 'people sought children with sweat and blood.' Yet many Haya believed that the infertile were usually regarded with sympathy. Few families after all were unaffected. Nonetheless old beliefs that sterility was contagious, or the consequence of moral failure or of witchcraft heightened tensions. Childless women 'could be hated' by their husbands or in-laws. Desperation drove men to pauper themselves by marrying woman after woman, or to seek out women from districts such as Ngara or Bugufi that were renowned for their high fertility. Wives were pressed to seduce

[41] Int. EK, 7 Aug. 2000, Kanyangereko Nkimbo, F.

[42] Int. A. CM, Busindi, 11 Aug. 2000, M; Int. KK, 15 June 2000, Bibanja, F; Int. N, 23 July 1998, Katongo, M; Int. EFC, 23 July 1998, Katongo, F; Int. FM, 21 July 1998, Rubya, M; Int. MM, 12 Aug. 2000, Kamachumu, F. Cf. B. Weiss, 'Good-for-nothing Haya *names*: powers of recollection in Northwest Tanzania', *Ethnos*, 64, 3 (1999), p. 404.

[43] Int. FM, 21 July 1998, Rubya, M; Int. KK, 15 June 2000, Bibanja, F; Int. AC, 9 Aug. 2000, Rubaa-Rubya, F; Int. AM, 11 Aug. 2000, Busindi, F; Int. PMJ, 9 Aug. 2000, Rubya, F; Int. SG, 21 Aug. 2000, Nkindo, F; Int. FM, 21 June 2000, Rubya, F; Int. PK, Rubafu, 6 Sept. 1999, M; Int. JM, 12 Aug. 2000, Kanoni, M.

neighbours who had fathered several children. Infidelity and polygamy though were unacceptable to the most committed Christians, who bleakly endured their suffering. One woman prayed novenas, a series of Catholic devotions performed over nine days, for decades in hope of falling pregnant. A childless Lutheran pastor sometimes dreamt of his wife giving birth to a child who died soon afterwards, or that he was a midwife: 'Every woman I touched bore children.'[44]

Secondary and, to a lesser extent, primary sterility were the leading causes of Buhaya's low fertility. Culwick's large-scale 1938 survey showed that primary sterility had been a serious problem since at least the turn of the century. The proportion of women aged fifty and above who had had no live births was 18.5%, rising to 22% for those in their thirties and forties. The EAMS investigations suggested that, while still severe, primary sterility had become slightly less significant by the early 1950s, affecting 16% of women aged thirty to forty-nine. Such levels of absolute infertility, though high, were lower than those found in Ankole and Buganda in the 1940s, and were insufficient in themselves to account for the extremely low average family size in this area. On average women aged fourteen to forty-nine had only had around two live births in both the late 1930s and the early 1950s. Secondary sterility was Buhaya's greatest demographic problem. The most striking finding of the EAMS was the 51% of women in their twenties who had been pregnant in the past but had not conceived in the past eight years. The proportion rose to a startling 88% for women in their thirties. It was because the average woman's reproductive life came to a very premature end that fertility in colonial Buhaya was so devastatingly low.[45]

The most visible reason for this early cessation of reproduction was the extremely high incidence of divorce in colonial Buhaya. In a 1954 survey, only 50.6% of ever married women in their twenties were still with their first husbands. For women in their thirties the proportion was still lower, at 41.1%. Three-quarters of marriages that had ended had done so due to divorce. Not only was divorce extremely common, but remarriage was far from automatic. Fifty-eight percent of divorcees had not remarried at the time of this survey. What this meant was that even though almost all women over the age of twenty had been married, a quarter of women in their twenties and thirties

[44] Int. KM, 18 Aug. 2000, Kikuku-Kanyigo, F; Int. FK, 16 Aug. 2000, Kikukwe, F; K. Rwiza, 'Natal customs in Bukoba', *Tanganyika Notes and Records*, 50, 1 (1958), pp. 105, 117; Int. VPB, 9 Aug 2000, Busindi, F; Int. YK, 19 Aug. 2000, Kikukwe, F; Int. AM, 14 June 2000, Isikila-Irungami, F; Sundkler, *Bara Bukoba*, pp. 103–5.

[45] Culwick, 'Population problem'; EAMS, *1951 Report*, p. 66; W. Brass, 'The estimation of fertility rates from ratios of total to first births', *Population Studies*, 8, 1 (1954), pp. 74–87. The average number of births per woman was 1.97 in Culwick's survey, and ranged from 1.57 to 2.25 in various EAMS samples.

were currently unmarried. As in many African societies, divorce often followed from childlessness, but heightened anxieties about sterility in Buhaya meant that failure to conceive within the first year of marriage often resulted in precipitate marital breakdown. Separation was so common that it should be seen as a cause as well as a consequence of infertility. Facilitated by Buhaya's customary law which required the return of bridewealth to the husband, it brought an end, or at best a major interruption, to very many women's reproductive lives.[46]

Informants' life stories though indicate that reproductive problems were as often biological as social in nature. A large number of women reported that they had sought medical help for failure to conceive or for repeated miscarriages and stillbirths. Most women had received treatment for STD infections, which they typically blamed on their husbands' infidelity. For most of the colonial period European discussion of STDs fixated on syphilis, with some commentators believing that nine out of ten adults were syphilitic at some point in their lives. It was not until the EAMS began its work that diagnoses were systematically supported by serological tests. Influenced by local opinion the EAMS initially tested its subjects only for syphilis. Twenty-seven percent of women had positive Kahn test results, but as the average fertility of these women was only marginally lower than those with negative results—they had produced 23.4% of the sample's live births—the research team decided that syphilis was too weakly correlated with fertility histories to be of any significance. This outcome was perhaps unsurprising as it is now known that the Kahn test produces false positives in patients affected by a range of ailments common to the region, as well as pregnancy. The Kahn tests then probably exaggerated the prevalence of sexually transmitted syphilis, but underestimated its role in sub-fertility.[47]

Syphilis was no doubt of some importance, but it played only a supporting role in Buhaya's fertility problems. Syphilis affects fertility mainly by causing miscarriage and stillbirth, yet informants remember pregnancy failure as being less of an issue than the inability to conceive. Contemporary records support these assertions. Vital registration data from the 1920s indicate that around 11% of all births were stillborn, not a remarkably high level by regional standards, though the accuracy of such records should not be overestimated. Women surveyed by the EAMS in 1951 stated that 16.1% of their pregnancies had ended in miscarriage or stillbirth, which again is far from exceptional.[48] Attention should instead be focused on those diseases

[46] Laurie and Trant, *East African Medical Survey*; H. Cory and M. Hartnoll, *Customary Law of the Haya Tribe, Tanganyika Territory* (London: Cass, 1971 [1945]), p. 68.
[47] EAMS, *1951 Report*, p. 71.
[48] Int. SG, 21 Aug. 2000, Nkindo, F; Bukoba District Annual Report 1928, TNA 215/77/B; Bukoba District Annual Report 1929, TNA 215/77/C; EAMS, *1951 Report*, p. 71.

which caused sterility in both men and women. This was the conclusion reached by the EAMS when, in three villages surveyed in 1952, its researchers found that among 525 men who agreed to be examined, the prevalence of gonorrhoea was 6.7%, while that of syphilis was 1.4%. Doctors working at Bukoba district hospital in the early 1950s reinforced this link between gonorrhoea and infertility, reporting that the Haya suffered more destructive gynaecological sequelae of gonococcal infection than any other people amongst whom they had ever worked.[49]

Haya came to share the European belief that STD infection was exceptionally common in the district, so that almost every female informant stated that they had taken herbal medicines during their pregnancies to prevent or cure syphilis and gonorrhoea. Women in Buhaya were exposed to a wide array of organic compounds during pregnancy, for local medications were commonly used not only against STDs and a range of other illnesses, but also to soften the pelvis, and to guarantee a 'clean' baby, free of vernix. It was not unusual for informants to list eight or more herbal treatments they had taken while pregnant. It is unknown whether any of these treatments carried significant risk for the foetus. However, the practice of taking oxytocic medications to strengthen contractions, which seems to have been even more common in Buhaya than Ankole, was strongly associated by medical researchers with maternal exhaustion, ruptured uterus, the death of the baby, and subsequent fertility problems. Even informants who emphasized the value of clinic-based ante-natal care during the colonial period and acknowledged the efficacy of western medications such as penicillin, used oxytocics.[50] The enthusiasm for medicinal herbs among Haya women, moreover, preceded conception. Many informants also used herbs during intercourse, some as perfume, some to enhance pleasure, some to tighten the vagina, and some to prevent STD infection. Again it is not known whether the chemical properties of any of the six herbs mentioned would have reduced the likelihood of conception, but the insertion of a wad of herbs into the vagina prior to intercourse may have replicated the effect of barrier methods of contraception.[51]

[49] EAMS, *1952 Report*, pp. 58–69. No effective test for chlamydia, another STD associated with infertility, was available in East Africa before the 1980s.

[50] e.g. Int. KM, 18 Aug. 2000, Kikuku-Kanyigo, F; Int. EFC, 23 July 1998, Katongo, F; Int. FK, 16 Aug. 2000, Kikukwe, F; Int. VPB, 9 Aug. 2000, Busindi, F; Int. YK, 19 Aug. 2000, 27, F; Int. AM, 14 June 2000, Isikila-Irungami, F; Int. MK, Kikuku, Aug. 2000, Kikukwe, F; Int. AM, 11 Aug. 2000, Busindi, F; Int. WBK, 27 July 1998, Bugabo, M; Reining, 'The Haya of north-western Tanzania', pp. 220–3; Rwiza, 'Natal customs', pp. 113–4.

[51] Int. PB, 22 Aug. 2000, Maruku, F; Int. CN, 12 Aug. 2000, Kanoni, F; Int. SKN, 22 Aug. 2000, Maruku-Butailuka-Kasha, F; Int. MM, 14 Aug. 2000, Ruhija, F; Int. AK, 8 Aug. 2000, Rubya, F; Int. DT, 14 June 2000, Ntoma, F.

Another biological obstacle to successful reproduction may have been nutritional in nature. In 1952 the EAMS recorded the average height and weight of around 800 women aged twenty and above, revealing that Haya women overall were very slightly built, with a mean body mass index (BMI) of 20.6. Most significantly, women in their twenties had a BMI of 19.9, meaning that the average woman during the peak years of reproduction was, by some definitions, underweight. It is likely therefore that a significant proportion of women would have been severely underweight, and therefore likely to have been sub-fertile. A low BMI tends to reduce the number of live births a woman has over her lifetime, as low body weight is associated with problems such as anovulation and late menarche.[52] It was striking how many female informants in Buhaya claimed to have commenced menstruation at an advanced age compared to women in Ankole and Buganda. One stated that menarche at eighteen was normal, and indeed a large number of women first menstruated between seventeen and nineteen. Some women had their marriages delayed into their twenties because they began to menstruate so late, but a more common experience was to be married off around the age of sixteen without yet having reached sexual maturity. It seems likely that the frequency of premature marriage partly accounted for Buhaya's high levels of infertility, as early sexual debut is associated with the development of pelvic inflammatory disease. The experience of one informant was far from unusual. Married at fourteen she had a stillbirth, then a miscarriage and then never conceived again. Other women married in their mid-teens but were well into their twenties before having their first child.[53]

[52] M. Jokela, M. Elovainio and M. Kivimaki, 'Lower fertility associated with obesity and underweight: the US National Longitudinal Survey of Youth', *American Journal of Clinical Nutrition*, 88, 4 (2008), pp. 886–93; R. Frisch, 'The right weight: body fat, menarche and fertility', *Proceedings of the Nutrition Society*, 53 (1994), pp 113–29; The definition of underweight is a BMI below 20 according to the British Nutrition Foundation, or below 18.5 according to the WHO. The EAMS also found that goitre affected 4.9% of Haya women in 1952. Goitre is associated with iodine deficiency, which in turn negatively affects fecundity, foetal survival and infant survival. It was believed that the extremely high level of goitre in Buhaya was a result of the area's mineral deficient soils and women's restricted access to iodine-rich foodstuffs such as eggs, meat and milk. H. Trant, 'Adult health in Nyakato', Appendix to Reining, 'Agrarian system', p. 342. Cf. J. Dunn and F. Delange, 'Damaged reproduction: the most important consequence of iodine deficiency', *The Journal of Clinical Endocrinology and Metabolism*, 86, 6 (2001), pp. 2360–3.

[53] Int. AM, 14 June 2000, Isikila-Irungami, F; Int. YK, 19 Aug. 2000, Kikukwe, F; Int. CB, 13 Aug. 2000, Busindi, F; Int. LN, 19 Aug. 2000, Kikukwe, F; Int. FK, 16 Aug. 2000, Kikukwe, F; Int. AM, 24 June 2000, Kashambya, F; Int. PKK, 18 Aug. 2000, Mshumba-Byazi, F; Int. CM, 11 Aug. 2000, Rubya, F; Int. LM, 12 Aug. 2000, Kanoni, F. Cf. M. Gray-Swain and J. Peipert, 'Pelvic inflammatory disease in adolescents', *Current Opinion in Obstetrics and Gynecology*, 18, 5 (2006), pp. 503–10. The frequency of late sexual maturation indicates that age at marriage should not be assumed to equate automatically to first exposure to the risk of conception.

The final aspect of Haya sub-fertility that must be considered is Reining's implication that small family size was tolerated due to the exceptional population density of Buhaya's long established village lands. In 1931, two of Buhaya's sub-counties carried more than 400 people per square kilometre, far in excess of anywhere else in Tanganyika. Some informants, perhaps influenced by decades of out-migration and declining returns from the land, supported Reining's view. 'Before there was no problem, because at that time a family was just made up of a wife and a husband with their two children, one son and one daughter. They were actually satisfied with what they had . . . There was no shortage of food as there is today.' When Reining asked young women what their ideal family size was, most answers fell between two and six. This was unusually low for colonial Africa, but as Reining herself notes it was impossible for women to consider this issue in the abstract. In the context of early 1950s Buhaya, hoping for six children must have seemed wildly ambitious. By contrast, when elders interviewed for this book were asked about ideal family size, typical answers were ten or twelve. Only childless individuals gave responses such as 'four' which had been considered ideal during Reining's period of research. Reining's thesis was in part that Haya in the early 1950s did not desire large families because parents had little enthusiasm for despatching their surplus sons to Buhaya's empty but unserviced interior. Another interpretation would be that Haya were not fundamentally opposed to larger families in the 1950s—they simply could not imagine having them. Buhaya today carries a population four times greater than in the 1950s yet ideal family size is larger. It seems likely that desired family size increased as a result of improved reproductive health and marital stability, as well as in response to the infrastructural investment in Karagwe and the central depression, which could be interpreted as removing a major deterrent to fertility maximization.[54]

Buhaya's population growth was due above all to a decline in the prevalence of sterility. According to the 1973 NDS 10.3% of women in their thirties and 15.1% of those in their forties had never had a child. The levels of primary sterility recorded in this survey were therefore around 20% lower than those reported by the EAMS in the early 1950s, and 42% lower than those observed by the Culwicks in 1938. Much more significant was the decline in secondary sterility. In 1973 the proportion of ever-pregnant women in their twenties who had not conceived in the past five years was 8%, while for women in their thirties the proportion was 36%. The equivalent rates in the early

[54] Culwick, 'Population problem'; Int. B, MM, 26 Aug. 1999, Katoma-Irogero, M; Reining, 'The Haya of northwestern Tanzania', pp. 218–9; Int. YK, 19 Aug. 2000, Kikukwe, F; Int. PB, 22 Aug. 2000, Maruku, F; Int. JNK, 11 Aug. 2000, Ijumbi, M; Int. SK, 21 June 2000, Rubya, M; Int. N, 23 July 1998, Katongo, M; Int. GK, Nkindo, 21 Aug. 2000, F.

1950s were 51 and 88%. Buhaya's transition to rapid population growth was driven above all by the increased longevity of women's reproductive lives.[55]

Within Buhaya, informants universally credited the reduction in the prevalence of gonorrhoea and syphilis since the 1950s as the primary reason for the increase in fertility. As the next chapter will show, the attempt to control STD infection in the 1950s in Buhaya was remarkable for the intensity with which public health messages were delivered and the universality of treatment. The latter factor was of particular significance because in 1952 the EAMS had found that men made up 93% of those infected with gonorrhoea in the villages surveyed, yet that year only 11% of those treated for gonorrhoea at Bukoba's STD clinic were male. The STD campaign of the mid-1950s not only ensured that the larger part of the adult population was treated with penicillin, but also reportedly resulted in a new openness about STD infection within relationships, so that couples began to come for treatment together.[56] In reality though the STD campaign was only part of a wider expansion of medical services which resulted in a major improvement in reproductive health in Buhaya. In 1929 only forty-two babies were delivered in a medical facility in the district. In the years that followed sustained pressure through chiefs, schools, and missions diminished the suspicion with which maternity services were viewed. Medicalized deliveries increased significantly from the mid-1930s, while by 1959 Buhaya's twelve Native Authority mother and baby clinics were so overwhelmed that the district medical officer proposed that fees should be introduced 'to discourage mothers not in need of institutional care'. Given that Bukoba district hospital also provided maternity facilities, and that the majority of institutional deliveries occurred in mission rather than Native Authority centres, it is clear that giving birth in the clinic had become immensely popular.[57]

Informants spoke more positively of the benefits of clinic delivery than did women in Ankole, their attitudes shaped by the severity of the reproductive health problems and the anxiety they had endured. Some women, for example, desired ante-natal care so they could be reassured that their babies were growing well and were correctly positioned. But a remarkably high

[55] Henin, *National Demographic Survey*, Vol.1, pp. 215–38, Vol. 3, pp. 1–134, and Vol. 6, p. 75; U. Larsen, 'Childlessness, subfertility, and infertility in Tanzania', *Studies in Family Planning*, 27, 1 (1996), pp. 20–7. The EAMS had used eight rather than five years as the measure of subsequent sterility, but the change is unlikely to have affected the results significantly.

[56] EAMS, *1952 Report*, pp. 58–67; Int. MM, 14 Aug. 2000, Ruhija, F; Int. TM, Busindi, Aug. 2000; Int. WBK, 27 July 1998, Bugabo, M. It is likely that the prevalence of gonorrhoea in women was underestimated to some extent, due to the greater difficulty of diagnosis in females.

[57] Walters, 'Fertility', p. 47; Tanganyika Territory, *Annual Medical Report 1929*, p. 108; Bukoba District Annual Report 1934, TNA 215/1136; Lake Province Annual Report 1935, TNA, 215/1246; Bukoba District Annual Report 1948,TNA 215/2237; District Medical Officer to Secretary of the Council of Buhaya, 18 Aug. 1959, MPA, M20/8 Maternity 1959–72.

number stated that they would have been childless if they had not benefited from medical intervention. Many who had suffered repeated miscarriages gave birth safely following treatment with penicillin or effective anti-malarials, or on undergoing surgery to resolve cervical incompetence. Other informants had been unable to conceive until they received medical help. One woman who had not become pregnant fifteen months after marrying sought help from Kagondo missionary hospital. Being diagnosed with gonorrhoea, she and her husband were treated and then went on to have six children. Other infertile women became pregnant following minor gynaecological operations for problems such as fibroids. Even those who had no problems seeing pregnancies through to term and preferred to deliver at home benefited from the expansion of maternity services. By the 1960s traditional birth attendants had been instructed, it seems with some success, to wear surgical gloves and to refer difficult cases to a hospital, while ante-natal care had persuaded expectant mothers of the importance of hygiene at the time of delivery. Some informants even claimed that the use of herbs during sexual intercourse declined around the time of independence, due to growing familiarity with the mechanics of conception. 'We realised they were like condoms.'[58]

The increase in fertility levels was also the result of wider changes in Haya society. The post-1945 surge in coffee prices brought a more complex economy as well as greater prosperity to Buhaya. The EAMS found that by the early 1950s four in ten householders were traders or employed in clerical and artisanal occupations. These households with off-farm income had 22% more children than those that relied solely on the land, most likely because their regular diet and ready access to marketed goods ensured more consistent access to high-quality foodstuffs than the typical farming family, whose consumption was shaped by alternating cycles of feasting and debt. Imports of slaughter cattle peaked during the coffee harvest, but the improvement in dietary standards over much of the year was based on the diversification of Buhaya's economy, and on rapidly expanding education. Schooling and antenatal information gradually broke down traditional restrictions on female consumption of high-value foods such as eggs, which would have benefited pregnant women above all.[59]

Of perhaps greater importance was the decline in the frequency of marital breakdown (see Chapter 6). Compared with the EAMS survey results of the

[58] Int. VPB, 9 Aug. 2000, Busindi, F; Int. KK, 15 June 2000, Bibanja, F; Int. EK, 7 Aug. 2000, Kanyangereko Nkimbo, F; Int. VM, 16 June 2000, Kanyangereko, F; Int. PB, 22 Aug. 2000, Maruku, F; Int. KM, 18 Aug. 2000, Kikuku-Kanyigo, F; Int. AR, 15 Aug. 2000, Ihagiro, F; Int. PKK, 18 Aug. 2000, Mshumba-Byazi, F; Int. SKN, 22 Aug. 2000, Maruku-Butailuka-Kasha, F; Int. TM, 13 Aug. 2000, Busindi, F; Int. MM, 12 Aug. 2000, Kamachumu, F; Int. AM, 11 Aug. 2000, Busindi, F; Int. DT, 14 June 2000, Ntoma, F.

[59] EAMS, *1952 Report*, p. 31; Int. WBK, 27 July 1998, Bugabo, M.

early 1950s, the 1973 NDS found that ever married women in their twenties were less than half as likely to be divorced, and women in their thirties were 50% more likely to be still married to their first husband. Moreover, the proportion of women of reproductive age who were widows fell over the same period from 8 to 5%, presumably due to declining adult mortality. It is highly likely that the proportion of couples who remained alive and together until the wife reached the age of menopause increased substantially after 1950. The increased longevity of marriage more than compensated for a modest rise in female age at first union around the time of independence. The rapid expansion in female education from the 1950s (see Table 7.2) meant that a steadily increasing proportion of women deferred marriage until their schooling was completed and, in some cases, employment was secured. The Bukoba parish register indicates that the female average age at first marriage rose by fourteen months between the early 1950s and the late 1960s. By 1973, while marriage was still almost universal among women aged twenty-five and above, 7.4% of women aged 20–24 had not yet married, a significant change since the EAMS survey.[60]

Table 7.2 Proportion of females with education by year of birth in Buhaya[61]

Year born	Before 1924	1924–33	1934–43	1944–48	1949–53	1954–58
Percentage with schooling	7.8	24.0	32.2	54.3	62.5	77.1

Female education may have delayed the onset of childbearing,[62] but it is likely to have contributed to the acceleration of the pace of reproduction. Informants believed that the shortening of the normal period of breastfeeding to less than a year after independence was partly due to the greater autonomy of young women, especially those with schooling, and partly down to the growing availability of higher quality foodstuffs, which made it easier to wean children earlier and enabled women to shorten their birth intervals without damaging their own health. Certainly follow-on foods such as Lactogen were widely available in Buhaya by the 1960s. But the length of breastfeeding may have started to shorten long before independence, for missionaries had

[60] Henin, *Survey*, vol. II, p. 32; Laurie and Trant, *East African Medical Survey*, pp. 37–8.
[61] Henin, *Survey*, vol. II, p. 21.
[62] Reining found nothing to indicate that female education had as yet caused an increase in premarital pregnancy by the early 1950s. A. Richards and P. Reining, 'Report on fertility surveys in Buganda and Buhaya, 1952', University of Dar es Salaam library (UDSM), Cory 373.

discouraged breastfeeding beyond twelve months since at least the 1930s.[63] Certainly birth intervals had begun to shorten long before girls' education had become at all common. Priscilla Reining found that 91% of women surveyed in the early 1950s were illiterate, yet the Bukoba baptism register data show that birth intervals began to shorten from the early 1940s, falling by 4.6 months by 1959. It is likely that the initial reduction in birth spacing was due to limited improvements in reproductive health and child survival, as well as pressure to limit breastfeeding. Retrospective data gathered by the EAMS indicated that infant and child mortality had declined substantially in recent decades (see Chapter 8). Maternal optimism about child survival must have increased still faster between 1951 and 1973, for the risk of a baby dying in its first year of life fell from one in four to one in twelve. The sense of danger associated with curtailed breastfeeding presumably diminished as a result.[64]

The final factor to consider is whether changing attitudes regarding ideal family size over this period directly affected reproductive decision making. Haya in the early 1950s, according to Reining, had had little need for more than two children, provided at least one was a boy, due to their limited labour requirements and inability to provide land for a large number of sons on the long-settled lakeshore lands. As the 1950s progressed, however, the district administration created the infrastructure which made migration from the crowded ridges near Lake Victoria towards the largely empty but fertile lands of Karagwe and western Kianja and Ihangiro an attractive option. New roads made the marketing of produce cost-effective, new schools and clinics reduced the relative advantages of coastal life, and agricultural support helped farmers grow coffee and bananas on land long regarded as too arid for such thirsty crops. If the problem of the landless son had ever acted as a limitation on fertility in Buhaya, it no longer did so after 1950, for tens of thousands of young families moved westwards in the years after Reining's fieldwork.[65] Nor, according to informants, did the low fertility of the Haya before the 1950s

[63] Int. AMA, 15 Aug. 2000, Rwagati, F; Int. PMJ, 9 Aug. 2000, Rubya, F; C. Kamuzora, 'Formation of a low fertility culture in Kigarama village, Tanzania: cultual materialism versus idealism', (University of Dar es Salaam Department of Statistics Demographic Unit, Occasional Paper no. 9, 1997), p. 1; A. Culwick and G. Culwick, edited by V. Berry, *The Culwick Papers 1934–1944: Population, Food and Health in Colonial Tanganika* (London: Academic Books, 1994), p. 165.

[64] Richards and Reining, 'Report on fertility surveys 1952'; EAMS, *1951 Report*, pp. 64–8; Henin, *Survey*, vol. II.

[65] Bukoba District Annual Report 1953, TNA 215/2700; D. McMaster, 'Change of regional balance in the Bukoba district of Tanganyika', *Tanganyika Notes and Records*, 56 (1961), pp. 85–92; Int. FR, 30 Aug. 1999, Kitobo, M; Int. MM, 20 June 2000, Karwoshe, M; Int. WK, 31 Aug. 1999, Igurati-Bugandika, M.

reflect the entrenched attitudes of a mature demographic system. Indeed, interviewees who started families in the 1950s and 1960s remembered being put under intense pressure from their parents' generation to have large numbers of babies, to compensate for the children they themselves had failed to bear.[66]

Changing attitudes towards the risk of child mortality, birth spacing, and family size were significant in Buhaya's movement from demographic stability to rapid growth, but in this case it was the dramatic improvement in fecundity after the Second World War that transformed this society's population history. The increase in Haya birth rates appears not to have been the product of a reduction in the age of marriage, and was only influenced to some degree by the shortening of birth intervals. What seems to have been crucial was the decline in primary and secondary sterility, due to improved reproductive health and marital stability. The data available for this study are too imperfect for definitive conclusions to be drawn, but the weight of evidence suggests that in Buhaya, as in Ankole, the key proximate determinants of high fertility were those that influenced the duration not the inception or pace of reproduction.

Buganda

The story of fertility change in Buganda differs from that of its neighbours to the west and south. Ankole was representative of Africa's higher fertility cultures such as Kikuyuland, where a relatively large number of births per woman already seems to have been the norm before the Second World War. Buhaya's experience by contrast was typical of those societies such as Bunyoro in western Uganda where fertility levels remained unchanged or even declined until the end of the colonial period before undergoing a remarkable and sustained increase in the second half of the twentieth century.[67] Buganda was much more unusual. Here fertility levels seem to have increased modestly between the 1920s and 1940s, rose rapidly from the 1950s, and then, as will be discussed in Chapter 9, began to stabilize in the late 1960s as a result of birth control before experiencing a steady decline from the 1980s. Fortunately Buganda is blessed with exceptionally rich demographic data for much of this period which enable the causes of this distinctive process of fertility change to be analysed with greater precision that is possible elsewhere in the region. Admittedly Buganda did not enjoy quite the same number of fertility surveys

[66] Int. WR, 21 June 2000, Rubya, M. See also Int. VPB, 9 Aug. 2000 Busindi, F; Int. KK, 15 June 2000, Bibanja, F.

[67] R. Kuczynski, *Demographic Survey of the British Colonial Empire, Vol. II* (Oxford: Institute of International Affairs, 1949), pp. 188–90, 222–7; S. Doyle, 'Population decline and delayed recovery in Bunyoro, 1860–1960', *The Journal of African History*, 41 (2000), pp. 429–58.

as Buhaya, but other sources more than compensate for this one weakness. In particular the presence of East Africa's premier institution of medical research, Mulago Hospital, within the city of Kampala meant that the reproductive health, attitudes, and practices of the local population were monitored and recorded in exceptional detail. Mulago's experimental health centre at Kasangati, for example, ensured that this peri-urban area housed one of the most intensely studied communities in post-war Africa. Medical researchers' access to external funding and need for demographic information of unusual precision caused Uganda's census officers in 1959 to collect detailed fertility histories from a quarter of the population of Kyaddondo, the county surrounding Kampala. Elsewhere in Uganda, only one in twenty people were sampled. Buganda's censuses were superior too because female literacy and numeracy were sufficiently common to enable age-specific questions to be asked. Kampala moreover was the headquarters of various missions and so was home to non-state hospitals such as Mengo and Nsambya which specialized in maternity care and carefully archived patient records. Changes in parity, birthweight, and birth outcome can therefore be tracked at regular intervals from the 1920s until 1939 in Mengo, and from 1939 to 1969 at Nsambya.[68]

Inevitably though the conditions which created these sources raise questions about the representativeness of the individuals whose reproductive experiences were recorded therein. The population of Kampala, and the small county of Kyaddondo, much of which was a peri-urban extension of the city, had better access to educational and healthcare facilities than the rest of Buganda. Greater Kampala, moreover, was characterized by an unusual family structure, with female-headed households and men living alone being much more common there than elsewhere. Yet Kampala and its environs should not be regarded as a distinct area, remote from a rural hinterland. The city's population was highly unstable before the 1960s, often housing individuals for relatively short periods of education or employment before their return to Buganda's small towns and villages.[69]

Moreover, Kampala's medical facilities drew in patients from a radius of up to sixty miles in the 1940s and somewhat further by the 1960s.[70] Many of these patients from outside Kampala appear in the archive because they were atypical, often being referred to urban hospitals by these institutions' network

[68] Uganda, *Uganda Census 1959*, pp. 19–20, 57. Mengo's maternity records were only available up to 1939, and Nsambya's registers only started in that year.

[69] See Chapter 4 for an extended discussion of the interconnectedness of the rural and urban in Buganda.

[70] H. Welbourn, 'First impressions' (unpublished TS in the possession of the author, 1946); C. Crocker et al., 'A study of knowledge, attitudes, and practices of family planning in Uganda, East Africa', *Journal of Reproductive Medicine*, 7, 5 (1971), pp. 235–8.

of satellite dispensaries, health centres, and maternity clinics due to their medical condition being defined as high risk. Mengo, Mulago, and Nsambya all had efficient referral systems, so that infertile people who required surgical intervention, women whose ante-natal checks predicted a difficult labour, or deliveries which developed complications were transferred from the dozens of rural medical centres dotted around Buganda to the great urban hospitals. As a result, the incidence of gynaecological problems, stillbirth, and maternal death was much higher in urban hospitals than in the far less sophisticated rural medical institutions.[71] The central issue, in terms of the analytical viability of the hospital maternity data, is whether this referral system was sustained consistently from the 1920s through to the 1960s. It seems that this was largely the case. Patients who were transferred from rural clinics run by the Catholic Franciscan Sisters appeared regularly in the maternity registers of Nsambya Hospital from the 1930s through to the 1970s. The Church Missionary Society's 'country centres' were already so efficient at relaying problem maternity cases to Mengo by the 1930s that their rates of stillbirth, maternal mortality, and neo-natal death matched those of England and Wales. Moreover, the gap between urban and rural outcomes was maintained through to independence, despite the improved technology enjoyed by the referral hospitals after the Second World War.[72]

Yet the prominence of difficult cases did recede with time, partly because of overall improvements in general and reproductive health, partly because institutionalized birth became so remarkably common in both rural and urban Buganda. No doubt the exceptional availability and visibility of maternity services facilitated the growth in attendances. As early as 1926 there were nineteen maternity centres, state and mission, in rural Buganda. By 1959 Buganda had 969 maternity beds in forty-five centres. Ankole had only seven centres with seventy-seven beds.[73] In Buganda by the middle decades of the twentieth century, earlier than in most of Africa, giving birth in the clinic lost its novelty. Once primarily associated with the elite and the desperate, obstetric facilities all over Buganda now struggled with the consequences of their success. The Mengo hospital records show that the number of maternity cases grew rapidly through the 1930s, it seems due to coercion by Buganda's chiefs, concerned about depopulation, as well as sustained government and missionary propaganda against unhygienic home birth.[74] The Nsambya records

[71] Grech, Galea and Trussell, 'Maternal', pp. 263–78.

[72] In 1958 rural state-run maternity centres referred 6.3% of patients, defined as high risk, to Mulago. Annual Medical Report Mengo District 1958 (Albert Cook Archive, Kampala).

[73] Buganda Annual Report 1926, ESA, A46/428; Ministry of Health, 'Medical Services Statistical Records, 1959' (unpublished TS, Ministry of Health library, Kampala).

[74] A. Cook, 'Report of the Lady Coryndon Maternity Training School, Namirembe, 1931', CMS Archive, Birmingham, M/Y/A7 1931–5.

indicate that the next surge in maternity cases began in the early 1950s, coinciding with an enormous expansion in ante-natal and mother and child services throughout Uganda. The number of deliveries at Nsambya almost trebled between 1949 and 1954, and then increased by 133% over the following decade. Mulago meanwhile experienced a later but greater transformation, delivering around 1,700 babies in 1954 and 14,500 in 1969.[75] Even in individual rural health centres more than a thousand births a year were registered by the 1960s.[76] The proportion of all births which took place in a medical facility in Buganda rose from approximately 20% in 1947 to 30% in 1958 and 40% in 1967.[77] Many more women were exposed to medical advice during pregnancy than delivered in an institution. As early as 1948 approximately 60% of pregnant women in Buganda attended state-run ante-natal clinics. By 1967 around 90% attended ante-natal clinics run by the state or missions, a remarkable level of contact.[78]

In Mengo, the first maternity hospital in Uganda, surgical intervention and neo-natal death became less common in the 1930s.[79] Nsambya, established much later, was still dominated by maternity crises in 1939, but not from 1949. Mulago delivered so many 'normal' pregnancies in the late 1950s that the mission hospitals at Mengo and Nsambya were paid to take 1,500 of its uncomplicated cases each year. Nsambya's patient body therefore changed significantly after 1960, as around half of its intake was pre-selected as low risk. That Nsambya's birth outcomes and birthweight figures improved only slightly between 1959 and 1964 is initially surprising, but can be explained by the differing social profiles of women who chose to deliver within the state and mission sectors. Mulago and other state maternity centres did not charge

[75] 'The history of our mission work', p. 6, Franciscan Missionary Sisters of Africa Archive, Dundalk (FMSA), Box 6; Uganda Protectorate, *Annual Report of the Medical Department, 1958* (2 vols., Entebbe: Government Printer, 1959), vol.II; C. Rendle Short, 'Health education for the expectant mother' (Report of a seminar 'Health education and the mother and child in East Africa', Makerere Medical School, Kampala, Nov. 1961), p. 14; B. Marasha, 'Causation and prevention of stillbirths and postnatal deaths at Mulago hospital, 1970–71' (unpublished DPH dissertation, Makerere University Kampala, 1972–3), p. 20.

[76] H. Gbejuade, 'Review of the problems of a rural health centre in Uganda' (unpublished DPH dissertation, Makerere University Kampala, 1969) p. 37.

[77] Uganda Protectorate, *Annual Report of the Medical Department, 1947* (Entebbe: Government Printer, 1948); Uganda Protectorate, *Annual Report of the Medical Department, 1958* (2 vols., Entebbe, 1959), vol.II; Grech, Galea and Trussell, 'Maternal', pp. 263–78. The 1947 report estimated that more than a third of all births were in an institution, but this figure was based on registered births. The 1948 census demonstrated that 40% of births were unregistered.

[78] Uganda Protectorate, *Annual Medical Report 1948* (Entebbe: Government Printer, 1949); Uganda Ministry of Health, *Annual Report 1967–8* (Entebbe: Government Printer, 1968).

[79] A. Cook, 'Report of the Lady Coryndon Maternity Training School, Namirembe, 1932' (Albert Cook Archive, Kampala).

their patients, whereas mission clinics like Nsambya did. It was thought at the time that the women who were transferred from Mulago to Nsambya were from a lower income group compared to those women who had planned to deliver at the Franciscans' hospital. To give a sense of the variation between the two hospitals' patients, at the end of our period the incidence of low birthweight, a marker of maternal health and nutritional status, was three times higher at Mulago than Nsambya. It should not be assumed though that the women who elected to deliver in Nsambya's main labour ward were in any sense of the Ganda upper class. Nsambya's basic charges were relatively modest, many Ganda women from Kampala's less desirable neighbourhoods in the 1950s chose Nsambya over Mulago, associating the latter hospital with low status immigrants, while the truly wealthy attended Nsambya's private maternity wing, whose records were maintained separately. Patients in Nsambya's main labour ward were not perfectly representative of the larger population, but nor were they remarkably different from the mass of Ganda pregnant women.[80]

In the 1950s some Ganda still worried that their ethnic group faced extinction due to low fertility. At first sight this seems surprising given that Buganda's population was 2.6 times higher in 1959 than 1911 (see Figure 7.3). However, as Ganda knew well, most of this growth was due to immigration from other parts of East Africa, and the anxieties of the late colonial period were in essence about being swamped by incomers with higher fertility. Audrey Richards was told by one chief in 1951 that immigrants had 'five children to one child of Baganda parents. If the government do not take steps there will be no land left for Baganda.' By 1959 immigrants officially made up 45% of Buganda's total population, but various sources indicate that many people who were defined as Ganda in fact had another ethnic origin. Local chiefs deliberately redesignated as Ganda the Nyoro inhabitants of the 'Lost Counties', the territory transferred from Bunyoro to Buganda at the end of the nineteenth century. According to the 1911 census there were 106,074 Nyoro in the Lost Counties. The 1931 census in this area though recorded only 2,301 Nyoro, who appear to have been recently arrived migrants, judging by their skewed age and sex profiles. All indigenes had been redefined as Ganda.[81] The numbers of Ganda in Buganda were also inflated by immigrants assigning to their children the ethnic identity of the host community. In the Catholic parish register of Kisubi 27% of the 2,600 babies who were baptized by immigrants during the colonial period were given names belonging to Ganda clans, in a

[80] Marasha, 'Causation', p. 40; Nsambya Maternity Registers.

[81] M. Southwold, 'The Baganda of central Uganda', in Molnos, *Cultural II*, pp. 171–80; Notes on conversation with Mut. III chief, Busiro, 28 Jan. 1951, A. Richards papers, LSE, 6/18; Uganda, *1921 Census*; Uganda, *1931 Census*.

clear attempt to accelerate their assimilation. Such well known practices enabled the Ganda to avoid becoming a minority in their own kingdom, but they added to the sense that that they were unable to sustain themselves without artificial assistance.[82]

Ganda fears of their imminent demise were much exaggerated. Ganda fertility was low for much of the colonial period, but their mortality was lower still. Evidence relating to fertility levels in the early colonial period is scanty and conflicting. A retrospective survey in 1952 found that women aged sixty and above had had 10% more live births than those aged between forty-five and fifty-nine, suggesting that Ganda fertility fell between around 1910 and 1935. Yet vital registration data indicates that the proportion of babies who were stillborn fell steadily from 7.1% in 1925, to an average of 3.8% in the 1930s, and 1.2% in the 1940s. Moreover the average parity of women who gave birth in Mengo hospital rose from 2.4 in 1924 to 2.8 in 1939. The Mengo data are of uncertain accuracy, however, as indications within the registers suggest that in some years miscarriages may have been included in parity calculations. The 1948 sample census found that female sterility was relatively high, at around 25% for women aged in their mid-thirties and above, but had not worsened significantly in the recent past. The average female age at first marriage, according to the Kisubi Catholic parish registers rose slightly between 1925 and 1939. The 1931 census supports this finding, as the proportion of Ganda women who were single had increased since 1921 from 22% to 26%, presumably as a result of the growing crisis in Ganda marriage (see Chapter 4). The effect of this on fertility levels, however, would have been outweighed by the reduction in the average birth interval over this period. According to the Kisubi registers, Ganda birth spacing fell rapidly from 1920, so that from 1930 birth intervals here were lower than in Ankole and Buhaya, a situation that would continue until the end of our period (see Figure 7.4).[83]

The size of the fall in birth intervals in Kisubi, from 32.5 months in 1920–24 to 30.5 months in 1935–39, is significant but, as is so often the case in the demographic history of Africa before the Second World War, difficult to explain with confidence. Few documentary sources relating to the duration of breastfeeding or post-partum sexual abstinence are available for these

[82] Kisubi Parish Registers; S. Doyle, 'Immigrants and indigenes: the Lost Counties dispute and the evolution of ethnic identity in colonial Buganda', *Journal of Eastern African Studies*, 3, 2 (2009), pp. 284–302.

[83] Richards and Reining, 'Report on fertility surveys, 1952'; Uganda Protectorate, Annual Medical Reports 1925–48, NA, CO/685; Uganda, '1948 Sample Census'; Uganda, *1931 Census*; Mengo Hospital Maternity Registers; Kisubi Parish Registers. The later vital registration figures relating to stillbirth were substantially lower than rates from hospital deliveries, but that is perhaps unsurprising given that many women gave birth in hospital due to difficulties in childbirth.

years, and only a handful of oral informants were old enough to have had children before 1940. What evidence exists indicates that post-partum abstinence typically continued to be reasonably long, by regional standards, at one to three months, but that the expected duration of breastfeeding at this time had reduced to around two years, rather than the three and a half of the pre-colonial period.[84] It is likely that missionaries would have preached against prolonged breastfeeding in Buganda as they did in Ankole and Buhaya. More importantly, Ganda mothers would presumably have been more willing to consider shortening their birth intervals in the mid-colonial period than their Nkole and Haya counterparts because child survival rates seem to have improved here unusually early. Mengo hospital records indicate that the level of previous child mortality experienced by expectant mothers almost halved between 1924 and 1939, and while data of this type and period should be viewed with caution, the scale of the change suggests that it should not be dismissed entirely. It is likely that child survival would also have improved around Kisubi, which possessed its own mission hospital, and was equidistant between the larger institutions of Kampala and Entebbe. The need to delay conception for as long as possible seems to have lessened after 1924.[85]

The pace of reproduction quickened early in Buganda, but overall fertility levels remained low until the 1950s, when they seem to have increased rapidly. Buganda's CBR was 30 per 1,000 at the 1948 census, a very low level by post-war African standards, but 36 in 1959. Buganda's CBR however was always artificially low due to the large numbers of male immigrants living alone, and it was not until 1959 that a more useful fertility measure, the total fertility rate (TFR) was published. The TFR was 4.9 in that year and 5.3 in 1969. Hospital parity data compensate for some of the limitations of Uganda's colonial censuses, though as previously discussed, all such medical records should be viewed with a degree of scepticism, given that the representativeness of women who elected to give birth in a medical institution increased over time. Nsambya's maternity registers show that the average parity of current patients increased sharply from 2.3 in 1949 to 2.7 in 1959 and 4.1 a decade later (see Figures 7.9 and 7.10). Unfortunately women in this period were not asked

[84] Int. FN, 29 Aug. 2004, Butanga, F; Int. MMA, 24 Aug. 2004, Kyanakase, F; Dr. P. Evans' diary of 1953 visit to Uganda, Wellcome Archive, A.3/1 PP/PRE; Birth customs, Maryamu, Kisozi village, 20 Oct. 1954, A. Richards papers, 7/16; J. Roscoe, *The Baganda: An Account of their Native Customs and Beliefs* (London: Macmillan, 1911), pp. 55–6.

[85] Mengo Hospital Maternity Records. Retrospective data on child mortality gathered for the 1948, 1959, and 1969 censuses also indicate that child mortality began to fall between the wars. K. Hill, 'Demographic estimation from deficient or defective data', in B. Fetter (ed.), *Demography from Scanty Evidence: Central Africa in the Colonial Era* (London: L. Rienner Publishers, 1990), p. 141; M. Semwogerere-Serunjogi, 'Population dynamics in Uganda for period 1959–1969', (unpublished PhD, University of London, 1980), pp. 100–101.

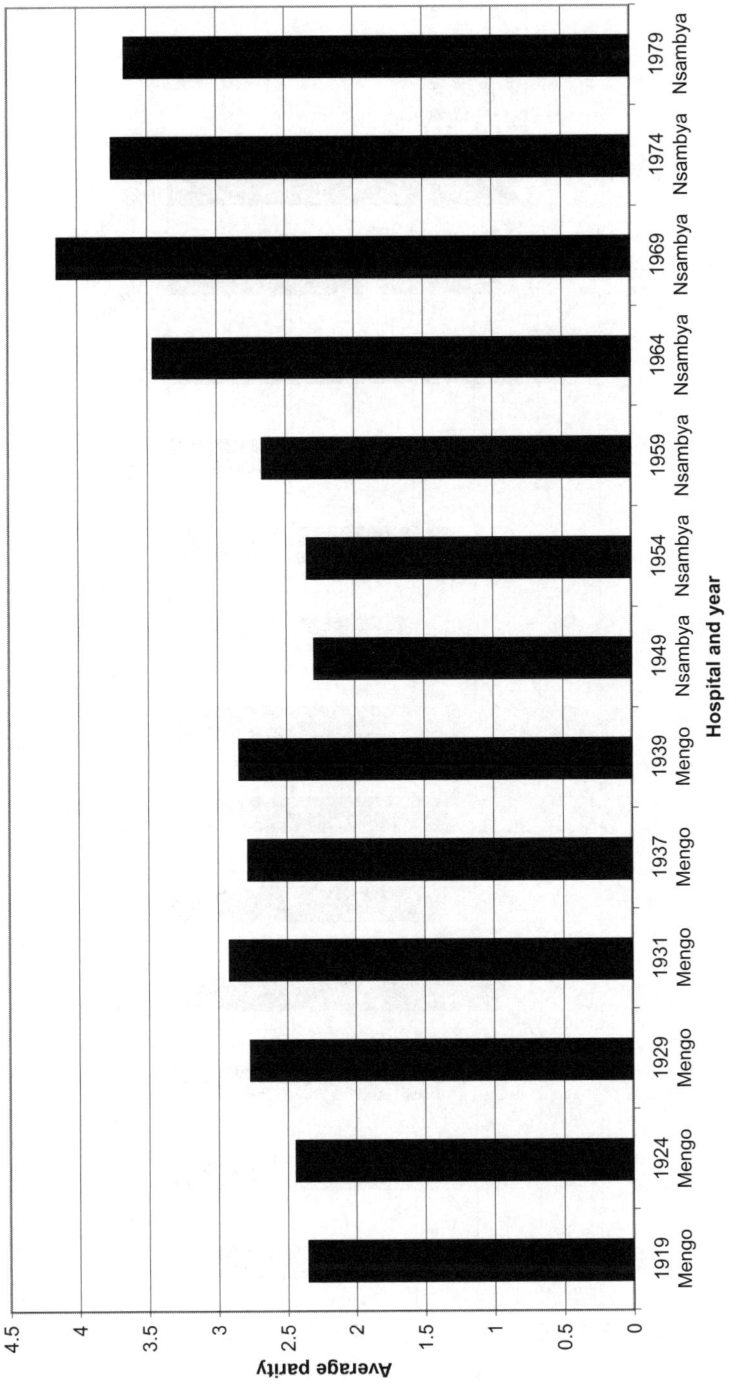

Figure 7.9 Average parity of Ganda mothers who delivered in Mengo and Nsambya Hospitals, Kampala, 1919–79

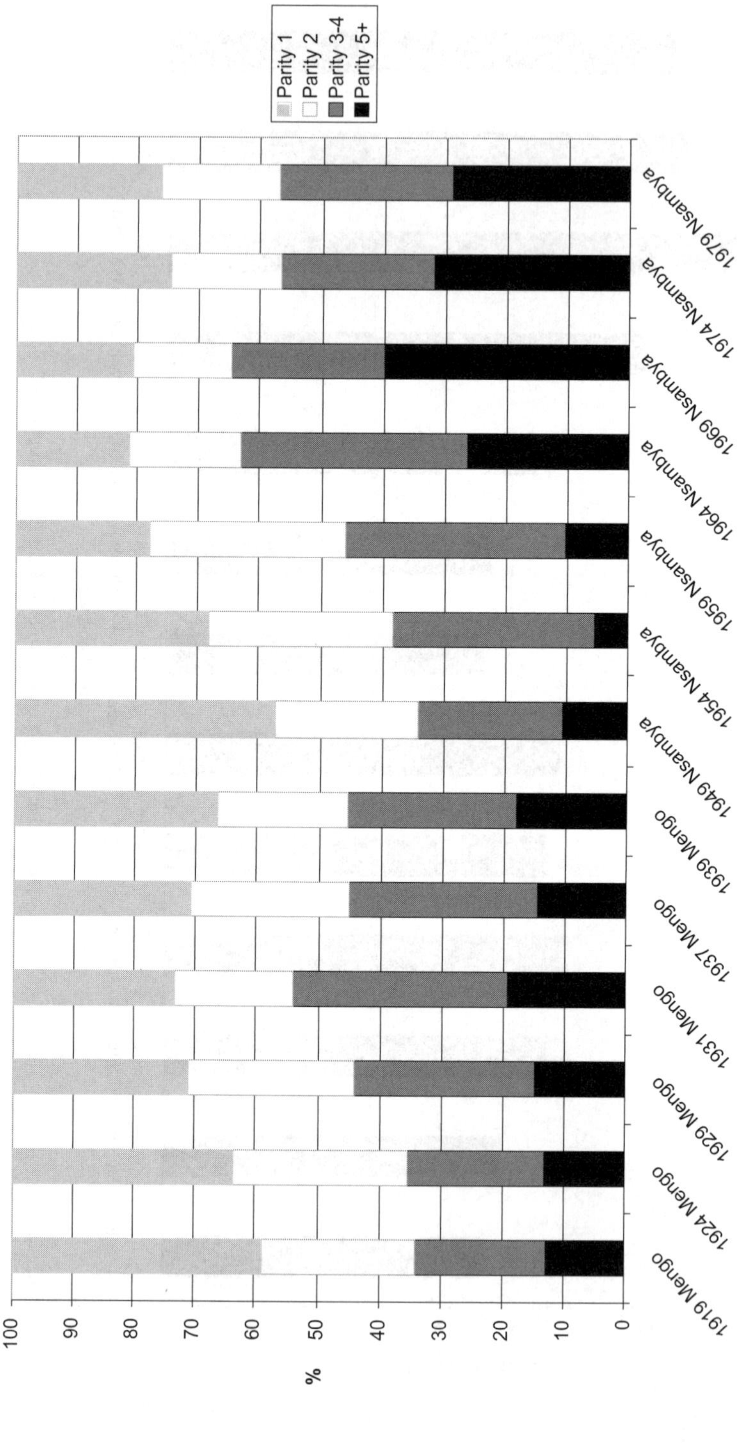

Figure 7.10 Percentage of mothers by parity, Mengo and Nsambya Hospitals, Kampala, 1919–79

their ages, so the possibility exists that rising mean parity simply reflected an increase in the average age of women who came to the clinic, so that, as medicalized childbirth became the norm, higher-risk, young, low-parity women formed a smaller proportion of admissions. As Chapter 9 shows, however, the average parity of women at Nsambya fell in the 1970s, even though the numbers of women attending the maternity ward continued to rise, suggesting that the entrenchment of hospitalized birth alone did not result in changes in average parity. Only in 1979 were expectant mothers' ages recorded, but what they showed was that 88% of women were under thirty years old, which suggests that the age profile of Nsambya's intake may not have changed radically over the decades, and that older women preferred to deliver at home.

Parity data though say nothing about the significance of primary sterility. A 1952 comparative survey found that the number of live births per woman aged forty-five and above in Buganda was, at 3, even lower than that reported in Buhaya, primarily because 31.6% of these women were childless. Sterility was higher in the surveyed community than in Buganda in general, whose childlessness rate was 25.1% in 1948, presumably because it was home to many single women who had lived much of their adult lives in nearby Kampala. By the late 1960s sterility in general had reduced sharply, and the differential between peri-urban and rural Buganda had almost disappeared. The 1969 census found that the sterility rate for women aged forty-five to forty-nine in Buganda had fallen to 18.4%, while in a 1967 survey in Kasangati, another community near Kampala with many single women, only a fifth of women aged over forty-four had never had a child.[86]

Ganda fertility was low not only because so many women never gave birth at all, but also because many women's reproductive lives were cut short. The 1959 census found that female fertility levels fell off rapidly over the age of thirty-four. Such figures are notoriously problematic due to under-reporting of births, but comparing the same type of data gathered in the same manner in successive censuses should enable some tentative conclusions to be drawn. The 1969 census indicated that the age specific fertility rate for 35–39 year olds had risen by approximately two-thirds over the intervening decade. This cohort of women born between 1930 and 1934 had not been characterized by noticeably high fertility at the time of the 1959 census. Women's reproductive

[86] Uganda Protectorate, *African Population of Uganda Protectorate: Geographical and Tribal Studies* (Nairobi: EAHC, 1953); Uganda, *Uganda Census 1959*; Uganda, *Report on the 1969 Population Census* (Entebbe: Ministry of Planning and Economic Development, 1971); Richards and Reining, 'Report on fertility surveys, 1952'; E. Kibukamusoke to A. Richards, 31 May 1967, A. Richards papers, LSE, 16/48.

lives seem to have lengthened in the late 1950s and through to the 1960s.[87] Part of this apparent elongation of the period of childbearing seems to have been due to social rather than biological changes. Marital instability had dampened female fertility levels to some extent into the 1950s, even though women were more willing to have children outside marriage in Buganda than in neighbouring societies. By the 1960s, by contrast, in Kampala and surrounding areas at least, women who were currently unmarried constituted a large minority of all mothers delivering at hospital. Divorcees and in particular never-married women were less obviously characterized by sub-fertility than they had been in the past. The link between marriage and reproduction had been fundamentally weakened.[88]

It is possible that more important causes of the reduction in sub-fertility in Buganda were associated with improvements in medical care. The early expansion of ante-natal and maternity services reduced the incidence of unattended difficult deliveries, lowering the risk of sterility consequent on post-partum infections. Similarly, the exceptionally large number of medical facilities in Buganda ensured that treatment with penicillin for STDs was accessible to the entire population more quickly than was the norm in Uganda. Gonorrhoea still affected the fertility of a significant number of women in the 1960s, but syphilis no longer seems to have been a major cause of miscarriage and stillbirth.[89]

Few areas in tropical Africa can match the level of detail which exists in Buganda regarding the impact of medical care on reproductive outcomes. Records of changing birthweight over time give a clear sense of how the nutritional status and disease burden of pregnant women improved significantly between 1924 and 1969. As Figures 7.11 and 7.12 show, at the start of

[87] Uganda, *1959 Census*; Uganda, *1969 Census*; M. Semwogerere-Serunjogi, 'Population dynamics in Uganda for period 1959–1969' (unpublished PhD, University of London, 1980), p. 89; Ntozi and Kabera, 'Patterns', p. 96. This finding goes against received wisdom about the shape of fertility patterns in Africa, and should be viewed with caution. It does, though, seem to fit with other local evidence of reduced secondary sterility and rising post-marital fertility during this period. Cf. e.g. T. Moultrie, T. Sayi and I. Timæus, 'Age and parity effects on birth intervals in the African fertility decline', (unpublished paper, Population Association of America Annual Meeting, 2010).

[88] P. Gutkind, 'African urban family life: Comment on and analysis of some rural-urban difference', *Cahiers d'Études Africaines*, 10 (1962), p. 202; C. Crocker, 'A study of knowledge, attitudes, and practices of family planning in Uganda, East Africa', *Journal of Reproductive Medicine*, 7, 5 (1971), pp. 235–8.

[89] Uganda Protectorate, *Annual Medical Report 1950* (Entebbe: Government Printer, 1951); R. Trussell, 'Pelvic inflammatory disease', *Proceedings of the Royal Society of Medicine*, 61 (1968), pp. 365–8; E. Grech, 'Stillbirths in Uganda', *Obstetrics and Gynecology*, 29, 6 (1967), pp. 764–73; E. Grech, J. Everett and F. Mukasa, 'Epidemiological aspects of acute pelvic inflammatory disease in Uganda', *Tropical Doctor*, 3, 3 (1973), pp. 123–7; Uganda, *1969 Census*.

this period the average birthweight of hospital-born babies in Kampala was 2,785 grams, with 27.9% weighing below 2,500 grams and therefore being classified as low birthweight, a condition which is strongly associated with a higher risk of stillbirth. By 1937 the average had climbed to 3,063 grams with only 10.6% being classed as low birthweight, levels which remained largely stable until the 1960s when the average rose by another 100 grams, and the proportion of low birthweight babies fell to around 5%. Researchers found that low birthweight in Kampala was associated with poor diet, malarial infection, poverty, and illiteracy. Its reduction over time was a function not only of broad improvements in income and the availability of high-value foodstuffs, but also reflected decades of sustained nutritional health education and a highly successful attempt to eradicate mosquito breeding sites in urban and peri-urban Kampala.[90]

Other medical interventions had a more immediate effect on pregnancy outcomes. The Mengo hospital records show that between 1924 and 1939 the proportion of maternity cases whose current pregnancies ended in miscarriage fell significantly from 9.3% to 5.2%, whereas these patients' reported experience of previous miscarriage remained unchanged. This suggests that improved ante-natal care had an immediate beneficial impact on the likelihood of seeing a pregnancy through to term.[91] The frequency of previous miscarriage, as reported by Mengo patients, subsequently fell by two-thirds between 1940 and 1955, presumably because ante-natal care became ever more common and the incidence of undernutrition, syphilis, and malaria reduced. Levels of stillbirth in mission hospitals meanwhile remained stable

[90] Nsambya Hospital Maternity Registers; C. Rendle Short, 'Health education for the expectant mother' (Report of a seminar 'Health education and the mother and child in East Africa', Makerere Medical School, Kampala, Nov. 1961), p. 14; H. Welbourn, 'Backgrounds and follow-up of children with kwashiorkor', *Journal of Tropical Paediatrics*, 5, 3 (1959), p. 86; T. Watts, 'Some observations on birth weights and nutritional changes during pregnancy: a prospective study of a self-selected group of mothers at an ante-natal clinic in West Mengo District Uganda'(unpublished DPH dissertation, Makerere University Kampala, 1969), pp. 32–3, 46–9; P. Akingbehin, 'Causes of neonatal morbidity and mortality in New Mulago Hospital' (unpublished DPH dissertation, Makerere University Kampala, 1970), p. 25; Dr. A. Alderdice papers, RHO, MSS.Afr.s.1872 (3). As birthweight increased with parity, the rising fertility of patients over time would of itself have increased birthweights slightly.

[91] Mengo Hospital Maternity Records. It is surprising that levels of miscarriage experienced by Mengo's patients did decline, given that the hospital routinely provided women attending ante-natal sessions with a mercury solution which they were advised to drink throughout their pregnancies as a treatment for syphilis. Mercury is now known to increase the risk of miscarriage. M. Tuck, 'Syphilis, sexuality, and social control: a history of venereal disease in colonial Uganda' (unpublished PhD dissertation, Northwestern University, 1997), p. 285; P. Goering et al., 'Toxicity assessment of mercury vapor from dental amalgams', *Fundamental and Applied Toxicology*, 19, (1992), pp. 319–29.

[92] Mengo Hospital Maternity Registers, Sir Albert Cook Library, Mulago, Kampala; Nsambya Hospital Maternity Registers. Babies who were identified as premature were excluded from the birthweight calculations.

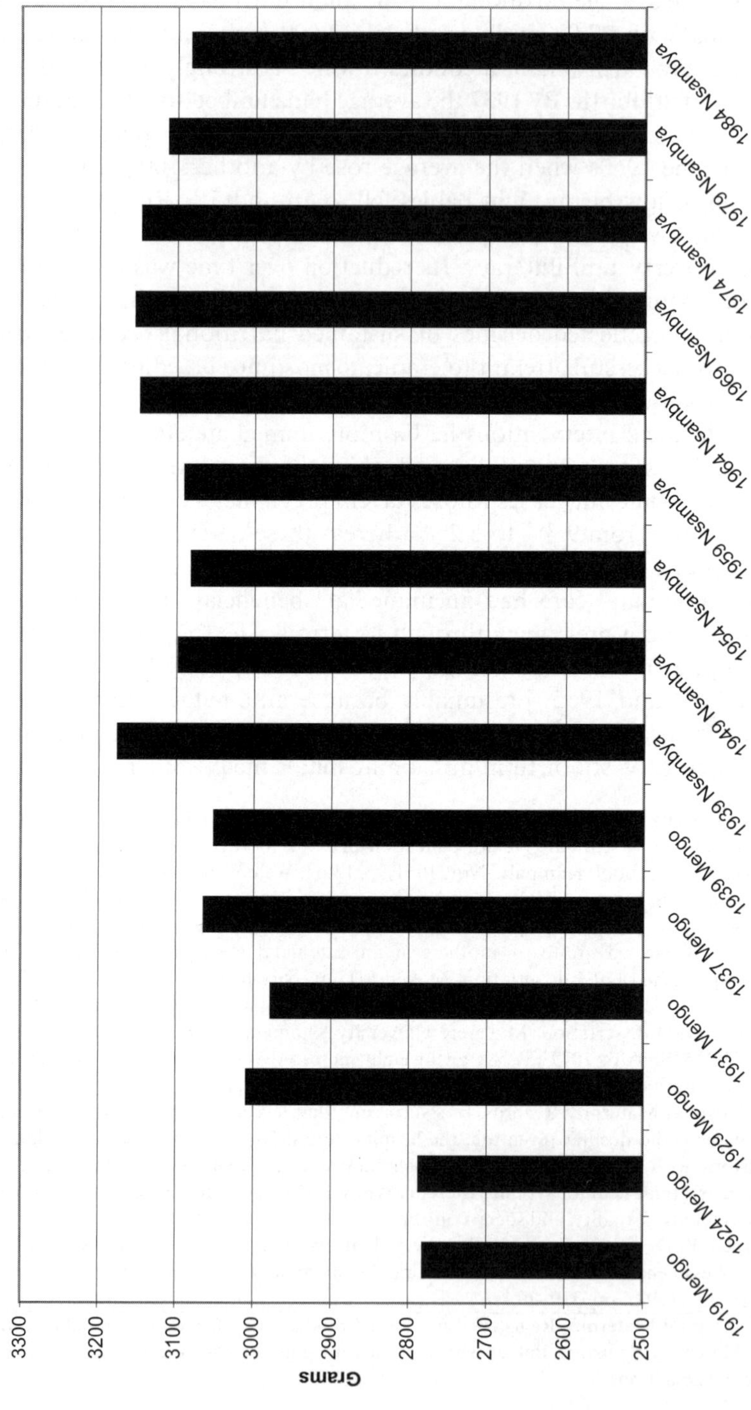

Figure 7.11 Average birthweight of babies born in Mengo and Nsambya Hospitals, Kampala, 1919–84

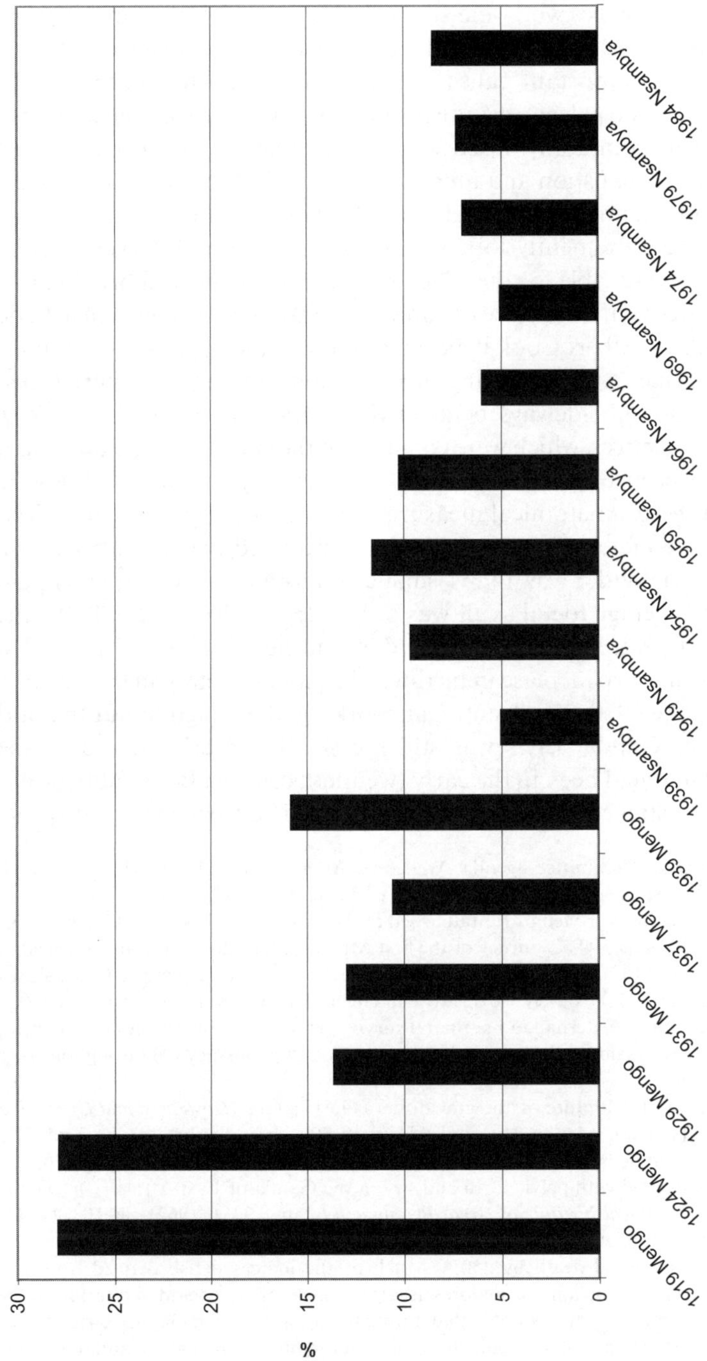

Figure 7.12 Percentage of babies born in Mengo and Nsambya Hospitals, Kampala, 1919–84 who were of low birthweight (<2,500g)[92]

until the 1950s when they experienced a remarkable improvement. The proportion of babies who were stillborn averaged 13.1% before 1950 and 3.4% in the 1950s and 1960s. Maternal mortality fell just as fast (see Chapter 8).[93]

The most important cause of maternal death and stillbirth before the 1950s, in hospital at least, was disproportion. Women experiencing obstructed delivery were commonly dosed with oxytocic herbs, increasing the likelihood of maternal exhaustion and uterine rupture, which occurred more frequently in Buganda than anywhere else in the world. Shock, haemorrhage, and infection were frequently followed by death. Surgical interventions between the wars were notable for their lack of success. Babies stillborn due to cranial injury consequent on the use of forceps appeared in the registers with depressing regularity. Albert Cook believed that the Ganda pelvis was compressed in childhood due to girls carrying heavy weights and being required to sit with their legs tucked sideways beneath them. Later research though suggested that these practices, which were common to the entire region, had an unusually grave impact in Buganda because of the severity of female adolescent malnutrition there. Anatomical measurements in the early colonial period found that 18% of maternity patients had a contracted pelvis, and that while the Ganda pelvic outlet was 14.3% smaller than that of women in England and Wales, the average foetal skull was only 5.2% smaller. In the 1930s the crisis reached its peak, as the improved diet and health of small-framed women resulted in a sharp increase in birthweights, and therefore in the size of babies' skulls. By the 1960s an obstetrician working at Mulago found that although the average Ganda pelvis was still the smallest ever recorded, it was 14% bigger than it had been in the early twentieth century. Better nutrition *in utero* had been sustained through to adulthood.[94] The frequency of disproportion

[93] Uganda Frazer Committee agenda, Wellcome Archive, PP/CDW E.3/1; Nsambya Hospital Maternity Registers; Marasha, 'Causation', p. 20; C. Olayiwola Akerele, 'Review of present M.C.H. services in West Mengo' (unpublished DPH dissertation, Makerere University Kampala, 1971), p. 23; N. Musisi, 'The journey of the first African female doctor through tropical medicine, international health and global health: Josephine Namboze of Uganda', (unpublished paper presented at the WHO Conference on African Health History, Nairobi, 6–8 Feb. 2007). Some of the improvement in maternal and perinatal survival was due to the transfer of low-risk patients from Mulago to Nsambya, but mortality associated with pregnancy fell throughout Buganda in this period.

[94] C. Rendle-Short, 'Rupture of the gravid uterus in Uganda', *Obstetrics and Gynecology*, 79, 6 (1960), pp. 1114–20; Mengo Hospital Maternity Records; Report of the Lady Coryndon Maternity Training School, Namirembe, 1932 (Albert Cook Archive); D. Allbrook 'Some problems associated with pelvic form and size in the Ganda of East Africa', *The Journal of the Royal Anthropological Institute of Great Britain and Ireland*, 92, 1 (1962), pp. 103–13. The use of oxytocics was associated with a fourfold increase in the incidence of stillbirth and raised the likelihood of maternal death by 250%. Much of the increased risk derived from underlying problems of disproportion or malpresentation which often caused oxytocics to be given. Interestingly, some informants stated that during the colonial period Ganda started to discourage pregnant women from eating carbohydrates in order to limit foetal growth and reduce the risk of disproportion. Female FGD, Takajunge, 26 Aug. 2004.

reduced from the 1950s, but just as importantly the medical response to the problem improved radically. Women of small stature were automatically identified during ante-natal checks as requiring assisted delivery, while the introduction of the lower segment caesarean section in the 1950s, and vacuum extraction in the 1960s, dramatically reduced the risk that disproportion would end with maternal death and stillbirth. The increased duration of women's reproductive lives after 1950 was in part due simply to a sharp reduction in the risk of death during childbirth.[95]

Improved healthcare impacted on fertility levels after 1940 in one other major area, birth spacing. Average birth intervals, according to the Kisubi parish baptism registers, declined by four and half months between 1940 and 1969.[96] The enormous improvement in the chances of child survival, which had begun between the wars and accelerated after 1945 (see Chapter 8), was likely to have affected maternal decision-making about breastfeeding strategy, though other factors also encouraged bottle-feeding and early weaning. The concentration of wealth, industry, and social services in Buganda meant that female education and employment were far more advanced here than elsewhere in the region. In 1959, 34% of females aged five and over had some schooling, twice the national average. By 1969, Buganda's female education rate had risen to 47%, and in some areas more girls than boys were in school. Schooling helped give women the confidence to reject pressure to maintain traditional breastfeeding practices, while the requirements of the workplace provided the impetus for many to do so. The sharpest fall in birth intervals, of 2.8 months, came in the early 1950s, coinciding not only with the dramatic improvement in health services, but also with the rapid take-up of bottle feeding, especially in the area around Kampala, where by 1960 42% of Ganda babies were bottle-fed.[97] Surveys of women in the 1950s who attended child welfare clinics, and therefore lived primarily in urban or peri-urban areas, found that the typical period of breastfeeding had halved in the recent past to around twelve months, with literate women stopping four months earlier than

[95] R. Billington, *A Tune on Black and White Keys. Partnership in Healing: the Story of Mengo Hospital* (London: Janus, 1993), pp. 13, 92–7; Int. HW, 31 July 2008, Bristol, F; C. Rendle Short, 'Causes of maternal death among Africans in Kampala, Uganda', *British Journal of Obstetrics and Gynaecology*, 68, 1 (1961), pp. 44–51; V. Everett, 'Causes of stillbirth in Mulago hospital, Kampala, and their prevention', *Uganda Medical Journal*, 1 (1972), pp. 45–7; Marasha, 'Causation', p. 32; E. Grech, 'Review of the treatment of ruptured uterus and Mulago hospital, Kampala', *East African Medical Journal*, 45, 7 (1968), pp. 508–15.

[96] C. Martin, 'Some estimates of the general age distribution, fertility and rate of natural increase of the African population of British East Africa', *Population Studies*, 7, 2 (1953), pp. 195–6; Uganda, *1959 Census*; Semwogerere-Serunjogi, 'Population dynamics', pp. 100–126.

[97] Richards and Reining, 'Report on fertility surveys, 1952'; Uganda, *1959 Census*; Uganda, *1969 Census*; Gbejuade, 'Review', p. 27; Uganda Protectorate, *Annual Report of the Medical Department, 1956* (Entebbe: Government Printer, 1957); H. Welbourn, 'Weaning among the Baganda', *Journal of Tropical Paediatrics*, 9, 1 (1963), p. 17.

those who had not been to school.[98] Interviewees, most of whom raised families in rural Buganda in the middle decades of the twentieth century, breastfed their babies for slightly longer than the urban rates, but very few lasted longer than eighteen months.[99]

It might be assumed that Buganda's high levels of female education after the Second World War would have delayed the onset of reproduction. In fact there is little evidence of that before the late 1960s. Successive censuses showed that women started their reproductive lives earlier in Buganda than in Uganda as a whole. Interestingly, the 1959 census showed that women in Kyaddondo —Kampala and its hinterland—enjoyed significantly higher levels of fertility than the rest of Buganda until age thirty, reinforcing the sense that high levels of education and healthcare, initially at least, increased birth rates. By contrast, average female marriage age, according to the Kisubi registers, rose by two and half years between 1945 and 1969, though it still remained lower than in Ankole. Education and employment seem to have had more impact in causing women to defer marriage than to delay the onset of sexual activity. This was seen most clearly in the area around Kampala, where retrospective reproductive histories found that in the late 1960s the average age at first birth, 18.7, was 1.3 years lower than the age at first marriage. Fertility rose in Buganda then partly because of the increased duration of women's reproductive lives, partly because they reproduced more quickly, and partly because of their improved health. The story of fertility decline, which will be told in Chapter 9, will be equally complex.[100]

CONCLUSION

Previous attempts to explain the origins of rapid population growth in Africa have been hampered by the weakness of fertility data for the period before the Second World War. In this region, however, the early development of complex bureaucracies, missions, and hospitals ensured that sufficient information

[98] Dr. P. Evans' diary of 1953 visit to Uganda, Wellcome Archive, A.3/1 PP/PRE; H. Welbourn, 'Notes on differences between Baganda and Luo children in Kampala', *East African Medical Journal*, 32, 7 (1955), pp. 291–8; H. Welbourn, 'Childhood in a changing world' (unpublished TS, n/d, Hebe Welbourn papers).

[99] e.g. Female FGD, Kagezi, 25 Aug. 2004; Female FGD, Takajunge, 26 Aug. 2004; Int. NNFW, 28 Aug. 2004, Kaswa, F; Int. HGN, 10 Sept. 2004, Kiiso, F.

[100] Uganda, '1948 sample census'; Uganda, *1959 Census*; Uganda, *1969 Census*; Kisubi Parish Registers; Semwogerere-Serunjogi, 'Population dynamics', pp. 40–1, 89; Ntozi and Kabera, 'Patterns', pp. 48, 73; Watts, 'Some observations', p. 32; Uganda Ministry of Health and Macro International, *Uganda Demographic and Health Survey 1988/89* (Entebbe and Calverton, Md: Statistics Department, Uganda and Macro International Inc., 1989), p. 15.

about the key life events of local people was recorded and archived to enable some changes in fertility patterns to be traced and explained. The most significant finding of this chapter is that fertility increase does seem to have begun prior to the Second World War, in Ankole and, less clearly, in Buganda. The 1950s saw birth rates begin to rise in Buhaya, and increase much more rapidly in the former two societies.

In few aspects of modern African history must the establishment of the chronology of change still take centre stage, but this is one. Just as important as identifying when fertility increased in these three societies is explaining how and why it did so. In none of the case study areas do church records indicate that a decline in age at first marriage enabled women to have larger families. Neither cash cropping nor labour migration reduced male marriage ages, while female marriage age rose due to schooling and missionary pressure. The relative insignificance of marriage age is indicated by the fact that in Ankole, where fertility was highest, women married latest. The hypothesis that rising birth rates stemmed from an economic desire for increased family labour was supported to some extent by evidence from Ankole, but not Buganda or Buhaya where greater cash wealth enabled farmers to adopt the alternative strategy, which brought more immediate benefits, of marrying extra wives or recruiting migrant labour.[101] But overall interviewees in Ankole gave little indication that the desire for children had heightened over the colonial period. Rather, what seems significant here is how the intensely pronatalist culture that characterized Ankole's agriculturalist majority at the start of the twentieth century survived largely intact through to independence. What did change was that the proportion of women in Ankole who were married increased in the 1920s, from which point marriage remained almost universal and exceptionally durable. Buhaya's increased fertility from the 1950s was also associated with a changing marriage pattern, in this case caused by a dramatic decline in the incidence of divorce, whereas in Buganda it was the increasing willingness of women to have children outside marriage that proved most significant.

In all three societies a crucial cause of higher fertility was an increase in the duration of women's reproductive lives, partly due to changes associated with marriage but, more importantly, consequent on improvements in women's health. Better maternal nutrition was a significant factor in Buganda from the interwar period and in Buhaya from the 1950s. After the Second World War penicillin limited the impact of STDs and post-partum infections on female fecundity across the region. Improved healthcare also reduced the prevalence of primary infertility, as did education and missionary criticism

[101] Female FGD, Takajunge, 26 Aug. 2004; Int. FN, 29 Aug. 2004, Butanga, F; Int. MMA, 24 Aug. 2004, Kyanakase F.

which reduced the frequency with which girls suffered reproductive damage consequent on premature marriage. Pregnancy outcomes improved most dramatically in Buganda, it seems, where the exceptional quality of maternity provision brought about a remarkable reduction in the frequency of miscarriage, stillbirth, and maternal mortality, though Ankole and Buhaya also benefited to a lesser degree.

The final factor which was of major importance was the reduction in the length of birth intervals, which began in Buganda in the 1920s, in Ankole in the 1930s, and Buhaya in the 1940s. The decline in birth spacing was it seems the result of improved maternal health and nutrition, and the shortening of the period of breastfeeding, due to female education and employment, and greater parental confidence in the likelihood of child survival.

For African historical demography as a whole, the significance of these case studies is above all that some factors which have frequently been assumed to have been of primary importance in stimulating higher fertility in the colonial period were largely irrelevant in each of these three societies. Moreover, the example of Buganda in particular demonstrates that it is dangerous to think of a smooth transition to a high fertility regime, for birth intervals declined extremely early here but the impact of this reduction in birth spacing was cancelled out for several decades due to the severity of marital instability and reproductive health problems in this kingdom. More specifically, southern Uganda and northwest Tanzania have been considered by some scholars to belong to the band of sub-fertility that stretched across equatorial Africa, encompassing much of southern Sudan, Central African Republic, both Congos, Cameroon and Gabon. Previous reviews have tended to identify STDs, often associated with prolonged post-partum abstinence, labour migration, or social disruption arising from the colonial takeover, as the pre-eminent cause of this enduring pattern of low fertility. STDs were also important in Buganda and Buhaya, though they were associated more with commercialization than migration and abstinence. But these case studies indicate that other health problems as well as marital breakdown contributed significantly to the sub-fertility of the Ganda and Haya. It seems likely that future research will add further complexity to our understanding of Africa's distinctive regional demographic histories.[102]

[102] O. Frank, 'Infertility in sub-Saharan Africa: Estimates and implications', *Population and Development Review,* 9, 1 (1983), pp. 137–44; U. Larsen, 'Sterility in sub-Saharan Africa', *Population Studies,* 48, 3 (1994), pp. 459–74; J. Caldwell and P. Caldwell, 'The demographic evidence for the incidence and cause of abnormally low fertility in tropical Africa', *World Health Statistics Quarterly*, 36, 1 (1983), pp. 2–34.

8

Disease and Death, 1925–69

INTRODUCTION

In the early colonial period mortality loomed large in East Africans' minds. Traditionally viewed as a malicious autonomous agent, death was thought to take pleasure in separating spouses, driving the childless to despair, and depriving children of their siblings. Death brought an end to familial happiness, personal ambition, and the lineal transfer of property. Many informants spoke of their tragic personal experience of repeated child loss or of seeing their siblings swept away by disease. Elderly interviewees had often been given names which memorialized the traumas of the past. One was called Bitorotoorwa, 'the chosen one', because he, unlike five older siblings, did not die within a few days of being born. Another was named Byabusha, 'for nothing', because his parents had seen their previous children all die later in infancy, and wished to prepare themselves for further pain. By the end of the 1960s, conceptions of death had begun to shift through conversion to one of the world religions and formal education.[1] The experience of death had changed even more radically. Now parents could reasonably hope that all of their children would survive to adulthood. Certainly they would be unlucky to lose more than one. This was one of the great transformations of modern African history.

Yet our understanding of when and how mortality declined is still unclear. It is generally accepted that the eradication of serious famine and the containment of some epidemic diseases through inoculation lowered the peaks of mortality between the wars, but the impact of colonialism on endemic disease is less certain. Many scholars emphasize the importance of the new medications and public health interventions introduced after the Second World War which enabled colonial and post-colonial medical systems to

[1] See for example Kiyungu Shema Focus Group Discussion (FGD) Male, 21 Aug. 2004; Int. RMR, 13 Aug. 2000, Byabusha, Busindi, M; Int. MPM, 10 Aug. 2000, Ibare, F, Int. FK, 16 Aug. 2000, Kikukwe, F, Int. GK, 21 Aug. 2000, Nkindo, F; Int. YK, 19 Aug. 2000, Kikukwe, F. Cf. S. Doyle, '"The child of death": Personal names and parental attitudes towards mortality in Bunyoro, Western Uganda, 1900–2005', *The Journal of African History,* 49, 1 (2008), pp. 361–382.

lower mortality caused by the most common ailments.[2] Others claim, by contrast, that any such benefits were outweighed or counterbalanced by the role of colonial taxation, regulations, and demands for labour in raising levels of endemic illness in the first place by draining rural wealth, impoverishing diets, and producing an economic system that took workers away from their families and local disease environments.[3] Again, while there is little doubt that the greatest fall in death rates typically occurred among young children, it is far from certain whether the earliest or fastest declines occurred among neonates (babies less than twenty-nine days old), infants (babies aged less than one year), or young children aged one to four. Nor is it agreed whether education was more important than healthcare in improving the likelihood of child survival.[4]

As with all demographic history in Africa, the weakness of the data relating to mortality fosters disagreement. Unfortunately the church registers in this region provide no new insights into patterns of mortality change. None of the Catholic parishes used for this study maintained a separate burial register, and in fewer than 5% of cases were the baptism registers updated with the details of parishioners' deaths. Confirmation dates were commonly recorded but not often enough to serve as a proxy for survival to late childhood.[5] However, in general Ankole, Buganda, and Buhaya possess demographic data of unusual wealth. Uganda's sample census in 1948 collected retrospective data on infant mortality, while in 1959 differences in mortality patterns according to urbanization and ethnicity were recorded in Buganda. Buhaya's 1969 census broke down the experience of mortality by education and locality. Civil death registration records were of some value in all three

[2]These range from the more triumphalist accounts such as D. Clyde, *History of the Medical Services of Tanganyika* (Dar es Salaam: Government Printer, 1962) to the more measured analysis of John Iliffe's *East African Doctors* (Cambridge: Cambridge University Press, 1998) or J. Caldwell, 'The population factor in African change', in A. Mafeje and S. Radwan (eds.), *Economic and Demographic Change in Africa* (Oxford: Clarendon Press, 1995), pp. 11–35.

[3]See for example M. Turshen, 'Population growth and the deterioration of health, mainland Tanzania 1920–1960', in D. Cordell and J. Gregory (eds.), *African Population and Capitalism* (Boulder: Westview Press, 1987), pp. 187–200; R. Packard, 'Maize, cattle and mosquitoes: The political economy of malaria epidemics in colonial Swaziland', *The Journal of African History*, 25, 2 (1984), pp. 189–212.

[4]Compare for example J. Caldwell, 'Routes to low mortality in poor countries', *Population and Development Review*, 12, 2 (1986), pp. 171–220 and G. Pison, J. Trape, M. Lefebvre and C. Enel, 'Rapid decline in child mortality in a rural area of Senegal', *International Journal of Epidemiology*, 22, 1 (1993), pp. 72–80.

[5]Cf. S. Walters, 'Fertility, mortality and marriage in northwest Tanzania, 1920–1970: A demographic study using parish registers' (unpublished PhD dissertation, University of Cambridge, 2008); V. Notkola, I. Timaeus and H. Siiskonen, 'Mortality transition in the Ovamboland Region of Namibia, 1930–1990', *Population Studies,* 54, 2 (2000), pp. 153–167 for examples of valuable work that has been done where church burial records are well maintained.

societies, most especially in Buhaya, where they appear to have been exceptionally comprehensive. These societies were also fortunate in the frequency with which they were selected as sites for in-depth, large-scale demographic and medical surveys, the best of which correlated mortality patterns with education, occupation, marital status, duration of breastfeeding, and usage of medical services. Hospital maternity records, moreover, provide information on mothers' previous experience of child loss as well as maternal and neo-natal mortality, the latter being particularly important as the deaths of newborns outside of hospital were relatively unlikely to have been registered by civil or religious institutions, and were not always mentioned during demographic surveys or censuses.

These sources will be used first to narrate a basic chronology of variations in mortality patterns and then will be employed in conjunction with medical records and oral interviews in an attempt to explain why these changes occurred when they did. The evolving story of healthcare in the region will focus on one particular group of diseases, STDs, because they were researched so intensely in the colonial and immediate post-colonial periods, and because they were so closely related to changes in fertility and sexuality, the other major themes of this study.[6]

MORTALITY ESTIMATES

East African governments possessed no accurate knowledge of overall mortality levels until the 1959 census in Uganda and the 1967 census in Tanzania. Before then governments had relied on the civil registration system and occasional surveys to give some sense of the direction of mortality change among the general population, though infant and child mortality data were gathered for the 1948 Uganda census. Unfortunately the civil registration of deaths in Uganda was far from complete. Between 1925 and 1949 the crude death rate (CDR), that is, the number of deaths recorded at all ages, averaged 18.8 per 1,000 in both Buganda and Ankole (see Figure 8.1). Yet within the province of Buganda, Mubende district had the lowest average CDR at 13.9 per 1,000 while Mengo had the highest at 21.5. Given that Mengo district had the best

[6] This approach is not without its disadvantages, of course. It will potentially create a slightly exaggerated impression of the significance of STDs within the medical community after 1945, and it underplays the scale and complexity of research into other medical conditions, and their contribution to morbidity and mortality patterns. Uganda, for example, became a global leader in malnutrition research, one consequence of which was the rapid expansion of preventive and community medicine from the late 1940s. But a fully comprehensive study of medical change over this period would fill several volumes, and would obscure the interlinkage of disease, sex, and demographic change.

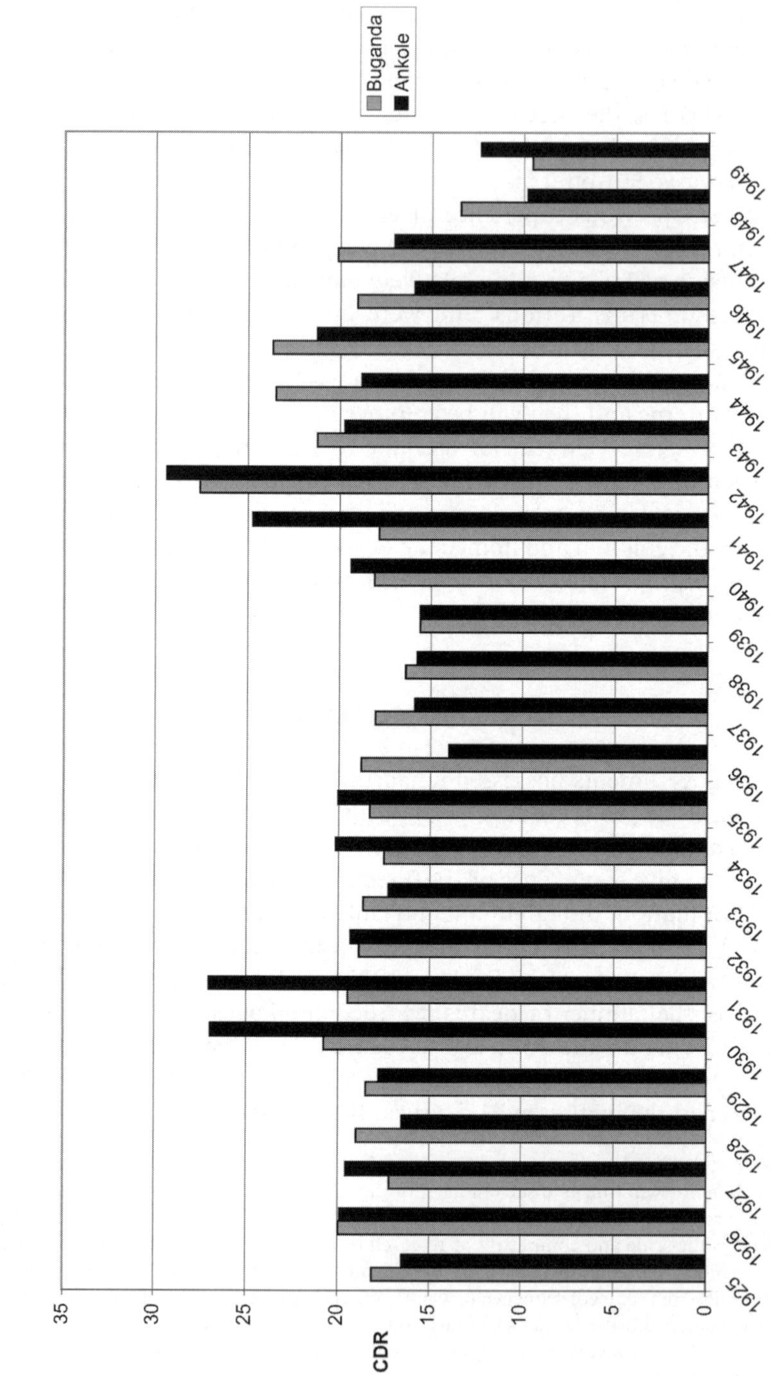

Figure 8.1 Crude death rate per 1,000 in Ankole and Buganda 1925–49, from vital registration records

medical care and the most efficient civil administration in Buganda, it seems likely that the apparent longevity of Mubende's notoriously sickly population was in reality a marker of widespread non-compliance with the registration system due to Ganda chiefs' unpopularity among the indigenous Nyoro population of the 'Lost Counties'.[7] The largely reliable 1959 Uganda census found that Mubende's CDR was in fact 24 per 1,000 compared to West Mengo district's 16. Buganda as a whole had a CDR in 1959 of 18 compared to Ankole's 24.[8] Given that Uganda's officials failed to update population totals to take account of immigration, only in census years can CDRs calculated from vital registration records be compared with any degree of reliability. If the rather risky assumption is made that Mengo's system of recording deaths was as accurate in 1948 as it had been in 1931, then, according to the registration data, overall mortality in the heart of Buganda fell by 37.3% during this seventeen-year period. Alternatively Mengo district's 1931 civil registration CDR of 22.2, which almost certainly was an underestimate, could be compared with West Mengo's census-based CDR of 16 in 1959, giving a minimum decline in mortality rates of 28.1% over the second half of the colonial period. A sense of how rapidly life expectancy was rising in the era of independence is provided by West Mengo's CDR at the 1969 census which, at 8 per 1,000, was half that of 1959.[9]

The East African Medical Survey (EAMS) considered that Buhaya's civil registration system was more accurate than that of Buganda. In 1931 Buhaya's CDR was 19.3 per 1,000, around the same as Buganda but significantly lower than Ankole's, which stood at 27.0. Buhaya's average CDR calculated from the 1948–1952 registration records was 17.0. It seems unlikely that the decline was simply the result of deteriorating data accuracy, given that the Medical Survey found that registered child mortality figures for the latter period tallied closely with those recorded in their own contemporaneous investigations.

[7] Uganda Protectorate, Annual Medical Reports 1924–49, National Archives [NA], CO/685. See S. Doyle, 'From Kitara to the Lost Counties: Genealogy, land and legitimacy in the kingdom of Bunyoro, Western Uganda', *Social Identities*, 12, 4 (2006), pp. 457–70; S. Doyle, 'Immigrants and indigenes: The Lost Counties dispute and the evolution of ethnic identity in colonial Buganda', *Journal of Eastern African Studies*, 3, 2 (2009), pp. 284–302 for further detail on this disconnect between ruler and ruled in Mubende. The CDR calculated from the civil registration records in Uganda suffered from two major flaws, the frequency with which deaths were not recorded and the failure to update the population total between censuses in response to immigration. These two inadequacies worked in opposite directions but require that the results be viewed with scepticism.

[8] Uganda Protectorate, *Uganda Census 1959: African Population* (Entebbe: Ministry of Economic Affairs, 1960).

[9] C. Olayiwola Akerele, 'Review of present M.C.H. services in West Mengo' (unpublished DPH dissertation, Makerere University Kampala [MUK], 1971), p. 20.

The Survey's report also emphasized the longevity of Haya adults, noting that half of all adults in this population were aged over forty.[10]

The CDRs produced from the vital registration records in these societies vary widely, ranging as they do from 9 to 33 per 1,000, but not wildly. The infant mortality rates (IMRs) derived from civil registration by contrast immediately appear unreliable (see Figure 8.2). Ankole's average IMR between 1925 and 1948 of 170 was entirely believable, but the rate of change was not. In 1925, 370 out of every 1,000 live-born children were reported to have died before their first birthday. The IMR supposedly then halved by 1933 and then again by 1943, finally reaching 58 in 1948. The much more reliable sample census of that year, however, reported that women in Ankole aged between thirteen and forty-five had lost 189 out of every 1,000 children in infancy, compared to 241 for women aged over forty-five. Ankole's IMR was 170 per 1,000 according to the 1959 census, and 116 in 1969. Clearly infant mortality had fallen substantially since the 1920s but the declining accuracy of the vital registration system, which by 1948 seems to have missed perhaps two-thirds of infant deaths in Ankole, exaggerated the scale of this change. The numbers of infant deaths registered fell much less steeply in Buganda, but the vital registers' IMR in 1948 of 57 per 1,000 was almost identical to that of Ankole. The retrospective data collected for the 1948 sample census though reported that women of reproductive age in Buganda had experienced infant mortality of 207 per 1,000, compared to 243 among older women. Infant survival seems to have been of similar severity in the early colonial period in both Ugandan societies, but improved more in Ankole in the 1930s and early 1940s. Yet, according to the 1948 census, Buganda's current IMR was only 182 per 1,000, and this dropped rapidly to 140 in 1959 and 98 in 1969. After the Second World War Buganda became the healthiest society in the region for infants.[11]

[10] W. Laurie and H. Trant, *East African Medical Survey, Monograph no. 2, A Health Survey in Bukoba District, Tanganyika* (Nairobi: EAHC, 1954), p. 63. Buhaya's civil registration records from 1948–52 have not been archived but the average totals were published by Laurie and Trant. The average population during these years was estimated to be 313,811 based on an intercensal growth rate of 2.274%. No CDR data for Buhaya were published in subsequent censuses within this period, though the 1967 census recorded a CDR of 17.6 per 1,000 for West Lake Region. Buhaya made up two-thirds of West Lake's population, and probably had lower mortality levels than the regional average. R. Henin and B. Egero, '1967 population census of Tanzania: A demographic analysis' (BRALUP Research Notes 19, UDSM, 1972), p. 6.

[11] Uganda Protectorate, Annual Medical Reports 1925–48, NA, CO/685; Uganda Protectorate, '1948 Sample Census' (I am grateful to Sarah Walters for sharing this document with me); Uganda, *1959 Census*; C. Costello, 'Maternal and child health in rural Uganda: the role of nutrition' (unpublished PhD dissertation, University of Pennsylvania, 1986), p. 69; Uganda, *Report on the 1969 Population Census* (Entebbe: Ministry of Planning and Economic Development, 1971). Age-specific questions asked in the 1948 sample census mean that only educated women participated, and therefore that the reduction in child mortality recorded was possibly greater than that experienced by these societies as a whole.

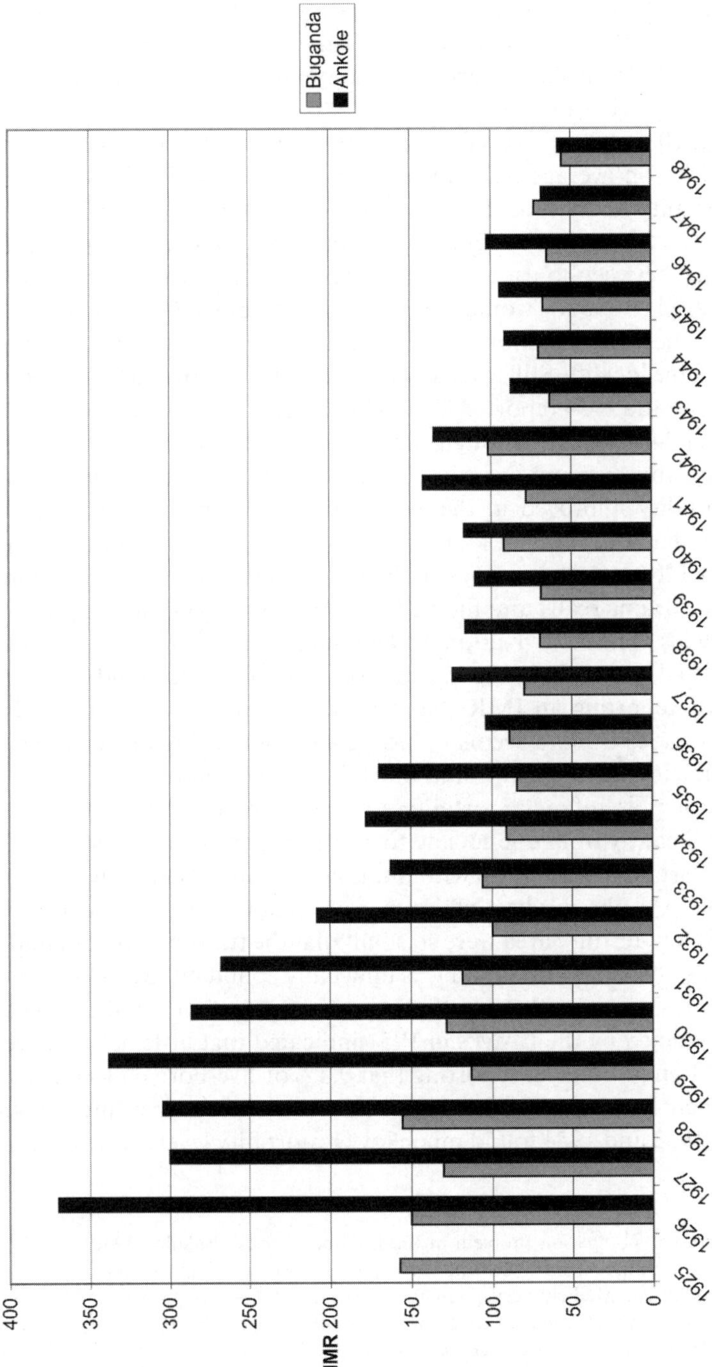

Figure 8.2 Infant mortality rate per 1,000 live births in Ankole and Buganda 1925–48, from vital registration records

Buhaya in marked contrast experienced extremely high infant mortality until at least the final years of colonial rule. Neither civil registration nor censuses recorded IMRs for Buhaya during the colonial period but two major retrospective surveys give a sense of the scale and trajectory of mortality change. In 1938, 3,510 women surveyed in Kanyangereko reported that of their live-born children on average 322 out of every 1,000 had died in infancy. That infant mortality had lessened somewhat in severity since the 1920s was suggested by the lower rates reported by younger women, 247 per 1,000 for women aged between fourteen and nineteen and 281 for those in their twenties, compared to 335 for women aged thirty and above. The post-war EAMS operated in the same lakeshore environment of Buhaya, though unfortunately not in the same locality. Still, each of the three retrospective surveys conducted between 1951 and 1954 reported lower IMRs than that recorded in 1938, varying between 248 and 286, though there was no indication in the age-specific rates of any improvement over time. Tentatively then it can be suggested that infant mortality improved in the 1920s and 1930s and then stabilized at a higher rate than was found in southern Uganda. That the 1967 census reported an IMR of 120 per 1,000 for West Lake Region suggests that infant mortality had reduced dramatically among the Haya, West Lake's dominant group since the mid-1950s. The 1973 National Demographic Survey, a less reliable but more localized source, gave broad support to this apparent trend, the parishes under study reporting an IMR that ranged from 65 to 95 per 1,000. In less than two decades Buhaya seems to have gone from having one of the highest to one of the lowest levels of infant mortality in the region.[12]

Levels of post-infancy mortality among young children appear to have varied significantly from one society to another. Compared to its severe levels of infant mortality, death rates within this age group in Buhaya were very low, perhaps because the weakest children had already died, or because family sizes in this low-fertility area were so small that the transmission of childhood diseases was obstructed and food was unusually abundant. In 1938, only 9.9% of babies in Kanyangereko died between the ages of one and six. The first survey conducted by the EAMS in 1951 indicated that little had changed for young children in Buhaya, reporting that 9.5% of live-born children had died between their first and fifth birthdays. However, two larger, more complex surveys in 1952 and 1954 found much lower mortality levels in this age group,

[12] A. Culwick, 'The population problem in the Bukoba district' (Bukoba, 1938, UDSM, EAF CORY 239), p. 15; East African Medical Survey, *Annual Report, 1951* (Nairobi: EAHC, 1952), pp. 65–6; East African Medical Survey, *Annual Report, 1952* (Nairobi: EAHC, 1953), pp. 18–37; Laurie and Trant, *East African Medical Survey*, pp. 55–9; Henin and B. Egero, '1967 population census'; R. Henin, *National Demographic Survey of Tanzania, 1973: Volume II, Data for Socioeconomic Groups* (Dar es Salaam: Tanzania Bureau of Statistics, 1973).

at 5.1% and 5.3% respectively, suggesting that a substantial improvement in child health had occurred between the late 1930s and the mid-1950s.[13] For Ankole data on young child mortality during the colonial period are very limited. One survey of Hima women in the mid-1950s found that 11.1% of live-born children died between one and five. The 1969 census collected retrospective data in Ankole which showed that past mortality in the one to five age group was lower than the western province average for women aged fifteen to twenty-nine but higher among women aged thirty-five to forty-nine, suggesting that child survival had significantly improved there at some point in the 1950s. A researcher involved in a major survey in Ankole in the mid-1960s estimated that between 6.5% and 12.7% of children died between one and five.[14]

For Buganda, there exist important though problematic data on child mortality from the mid-colonial period. At Mengo hospital in Kampala expectant mothers were asked over a period of decades about the outcome of their previous live births. Surviving data show that the proportion of women who had experienced the death of one of their previous children fell from 53.3% in 1924 to 37.1% in 1939 and 17% in 1955. No doubt part of this decline resulted from the changing nature of the sample, as the growing popularity of medicalized childbirth reduced the numerical dominance of women with tragic reproductive histories. Nonetheless, the scale of this change is highly suggestive. Many of the deaths reported by these women would have occurred under the age of one and over the age of four. Narrowing the sample to those mothers who had had only one previous live birth would in most cases at least exclude older child mortality. The percentage of Ganda women whose first child had died before the birth of their second baby declined dramatically from 54.8 to 23.2 between 1924 and 1939.[15] It is reasonable to assume that women attending a maternity ward would have been particularly likely to have benefited from any improvements in medical provision over this period. The 1948 sample census also gathered important data on child mortality, though the information unfortunately was not limited only to the one to four age group. Overall women in Ankole had lost 9.1% more children than those in Buganda. As Buganda's infant mortality was higher than Ankole's in 1948, it was superior survival rates among the over-one age group that was

[13] Culwick, 'Population problem' (Cory 239), p. 4; EAMS, *Annual Report 1952*; Laurie and Trant, *East African Medical Survey*, p. 57.

[14] 'Population composition by age and sex of ten kraals: Bahima live births and survivorship', Derrick Stenning papers, Cambridge University Library, D2, C4; Costello, 'Maternal', p. 61; R. Cook, 'Child health in Ankole, Uganda: A programme of immunization and health education and its evaluation' (unpublished DMed dissertation, University of Oxford, n/d [*c.*1968]).

[15] Mengo Hospital Maternity Records; Uganda Frazer Committee agenda, 'Information concerning Mengo CMS hospital, Oct. 1955', Wellcome Trust Archive, PP/CDW E.3/1.

key. However, there is reason to assume that Buganda's post-infancy advantage declined after the Second World War. In 1948, child mortality was 21% lower among women aged 43–47 in Buganda compared to those from Uganda's Western Province, which included Ankole, but only 13% lower among Buganda's 18–22 year olds. By 1959 Buganda's ascendancy had been lost. Mortality among one to two year olds was 65 per 1,000 in Buganda but 45 in Western Province. Ten years later the rate in Buganda was 45, that in Western Province 31. In 1969 in Kampala, Buganda's capital, 7.5% of children died between their first and fifth birthdays, meaning that a newborn child was as likely to die during these years as in infancy. This demographic shift was reflected in the focus of medical research and interventions, which came to view infancy in Buganda as a less vulnerable life stage than the second and third years of life, a period which became associated with the onset of kwashiorkor (protein-energy malnutrition).[16]

The Causes of Mortality Change

A summary of the developments detailed above for each of the three case study areas makes it clear that the pattern of mortality change was not consistent across the Great Lakes region. Mortality among Buhaya's adults seems to have been very low throughout this period. Child mortality was also reasonably low in the 1930s, and had seen substantial improvement by the early 1950s. By contrast the Haya suffered very high levels of infant mortality around 1925, and while these seem to have reduced somewhat by the 1930s, they remained more or less constant at a high level until at least the mid-1950s after which a dramatic increase in infant survival rates began.

Infant mortality in Buganda at the start of our period was probably lower than in the other societies. It seems to have fallen gradually until 1948, and then ever more rapidly through the 1950s and 1960s. Child survival in Buganda appears to have improved substantially between the wars, but the rate of improvement slowed down after 1940. It seems likely that Buganda had the highest one to five mortality of all three societies by the 1960s. Adult mortality here probably declined gradually until the 1950s but then seems to have fallen sharply in the 1960s.[17]

[16] Uganda Protectorate, '1948 Sample Census'; C. Martin, 'Some estimates of the general age distribution, fertility and rate of natural increase of the African population of British East Africa', *Population Studies*, 7, 2 (1953), p. 196; Uganda Protectorate, *1959 Census*; Uganda, *1969 Census*; I. Sembajwe, 'Impact of urbanization on fertility and child mortality. The case studies of Tanzania and Uganda' (unpublished MA dissertation, UDSM, 1973), p. 186; R. Dean, 'Health education and protein-calorie malnutrition' (Report of a seminar 'Health education and the mother and child in East Africa', Makerere Medical School, Kampala, Nov. 1961), pp. 10–11.

[17] Semwogerere, 'Population', p. 134; E. Grech et al., 'Maternal mortality in Uganda', *International Journal of Gynecology and Obstetrics*, 7, 6 (1969), p. 26.

Ankole's infant mortality seems to have reduced significantly between 1925 and 1948, relatively slowly through the 1950s, and then very sharply again in the 1960s. Child mortality in Ankole was relatively high before the 1940s, but steady improvement thereafter saw survival rates surpass those of Buganda in the 1950s. What little is known about adult mortality suggests gradual improvement but that Buganda had a substantial advantage.

It is initially surprising that Buhaya and especially Buganda did not enjoy substantially lower levels of mortality than Ankole. For most of this period Ankole had much lower levels of cash income, education, and medical provision than the other societies. In 1959, for example, average income in Buganda was more than five times higher than in Ankole, the literacy rate among women of child-bearing age was twelve times higher, and annual medical attendances per capita were 79% higher.[18] Such developmental markers are significant, but their impact in this region was mediated by other environmental and social factors.

That development, loosely defined, did in general tend to reduce mortality rates can best be shown by looking within societies rather than comparing one with another. Towns and cities, for example, were this region's most developed areas, with the densest network of schools, medical facilities, and opportunities for skilled employment. It was not surprising then that in 1969 under-five mortality in the small town of Bukoba was, at 129 per 1,000, almost half that of the rest of Buhaya. The city of Kampala never enjoyed such an advantage over rural Buganda, partly because schooling and quality healthcare were less concentrated in Buganda, partly because Kampala contained a substantial underclass of the semi-employed who lived in unplanned slums. Nonetheless the 1959 sample census found that the experience of child mortality was 26% lower in the area around Kampala than in Buganda as a whole. A sense of how rapidly child survival had increased can be obtained from the much lower rates of infant death reported by younger women in 1959 compared to the older generation. Ganda women of childbearing age had lost only 8% of their children in infancy compared to 13.3% for those aged forty-five and above, though of course as some children belonging to younger women would not yet have reached their first birthday, their reported IMR would have been slightly underestimated. The benefits of urban residence seem to have increased rapidly in the period leading up to the 1959 census, for Greater Kampala's advantage in child survival over the rest of Buganda rose from 15% in mothers aged between forty-five and forty-nine to 66% for women aged between fifteen and nineteen. By 1969, however, overall child mortality rates were only 22% lower in the city, most likely because of the upgrading of rural

[18] Uganda Protectorate, *Medical Department and Statistical Office Annual Reports for 1959* (Entebbe: Government Printer, 1960).

health units but perhaps also due to Kampala's rapid expansion during the 1960s.[19]

A sense of which aspect of urban living was most likely to have lowered mortality rates can be obtained from examining the ethnic differences in death rates within Buganda, as measured by the 1959 census. Overall non-Ganda living within Buganda experienced an IMR of 170 per 1,000, 42% higher than the Ganda rate. Whereas Ganda women of childbearing age had experienced levels of infant mortality that were 12% lower than those suffered by Ganda women aged over forty-five, the differential between the IMRs experienced by younger compared to older non-Ganda women was only 4%. Yet the children of older immigrant women were likely to have spent their infancy outside of Buganda, in most cases in areas which suffered higher IMRs. In general then, non-Ganda women were unable to take full advantage of the increasing potential for improved infant survival that was available in their host society. But within Greater Kampala immigrants' IMR was 130, still 44% higher than that of local Ganda, but nonetheless one of the lowest rates reported by any group in Uganda. As urban immigrants' advantage over migrant labourers in Buganda's countryside in terms of real income and educational levels was very modest, it seems most probable that it was the density of medical, and especially maternity, services that advantaged immigrants' children in the city. Immigrants contributed a higher proportion of Mulago Hospital's deliveries and in- and out-patients than they did to the urban population as a whole. They also appeared surprisingly regularly in the records of urban child welfare clinics. It seems that immigrants in rural Buganda, where medical provision was less visible, public information less readily available, and social differentiation much more intense, were less likely to seek medical attention for their children. Comparing the maternity registers of Nsambya Hospital in Kampala with those of Nkokonjeru Hospital, located in a rural area of Buganda which possessed a large immigrant population, it is striking how rarely non-Ganda came to the clinic in the countryside. Given that both institutions were run by the same Catholic order, and presumably maintained a similar admissions policy, and given that non-Ganda in Kampala were known to prefer Mulago's free service to that provided by mission hospitals, it is reasonable to argue that urbanization increased immigrants' awareness of the benefits of western biomedicine.[20]

[19] Martin, 'Some estimates', pp. 195–6; Uganda, *1959 Census*; M. Semwogerere-Serunjogi, 'Population dynamics in Uganda for period 1959–1969', (unpublished PhD dissertation, University of London, 1980), pp. 100–126. The 1959 Census provided data on Kyaddondo, the county within which Kampala was situated. The population of this county was predominantly urban or peri-urban. By 1969 the city limits had been expanded to incorporate much of Kampala's peri-urban fringe.

[20] Uganda, *1959 Census*; Semwogerere-Serunjogi, 'Population dynamics', pp. 100–126; H. Welbourn, 'Backgrounds and follow-up of children with kwashiorkor', *Journal of Tropical Pediatrics*, 5, 3

Development though also impacted negatively on mortality levels in some ways, meaning that Buganda and Buhaya could not take maximum advantage of their superior medical and educational provision. For example, the commonplace practice in Buganda of fostering out children to relatives, which was often associated with some degree of neglect and heightened risk of malnutrition, was reinvigorated by the desire of parents to place their children with relations who lived near a good school.[21] Malnutrition was particularly severe in Buganda for a variety of reasons, including female food taboos and weaning practices, but one new factor that emerged in the late 1940s was the adoption of bottle feeding by many semi-educated urban and peri-urban Ganda women. It was thought that such women, 42% of Ganda attendees at Greater Kampala's child welfare clinics in the early 1960s, bottle-fed their babies partly in order to emulate what they believed was the most modern western practice, and partly in order to facilitate their return to the workplace. Medically trained critics of bottle feeding in Uganda argued that many mothers could not afford to provide their babies with the appropriate ratio of formula milk to water, in some cases creating a solution that was described as homeopathic. The lack of facilities to make up and keep the formula in hygienic conditions was also frequently criticized. In the early 1950s it was claimed that almost all bottle-fed babies died, but later accounts were much less cataclysmic, perhaps a sign that public health messages about correct dosage and cleanliness in preparation had had some success.[22]

While relatively few women in this region abandoned breastfeeding entirely, the general trend was for the duration of breastfeeding to reduce over time. The impact of the resultant shortening of birth intervals on child

(1959), p. 86; Uganda Protectorate, *The Pattern of Income, Expenditure and Consumption of African Unskilled Workers in Kampala, September 1953* (Nairobi: EAHC, 1954), pp. 1–8; Uganda Protectorate, *1951 Annual Medical Report* (Entebbe: Government Printer, 1952); Nkokonjeru Maternity Registers. In 1959 the age profile of Ganda and non-Ganda females was almost identical.

[21] H. Welbourn, 'Weaning among the Baganda', *Journal of Tropical Pediatrics*, 9, 1 (1963), pp. 14–24; H. Welbourn, 'Childhood in a changing world' (unpublished TS, n/d, Hebe Welbourn papers); J. Butler, 'Willingly to school: the day student in Uganda', *Transition*, 9 (1963), pp. 27–9.

[22] H. Welbourn, 'A comparison between children attending child welfare clinics in 1950 and in 1955', *East African Medical Journal*, 34, 2 (1957), pp. 47–54; 'Children's Doctor' (transcript of a monthly radio programme, *c.*1962, H. Welbourn personal papers); D. Jelliffe, 'Pediatrics in Uganda', *Clinical Pediatrics*, 5 (1965), p. 58; H. Welbourn and G. De Beer, 'Trial of a kit for artificial feeding in tropical village homes', *Journal of Tropical Medicine and Hygiene*, 67 (1964), pp. 155–9; D. Jelliffe, 'Village level feeding of young children in developing tropical regions, with especial reference to Buganda', *Journal of the American Medical Women's Association*, 17, 5 (May 1962), p. 413. Cf. John Knodel, *Demographic Behaviour in the Past: a Study of Fourteen German Village Populations in the Eighteenth and Nineteenth Centuries* (Cambridge: Cambridge University Press, 1988), p. 44. It is of course likely that mothers attending child welfare clinics would have been more likely than non-attendees to bottle-feed, because their children were ill or because they were more self-consciously modern.

mortality rates was inconsistent, and difficult to unravel, though very short intervals seem to have been damaging everywhere. In Buhaya in the early 1950s a large-scale survey found that infant mortality for women with mean birth intervals of less than two years was 19% higher compared to women with birth intervals of between two and four years, and over two and half times higher compared to those whose births were spaced more than four years apart. Women who had had seven or more live births by the age of thirty had seen 56% of their children die in infancy, whereas women with just one child before they turned thirty had lost only 18% as infants. Of course though the relationship between fertility and child mortality works in both directions, so that high infant mortality in a family would have potentially fostered high fertility, due to the repeated curtailment of breastfeeding. This factor, along with problems of underreporting, must be taken into account, but their significance is reduced to some degree when comparative data show that substantial differences existed between societies in the association between birth spacing and mortality. In Ankole at the end of our period, another major survey found that women whose birth intervals averaged less than eighteen months had suffered levels of child mortality that were around 60% higher than those experienced by women with mean birth intervals of between eighteen and thirty-five months, but only 3% higher than among women with birth intervals of three years and above. The impact of shortened birth spacing on the likelihood of child survival seems to have been greater in Buhaya than Ankole, and in Ankole particularly long birth intervals appear to have been associated with an elevated rather than reduced risk of child death. It can be hypothesized that because Buhaya's rate of infant mortality was so immense in the early 1950s, children there required a particularly high level of attention and nutrition. Levels of disease were so much lower in Ankole by 1970 that moderate birth spacing was sufficient to maximize survival chances. It seems probable that longer birth intervals here were a marker of sub-fertility, and that some of the factors which contributed to maternal morbidity also damaged the health of children.[23]

In the case of 1950s Buhaya, one of the defining influences on the ability of mothers to care for their children was their marital condition. While no significant difference in child survival could be detected between monogamous and polygamous marriage, the EAMS found that the ending of a mar-

[23] Laurie and Trant, *East African Medical Survey*, pp. 55–60; Costello, 'Maternal', p. 174. Cf. Walters, 'Fertility, mortality and marriage', p. 241. The role of short birth intervals in child mortality is exaggerated by such figures, as the death of a child tends to bring forward the subsequent conception. It should also be noted that it is possible that the low reported IMR among Haya women with long birth intervals was in some cases due to women failing to report the birth and subsequent death of one of their children.

riage substantially increased mortality levels under age five. Women who were still married to their first husband had lost 24% of their children before their fifth birthday. Widows had lost 31%, remarried women 39%, and women who were divorced or separated 40%. Orphanhood clearly had a negative impact on children's survival chances, but the higher mortality rates for divorced, separated, and remarried mothers suggests that spousal neglect or conflict carried additional risks to the obvious problems arising from the absence of the birth-father. No other study considered the role of marital condition, but it can be assumed that the rapid decline in the frequency of marital breakdown in Buhaya in the decades after the EAMS would have contributed to the reduction in levels of child mortality over this period. Buganda had similarly high levels of marital breakdown, which seem to have remained unchanged through to the 1970s. Perhaps this helps explain why child mortality continued to be relatively severe in Buganda through the 1950s and 1960s, though it is possible that the impact of divorce and separation was lessened here by the relative ease with which single women could secure fraternal support, land, and independent income (see Chapter 4).[24]

In a large-scale comparative study, Jack Caldwell demonstrated that the most important factor in the decline of child mortality in low-income societies after the Second World War was female education. Within Nigeria, for example, he found that the gain in life expectancy at birth was 20% when illiterate mothers gained access to adequate health facilities, 33% when women were educated but no health facilities were available, and 87% when both female schooling and medical provision were provided. In the Ghanaian census in 1960 it was observed that uneducated mothers had lost twice as many children as those with elementary schooling and over four times as many as those with secondary education. Scholars have hypothesized that female education reduced child mortality by increasing faith in scientific medicine, helping mothers appreciate the importance of hygiene and sanitation, and increasing the likelihood that medical advice would be sought and followed when children became ill.[25] It seems, however, that the correlation between schooling and child survival was not so strong in the Great Lakes region of East Africa. Buganda and Buhaya were two of East Africa's best educated societies between 1925 and 1969, whereas Ankole lagged far behind the Ugandan average until after independence. Yet infant and child mortality rates were not radically inferior in Ankole compared to its neighbours. That education in general, and that of girls in particular, was so advanced in Buganda and

[24] Laurie and Trant, *East African Medical Survey*, pp. 72–3; Uganda, *Census 1969*, Vol. III, p. 69; Henin, *National Demographic Survey Volume II*, pp. 78, 32.

[25] Caldwell, 'Routes to low mortality', pp. 171–220; J. Iliffe, *Africans: the History of a Continent* (Cambridge: Cambridge University Press, 1995), p. 252.

Buhaya was related in the first place to the rapidity with which Christianity spread there, because missions dominated schooling across the region until the 1950s. In addition the wealth of these two societies facilitated the employment of agricultural labour, so that it was relatively easy to release girls from the expectation that they should work constantly on the family farm until marriage. As the colonial period progressed the education of daughters, especially in Buganda, was increasingly viewed by parents as a marker of social status and as a route to greater material prosperity. A highly educated woman reportedly could command a bridewealth a hundred times higher than that typically obtained for an illiterate wife, and was thought to be more likely to share her income with her parents than a son with an equivalent education.[26]

Ankole, like most East African societies before the 1950s, was condemned to relative poverty by its designation as a reservoir for migrant labour, and saw Christianity spread slowly from the founding missions. Accordingly the 1959 census reported that only 1.6% of women aged over forty-five had had any education. For women of childbearing age the proportion was 5.4%. The experience of education among adult males was six times higher. Female schooling did expand rapidly from around 1950 so that by 1969 the gender gap had narrowed, with 18.3% of women aged between fifteen and forty-four having been to school. Within Buganda the 1959 census found that the female experience of education above the age of forty-five was, at 4%, little higher than the Ugandan average. But girls began to go to school in large numbers here from the 1920s so that by 1959 36.3% of women of childbearing age had been educated. By 1969 the level of education in this age group had reached 46.6%. In the colonial period men were approximately 50% more likely to be educated than women, but by the 1960s as many girls as boys went to primary school, though males still dominated secondary education. Equivalent data do not exist for Buhaya, though other evidence suggests that its experience was midway between that of Ankole and Buganda. Figures on school attendance showed that boys were three times more likely than girls to go to school there, while retrospective data gathered in 1973 indicated that one in four women born around 1925 had some education.[27]

Some elderly female informants were sceptical of the notion that the children of educated women survived in greater numbers than those with illiterate mothers, asserting that women who had been to school sometimes valued their

[26] A. Maleche, 'Sociological and psychological factors favouring or hindering the education of African women in Uganda' (unpublished TS, EAISR seminar paper 1961, African Studies Centre Library, Cambridge), pp. 6–7; 'Women's advancing status in Uganda', June 1955 (ASC Cambridge, reprint from *The Times British Colonies Review*, Spring 1955).

[27] Uganda, *1959 Census*; Uganda, *1969 Census*; Henin, *National Demographic Survey, Volume II*; A. Culwick and G. Culwick, edited by V. Berry, *The Culwick Papers 1934–1944: Population, Food and Health in Colonial Tanganika* (London: Academic Books, 1994), pp. 231–2.

jobs above their children.[28] The majority though thought that schooling meant that women were more likely to associate the signs of fever with illness, to prioritize basic hygiene such as handwashing and the use of latrines, and to understand the principles of nutrition and chemotherapeutics.[29] Generally the statistical evidence supports this latter view. In the 1950s rates of kwashiorkor and child mortality in Buganda declined significantly in relation to maternal education.[30] In Ankole in 1970 one study found that uneducated women suffered 73% more neonatal deaths than women who had been to school. Another community survey found that maternal education had lowered child mortality by 11%, but within the sub-sample of women who volunteered for a medical examination child mortality was 29% lower among those who were educated. The implication is that education was most effective when combined with a willingness to access medical care. Further analysis of this survey revealed that the benefits for child health associated with maternal education were in fact partly achieved through the increased likelihood that women who had been to school would marry men with good education and high incomes.[31] Other surveys indicated that female education alone did not determine child mortality levels, as of course Caldwell has noted. Uganda's 1948 sample census was based on information provided only by women who knew their precise ages, and therefore had been educated. But instead of showing that educated women everywhere suffered similar levels of child loss, it found that child mortality was 27.5% lower in Buganda than the national average. In 1952 a comparative study found that maternal education was associated with a reduction in child mortality of 60% in Buganda, but only 20% in Buhaya. It may be that Buganda's superior medical services permitted schooling to have maximum impact, but it is equally possible that it was the greater duration of female education in colonial Buganda that was key. In Buhaya in 1967 the census found that it was only when women had five or more years of schooling that there was any noticeable decline in child mortality. Informants recounted that information on childcare was not part of the curriculum in the first four years of primary school, which in part explains why child mortality fell fastest among mothers with longer periods of schooling.[32]

[28] e.g. Int. VM, 16 June 2000, Kanyangereko F; Int. AM, 24 June 2000, Kashambya, F; Int. MM, 12 Aug. 2000, Kanoni, F; Int. CB, 13 Aug. 2000, Busindi, F; Int. TM, 13 Aug. 2000, Busindi, F.

[29] e.g. Int. YK, 19 Aug. 2000, Kikukwe, F; Int. CKM, 17 Aug. 2000, Kibanda, F; Int. AC, 9 Aug. 2000, Rubaa-Rubya, F; Int. MM, 11 Aug. 2000, Ijumbi, F; Int. PKK, 18 Aug. 2000, Mshumba-Byazi, F; Int. SKN, 22 Aug. 2000, Maruku-Butailuka-Kasha, F.

[30] Welbourn, 'Backgrounds', p. 86.

[31] K. Masters and J. Iraka, 'The influence of custom and tradition on maternity care in Ankole district', *East African Medical Journal*, 47, 11 (1970), p. 553; Costello, 'Maternal', pp. 136–97.

[32] Martin, 'Some estimates', p. 196; A. Richards and P. Reining, 'Report on fertility surveys in Buganda and Buhaya, 1952' (University of Dar es Salaam [UDSM], Cory 373); Uganda, *1959*

Education, then, was important not only in terms of the breadth of its coverage, but also in terms of its quality. This is well known.[33] But it seems that the same is true of healthcare. Buhaya, for example, enjoyed an exceptional density of medical facilities in the interwar period. As well as the state district hospital in Bukoba town, there existed three mission hospitals and twenty-two dispensaries, scattered across the countryside. Haya made use of their services in large numbers. As early as 1923 attendances at the medical institutions of the Catholic mission alone totalled 180,000, including repeats, a remarkably high number given that the population of the district was only 256,000. But between the wars all but two of Buhaya's dispensaries were staffed by tribal dressers or sanitary inspectors who typically had received only a few months training, and whose treatment options were based on an extremely limited repertoire of drugs. The mission hospitals, though highly regarded, were small and mainly served their local rural communities. The district hospital was larger but in 1925 was found to be in a sorry state of disrepair, run by a sub-assistant surgeon rather than a fully qualified doctor.[34] The rapid expansion of medical services in Buhaya in the 1910s and 1920s was followed by two decades of stagnation. By the mid-1940s Buhaya, first or second among Tanganyika's districts in terms of income and educational provision, lay only around fifth in the rankings of total medical provision, and far lower in terms of health facilities per capita.[35] Healthcare within Tanganyika as a whole, meanwhile, slipped far behind its East African neighbours in the 1930s and 1940s. Just after the Second World War, Tanganyika's doctor:patient ratio was a third lower than Uganda's. By 1946 only five Tanganyikans had qualified as doctors, with four more currently being trained. In Uganda, the equivalent figures were fifty-seven and fifty-two. As Tanganyika's Director of Medical Services observed, the country was on track to have Africanized its medical system in around 500 years.[36] From the late 1940s

Census; Sembajwe, 'Impact', p. 49; Advisory Committee on Public Health, 'Minutes of meeting, 14 Apr. 1947, Medical instruction in school curricula—inclusion of', Tanzania National Archives [TNA], 36433; e.g. Int. AM, 24 June 2000, Kashambya, F.

[33] J. Caldwell and P. McDonald, 'Influence of maternal education on infant and child mortality: Levels and causes', *Health Policy and Education*, 2, 3–4 (1982), pp. 251–67; J. Cleland and J. van Ginneken, 'Maternal education and child survival in developing countries: The search for pathways of influence'. *Social Science and Medicine*, 27, 12 (1988), pp. 1357–68.

[34] Lake Province Annual Report 1935, TNA, 215/1246; Bukoba District Annual Report, TNA, AB/1–1733/8; A.R.M. for DMS to C.S., 18 October 1943, Minute 2, 'Yaws', TNA, 31732; R. Kuczynski, *Demographic Survey of the British Colonial Empire, Vol. II* (Oxford: Institute of International Affairs, 1949), pp. 382–3. Cf. Iliffe, *East African Doctors*, pp. 41–5.

[35] P. A. T. Sneath, 'Memorandum. Post-war development of the Tanganyika Medical Service: Optimum and sub-optimum objectives, 9 Apr. 1946', in Tanganyika Territory, *Post-war Development: Medical Department* (Dar es Salaam: Government Printer, 1947).

[36] Uganda Protectorate, Annual Medical Report 1948, NA, CO/685/31; A. Williams, 'Report on Health Sevices in Tanganyika' (*c.*1962), p. I/26, A. Williams papers, Rhodes House Oxford

though the proportion of government expenditure devoted to healthcare increased sharply, so that by the mid-1950s it was, at 9%, higher in Tanganyika than Uganda, though per capita spending on health remained higher in the latter country, due to its much greater wealth. Improved training for rural healthworkers was one of the most obvious benefits of Tanganyika's increased investment.[37] Within Buhaya too the early 1950s brought a radical change in the nature of medical care. The recommendations of the EAMS for a sustained campaign against STDs and poor maternal and infant health were broadly accepted, so that long-standing problems of drug and staff shortages were overcome, and public health and maternity and child welfare services took a much more prominent place within the local medical system than had previously been the case.[38] Only in the last decades of colonial rule then did the efficacy of Buhaya's healthcare match its scale.

Medical services in Ankole were much more sparse than Buhaya until the 1950s. It did have one of the larger district hospitals in Uganda at Mbarara, but only in 1950 did a mission hospital open while the construction of a second state hospital to serve the needs of the densely settled western half of Ankole had to wait until after independence. Only a handful of dispensaries and maternity centres were maintained by missions, and state-run dispensaries were relatively rare for most of the colonial period. In the late 1950s, there were only three government doctors in the district, the number of maternity beds per capita was less than a third that found in Buganda, while the Haya were more than three times as likely to go to a government dispensary as the Nkole.[39] Only in the last years of colonial rule did Ankole's local government, energized by sub-ethnic and religious rivalry, turn this competition into creative energy in the form of increased investment in medical provision. In the mid-1960s Ankole was home to the largest programme of rural vaccination ever launched in Uganda, as well as a sustained campaign to improve maternal health.[40] Ankole's disadvantages diminished rapidly in the last fifteen years of

[RHO], MSS. Afr. s. 1872 (153), Box XXXVIII; Governor to Secretary of State, 11 May 1946 and Director of Medical Services to Chief Secretary, 3 Aug. 1946, 'Higher Medical Training For Non-Europeans', TNA, 34929; P. A. T. Sneath to Chief Secretary, Memorandum, 19 Sept. 1945 and Sneath, 'Memorandum'.

[37] A. Williams, 'Report on Health Sevices in Tanganyika', *c.*1962, p. I/26, A. Williams papers, RHO, MSS. Afr. s. 1872 (153), Box XXXVIII; Frazer Committee, Minutes of meeting, 30 Aug. 1955, Wellcome Archive, London, PP/CDW E.3/2.

[38] Laurie and Trant, *East African Medical Survey*, pp. 139–42; Bukoba District Annual Report 1955, TNA, 215/3101; West Lake Province Annual Report 1960, TNA, 967.822.1.

[39] Survey of Catholic Dioceses, 1956, Rubaga archives, Kampala; Uganda Protectorate, *Annual Medical Report 1956* (Entebbe: Government Printer, 1957); Uganda Protectorate, *Annual Medical Report 1957* (Entebbe: Government Printer, 1958); Bukoba District Annual Report, 1946, TNA, 215/2070.

[40] Cook, 'Child health'; Masters and Iraka, 'The influence'.

our period, especially after 1966 when local administrations invested heavily in preventive healthcare in all areas of Uganda except Buganda, which suffered some degree of discrimination after its king, who was also Uganda's first President, was deposed in 1966.[41]

Buganda had a slightly smaller number of health units per capita than Buhaya between the wars, but they differed markedly in terms of their focus and quality. In 1927 Buganda had twenty-two government dispensaries, about the same number as Buhaya, serving a population that was 2.7 times higher. But the training available for rural medical staff in Uganda between the wars was both superior and on a larger scale to that offered in Tanganyika. Moreover, Ganda dominated the intake of the mission and state training programmes. Of equal importance, rural Buganda in the 1920s was home to twenty-four mission maternity centres, which advised on child welfare as well as offering ante-natal care and performing deliveries.[42] In the late 1930s growing financial pressure forced the Church Missionary Society to close a number of its maternity centres, but by the 1940s deliveries at state hospitals and rural dispensaries were becoming increasingly common.[43] Buganda's third major institutional advantage was the large number of hospitals established in the kingdom. In Kampala the government and the three main missions had each opened a hospital before the First World War. By the end of the 1930s mission or state hospitals had been established at Entebbe, Kisubi, Masaka, Mubende, Mukono, and Villa Maria, and over the next two decades new, small hospitals opened in Bombo, Kitovu, Mityana, and Nkozi. Many of these institutions were poorly resourced in their early years, but they were all led by qualified doctors. In the 1950s the doctor:patient ratio in Buganda, buoyed by a large number of private practitioners, was seven times higher than in Ankole. Accordingly in Buganda in 1955 44% of new medical cases were treated at hospital rather than a dispensary, compared to 27% in the rest of Uganda. Moreover, patients were 9% more likely in Buganda than in the rest of the country to reattend for further treatment and consultation. The accuracy of diagnosis and the provision of treatment must have been far superior overall in Buganda than Ankole or Buhaya.[44]

[41] S. Scheyer and D. Dunlop, 'Health services and development in Uganda', in C. Dodge and P. Wiebe, *Crisis in Uganda: The Breakdown of Health Services* (Oxford: Pergamon Press, 1985), pp. 27–8.

[42] Buganda Annual Report 1927, Entebbe Secretariat Archives [ESA], A46/433; Iliffe, *East African Doctors*, pp. 42–5; D. Zeller, 'The establishment of western medicine in Buganda' (unpublished PhD dissertation, Columbia University, 1971), pp. 254–8.

[43] Uganda Protectorate, Annual Medical Report 1948, NA, CO/685/31. In 1948 38.5% of all registered births took place in a medical institution.

[44] Uganda Protectorate, *1951 Annual Medical Report* (Entebbe: Government Printer, 1952); Uganda Protectorate, *1955 Annual Medical Report* (Entebbe: Government Printer, 1956).

The most important of Buganda's fourteen hospitals by far was Mulago, the national referral hospital and home to East Africa's medical school. During the Second World War, as specialization was encouraged by the suspension of home leave and the arrival on military service of a number of consultants from Britain, Mulago began to acquire a reputation for research excellence. Over the next two decades a remarkable group of clinicians gathered at Mulago, making breakthroughs of global significance in a number of fields including malnutrition, cancer, and heart disease.[45] What was of immediate benefit to Buganda was that for many of these researchers, Greater Kampala was their laboratory. The most valuable outcome of the various epidemiological investigations and experiments with outreach was the renewed attention devoted to child welfare. Previous attempts to open child welfare clinics had collapsed due to the lack of interest shown by mothers in averting rather than curing childhood illness. This changed in 1950 when Hebe Welbourn was charged with improving child health in peri-urban Kampala. By the end of the 1960s her mobile clinics had gathered data which helped explain why the health of young Ganda children was relatively poor, compared to that of infants, and showed that mothers absorbed preventive advice when adequately explained and linked to curative provision. Her Mwana Mugimu [Healthy Child] clinic in Kampala would be the model for nutritional rehabilitation efforts throughout Buganda and later Uganda. Her work also contributed to the development of health centres, an attempt to counterbalance the ever-increasing investment in high-level medical care at Mulago. The first health centre opened in 1959 at Kasangati, a dormitory village sixteen kilometres from Kampala, which had the primary function of training Uganda's medical students in healthcare in a semi-rural environment. In the years that followed the 12,000 people who lived in the area surrounding Kasangati became perhaps the most closely monitored, and medicalized, community in East Africa. A series of interventions such as comprehensive ante-natal care, immunization, child welfare clinics, and advice on diet and hygiene had by 1969 brought the local IMR and CDR down to 22 and 5 per 1,000 respectively, which, if accurate, meant that life expectancy was greater here than in many contemporary European countries.[46]

Kasangati's achievement was not matched elsewhere in Buganda. No other rural unit could command the same quality and quantity of staffing

[45] East African Notes, A. Williams papers, RHO, MSS. Afr. s. 1872 (153A), Box XXXVI; Iliffe, *East African Doctors*, pp. 87–9, 141–4.

[46] H. Welbourn, Reminiscences, RHO, MSS.Afr.s.1872.152; H. Welbourn interview, Bristol, 31 July 2008; N. Musisi, 'The journey of the first African female doctor through tropical medicine, international health and global health: Josephine Namboze of Uganda', (unpublished paper presented at the WHO Conference on African Health History, Nairobi, 6–8 Feb. 2007).

and resources. But the value of public health, particularly in the prevention of childhood disease, had become widely recognized within the Ugandan rural medical system.[47] This reflected not only the recent success of Kasangati but the longer-term prominence given to preventive medicine in Uganda since the 1930s. The way in which medical budgets were cut in response to the great depression varied across East Africa. In Tanganyika it was considered that resources were so stretched that attention had to focus almost entirely on maintaining a basic level of coverage for curative services. In wealthier Uganda expenditure could be sustained at a higher level, so that such a single-minded approach was unnecessary. But more than this, the depression was viewed by the leading officials in Uganda's medical department as an opportunity to reshape the health service. On the basis that investing in preventive work would save money in the long run, a quarter of the medical budget in the decades that followed was devoted to the intensification of public health efforts, with a particular focus on mother and child health. The public's response to the medical care and advice made available for these groups was far from overwhelming in the 1930s, but ante-natal care became popular in Buganda in the 1940s, and the remarkable success experienced by child health and especially maternity services in the 1950s was built on the foundations laid in earlier years. Through the 1940s assistant health inspectors and hygiene orderlies, proselytizers of 'the gospel of preventive medicine', had significant success in protecting sources of drinking water from contamination. They also ensured that thousands of latrines were dug each year, although evidence that these were consistently used at first was mixed. In practice, the most impressive achievements of the public health lobby in the 1930s and 1940s in Buganda were urban rather than rural in focus. By 1950 the population of Masaka town lived in an environment that had been entirely free of malaria for several years, that had an effective sewerage system, and had ready access to a chlorinated water supply. Only in the 1950s did popular scepticism about the logic and value of public health at home seem to recede in Buganda, as evidenced by such signs as the mass construction of well-ventilated homes and the redefinition of soap as a necessity rather than a luxury.[48] There are

[47] J. Goodall, 'The hospital care of East African children', *Journal of Tropical Paediatrics*, 18, 1 (1972), p. 48.

[48] A. Crozier, *Practising Colonial Medicine: The Colonial Medical Service in Colonial East Africa* (London: I. B. Tauris, 2007), p. 82; A. Williams, Report on Health Sevices in Tanganyika, *c.*1962, p. I/10, A. Williams papers, RHO, MSS. Afr. s. 1872 (153), Box XXXVIII; W. Kauntze, 'Memorandum on Departmental Policy, 1934', in A. Williams papers, RHO, MSS. Afr. s. 1872, Box XXXVII; Uganda Protectorate, 1942 Annual Medical Report, British Library, B.L.SPR. MicB, Group 5, Reel 281; Uganda Protectorate, *1946 Annual Medical Report* (Entebbe: Government Printer, 1947); Uganda Protectorate, *1955 Annual Medical Report* (Entebbe: Government Printer, 1956). Only in the late 1940s did Tanganyika begin to invest significantly in preventive medicine and maternity care. R. Kuczynski, *Demographic Survey Vol. II*, pp. 382–3; Walters, 'Fertility', p. 49; Clyde, *History*, pp. 168, 199–203.

several possible reasons for this growing acceptance of the value of medical information relating to sanitation and disease causation among the Ganda. Interviews showed very clearly that the influence of the older generation on health-related decision-making remained powerful in Ankole throughout the colonial period, but not in Buganda. This seems to have been related to the uneven expansion of Christianity and formal education, factors which tended to encourage faith in new forms of knowledge, and challenge the basis of elders' wisdom. There are, moreover, some indications in oral accounts that there was a growing sense of family autonomy during this period in Buganda, and that mothers were more important in decision-making about health in this society than the stereotype of wifely submissiveness would suggest. Finally, in Buganda female interviewees' memories of the medical care they and their children received during the later colonial period were generally positive, a reflection of the quality and availability of medical care. By contrast, in Ankole informants not infrequently emphasized the poor care they and their families had received from medical staff until the late 1960s, which seems to have obstructed the strengthening of faith in biomedical advice.[49]

Buganda enjoyed medical care which was far more impressive than that found in Ankole or Buhaya. But using data on disease patterns in order to demonstrate that Buganda's superior provision was translated into superior health is problematic, as comparable figures exist only within Uganda for the last years of the colonial period, and only for government dispensaries. It is likely that the difference between Ankole and Buganda would have been greater earlier, and it is probable that patients would have been more likely to go to a hospital than a dispensary with the most serious conditions, a factor that would skew the data more in Buganda.[50] Moreover, diagnoses by dispensary staff are of uncertain reliability. Still, the number of new dispensary cases per capita was more or less the same in both areas and the figures do seem to tell a significant story. Between 1959 and 1962 children under six made up 28.3% of dispensary patients in Buganda, but only 23.7% in Ankole. Given that children made up a much larger proportion of Ankole's population than that of Buganda in 1959 (49% compared with 36%), this strongly

[49] For Buganda see e.g. Int. AN, 25 Aug. 2004, Kagezi, F; Int. KN, 31 Aug. 2004, Bukande Kande, F; Int. EM, 28 Aug. 2004, Kyansi, M; Int. TNN, 3 Aug. 2004, Kitala, F; Male FGD, Bukoto, 24 Aug. 2004. For Ankole see Kiyungi FGD Female, 21 Aug. 2004; Kyenjenyi FGD Female, 22 Aug. 2004; Female FGD Ruti, 2004.

[50] The assumption that the seriously ill would have been more likely to attend hospitals rather than dispensaries is based on evidence from the post-colonial period that patients believed, correctly, that the medical staff at Mulago Hospital possessed superior diagnostic skills and curative capacity. Dr. P. Evans, 'Notes on 1970 visit', Wellcome Archive, London, PP/PRE A.3/3. There is though a gap in our knowledge about local perceptions of how to categorize and best respond to different illnesses during the later colonial period.

suggests that either Ganda parents took a more active interest in their children's health or that Ganda children were less healthy. The breakdown of disease incidence gives some support to both explanations. For example, the incidence of malaria, a disease that was most dangerous in young children, was 57% higher in Buganda than Ankole, whereas the incidence of worms and diarrhoea in the 0–5 age group was 39% and 31%, respectively, higher in Ankole. It was well known that malaria was more common in Buganda than Ankole, most of which was drier, had more freely draining soils, and lay at a higher altitude. At a time when bednets, screens, and antimalarial prophylaxis were not readily available in rural Uganda, malaria could not be regarded as an easily preventable disease. Worms and diarrhoea, however, were.[51] Medical surveys reinforced the link between an increased risk of child mortality and both unsanitary living conditions and a mother's inability to secure appropriate treatment for curable diseases. Women studied in Ankole in 1970 who had active malaria had experienced child mortality that was 15% above the norm, while in 1954 in Buhaya the 10% of women who tested positive for helminthic infection had lost 26% more children than average.[52] It seems likely then that the high regard for medicine within Buganda, as well as its high quality, would have had a very significant impact on mortality levels.

This can be seen most clearly in the two groups who were the subjects of medical supervision most regularly, expectant mothers and newborns. Overall in Uganda death rates among in-patients within medical units run by a doctor improved dramatically over the course of the colonial period. Hospital mortality was initially high at an average of 8.4% between 1906 and 1924, at which point a clear step change, presumably linked to patients securing earlier treatment due to the rapid expansion of rural health units and a growing willingness to seek treatment before illnesses became acute, brought average death rates down to 5.4% between 1925 and 1939. Another step change, this time probably connected in the first place to the introduction of effective antibiotics, saw mortality rates fall to an average of 3.6% between 1940 and 1962. Maternal and neonatal mortality rates within hospital though remained stubbornly high for most of the colonial period. According to the Mengo and Nsambya mission hospital registers, levels of maternal mortality changed little until the 1950s when they enjoyed a massive and sustained improvement. Maternal mortality per 1,000 fell from an average of 45 between 1924 and 1949 to 5 from 1954 to 1969. Some of this improvement was down to the

[51] Uganda Protectorate, *Annual Medical Report 1959* (Entebbe: Government Printer, 1960); Uganda Protectorate, *Annual Medical Report 1960* (Entebbe: Government Printer, 1961); Uganda Protectorate, *Annual Medical Report 1961* (Entebbe: Government Printer, 1962); Uganda Protectorate, *Annual Medical Report 1962* (Entebbe: Government Printer, 1963).

[52] Costello, 'Maternal', p. 174; Laurie and Trant, *East African Medical Survey*, p. 76.

transfer of low-risk patients from Mulago to Nsambya from 1960, but the same broad trends were observed at the latter hospital, and at Kasangati Health Centre, albeit somewhat later.[53] Maternal mortality declined so rapidly in the 1950s because penicillin and a blood transfusion service averted deaths due to post-partum infections and haemorrhage. Such interventions resulted in the proportion of ruptured uterus cases at Mulago which resulted in maternal death falling from 90% in 1951 to 29% in 1959 and 26% by the late 1960s.[54] Uganda's 1969 census found that Ankole children of all ages were more likely than their counterparts in Buganda to still have their father alive, but less likely to have their mother alive. Variations in marriage age were inadequate to explain the difference, so the most likely explanation for this phenomenon is that adult mortality was lower in Ankole in general, but that Ankole women had not yet benefited from the reduced risk of dying in childbirth associated with high quality maternity care. Comparative data support this hypothesis. In the late 1960s Buganda had the lowest maternal mortality rate in Uganda, at 3.6 per 1,000. Ankole, at 10.1, had Uganda's highest rate.[55]

Deaths of newborns within Buganda's mission hospitals also became much less frequent after 1949, falling from an average of 7.7% of all live births before this date to 2.8% during the 1950s and 1960s. There is no indication in the records that new mothers were discharged more quickly as the decades passed. Instead it seems that the primary causes of this transformation in survivorship were a huge increase in the incidence of caesarean sections, which reduced birth trauma and asphyxiation, the development of blood transfusion and tube feeding, and a steady rise in birthweight (see Figure 7.11). After 1939, moreover, a sharp decline in the numbers of babies who were delivered before reaching the hospital indicated that mothers had begun to plan their deliveries more carefully.[56] Presumably this change was

[53] Uganda Protectorate, Annual Medical Reports 1906-62, NA, CO/685; Mengo Hospital Medical Records; Uganda Frazer Committee agenda, Wellcome Archive, PP/CDW E.3/1; Nsambya Hospital Medical Records; B. Marasha, 'Causation and prevention of stillbirths and postnatal deaths at Mulago hospital, 1970–71' (unpublished DPH dissertation, MUK, 1972–3), p. 20; C. Olayiwola Akerele, 'Review of present M.C.H. services in West Mengo' (unpublished DPH dissertation, MUK, 1971), p. 23; Musisi, 'The journey'.

[54] R. Billington, *A Tune on Black and White Keys. Partnership in Healing: the Story of Mengo Hospital* (London: Janus, 1993), pp. 13, 92–7; Int. HW, 31 July 2008, Bristol, F; C. Rendle Short, 'Causes of maternal death among Africans in Kampala, Uganda', *British Journal of Obstetrics and Gynaecology*, 68, 1 (1961), pp. 44–51; V. Everett, 'Causes of stillbirth in Mulago hospital, Kampala, and their prevention', *Uganda Medical Journal*, 1 (1972), pp. 45–7; Marasha, 'Causation', p. 32; E. Grech, 'Review of the treatment of ruptured uterus and Mulago hospital, Kampala', *East African Medical Journal*, 45, 7 (1968), pp. 508–15.

[55] Semwogerere, 'Population', p. 134; E. Grech et al., 'Maternal mortality in Uganda', *International Journal of Gynecology and Obstetrics*, 7, 6 (1969), p. 26.

[56] Mengo Hospital Maternity Registers; Nsambya Hospital Maternity Registers; Mengo Maternity Records, CMS Archives [CMSA] M59 Y A7 1955–6. Premature births were excluded

associated with the rising popularity of ante-natal care, one of whose main functions was to pre-select women for medicalized delivery due to anticipated complications. The maternity records of Nkokonjeru Hospital indicate that medical units in rural Buganda experienced even lower rates of death among newborns than the urban hospitals, a clear sign of the effectiveness of the referral system. Nkokonjeru's newborn death rate was half that of Nsambya, its referral hospital, during the 1950s and 1960s.[57] Outside of hospital too the causes of neonatal death seem to have changed sharply around independence. In the early 1960s deaths among neonatal admissions to Mulago were due primarily to tetanus neonatorum and gastro-enteritis, both linked with poor hygiene. In 1963, 94% of neonatal admissions across Uganda had diarrhoea. By the end of the 1960s Mulago's records showed that mortality among newborn admissions due to tetanus neonatorum, diarrhoea, birth injuries, and pneumonia had all declined sharply, suggesting that delivery techniques and standards of cleanliness for homebirths had greatly improved, presumably in response to medical advice. Similar data are unavailable for Buhaya for this period but if the same pattern of improvement held true there then this would go a long way to explaining the impressive fall in IMRs recorded after 1955, because according to a 1938 survey one in four live-born Haya children died in the first week of life.[58]

SEXUALLY TRANSMITTED DISEASES

European observers during the colonial period were troubled that the superiority of income and medical and educational provision enjoyed by Buganda and Buhaya did not translate directly into equally superior levels of health and longevity. The EAMS final report in 1954 began with the observation that 'in spite of the favourable conditions the Bahaya are not reproducing themselves.' It ended with a familiar refrain, that uncontrolled westernization had undermined local moral codes but had not yet replaced them with European standards of sexual probity. Easy money, widespread schooling, and good communications had fostered disrespect for authority and encouraged the expansion of sexual networks and STDs.[59]

---

from these data. Cf. P. Akingbehin, 'Causes of neonatal morbidity and mortality in New Mulago Hospital' (unpublished DPH dissertation, MUK, 1970), p. 121.

[57] Nkokonjeru Hospital maternity registers, 1954–69.

[58] L. Musoke, 'Analysis of admissions to the paediatric division, Mulago Hospital', *Archives of Disease in Childhood*, 36 (1961), pp. 305–15; Marasha, 'Causation', p. 47; A. Culwick, 'The population problem in the Bukoba district' (Bukoba, 1938. UDSM, EAF Cory 239), p. 15.

[59] F. Lambkin, 'An outbreak of syphilis on virgin soil', *The Lancet* (1908), p. 1022; Lambkin, Mission to the Uganda Protectorate on the prevalence of venereal diseases. Summary of evidence,

Such arguments were commonly made in Buhaya until independence, but, as was shown in Chapter 2, were encountered less frequently in Buganda after 1925. European doctors in Uganda began to lose confidence in the accuracy of their diagnoses of sexually transmitted syphilis from the early 1920s, as their assumptions, evidence, and practices were questioned from the metropolis on clinical, humanitarian, and political grounds. But decades of medical, missionary, and government propaganda had become absorbed by the general population and dispensary staff, so that rural medical records sustained the sense of uncontrollable levels of syphilis until well after the Second World War. Even in Kampala the mission hospital at Mengo detected much more syphilis in the local population than did the government doctors at Mulago. Mengo's founder, Dr. Albert Cook, had been key in the development of the stereotype of the syphilitic Ganda, and had struggled to abandon his preconceptions about the disastrous impact on health of Ganda sexual immorality. In the early 1930s, even though he acknowledged that syphilis was more difficult to diagnose accurately than had earlier been realized, Cook still maintained that it was a highly prevalent disease. Yet Mengo's maternity records indicate that a more cautious approach to the diagnosis of syphilis was adopted during the 1930s. Between 1929 and 1939 the proportion of women who delivered in Mengo and were recorded as having a history of syphilis declined steadily from 44% to 33%. In 1929 the neonatal mortality rate among babies born to mothers with a history of syphilis was 7.1% compared to 6.5% for mothers with no such history. By 1939 the rates for the two groups were 7.3% and 4.0%. It seems likely that over this period the diagnosis of syphilis grew more accurate, so that the association between a negative pregnancy outcome and a history of syphilis, or, perhaps more precisely, of some serious illness, grew much stronger. Nonetheless, even in the mid-1940s Mengo's doctors still grossly overdiagnosed congenital syphilis, according to one recently arrived specialist in child health. Cook's assertions of the early colonial period were still being repeated almost verbatim. 'When I went out in '46 the first thing I was told was that c.80% of the population were syphilitic.'[60]

Dec. 1907, NA, CO/536/15; B. Larsson, *Conversion to Greater Freedom? Women, Church and Social Change in North-Western Tanzania under Colonial Rule* (Uppsala: University of Uppsala, 1991), pp. 107–8; A. Culwick, 'The population problem in the Bukoba district' (Bukoba, 1938, UDSM, EAF CORY 239), pp. 7–9; Bukoba District Annual Report 1948, TNA 215/2237; East African Medical Survey, *Annual Report, 1952*, pp. 23–32; Laurie and Trant, *East African Medical Survey*, pp. 1–4, 138–40.

[60] A.R. Cook, 'Report of the Lady Coryndon Maternity Training School, Namirembe, 1931', CMSA, M/Y/A7 1931–5; MHMR; H. Welbourn, 'First impressions' (unpublished TS in the possession of the author, 1946), pp. 4–5; Billington, *A Tune*, pp. 46–8; Hebe Welbourn Interview, Bristol, 31 July 2008.

It is tempting to suspect that the enthusiasm with which Mengo diagnosed syphilis related to the income which this cash-strapped hospital received in exchange for syphilis treatment. Diseases of immorality were subject to a surcharge, so that the fee paid by the patient was 400 times the cost of the medicine received. The hospital was warned in the 1930s that financial reliance on treatment for one particular disease raised ethical questions about diagnostic practice, but as late as the mid-1940s one of Mengo's doctors noted that she injected 600 patients supposedly suffering from syphilis in a day. This earned the hospital £90 (equivalent to £2,900 in 2011). It suggests moreover that the methods of diagnosis were extremely cursory.[61] The tendency towards overdiagnosis at Mengo was also due to the rarity with which patients from this hospital were tested for STDs during this period. But even at Mulago hospital, where serological testing for syphilis became standard practice after the Lamont scandal of the early 1920s, the incidence of the disease was exaggerated. In 1951, for example, half of all women attending ante-natal clinics around Kampala had positive Kahn test results for syphilis. But the Kahn and Wassermann tests that were used in Uganda before the 1950s were frequently inaccurate, in part due to problems of technique, uneven electricity supply, and other practical problems. In the mid-1950s a technical refinement of the Kahn test meant that the proportion of ante-natal patients who tested positive for syphilis incidence fell from one in two to one in five. Even this was now thought to overestimate the true level because of the frequency with which both Kahn and Wassermann tests produced false positives where patients had been recently inoculated or in cases of yaws, endemic syphilis, leprosy, malaria, anaemia, tropical ulcer, relapsing fever, trypanosomiasis, and, ironically, pregnancy. Accordingly doctors at Mulago in 1953 were only prepared to make a cautious diagnosis of syphilis in the 7% of ante-natal cases whose Kahn tests were strongly positive. The tendency of these tests to produce false positives was well known as early as the 1920s, but Michael Tuck has argued that in the interwar period racial prejudice influenced diagnostic decisions in Uganda, so that European patients with the same clinical signs and serology as Africans were at that time less likely to be diagnosed as syphilitic.[62]

[61] M. Tuck, 'Syphilis, sexuality, and social control: A history of venereal disease in colonial Uganda' (unpublished PhD, Northwestern University, 1997), p. 226; A. Cook, Memorandum before the sub-committee on policy and the financial position of the hospital, Dec. 1933, and Albert to Jack Cook, 1 May 1932, and Anon. [probably A. Cook], 'The treatment of ante-natal syphilis in Baganda women', a paper read before the Uganda branch of the British Medical Association, 22 Mar. 1929, CMSA, M/Y/A7 1931–5; J. Cook, Interview with DMS Kauntze, n/d [1930s], CMSA, Acc. 318 Z4, G. Hewitt papers; H. Welbourn, 'First impressions' (unpublished TS in the possession of the author, 1946), pp. 4–5.

[62] Anon. [probably A. Cook], 'The treatment of ante-natal syphilis in Baganda women', a paper read before the Uganda branch of the British Medical Association, 22 Mar. 1929, CMSA, M/Y/A7 1931–5; East African Notes, A. Williams papers, RHO, MSS. Afr. s. 1872 (153A), Box

By the 1940s a new generation of doctors, more research-oriented and liberal, questioned earlier assumptions, noting that rates of congenital syphilis and general paralysis of the insane, for example, were disproportionately low in relation to the supposed levels of sexually transmitted syphilis in the adult population. The real breakthrough came when the pathologist J. N. P. Davies re-evaluated a series of post-mortem examinations conducted in Kampala between 1931 and 1946. These revealed evidence of previous syphilitic infection in 11.8% of cases, a high level, but very similar to contemporaneous rates in the United States, and far lower than the estimates of prevalence based on serology or clinical signs. In a related study, Davies found that in Kampala most neo-natal deaths were due to birth-related infection, while infant deaths were mainly the result of pneumonia, malaria, meningitis, and malnutrition. Syphilis, which had previously been blamed for most child death, was in fact of marginal significance.[63] Levels of syphilis then had been consistently overestimated in Buganda before the late 1940s. The opposite was true of gonorrhoea. Medical authorities paid surprisingly little attention to gonococcal infection in Buganda before the 1950s, primarily it seems because Ganda sought medical attention for the condition relatively rarely. Yet a medical survey of a rural community in Buganda in 1933 found that one in eight adults showed clinical signs of gonorrhoea, a very high rate, even if some of the cases were probably misidentified non-specific urethritis. Gonorrhoea was described as 'the commonest disabling infection', but also 'the one most rarely treated in the sub-dispensaries', because no cure was on offer.[64]

This changed gradually from the 1930s with the introduction of sulphonamides and especially penicillin, a drug which revolutionized the treatment of STDs, not just because of its exceptionally high success rate, but also because

XXXVI; Uganda Protectorate, *1955 Annual Medical Report* (Entebbe: Government Printer, 1956); L. Harrison and T. Osmond, 'The uses and limitations of the serum tests for syphilis', *British Journal of Venereal Diseases*, 19 (1943), pp. 108–18; A. Adeoba, 'Interpretation of positive serological tests for syphilis in pregnancy', *British Journal of Venereal Diseases*, 43 (1967), pp. 249–58; W. Foster and L. Kerchan, 'Biological false positive Wassermann Reactions in Uganda', *British Journal of Venereal Disease*, 42 (1966), pp. 272–5; Dr. P. Evans' diary of 1953 visit to Uganda, Wellcome Archive, A.3/1 PP/PRE; Tuck, 'Syphilis, sexuality', p. 227. Only in 1954 did the number of Kahn tests conducted by government hospitals in Uganda exceed the number of diagnoses of syphilis.

[63] Hebe Welbourn Interview, Bristol, 31 July 2008; R. Billington, 'Neurosyphilis in natives of East Africa' (unpublished dissertation, University of Cambridge, 1945), p. 32; J. Davies, 'Pathology of central African natives: Mulago Hospital post mortem studies', *East African Medical Journal*, 24, 8 (1947), pp. 289–303; J. Davies, 'Causes of death in African children', *East African Medical Journal*, 25 (1948), p. 228. Subsequent research suggested that even Davies had misdiagnosed some cases of cardiovascular disease as having a syphilitic origin. I. Steiner, J. Thomas and M. Hutt, 'Aortopathies in Ugandan Africans', *Journal of Pathology*, 109, 4 (1973), pp. 300–1.

[64] A. Williams, 'Report on an investigation into the prevalence of serious disease in Buyaga county, Mubende district', Sept. 1933, RHO, MSS Afr. S. 1872/XXXIX.

of the speed and relative painlessness of the cure that was achieved. Penicillin's impact was limited at first because its high cost in the mid-1940s meant that it was used primarily for advanced sulfa-resistant or life-threatening cases. In 1951 though Uganda's medical department finally accepted that 'most of the treatment given for syphilis is largely a waste of drugs ... less than 1% of the patients who received treatment in Mengo completed the minimum course of injections', presumably of bismuth. In 1952 penicillin became the treatment of choice for STDs in state hospitals as its price came down, and as a new single-shot treatment for syphilis reduced the defaulter problem. However, restrictions on its use by dispensers remained in place for some years to come, and small rural mission hospitals such as Nkokonjeru were still treating syphilis with bismuth in 1953.[65] A demand for black market penicillin was stimulated by the pressure patients came under to change their sexual behaviour, and especially by medical professionals' insistence that they should bring their sexual partners for testing and treatment. One elderly man explained 'we used to fear telling our wives ... It was obvious that the infection was the result of adultery and it was shameful to tell the wife to be treated. It used to bring disagreements. You would keep quiet and you would not go back there [to the clinic].' Injectionists, typically using stock stolen from medical stores, were blamed for consistently underdosing their clients. Drug-resistant strains of gonorrhoea though also resulted from patients failing to complete a course of treatment if the visible signs of infection had already disappeared. As one elderly Ganda interviewee put it, 'I did not go back ... after three days I was no longer seeing the symptoms I had before. It was not necessary. I had completely healed.' By the early 1960s cases of gonorrhoea which failed to respond to penicillin were common enough to force local researchers to experiment with alternative antibiotic treatments. The impact of these problems during this period should not be exaggerated, for procaine penicillin in high dosage still had a 91% cure rate, while the best alternatives cured 96% of cases. The crisis came in the 1970s as gonococcal resistance to penicillin and tetracycline worsened and as sourcing and paying for more expensive antibiotics such as trimethoprim or sulphamethoxazole became increasingly difficult.[66]

[65] Hebe Welbourn Interview, Bristol, 31 July 2008; Uganda Protectorate, 1948 Annual Medical Report, NA, CO/685/31; Uganda Protectorate, 1951 Annual Medical Report (Entebbe: Government Printer, 1952); Uganda Protectorate, 1952 Annual Medical Report (Entebbe: Government Printer, 1953); Nsambya Hospital Maternity Registers.

[66] Int. RK, 26 Aug. 2002, Takajjunge, M; Male FGD, Bukoto, 24 Aug. 2004; Male FGD Kitala, 1 Sept. 2004; Male FGD Kisubi Kiwulwe, 4 Sept. 2004; O. Arya and I. Phillips, 'Antibiotic sensitivity of gonococci and treatment of gonorrhoea in Uganda', *British Journal of Venereal Diseases*, 46 (1970), pp. 149–53; O. Arya, C. Pearson, S. Rao and R. Blowers, 'Treatment of gonorrhoea with trimethoprim-sulphamethoxazole in Uganda', *British Journal of Venereal Diseases*, 46 (1970), pp. 214–6.

In Uganda as a whole, government data indicate that the proportion of new cases which were diagnosed as gonorrhoea increased by 161% between 1939 and 1948, whereas that of syphilis rose by 34% (see Figure 8.3). The number of new syphilis cases in Uganda peaked in 1949, when they accounted for 5.8% of all cases, and then fell rapidly over the next decade. By 1959 only 9,143 cases were diagnosed, less than a fifth of the 1949 figure, and only 0.9% of all diseases. Syphilis's absolute decline halted in the 1960s, with the number of cases fluctuating between 5,000 and 8,000, though in the context of rapid growth in population and medical attendance the disease was becoming increasingly insignificant. The number of gonorrhoea cases first peaked in 1948 at 33,160, representing 3.9% of all patients diagnosed. The number of new gonorrhoea cases then fell substantially over the next five years, before starting a gradual recovery, so that by 1955 they exceeded those of syphilis for the first time. The incidence of gonorrhoea then rose to a second peak of 3.7% in 1959, fell back during the early 1960s before undergoing another period of rapid growth, making up 3.5% of diagnoses in 1967–8 with 91,890 new cases, and 4.1% in 1968–9 when 127,667 people received treatment for the disease. Those diseases grouped as 'Other STDs' followed a similar trajectory, declining in relative frequency from a peak of 1% of all new cases in 1949 to a nadir in 1953 before recovering to make up around 0.7% of diagnoses through to the late 1960s when their incidence increased significantly to around 1%, with chancroid becoming increasingly prominent, perhaps because of growing resistance to penicillin and tetracycline.[67]

These incidence data must be treated with some caution given the frequency with which STDs were diagnosed either with no serology whatsoever, or on the basis of tests of limited accuracy. Only in the 1960s did relatively reliable tests for syphilis such as RPCF (Reiter protein complement fixation) become commonplace, and then only in Kampala.[68] Nonetheless these divergent and inconsistent trends are strong enough to suggest that they deserve explanation. It seems likely that it was the relative inferiority of treatment

[67] Uganda Protectorate, Annual Medical Reports 1938–62; Government of Uganda, Annual Reports of the Ministry of Health 1963–9 (Entebbe: Government Printer, 1964–70); J. Kibukamusoke, 'Venereal disease in East Africa', *Transactions of the Royal Society of Tropical Medicine and Hygiene*, 59, 6 (1965), p. 643.

[68] A. Masawe, G. Lomholt, K. Aho and A. Lassus, 'Unusual behaviour of serological tests for syphilis in Ugandan Africans', *British Journal of Venereal Diseases*, 48 (1972), pp. 345–9. Experiments with the most accurate test for syphilis available in the early 1970s, FTA–ABS, showed that mainstream testing, which had been refined in the late colonial period in order to reduce the frequency of false positive diagnoses of syphilis, failed to identify 12% of secondary syphilis cases. Incidence data from the 1960s therefore somewhat underestimated levels of syphilis infection, but were nonetheless probably much more accurate than those produced previously by Kahn or Wassermann tests.

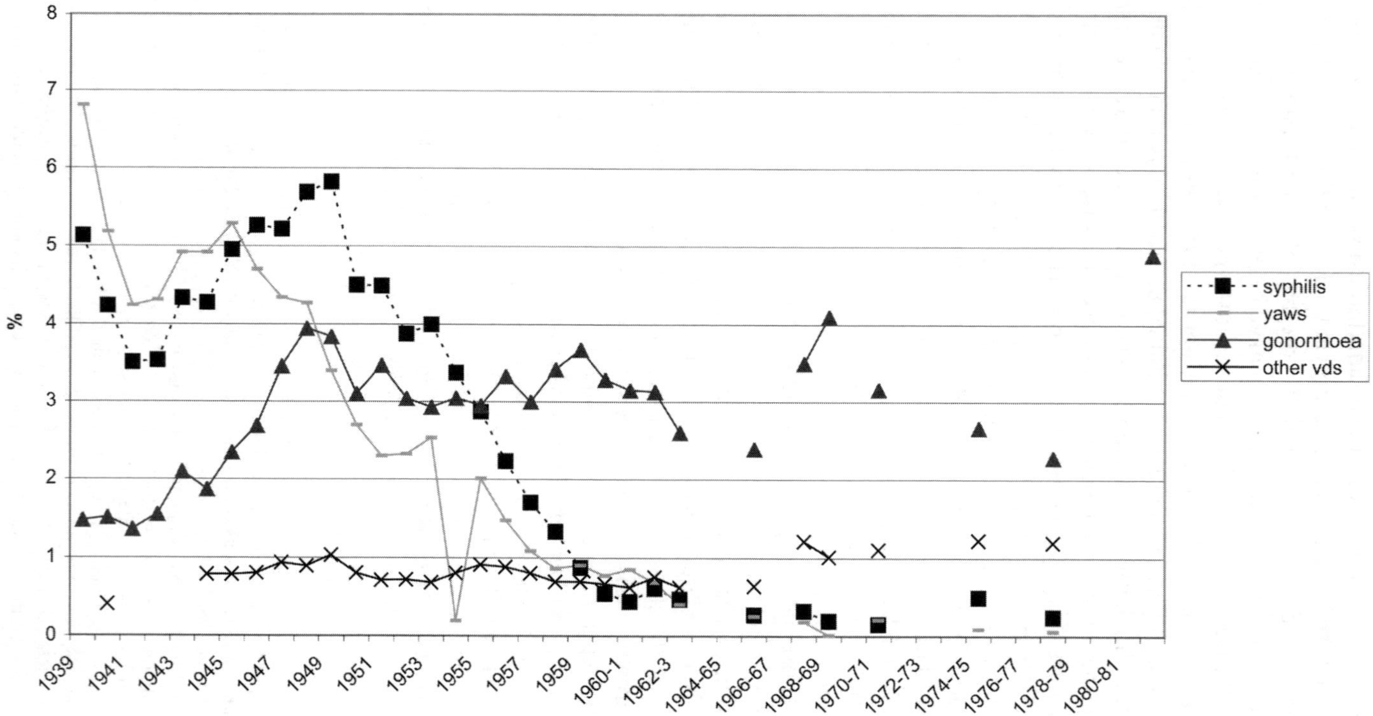

Figure 8.3 STDs and yaws as a percentage of all new outpatient cases at government hospitals in Uganda, for years with data (1939–82)

options available for gonorrhoea before the late 1930s that caused sufferers of that disease to come forward in such huge numbers once news of the miraculous cures achieved through the new antibiotics spread across Uganda. It is surely no coincidence that the incidence of both syphilis and gonorrhoea began to decline as penicillin's usage increased. That gonorrhoea's initial decline was reversed in the mid-1950s can probably be explained by three factors. The first is that reinfection with gonorrhoea was so common, primarily due to the relative rarity with which women sought treatment for the disease. Males formed the majority of patients seeking treatment for all STDs. STD clinics were acknowledged by medical personnel to be male spaces to such an extent that in 1971 Mulago created a separate female STD clinic. Moreover, most men refused to bring their contacts for treatment. In 1970 only one in six male patients at Mulago were accompanied by their wives or girlfriends. Many men became infected through sleeping with sex workers and barmaids, which helps explain why more males than females attended STD clinics, and why so few men brought their contacts with them. More men than women maintained a high-risk lifestyle. Non-cooperation on such a scale forced government policy to change at the end of our period, as doctors realized that the attempt to force men to ensure their contacts got treated deterred men from completing their own treatment or pushed them towards private practitioners who made no effort to bring about behaviour change. Reinfection was also frequent because, for anatomical reasons, women often failed to realize that they were infected with an STD. This was particularly so with regard to gonorrhoea, so that in the 1950s and 1960s males made up 68% of patients suffering from that disease, but only 58% of syphilitics. The second reason for gonorrhoea's resurgence was the growth of resistance to penicillin, which was first identified in 1961 if not earlier and then became extremely severe in the late 1960s, with 72% of gonorrhoea cases failing to respond to the standard dosage of this drug. A third possible factor is that the changes in sexual behaviour discussed in Chapters 4 and 6 increased the frequency with which individuals were exposed to the risk of STD infection.[69]

A deeper understanding of the evolving nature of STD infection in this period can be obtained from analysing data relating to Buganda, because Mulago Hospital and Kasangati Health Centre were the main centres of research into these diseases. Overall the medical sources indicate that STDs

[69] Masawe, Lomholt, Aho and Lassus, 'Unusual behaviour', pp. 345–9; Uganda Protectorate, *1952 Annual Medical Report* (Entebbe: Government Printer, 1953); A. Masawe, 'Syphilis in Uganda: The history, clinical features and cellular immunity' (unpublished MMed dissertation, Makerere University Kampala, 1971), pp. 29–31; Kibukamusoke, 'Venereal disease', p. 643; I. Phillips, 'A guide to antibiotic treatment of gonorrhoea in Uganda', *Makerere Medical Journal*, 1, 3 (1968), p. 105.

were more common in Buganda than in Uganda as a whole. The differential though was not as severe as was sometimes assumed. In 1948 the Annual Medical Report asserted that 'venereal disease ... is commonest in Buganda', on the basis that the kingdom accounted for approximately 35% of all new cases of gonorrhoea and syphilis, yet made up only 26.5% of Uganda's population. But Buganda had more medical facilities per capita than anywhere else in Uganda and incidence data provided in the report's previous paragraph had shown that the Eastern Province accounted for more than half of all STD cases in the country. The stereotype of the immoral Ganda was firmly entrenched. A survey of all medical units under the supervision of a doctor between 1959 and 1961 found that Buganda accounted for 31.3% of all gonorrhoea cases. The number of new cases of gonorrhoea per capita in Buganda was 9% higher than the national average. Not until the mid-1960s were disease incidence data again broken down by district, and then only for rural medical units, meaning that the accuracy of diagnosis was particularly questionable. The picture they showed was that in the second half of the 1960s the incidence of gonorrhoea was slightly higher in Buganda than the national average whereas that of syphilis and yaws was around 60% higher.[70]

It does seem then that compared to the Ugandan average after the Second World War Buganda had higher levels of STDs. More significant was what was happening around Kampala. In urban and peri-urban Buganda it seems that the frequency of STD infection was exceptionally high. In 1971 the gonorrhoea case rate per 100,000 was estimated to be 15,000 in Kampala and 2,760 in Kasangati. The American city of Atlanta, which was regarded as having perhaps the worst gonorrhoea problem in the western world, had a case rate of 2,474. Unusually in Buganda migrant labourers had far lower rates of STD infection than the host community. At Mulago Hospital in 1964 the frequency of complications of advanced syphilis and gonorrhoea among the Ganda was four times higher than among the Rwanda, and eight times higher compared to the Rundi.[71] Moreover, Buganda's high-risk culture was distinctive also because of the high incidence of other STDs apart from gonorrhoea and syphilis. In 1965–6 gonorrhoea and syphilis accounted for 80.6% of new cases of STDs nationally, compared to 70.5% in Mulago. This suggests

[70] Uganda Protectorate, 1948 Annual Medical Report, NA, CO/685/31; H. Griffith, 'Infertility and gonorrhoea in Uganda', *Eugenics Review*, 55, 2 (1963), pp. 104–7; Government of Uganda, Annual Reports of the Ministry of Health 1965–9 (Entebbe: Government Printer, 1966–70). Syphilis and yaws were grouped together by dispensary staff due to the problems of differential diagnosis. Ankole was believed to have more yaws than Buganda.

[71] O. Arya, 'Changing patterns in the organization of the venereal diseases and treponematoses service in Uganda', *British Journal of Venereal Diseases*, 49 (1973), p. 13; M. Hutt and A. Dulo, 'An analysis of diseases found in adults of the Baganda and Banyarwanda/Rundi tribes at autopsy in 1964', *Makerere Medical Journal*, 1 (1966), pp. 24–7.

that either diagnoses at Mulago were more accurate, or that the sustained use of penicillin among the population around Kampala, the most medicated in Uganda, gave STDs such as chlamydia, for which penicillin was not an effective treatment, a relative advantage. The latter hypothesis is supported by data from Makerere University's clinic and Kasangati Health Centre, as the communities they served probably received the best STD care in Uganda. Gonorrhoea and syphilis accounted for only 53.2% of new STD cases at Makerere in 1966 and 64.5% at Kasangati in 1972.[72] This increasing diversity in the pattern of STD incidence around Kampala received relatively little attention at the time. Medical concerns focused instead on the growing problem of drug-resistant gonorrhoea, even though in retrospect it seems likely that what they were observing was in some cases non-gonococcal urethritis. But such worries were dampened by the striking success which had been achieved in reducing the destructive consequences of late syphilis. Studies at Mulago found that the incidence of neurosyphilis declined from 0.3% in 1937–41 to 0.04% in 1960–64, while conditions linked to syphilis accounted for 27% of cardiac admissions in 1952, 12% in 1957, 6% in 1965, and 4% in 1970.[73] The true importance of the less-well-known STDs would only become clear when their role in facilitating HIV transmission was recognized in the 1980s.[74]

In the case of Buganda, attempts to control STDs in the early colonial period had relied on a combination of morality campaigns and coercive mass treatment. By 1925 the latter option was no longer available to Buganda's administrators and medical staff. The Lamont affair (see Chapter 2) ensured that STD policy in Buganda would be carefully monitored by British feminists and pressure groups who campaigned against proposals to make prostitution or infection with STDs a criminal offence. In 1941 though a law was passed by Buganda's chiefly council which defined a prostitute as a woman 'who habitually gives her body indiscriminately for profit or gain or who persistently indulges in promiscuous intercourse with men even though she derives no gain or profit thereby.' Unmarried women under the age of twenty

[72] Kibukamusoke, 'Venereal disease', p. 643; O. Arya and F. Bennett, 'Venereal disease in an elite group (university students) in East Africa', *British Journal of Venereal Diseases*, 43 (1967), pp. 275–9; O. Arya and F. Bennett, 'Role of the medical auxiliary in the control of sexually transmitted disease in a developing country', *British Journal of Venereal Diseases*, 52 (1976), p. 116.

[73] W. Billington, 'Neurosyphilis in Uganda: a comparison of two five-year periods', *East African Medical Journal*, 43, 11 (1966), pp. 469–73; A. Masawe, 'Syphilis in Uganda: the history, clinical features and cellular immunity' (unpublished MMed dissertation, Makerere University Kampala, 1971), p. 14.

[74] D. Fleming and J. Wasserheit, 'From epidemiological synergy to public health policy and practice: The contribution of other sexually transmitted diseases to sexual transmission of HIV infection', *Sexually Transmitted Infections*, 75 (1999), pp. 3–17.

were also forbidden from seeking employment which would keep them away from their parents' homes at night. This legislation was quietly approved by the colonial state as a wartime measure due to the fear that STDs would lower troops' efficiency unless measures were adopted to control prostitution. The law, it seems, remained largely quiescent until 1951 when male fears about the increase in female industrial employment resulted in a generalized assault on independent women in Buganda. Women travelling alone to Kampala were removed from buses and forced to return to the countryside, others were randomly arrested on the city's streets and carried off to be tested for STDs, and a number of schools were unable to open for the new academic year as so many unmarried schoolteachers had been charged with prostitution. The Mother's Union and the Association for Moral and Social Hygiene pressured the Colonial Office to intervene, but were satisfied with the assurance that no-one had been prosecuted in the previous year under the Venereal Disease legislation and that only twenty-four women had been convicted for breaking the law against prostitution. The imminent arrival of a new Governor, Andrew Cohen, well known for his interest in female advancement, reassured the pressure groups that harassment of women by the police would soon be brought under control. Unfortunately for Cohen, his authority collapsed when his decision to deport Buganda's king was ruled illegal in 1955, one result of which was a conservative backlash against independent women. Over the years that followed the rights of unmarried women to live and work in the city would be threatened periodically by local authorities on the ground that they undermined Ganda moral codes and spread STDs, but in practice such campaigns were rarely sustained for more than a few weeks, and had no discernible impact on the number of autonomous women in the city, prostitution, or STD prevalence.[75]

Colonial policy on STD control was in practice relatively inactive in Buganda after 1925. Occasional voices advocated the strict control of prostitution, and medical reports repeatedly complained about the frequency with which individuals became re-infected, and the difficulty of ensuring that patients' contacts were treated. The sense that penicillin's potential could only be realized if mass treatment was supported by targeted testing did revive notions of compulsion, but the rise of radical ethnic nationalism in Buganda in the 1950s made such a provocative policy impossible to support. In general European officials limited themselves to attempting to encourage Ganda society to adopt a more condemnatory attitude towards promiscuity, and to

[75] Anon. to M. Billson (AMSH), 1 Feb. 1951, F. Webber, CO, to General Secretary AMSH, 30 Oct. 51, Mary Stuart to Billson, 3 Apr. 1952, Uganda 1908–54, 3AMS/D/49, Women's Library, London; A. Southall and P. Gutkind, *Townsmen in the Making: Kampala and its Suburbs* (Kampala: East African Institute of Social Research, 1957), pp. 193–4.

pressure Ganda males to think of the destructive consequences of STD infection. Michael Tuck has argued that as colonial medicine became more secularized between the wars, so was the religious character of STD health education reduced. Instead the state attempted to convert the Ganda to what was defined as a more modern concept of the family, one where the male household head concentrated his expenditure within the bounds of the nuclear family, and prioritized its health and living standards. The 1951 Annual Medical Report explicitly tied STDs to a wider malaise in Ganda society: 'The medical aspect is only one part of a complex social and economic problem, involving defective ways of life and usage of land.' The most obvious attempt to Africanize this improving vision of modernity was the emphasis placed on the need to avoid STDs to satisfy the assumed desire for high levels of fertility.[76]

By the 1960s the goals of Uganda's medical department had become less ambitious. Rather than try to reshape Ganda culture, STD strategies now focused on attempting to understand how local patterns of sexual behaviour had changed, so that public health information on how to minimize the risk of infection could be best targeted.[77] In part this reflected a broader shift within Ugandan medicine which endeavoured to explain variations in the incidence of a range of conditions, such as Burkitt's lymphoma, strangulated hernia, and intussusception, on the basis of geographical and ethnic difference. Researchers therefore focused less on the moral causes of STD infection and more on social factors, such as the role played by alcohol usage and Buganda's changing age structure. One consequence of this increasingly pragmatic and responsive approach was the recognition that prostitutes and barmaids were not the only social group with high STD prevalence. The police, army, truck and bus drivers, and university students were also identified as having particularly high levels of infection. For example, in 1966 STDs accounted for 23% of all visits to Makerere's health centre by male students. Of the male undergraduate community as a whole 28% had at least one infection during that year, rising to 36% among Ganda students. Moreover, once it became well known that 15% of Mulago's STD cases were schoolchildren

[76] G. McElligott, 'Venereal Diseases in the Tropics', *British Journal of Venereal Diseases*, 27 *(1951)*, p. 125; Uganda Protectorate, *1951 Annual Medical Report* (Entebbe: Government Printer, 1952); Uganda Protectorate, *1952 Annual Medical Report* (Entebbe: Government Printer, 1953); M. Lyons, 'Sexually transmitted diseases in the history of Uganda', *Genitourinary medicine*, 70 (1994), pp. 141–2; Tuck, 'Syphilis, sexuality', pp. 164–9.

[77] Arya and Bennett, 'Venereal disease in an elite group', pp. 275–9; O. Arya and F. Bennett, 'Attitudes of college students in East Africa to sexual activity and venereal disease', *British Journal of Venereal Diseases*, 44 (1968), pp. 160–6; O. Arya and F. Bennett, 'What do the educated want to know about VD? An analysis of the questions asked by university and college students in Uganda', *Uganda Medical Journal*, 2 (1973), pp. 91–103.

and 70% were unmarried, the fixation with redefining Ganda marriage lost much of its relevance.[78]

Just as medical attitudes towards STDs changed after the Second World War, so it seems did those of the Ganda. According to oral interviewees, at the start of our period Ganda still associated gonorrhoea with the monarchy, and songs and proverbs reminded men that infection with gonorrhoea was a sign of bravery and sophistication. Throughout Buganda hospital in-patients receiving treatment for STDs were referred to as having gone to the heroes' ward, a term that survived through to independence. Yet the idea that men might have actively sought infection with gonorrhoea, or were admired for acquiring the disease, was defined by elderly informants as a mark of ignorance, a sign of the backwardness of the previous generation. A number of informants contrasted the supposed courage and potency of the infected with the grim reality of the advanced stages of the disease. 'Whenever women would move around the heroes' ward, these men would shout at them, accusing them of being responsible for their suffering.' 'One would hear men crying seriously.' By the 1950s gonorrhoea had an essentially negative image, 'a dirty disease' with repellent, agonizing symptoms, associated with promiscuity. Moreover, male and female informants agreed that even though the Ganda state before the 1960s had targeted independent women in its campaign to rid the kingdom of STDs, it had been men who were primarily responsible for spreading gonorrhoea.[79]

Syphilis by contrast was regarded by Ganda in a slightly less negative light during the colonial period. Its symptoms were thought to be less severe, and it was not automatically assumed to be the produce of immoral sexual behaviour. Informants were clear that there were two forms of syphilis, 'that one which you get from sex, and that which is inherited'. 'It would be difficult for syphilis to completely get cured. That was a very terrible disease. That's why expectant women were all given herbal treatment against syphilis. Syphilis remains in the body, syphilis remains in the bones, syphilis remains in the blood and it brings about many other illnesses.' 'Syphilis was difficult to treat [laughs], even as you see me here, I have syphilis [all laugh]. It's inherited, I was born with it. Even my children have inherited it because it's in the

[78] Denis Burkitt to Sir Harold Himsworth (MRC), 21 Jan. 1963, External scientific staff, Mr. D. Burkitt, Makerere College Medical School, NA, FD12/882; F. Bennett, 'The social determinants of gonorrhoea in an East African town', *East African Medical Journal*, 39 (1962), pp. 332–42; V. Ongom, Prevalence and incidence of venereal diseases in military communities in Uganda, *East African Medical Journal*, 47, 9 (1970), pp. 479–83; Masawe, 'Syphilis in Uganda', p. 34; Arya and Bennett, 'Venereal disease in an elite group', pp. 275–9; Uganda Protectorate, *1952 Annual Medical Report*.

[79] Male FGD Kitala, 1 Sept. 2004; Male FGD Bukoto, 24 Aug. 2004; Int. KJK, 31 Aug. 2004, Kitala, M; Int. JN, 29 Aug. 2004, Butanga, F; Male FGD Kisubi Kiwulwe, 4 Sept. 2004.

blood.'[80] Presumably the sense that syphilis was almost universal must have been strengthened by the repeated assertions of medical personnel, clergy, and other authority figures that 80% of Ganda had syphilis at some point in their lives. Until at least the 1940s patients freely admitted to having syphilis with no sense of shame, if they did not believe they had acquired the disease through sexual immorality. One British doctor remembered that patients would attend mobile clinics in the villages and 'with a beaming smile say "I've got syphilis"'. Medical personnel were warned not to trust patient histories of syphilis since Ganda associated a variety of symptoms with the supposedly inherited form of the disease. Over the past century or so it seems that Ganda have gradually shifted from a perception that syphilis was predominantly a non-sexual infection towards the assumption that syphilis is an STD, in part presumably because of the decline in incidence of the endemic treponematoses, and in part because of their sustained exposure to missionary, administrative, and medical assertions that the disease was typically sexually transmitted. The problem, as medical staff in the middle decades of the twentieth century saw it, was that during this prolonged attitudinal evolution, syphilis enjoyed an ambiguity which facilitated its sexual transmission.[81]

European doctors frequently expressed concern that penicillin would weaken Ganda prohibitions against high-risk sexual behaviours even further. This was not universally true, and for some Ganda the horror of the infection rather than the speed of the cure made a bigger impression. One remembered that the trauma of developing gonorrhoea deterred him from committing adultery again. 'You would stop. I for one, I didn't at any time wish to get re-infected. So I avoided such habits.' It was more common however for informants to agree that the development of an effective cure did transform individuals' perception of risk. 'People didn't fear gonorrhoea very much because they could be treated and go back home, get infected again and go back for more treatment.' 'We all suffered from the disease, but would go and get treatment for it.' 'Male promiscuity even increased because after whites came, the STDs could be healed.' In the 1960s university students' attitudes towards STDs were studied. What was striking was that while male students did express anxiety and shame when discussing STDs, one of their primary concerns was how to work out what kinds of women were least likely to infect them. Two of the questions asked of medical staff were 'Are high school girls

[80] Int. NNFW, 28 Aug. 2004, Kaswa, F; Female FGD Kagezi, 25 Aug. 2004; Int. IST, 21 August 2004, Kagezi village, Masaka, M.

[81] Anon. [probably A. Cook], 'The treatment of ante-natal syphilis in Baganda women', a paper read before the Uganda branch of the British Medical Association, 22 Mar. 1929, CMSA, M/Y/A7 1931–5; Hebe Welbourn Interview, Bristol, 31 July 2008; Uganda Protectorate, *1952 Annual Medical Report*.

often infected?' and 'Are there any women free from gonorrhoea in Kampala?' This was not the kind of health education the doctors who conducted the survey wanted to provide, and suggested that some Ganda at least had become more interested in managing rather than avoiding risk.[82]

Fewer disease data exist for Ankole than Buganda. Early in our period it was claimed that the 'great majority of deaths are due to syphilis' in Ankole, and that the Nkole, like the Ganda were 'syphilitized to an extraordinary degree'. Such assertions were unsupported by any testing, though, and seem unlikely to have been accurate. Between 1959 and 1961 the number of new cases of gonorrhoea per capita recorded at medical units supervised by a doctor in Ankole was 24% lower than the national average. At rural medical units in the second half of the 1960s the incidence of syphilis and yaws combined was around 230% higher than the national average in Ankole, whereas that of gonorrhoea was around 40% lower. But as yaws made up two-thirds of treponemal disease in Ankole as late as 1958, it is likely that the incidence of syphilis was little higher than the Ugandan average.[83] Retired medical personnel who worked in Ankole in the late colonial period indicated that STD testing was the exception rather than the rule there, in contrast to much of Buganda. 'Gonorrhoea is self-evident. You see if the person has pus in the penis. The person is urinating, getting burning sensations ... It was the same thing with syphilis. If they had sores around the ... you know ... It was very rare to test them.'[84] Only at the end of our period did more reliable data emerge from Ankole. In 1971, as part of a demographic survey of rural Ankole, 416 adult volunteers were medically examined and tested for STDs. Of 250 women 2.4% tested positive for gonorrhoea, 5.9% suffered salpingitis, 8.9% experienced lower abdominal pain, and 10% had a mucopurulent vaginal discharge, but none had pelvic inflammatory disease. Among the males 8% suffered from urethral discharge and 4.2% had gonorrhoea. Overall 13% of Nkole tested positive for past or current treponemal infection, but it is likely that many of these individuals had a history of yaws rather than syphilis. Given

[82] Uganda Protectorate, 1948 Annual Medical Report, NA, CO/685/31; Male FGD Kisubi Kiwulwe, 4 Sept. 2004; Int. KJK, 31 Aug. 2004, Kitala, M; Int. IST, Kagezi village, 21 August 2004, Masaka, M; Female FGD, Takajunge, 26 Aug. 2004; Arya and Bennett, 'What do the educated want', pp. 91–3.

[83] Western Province Annual Report, 1926, NA, CO/685/8; Anon. [A. Cook?], 'The treatment of ante-natal syphilis in Baganda women', a paper read before the Uganda branch of the British Medical Association, 22 Mar. 1929, CMSA, M/Y/A7 1931–5; Uganda Protectorate, 1948 Annual Medical Report, NA, CO/685/31; Griffith, 'Infertility', pp. 104–7; Uganda, *Annual Medical Reports 1965–9*; Uganda Protectorate, *Annual Medical Report 1958* (Entebbe: Government Printer, 1959). Syphilis and yaws were grouped together due to the problems of differential diagnosis by dispensary staff.

[84] Int. MM, 28 June 2004, Kampala, M; Int. YZ, 13 Aug. 2004, Mbarara, M.

that prevalence was believed to have been much higher around Mbarara than in the countryside this survey indicates that Ankole suffered significant levels of STD infection by the end of our period, but still probably not so high as in Buganda.[85]

Attitudes towards STDs seem to have differed significantly between Ankole and Buganda for most of this period. No Nkole informants admitted to having ever been infected, and interviewees spoke of the diseases with more fear and revulsion than their Ganda counterparts. 'One man I saw even broke a banana plant while urinating for the pain was too much.' In interviews people stated that they tried to avoid the infected, and would ensure they neither touched their clothing nor where they had sat. Men would be refused entry to beer drinks and no-one would consider having sex with a person believed to suffer from an STD. 'If someone found out that so and so had an STD, they would announce it throughout the whole area.' The infected 'were like an unwanted animal in the village'. The language of guilt was used much more frequently in Ankole than Buganda in relation to STDs. Embarrassment was, of course, not always beneficial. Some Nkole refused to seek treatment, or were too ashamed to inform their spouses of their condition. But oral sources suggested that most people worked around such difficulties. Retired medical personnel reported that they frequently agreed to treat the sick at their homes rather than in the clinic, to minimize the number of people who knew of the patients' condition. And it seems that it was common for infected men to instruct their wives to receive medical treatment without revealing the nature of their shared illness. 'A husband would never say it out loud lest you accuse him of adultery. So if he realized that he was sick, he would just take the wife for treatment without telling her why or for what.' No-one in Buganda mentioned such a practice, presumably reflecting the lesser degree of female subservience in that society. Even more remarkable, it seems that medical practitioners cooperated with husbands' demands. 'Some would just plan with their doctors. That when my wife comes, do not tell her anything just give her the injections.' 'My brother told his wife one time "let's go to the doctor for your injection". My sister-in-law kept asking why but he never said anything... the family doctors would help men out and be sworn to secrecy. They were not meant to tell the wives what they were suffering from.' Other men 'would just bring injections home and they would keep injecting their wives. And the women would never ask why ... A woman does not question

[85] O. Arya, S. Taber and H. Nsanze, 'Gonorrhea and female infertility in rural Uganda', *American Journal Of Obstetrics And Gynecology*, 138, 7 (1980), pp. 929–32; Costello, 'Maternal', p. 129. It is sensible to be wary of self-selected samples of this kind, though whether STD prevalence was overestimated due to the ill seeking treatment, or underestimated as embarrassment deterred attendance, is uncertain.

her husband's motives ... Also, as a woman, you feel he is helping you, by the mere fact he is administering treatment.' It is striking nonetheless that retired medical workers believed that the majority of men brought their partners for treatment, which was certainly not the case in Buganda. It may be that this reflected not only patriarchal authority and a local willingness to bend the rules of medical practice, but also the survival of old beliefs that sexual misconduct threatened the health of spouses and children unless reparative action was taken.[86] Only towards the end of this period did attitudes in Ankole change significantly. The coming of penicillin caused some people to lose their fear of infection. 'They knew they would get treatment. It was free medicine so people used to have sex anyhow', and people who lived in Mbarara 'who were more frequently infected, and then cured, grew less ashamed of the condition'.[87]

At the start of our period Buhaya, like Ankole and Buganda, was described by local Europeans as suffering from nearly universal syphilitic infection.[88] Whereas medical opinion grew much more cautious in Uganda from the mid-1920s, in Buhaya the belief that STDs were so prevalent that the population faced possible extinction was still expressed in the mid-1950s.[89] In part this simply reflected the relative absence of external critical analysis of medical policy, but the sense that the Haya suffered exceptionally high levels of STD infection did have some statistical basis, even if the statistics recorded were of uneven reliability. In 1925 syphilis accounted for 31% and gonorrhoea for 7% of all out-patient diagnoses at Bukoba hospital. In 1928, 42% of all cases treated in Buhaya's many dispensaries and dressing stations were diagnosed as syphilis, three and a half times the national average. By around 1940 the proportion of cases diagnosed as syphilis at Buhaya's dispensaries had fallen to around 20%, but this was simply the result of the willingness of the Haya to seek treatment for a wider variety of ailments. The number of syphilis cases per capita had risen significantly between the wars. In 1938 Bukoba treated by far the largest number of STD patients of all the hospitals in the Territory, accounting for 17.1% of Tanganyika's gonorrhoea cases and

[86] Female FGD Bumbire (Bushenyi), 23 Aug. 2004; Male FGD Namitanga, 19 Aug. 2004; Female FGD Kyenjenyi, 22 Aug. 2004; Int. MM, 28 June 2004, Kampala, M; Int. YZ, 13 Aug. 2004, Mbarara, M; Female FGD Nyamitanga, 19 Aug. 2004; Female FGD Ruti, 19 Aug. 2004; Kiyungi FGD Female, 21 Aug. 2004.

[87] Male FGD Namitanga, 19 Aug. 2004; Int. EM, 27 Sept. 2001, Kampala, M; Int. MM, 28 June 2004, Kampala, M.

[88] Bukoba District Annual Report 1923, TNA 1733/8 (AB10); Bukoba District Annual Report 1925 (Bukoba sub-district), TNA 1733/3:46 (AB40).

[89] Berry, Culwick and Culwick, *Nutrition*, p. 173 [quoting the 1937 annual district medical report]; Annual Report for the Bukoba District for the year 1948, TNA 215/2237; Laurie and Trant, *East African Medical Survey*, p. 142.

10.4% of all syphilis cases. In the early 1940s, 26.3% of 1,392 consecutive ante-natal cases had strongly positive Kahn tests, and 20% of 2,200 Haya recruits for military service were diagnosed as suffering from gonorrhoea. A third of all operations at Bukoba hospital were external urethrotomies to relieve strictures which were assumed to result from untreated gonorrhoea.[90] This was not simply a case of diagnosis following stereotype. The British Army's venereologist in East Africa travelled across the region and noted that during his brief stay in Bukoba he had encountered 'an amazing amount of gonorrhoea and many phagedenic penile lesions', the latter probably a reference to chancroid. The EAMS appears to have adopted extremely careful diagnostic methods, and found that 6.8% of men in three communities surveyed had gonorrhoea, and 17.1% of the entire population surveyed had strongly positive Kahn test results.[91] It seems clear that STDs were a much greater problem here than in Ankole and even Buganda. The intense mass treatment of STDs initiated by the EAMS appears to have caused STDs' prominence within medical reports to diminish after the mid-1950s. The EAMS pilot scheme treated 3,494 people for STDs in its first two years of activity and then made plans for 45,000 more cases to be treated over the next three years. The only formal indication though that this programme was sustained and had met with some success was an isolated comment in 1966 that the number of STD cases was steadily decreasing.[92]

The prevalence of syphilis was probably overestimated in Buhaya, especially in the earlier period when yaws was still common within the district, but gonorrhoea was almost certainly underestimated, given that males were five times as likely to be diagnosed with the disease as females, primarily because the symptoms were less obvious in women, and embarrassment was believed to be more of an obstacle for women than men.[93] That the response of the medical department and colonial and chiefly administrations to the STD problem was much more aggressive in Buhaya after 1925 than Uganda was due no doubt largely to the exceptional prominence of sexually transmitted

[90] Bukoba District Annual Report 1925 (Bukoba sub-district), TNA 1733/3:46 (AB40); Bukoba District Annual Report 1928, TNA 215/77/B; Tanganyika Territory, Annual Medical Report 1928, TNA Library; Berry, Culwick and Culwick, *Nutrition*, p. 173; Tanganyika Territory, *Annual Medical report 1938* (Dar es Salaam: Government Printer, 1940); Tanganyika Territory, *Annual Report of the Medical Department 1941* (Dar es Salaam: Government Printer, 1942); Tanganyika Territory, *Annual Report of the Medical Department 1943* (Dar es Salaam: Government Printer, 1944).

[91] W. Young, 'Extra-urethritic cases in an African venereal diseases hospital', *The British Journal of Venereal Diseases*, 20 (1944), pp. 143–4; Laurie and Trant, *East African Medical Survey*, pp. 119–34.

[92] Laurie and Trant, *East African Medical Survey*, pp. 135–41; Annual report Bukoba District Council Medical Services, 1966, 30 Jan. 1967, Mwanza archives, MISS/DN/53.

[93] Laurie and Trant, *East African Medical Survey*, pp. 135–41.

infections within the medical statistics. But in addition the belief that many Haya were unaware that gonorrhoea was transmitted sexually, in the 1920s and 1930s at least, may have given impetus to plans for disease control. Public health campaigns which focused primarily on correcting misinformation were always considered to have a reasonable likelihood of success. Moreover, in Buhaya, the circular movement of large numbers of sex workers in and out of the district provided the authorities with a constant target on which to concentrate their efforts. From the 1920s through to the 1960s proposals to prevent suspected prostitutes from boarding buses and ferries, or to require them to operate from licensed brothels, or simply to lock them up were periodically made.[94] Finally, Tanganyika's medical department had already provided a model for the mass eradication of treponemal disease in the form of its yaws control programme which treated 137,112 people in 1930 alone. As the same medication could theoretically cure syphilis and yaws together, it was hoped that both diseases could be controlled simultaneously. In fact bismuth was singularly unsuccessful as a syphilis treatment, due to the number of injections that were required over a period of several months. In 1948 the district medical officer found that nine dispensaries which had given 3,881 bismuth injections for syphilis that year had effected not one single cure because no patient had completed the course. The same problem meant that gonorrhoea had become widely resistant to sulphonamide as early as 1946.[95]

Before the age of penicillin then, mass treatment offered little hope of controlling STDs in Buhaya. Instead it was repeatedly stated that only a change of attitudes and behaviour could save the Haya. The district was targeted for a particularly intense public information campaign between the wars. STDs featured prominently in missionaries' sermons and school visits, the Lutheran church required adherents who wished to marry in church to seek medical confirmation that they were not infected with an STD, and the Haya Council ruled that a man could divorce his wife if she was found to be infected with syphilis. The Lutheran mission adapted this rule so that either partner could end a church marriage if the other became infected with any STD.[96] As was discussed in Chapter 5, in the late 1930s two of the Tanganyikan

[94] Bukoba District Annual Report, TNA 215/77/B 1928; Berry, Culwick and Culwick, *Nutrition*, p. 173; DC to PC, 10 Apr. 1951, in EAF Cory 21, Bukoba: Official Correspondence relating to constitutional matters, politics and land, including notes and memoranda by Hans Cory, 1950–8, UDSM; W. Laurie, 'A pilot scheme of venereal disease control in East Africa', *British Journal of Venereal Diseases*, 34 (1958), p. 21. See also Chapter 5.

[95] Iliffe, *Doctors*, p. 40; Bukoba District Annual Report 1948, TNA 215/2237; Bukoba District Annual Report 1948, TNA 215/2237; Annual Report for the Bukoba District for the year 1946, TNA, 215/2070.

[96] A. Donne, editor Mambo Leo, to Sec. of Native Affairs, 12 Sept. 1930, TNA, 19153 vol.1, Venereal Disease: Anti-venereal Measures; Larsson, *Conversion*, pp. 107–9; H. Cory and

administration's leading experts on indigenous society, Hans Cory and Arthur Culwick, were despatched to Buhaya to come up with solutions to the STD problem. Their proposals came to nothing in the short term, partly no doubt because the beginning of the Second World War disadvantaged any project which threatened expense and had the potential for unrest. Yet the suggestion that the healthy should be segregated from the sick and that a full course of treatment should be enforced on all who were ill influenced local opinion into the 1950s, and the cataclysmic picture they painted of a society threatened with moral, demographic, and economic decline ensured that Buhaya would be one of the sites chosen by the EAMS in 1950.[97]

It seems that the concept of mass compulsory STD treatment on a local scale took hold within the Tanganyika administration during the war. In 1943 the Director of Medical Services announced that it was 'the intention of this Department to carry out after the war campaigns against special diseases in selected areas of heaviest incidence, for example, against VD in Bukoba'. Wartime experience had demonstrated the advantages of compulsory STD treatment within a captive population.[98] Local opinion had also solidified around the idea of radical intervention to control STDs. The district administration came under intense pressure from Haya leaders during the late 1940s to enhance medical provision so that those infected with STDs could be cured, and to prevent Haya women from leaving for the cities. The colonial response that STDs were social diseases which required reform within Haya society and that freedom of movement was guaranteed for all subjects provoked sustained anger, being interpreted as a 'deliberate policy designed to reduce the population of the District'. The STD issue became associated with a wider debate about the use of Buhaya's coffee cess, a development tax which the colonial state had consistently employed to encourage Haya to improve their coffee cultivation. As this involved more work with no immediate returns the policy was deeply unpopular. The arrival of the EAMS offered the district administration a way out of the impasse. The success of its pilot scheme convinced the Haya that the mass use of penicillin could eradicate syphilis and gonorrhoea. The district commissioner hoped that the high cost of such a programme, if it was paid for from the coffee cess, would cause the Haya to

M. Hartnoll, *Customary Law of the Haya Tribe, Tanganyika Territory* (London: Cass, 1971), pp. 104–5; B. Sundkler, 'Marriage problems in the church in Tanganyika', *International Review of Missions*, 34 (1945), pp. 253–5.

[97] Hans Cory, The Haya tribe and the incidence of venereal disease, Bukoba 1938–48, TS. UDSM, EAF CORY 104, p. 10; Berry, Culwick and Culwick, *Nutrition*, pp. 44–50; A. Culwick, The population problem in the Bukoba District. Bukoba, 1938. UDSM, EAF CORY 239, p. 9. Cf. Annual Report for the Bukoba District for the year 1948, TNA 215/2237.

[98] A.R.M. for DMS to C.S., 18 October 1943, Minute 2, TNA 31732, Yaws.

take greater responsibility for their own health, and reform their sexual behaviour. 'If not, the Haya would learn at their own expense that a purely medical approach will not work, and they would in future have only themselves, instead of government, to blame.' At the very least, a programme on such a scale would require that the medical services of the district would all have to be upgraded, so that the health and efficiency of the Haya would inevitably improve.[99]

Despite some opposition from the provincial administration, the proposed campaign quickly took shape, partly because of the support of the EAMS. It seems that the EAMS gave at least implicit support to the concept of mass compulsory treatment because they rejected the local fixation with female immorality. The EAMS quickly came to the conclusion that while prostitution had to be controlled, in general terms women were the victims of Buhaya's STD problem. As one of the project leaders remembered 'the men spent most of their time womanizing and drinking ... The women were made to do all the work ... All the revenue from the coffee went to the husband ... It is not surprising that several of the women revolted at such treatment and ran away.' Most female infections were believed to stem from their husbands' infidelity, and, due to the difficulty of diagnosing gonorrhoea in women, the disease had typically already damaged the female reproductive system by the time women sought treatment.[100] A voluntaristic campaign then would leave most female sufferers untreated.

The relative success of the STD control programme lay in the decision to adopt a single-shot high dosage injection of procaine penicillin as the standard treatment for both gonorrhoea and syphilis. The initial strategy was to move quickly, treating all residents in the vicinity of each centre who reported any history of STD infection or low fertility, and dispensing with the time-consuming process of testing. The medical teams relied on forceful persuasion, calling on local chiefs and missionaries to encourage attendance. As one participant remembered, 'They brought the medicine there, and people were being injected compulsorily. I saw it ... There was really meaningful propaganda going on, and the force behind it in the villages was kind of hand in glove, but chiefs were encouraging their people. The force was there but it was never used.' Only in the mid-1950s, as the campaign matured, did testing begin to take on more prominence. The control programme in its early years

[99] T. Harris, *Donkey's Gratitude: Twenty-two Years in the Growth of a New African Nation—Tanzania* (Durham: Pentland Press, 1992), pp. 261–5; DC to PC, 10 Apr. 1951, in EAF Cory 21, Bukoba: Official Correspondence relating to constitutional matters, politics and land, including notes and memoranda by Hans Cory, 1950–8, UDSM.

[100] H. Trant, 'Not Merrion Square: Anecdotes from a Woman's Medical Career in Africa', RHO, MSS.Af.s.1872(143), p. 128; Laurie, 'Pilot', p. 18; Laurie and Trant, *East African Medical Survey*, pp. 4–5.

was peripatetic, aiming to cure all infections in a defined area before moving on. The early reliance on a few primary treatment centres backed up by a mobile clinic ended in 1957 with the decision to allow penicillin to be injected at all twenty-three of Buhaya's dispensaries. By this time around 7,000 cases were treated each year, as the campaign settled into a routine of offering easily available cures for all new infections. The popularity of the STD control programme rested in large part on the decision to send several of the best recently qualified Haya doctors to work in Buhaya, with instructions to use their social contacts to help bring down the prevalence of STDs. They were instrumental in persuading local sex workers to agree to voluntary registration and monthly doses of penicillin, and ensured that STD control became part of a wider push to improve public health in the district, so that significant investment was made in anti-malarial measures, water sanitation, and nutritional health education.[101]

Compared to the Ganda and Nkole what was particularly striking about elderly Haya informants was how knowledgeable they were about STDs. Interviewees referred to a wider range of diseases, and often gave textbook descriptions of their typical symptoms and complications. Some even expounded on the varying stages of urethral stricture: 'sometimes urine came very slowly in drops, "toi toi toi", sometimes in gushes, "choro choro choro", sometimes completely blocked ... then a man would cry like an angry baby.' Presumably this familiarity stemmed from the high prevalence of STDs in this society and the intensity of health information advocating behavioural change which Haya encountered over the decades.[102] Informants were also relatively open about having been infected with various STDs in their younger days. This does not mean that Haya in general felt no shame about STD infection. Some did downplay the diseases: 'we had no disease like now [AIDS]—we had only syphilis and gonorrhoea. We didn't worry about them.'[103] But it was more common for Haya to state that STDs were feared, and their victims were disliked, disrespected, or avoided. 'People hated those with STDs. If someone had syphilis they used to be confined at home. If a man with syphilis

[101] Laurie and Trant, *East African Medical Survey*, pp. 135–41; DC to PC, 10 Apr. 1951, in EAF Cory 21, Bukoba: Official Correspondence relating to constitutional matters, politics, and land, including notes and memoranda by Hans Cory, 1950–8, UDSM; Int. HL, 17 June 2000, Maruku, M; Int. JBK, Ijumbi, 11 Aug. 2000, M; Annual Report for the Bukoba District for the year 1953, TNA 215/2700; DMO to PMO, Monthly report, West Lake, May 1957, 6 June 1957, TNA, Acc.71 M.1/1 Medical general, Vol.2; West Lake Provincial Annual Report 1960, TNA 967.822.1; Annual Report for the Bukoba District for the year 1957, TNA 215/3449; Int. VK, 27 June 2000, Bukoba, M.

[102] e.g. Int. LN, 19 Aug. 2000, Kikukwe, F; Int. FK, 16 Aug. 2000, Kikukwe, F; FGD, 23 August 2000, F; Int. RMR, 13 Aug. 2000, Byabusha, Busindi, M.

[103] Int. TM, 13 Aug. 2000, Busindi, F; Int. VPB, 9 Aug. 2000, Busindi, F; Int. SKN, 22 Aug. 2000, Maruku-Butailuka-Kasha, F.

went to a bar, he was given a separate seat made of banana leaves. They gave him a drink and he left.'[104]

Prevalence levels were believed to be so high that some accepted that infection was 'normal'. 'A man with three or four wives could not avoid these diseases because not all the wives would be faithful to him.' Haya travelled so much on business that 'a great deal of sexual interaction was inevitable.'[105] But a more common theme in interviews was the attempt to manage the risk of infection. For some this involved little more than taking the most obvious precautions. 'We would run away from men with STDs, for fear of infecting our husbands if we slept with them.' Families and villages with a reputation for high levels of STD infection would struggle to find people willing to marry into them. Others employed traditional medicine to avert disease transmission. Most women used a range of drugs to prevent their children from becoming infected in utero. Some women inserted herbal medicine into their vaginas when having a sexual affair 'to prevent themselves from catching diseases'. With such attitudes it is hardly surprising that penicillin had such an immense impact here.[106]

CONCLUSION

The timing and causes of mortality decline in Africa are intensely disputed. This study cannot claim to have resolved these debates. The data which were recorded before the late 1950s are all problematic in various ways. Vital registration may have declined in comprehensiveness over time; early censuses were inaccurate and inconsistent in the information they gathered; and the many demographic surveys, even though they covered a significant proportion of a district's population and claimed to have secured a representative sample, were frequently affected by problems of self-selection, as of course were all hospital records. The wider importance of some of the findings of this chapter cannot be known until further comparative case studies produce similar results.

The conclusions that can be reached then must be tentative, but, if correct, they are significant. One of the more strongly evidenced findings is also

[104] Int. LN, 19 Aug. 2000, Kikukwe, F; Int. MM, 11 Aug. 2000, Ijumbi, F; Int. JM, 17 June 2000, Ntoma, F; Int. CM, 11 Aug. 2000, Rubya, F.
[105] Int. SK, 21 June 2000, Rubya, M; Int. RMR, 13 Aug. 2000, Byabusha, Busindi, M; Int. GI, 30 Aug. 1999, Igurugati-Bugandika, M.
[106] Int. PEK, 7 Aug. 2000, Nkimbo Bweramutima, F; Int. CM, 11 Aug. 2000, Busindi, M; Int. PB, 22 Aug. 2000, Maruku, F; Int. EK, 7 Aug. 2000, Kanyangereko Nkimbo, F; Int. YK, 19 Aug. 2000, Kikukwe, F.

one of the more surprising, that Ankole's mortality rates were very similar to those of Buganda and Buhaya, even though the latter areas were so much wealthier and had far superior levels of healthcare and female education. Most other regions in Africa, by contrast, seem to support the modernization thesis of mortality change, that societies that underwent the most development, broadly defined, would be where the earliest falls in death rates would occur.[107] Ankole though was perhaps unusual in several ways. Although cash poor, it was much richer in livestock than its neighbours, and, just as importantly, livestock were by the mid-colonial period distributed much more equitably within Ankole than Buganda and Buhaya, as colonial officials ended the Hima near-monopoly on cattle ownership. It is likely then that Nkole had a diet that was richer in animal protein than their wealthier neighbours, before the 1950s at least.[108] Ankole also suffered much less severely than Buganda and Buhaya from malaria, a disease on which colonial medicine had little impact outside the major towns before the 1950s. Finally, it is likely that Uganda's heavy investment in preventive medicine from the 1930s had a relatively greater impact in poorer districts such as Ankole than equivalent expenditure on curative care would have done, given that the latter tended to be heavily concentrated in the most developed areas. This region's exceptionalism though is as much about Ganda and Haya underperformance as Ankole's relative success. Modernization in the wealthier societies was a mixed blessing, due to the early uptake of bottle feeding, the role of schooling, and female employment in sustaining fostering, and the relationship between cash cropping and divorce, all of which were believed to increase child mortality.

These societies were unusual also in that female education seems to have been less significant in determining child mortality rates here than has been demonstrated in a number of previous studies elsewhere in the developing world. Maternal education, especially if it had lasted more than a few years, did increase child survival chances, but not as much as was expected. It seems that in this region paternal educational may have been relatively important, perhaps indicating that fathers played a significant role in maintaining the

[107] See e.g. S. Rutstein, 'Socio-economic differentials in infant and child mortality', *WFS Comparative Studies* 43. (London: World Fertility Survey, 1984); Cleland and J. van Ginneken, 'Maternal education'.

[108] Uganda Protectorate Department of Agriculture, 'A report on nineteen surveys done in small agricultural areas in Uganda with a view to ascertaining the position with regard to soil deterioration' (Entebbe, *c.*1938, TS, ASC, Cambridge). Livestock ownership increased enormously in Buganda during the 1950s, while Haya imports of slaughter cattle totalled nearly 19,000 in 1955. By 1947 agriculturalists owned 60% of Ankole's cattle. Uganda Protectorate, *Annual Reports of the Veterinary Department 1950–59* (Entebbe: Government Printer, 1951–60); Bukoba District Annual Report 1955, TNA 215/3101; Notes on meeting with Lord Hailey re Ankole, 31 Aug. 1947, NA, CO/1018/82.

health of their family here.[109] It also appears that where curative provision, maternity and child welfare services, and health information were sufficiently ubiquitous, the children of poor and unschooled women benefited proportionately almost as much as those of prosperous, educated mothers.

The role of curative medicine in triggering rapid demographic growth has been disputed globally by Thomas McKeown, who argued that improved living standards and nutrition were more significant, and within Africa more specifically by neo-Marxist historians such as Dennis Cordell and Joel Gregory, who maintained that rising fertility rather than falling death rates stimulated Africa's modern population explosion.[110] It is difficult to disentangle such interrelated factors, but medical records show clearly that hospital death rates fell sharply from 1924, as did the previous child mortality experienced by women who gave birth in a medical institution, which would suggest that a combination of exposure to medical advice and openness to biomedical treatment brought very significant benefits surprisingly early. The steady rise in birthweights recorded in Buganda's hospitals between 1924 and 1969 lends some support to McKeown's thesis, coinciding as it did with a major reduction in mortality levels. But Buganda became famous from the late 1940s as a society where malnutrition had become epidemic in a land of plenty. Ganda practices of weaning children onto a diet of bulky foods lacking in fat and protein appears to have been the key factor which prevented mortality levels in the young child age group from falling as fast as those of infants and adults. Only in the 1960s through sustained treatment and nutritional health education did the incidence of kwashiorkor reduce. Here improved nutrition depended not only on higher standards of living but also on the provision of medical information.[111]

The shape of mortality change is more difficult to ascertain than the date of its onset. It seems that infant mortality was falling significantly in the Ugandan societies in the 1930s and especially 1940s, but only really declined substantially in Buhaya from the 1950s. Child mortality probably fell in Buganda from the 1930s, and in Ankole from the 1950s. Only towards the end of our period, after remarkable declines in infant mortality, were children almost as likely to die between the ages of one and four as during infancy. Africa's distinctive distribution of child mortality may be of recent origin.[112]

[109] Costello, 'Maternal', p. 136.
[110] T. McKeown, *The Modern Rise of Population* (London: Arnold, 1976), pp. 152–63; Cordell and Gregory, *African Population*.
[111] Hebe Welbourn Interview, Bristol, 31 July 2008; Welbourn, 'Backgrounds', pp. 88–93; D. Jelliffe, 'Village level feeding of young children in developing tropical regions, with especial reference to Buganda', *Journal of the American Medical Women's Association*, 17, 5 (May 1962), pp. 409–18; Uganda, *Ministry of Health Annual Reports 1960–69* (Entebbe: Government Printer, 1961–70).
[112] Caldwell, 'The population factor', p. 22.

Hospital records indicate that neonatal and maternal mortality only fell after 1949. The onset of the decline in adult mortality more generally is less easily identifiable, but seems to have occurred before 1948, and then gathered strength in the 1960s. The pattern of mortality in this region therefore changed unevenly. The causes of these changes too were complex. This study would suggest that the quality of healthcare during the colonial period as well as the quantity of provision was significant. It also indicates that the tendency of the colonial state to focus its energies on targeted medical campaigns should be considered perhaps more positively than has often been the case. The attempt to encourage women to give birth in hospital had obvious direct benefits in terms of falling neonatal and maternal mortality, but it also exposed women to periods of intense health education relating to hygiene and nutrition which seem likely to have reduced subsequent infant and child mortality. The STD campaign in Buhaya no doubt reduced morbidity and mortality associated with syphilis and gonorrhoea, but it also transformed the nature of rural healthcare, resulting in dramatic improvements in preventive medicine and the treatment of endemic complaints such as worms and malaria. Finally, the kwashiorkor scare in late-colonial Buganda, which saw malnutrition displace syphilis as both the marker of Ganda moral failings and the primary explanation for child mortality, in fact produced broad-ranging improvements in child survival, not just due to better dietary practices, but also associated with improved sanitation, so that gastro-enteritis, which had increased hugely in incidence in the 1950s, fell away rapidly in the 1960s. One of the most interesting recent studies of indigenous responses to colonial medicine in this region emphasizes the suspicions which healthcare aroused. Some of my interviewees also discussed issues such as vampires and cannibalism, though these were elderly medical personnel recounting beliefs held by some patients in the past. Some female informants expressed a distaste for hospitalized birth; others complained of the negligence and corruption of some Ugandan medical personnel during the later 1970s and early 1980s. But overwhelmingly the response to questions about health was a positive appreciation of increased survivorship associated with western biomedicine, a position which was almost always maintained when the focus of enquiry shifted from broad perceptions to the personal experiences of informants and their families. It might be suspected that such responses were conditioned by the intensity of AIDS awareness programmes since the mid-1980s, which have sought, with significant success, to convince people in northwest Tanzania and southern Uganda, that compliance with public health advice can prevent HIV infection, and that HIV responds to chemotherapeutic treatment. But care should be taken not to exaggerate the novelty of health education in this region. Informants displayed impressive knowledge about the causes, symptoms, and treatment of conditions such as kwashiorkor and gonorrhoea, which had been the subject of sustained public information provision since the mid-colonial period. This was a heavily medicalized society by the 1970s, one that had become habituated to health campaigns advocating behavioural change. It seems likely that this heritage partly explains the relative success of AIDS control programmes in this region after 1980.[113]

[113] L. White, '"They could make their victims dull": Genders and genres, fantasies and cures in colonial southern Uganda', *American Historical Review*, 100, 5 (1995), pp. 1379–1402; Male FGD Bukoto, 24 Aug. 2004; Int. CM, 11 Aug. 2000, Busindi, M; Int. EM, 28 Aug. 2004, Kyansi, M; Int. NNFW, 28 Aug. 2004, Kaswa, F; Int. MM, 11 Aug. 2000, Ijumbi, F.

9

Sexuality, Mortality, Disease and Fertility in the 1970s

INTRODUCTION

Scholars seeking to explain the origins of the HIV epidemic in southern Uganda and northwest Tanzania have tended to focus on the 1970s and early 1980s as the key moment when sexual behaviour became much more high risk. Some researchers have emphasized the economic collapse associated with Idi Amin's regime in Uganda and villagization in Tanzania which in particular increased the sexual vulnerability of young women and heightened sexual opportunities for young men involved in smuggling; others prioritized the rise in coercive sex linked to Amin's military rule and the war between Tanzania and Uganda at the end of the 1970s; Uganda's liberation from Amin's tyranny has been identified as the point at which sexual freedom suddenly exploded in that country; finally, urbanization across the region has been associated with a new kind of economic degradation, the rapid spread of commercial sex, and heightened opportunities for partner exchange.[1] None of these explanatory factors are incorrect, and inequality and economic decline without doubt contributed to the rapid spread of HIV, but they tend to exaggerate the sense to which societies in this region descended into utter poverty and chaos, and they distract attention from evidence which suggests that sexual culture changed during these years as much due to new forms of aspiration as desperation. This chapter will argue that while the 1970s saw some of the gains in life expectancy achieved in previous decades being lost, it was not until the mid-1980s that medical provision and health standards reached their nadir. In addition it will suggest that the onset of fertility decline in central Buganda during the 1970s requires a re-evaluation not only of perceptions of Uganda during this decade, but also of the theoretical preconditions for the uptake of family planning. Changes in sexual behaviour and

[1] e.g. H. Pickering et al., 'Sexual behaviour in a fishing community on Lake Victoria, Uganda', *Health Transition Review*, 7 (1997), pp. 13–20; F. Kaijage, 'AIDS control and the burden of history in northwestern Tanzania', *Population and Environment*, 14, 3 (1999), pp. 279–300; G. Lwihula, L. Dahlgren, J. Killewo and A. Sandstrom, 'AIDS epidemic in Kagera region, Tanzania: The experiences of local people', *AIDS Care*, 5, 3 (1993), pp. 347–57.

attitudes during this decade moreover were in part simply the result of the deepening and widening of existing trends, ensuring that patterns of sexuality which had been initially associated with urban contexts dispersed far into the regions' rural communities. The existing scholarship has tended to focus on the grimmest aspects of life in this period, but interviewees on the whole present a contrasting picture. For them, sex had occasionally been coerced, more often it had been strategic, but primarily it had been pleasurable and exciting.

SEXUAL BEHAVIOURAL CHANGE

Buhaya

In the 1970s writing about Haya sexuality continued to be dominated by the role of the sex worker. This was also true when oral informants were asked about that decade, though the growing sexual freedom of unmarried girls and young women was almost as prominent in interview discussions.[2] Yet soon after the first cases of HIV were diagnosed in 1983 epidemiological research revealed that these fixations only partially explained the remarkable severity of the epidemic in this area. To some extent sexual behaviour had changed as a result of the Ugandan war and its aftermath, but many of the findings of the early work on AIDS, as earlier chapters of this study show, clearly applied to long-established patterns of sexuality. It seems reasonable then to utilize the first epidemiological studies on HIV to supplement sources from the 1970s.

One of the most striking changes to have occurred in Haya sexual life in the years around independence seems to have been a sharp increase in both the stability of marriage and likelihood of remarriage. A survey of 5,050 women in 1972 in Kiziba found that only 10.5% were currently divorced, compared to 15% in an equivalent survey in the early 1950s.[3] Yet the proportion of the

[2] M.-L. Swantz, *Women in Development: a Creative Role Denied. The Case of Tanzania* (London: Hurst, 1985); A. Ishumi, *Kiziba: The Cultural Heritage of an Old African Kingdom* (Syracuse:, Maxwell School of Citizenship and Public Affairs, 1980); Z. Bader, 'Women, private property and production in Bukoba district' (unpublished MA dissertation, University of Dar es Salaam [UDSM], 1975); I. Sembajwe, 'Impact of urbanization on fertility and child mortality. The case studies of Tanzania and Uganda' (unpublished MA dissertation, UDSM, 1973); Int. SN, 25 Aug. 1999, Katoma, M; Int. AC, 9 Aug. 2000, Rubaa-Rubya, F; Int. EK, 7 Aug. 2000, Kanyangereko Nkimbo, F; Int. YK, 19 Aug. 2000, Kikukwe, F.

[3] Ishumi, *Kiziba*, p. 86; W. Laurie and H. Trant, *East African Medical Survey, Monograph no. 2, A Health Survey in Bukoba District, Tanganyika* (Nairobi: EAHC, 1954), pp. 37–8. See also R. Henin, *National Demographic Survey of Tanzania, 1973: Volume II, Data for Socioeconomic Groups* (Dar es Salaam: Tanzania Bureau of Statistics, 1973), pp. 78, 32, which found that 11.5% of women were divorcees.

adult female population which was reported to have divorced or been widowed and then left for East Africa's cities was, at 8%, higher than during the mid-colonial period. More than ten times as many Haya divorcees in their thirties had gone to Mombasa, Kampala, and other distant cities as had stayed at home, presumably because opportunities for remarriage were lower than for younger women. It was not only divorcees who felt the pull of the city. Haya women continued to leave their homeland in high numbers even though the incidence of childlessness and divorce, the two major factors formerly believed to have pushed women into urban prostitution, had declined together. It seems that the potential profit and autonomy associated with sex work and barmaiding had become increasingly attractive to Haya women over time. Of course, not all Haya women who went to the city during this decade became sex or bar workers, but the sources suggest that most did. Certainly Haya dominated the sex trade in East Africa's urban areas right through to the early 1990s.[4] Informants emphasized that after independence sex workers became increasingly common within rural Buhaya as well. One researcher in 1973 reported that there were five active prostitutes within one rural community 'who often travel to other villages for this purpose in order to subsidize their meagre forms of subsistence'.[5] Prostitution was more firmly established within Bukoba town, though even here many women were part-time, relying on cash earned from sex work to supplement their income from serving in bars or hotels. The high-risk nature of these occupations meant that they were subject to occasional STD testing, which revealed in 1986 that twenty-nine of the town's seventy-eight barmaids were already HIV positive.[6]

By this time HIV had spread rapidly through Bukoba's densely settled hinterland, and had begun to devastate a series of villages strung along the area's major roads, north to Uganda, south towards Mwanza, and west towards Karagwe and Rwanda. Early researchers into HIV here were struck not so much by the high prevalence among urbanites, but by the narrow differential between urban and rural infection rates. In part this was explained

[4] A. Culwick, 'The population problem in the Bukoba district', Bukoba, 1938, UDSM, EAF CORY 239; W. Nkya et al., Sexually transmitted diseases in prostitutes in Moshi and Arusha, Northern Tanzania', *International Journal of STD and AIDS*, 2, 6 (1991), pp. 432–5; P. Piot et al., 'Retrospective seroepidemiology of *AIDS* virus infection in Nairobi populations', *Journal of Infectious Diseases,* 155 (1987), pp. 1108–12; A. Shorter, *East African Societies* (London: Routledge and Kegan Paul, 1974), p. 114.

[5] Int. AC, 9 Aug. 2000, Rubaa-Rubya, F; Int. BB, 2 Sept. 1999, Kenyana, M; Int. SN, 25 Aug. 1999, Katoma, M; Sembajwe, 'Impact', pp. 79–80. Cf. Lwihula, Dahlgren, Killewo and Sandstrom. 'AIDS epidemic in Kagera region', pp. 352–3.

[6] G. Lwihalu, 'Sexuality and HIV transmission in Kagera Region, Tanzania', *International Conference on AIDS*, 5 (1989), p. 878; D. Forthal et al. 'AIDS in Tanzania' (unpublished paper, Centers for Disease Control, Atlanta, 1986).

by the frequency with which Haya moved between town and village, but outside observers had long observed that much of rural Buhaya had distinctly urban characteristics. Many notionally rural wards had population densities exceeding 500 people per square kilometre, and 'most of the villages . . . have town-like centres, characterized by roadside shops and public drinking or meeting places.'[7]

Early HIV studies identified some key high-risk groups, most obviously sex workers, barmaids and soldiers, but also young entrepreneurs who profited from the closure of the Tanzania-Uganda frontier between 1978 and 1985. These young men shuttled from their bases in the smuggling villages near the border and the lakeshore to Bukoba and then to their home villages, reportedly using their wealth to maintain a series of sexual partners. Buhaya's rural economy had sunk into depression since the 1960s, though it seems the area fell into real poverty because of HIV, rather than before it. Surveys of sexual behaviour in the mid-1980s found that high levels of partner exchange were endemic in Buhaya. A largely rural sample reported that within the past two years men had had 7.4 different sexual partners on average, while women had had 2.3. Strikingly, given the strict control formerly maintained over female pre-marital sexuality, the early victims of AIDS were predominantly married men and unmarried women, though marital status rapidly became less important as a distinguishing factor as the disease became more widely dispersed. Another study concluded 'it seems almost irrelevant to talk about special risk groups. Everybody in this area is at risk of being infected with the AIDS virus and the stigmatization of special groups (even if relevant) may be a masquerade to hide the real magnitude of the HIV infection.' It was thought to be inadequate to focus on sex workers when so many situations in village communities were reported as commonly leading to unplanned sexual encounters: 'market places, night-time discos, over-night wedding ceremonies, all-night drinking spots, as well as all-night party and government functions'.[8] Buhaya's

[7] J. Killewo, 'Epidemiology towards the control of HIV infection in Tanzania with special reference to the Kagera Region' (unpublished PhD dissertation, University of Umea, 1994), p. 43; J. Killewo et al., 'Prevalence of HIV-1 infection in the Kagera region of Tanzania: a population-based study', *AIDS*, 4, 11 (1990), pp. 1081–6; J. Rudengren, 'A methodological study of population density and distribution: A case study of West Lake Region', (BRALUP Research Report 7, University of Dar es Salaam, 1974), p. 4; J. Killewo, L. Dahlgren and A. Sandström, 'Socio-geographical patterns of HIV-1 transmission in Kagera Region, Tanzania', *Social Science and Medicine*, 38, 1 (1994), p. 132. The OECD defines rural areas as having a population density of less than 150 people per square kilometre.

[8] J. Killewo et al., 'Incidence of HIV-1 infection among adults in the Kagera Region of Tanzania', *International Journal of Epidemiology, 22* (1993), pp. 528–36; Forthal et al., 'AIDS', p. 2; Lwihula, Dahlgren, Killewo and Sandstrom, 'AIDS epidemic in Kagera region', pp. 352–7; Killewo, 'Epidemiology', p. 49. Another study reported that between 1979 and 1987 urban respondents had had 9.2 sexual partners on average, rural respondents 6.1. Killewo et al., 'Incidence of HIV-1', pp. 528–36.

social environment had long proven conducive to sexual affairs but it seems that the 1970s and early 1980s had increased the frequency with which individuals were exposed to risk.

Ankole

The conservatism which characterized Ankole's sexual culture in the colonial period survived to some extent until the end of our period. Informants believed that while wife-sharing among Hima pastoralists was gradually declining in the 1970s, it remained common into the 1980s, and even among agriculturalists, who had begun to reject the practice much earlier than the Hima, it was only finally abandoned when it was identified as a risk factor for HIV transmission. A 1984 study reported that two-thirds of Hima women participated in the practice, compared to 8% of agriculturalists. Migrants to Kampala in the mid-1970s still glorified the virtue of Ankole's village women, while Ntozi and Kabera in the mid-1980s emphasized that pre-marital pregnancy remained a source of shame. Some informants claimed that murder remained a common response to the seduction of a man's wife until the Museveni regime took power in Uganda and insisted on monopolizing the use of violence. In the 1970s 'there were no laws'. Female interviewees insisted that the old stories about the execution of unmarried girls who fell pregnant still carried weight at the start of the 1970s, and even at the end of the decade it continued to be widely believed that for either spouse to engage in adulterous affairs during a pregnancy would damage the unborn child.[9]

Yet some long-established penalties lost much of their significance over the course of the 1970s. A survey in western Ankole in 1980, for example, found unanimous agreement that even banishment as a punishment for pre-marital pregnancy had been abandoned. New opportunities for socializing, almost universal schooling, and the shift from arranged marriage to a culture of dating and courtship had facilitated an increase in pre-marital sex in 1970s Ankole. One consequence of this was a marked increase in the number of cases where genitors refused to accept the responsibilities of fatherhood outside marriage. In the Nyamitanga parish baptism register the proportion of

[9] Male Focus Group Discussion (FGD) Ruti, 19 Aug. 2004; Int. HM, 16 Aug. 2004, Mbarara District Hospital, F; Int. JT, 16 Aug. 2004, Mbarara District Hospital, F; Female FGD Kyenjenyi, 22 Aug. 2004; J. Ntozi and J. Kabera, 'Marriage patterns in Ankole, South-Western Uganda', African Demography Working Papers no. 16, University of Pennsylvania, August 1988, pp. 21, 34; C. Obbo, 'Town migration is not for women' (unpublished PhD dissertation, University of Wisconsin-Madison, 1977), p. 156; Male FGD Kyangyenyi/Kiyungu, 22 Aug. 2004; Female FGD Kiyungi, 21 Aug. 2004; A. Kamugisha, 'Beliefs and customs connected with childbirth among the Banyankole, with special reference to utilisation of modern medical services' (unpublished BA Social Work and Social Administration dissertation, Makerere University Kampala [MUK], 1980), p. 54.

babies with no named father was never higher than 0.2% until 1969, but then rose during the 1970s to 0.8%. These babies almost certainly represented only a fraction of the children born outside a socially recognized marriage, but their increasing numbers suggest either that a growing number of males, presumably because of their immaturity, were in no position to claim their offspring for their clan, or that women were becoming less dependent on paternal involvement in childrearing. The young age of the mothers of these children as well as the fact that two homes for abandoned babies opened in Ankole in the early 1970s suggests the former explanation is more likely. Elderly informants agreed that pre-marital sex had become relatively common in the 1960s, but increased markedly in the 1970s.[10]

Narratives of moral decline emanating from the older generation of any society should always be viewed with some scepticism, but the consensus view among elderly Nkole informants fitted well with the chronology of change detectable in documentary sources. Moreover, interviews with medical personnel who had worked in Ankole at that time supported the assertion that the sexuality of the young had changed significantly during this decade. These doctors and nurses were generally younger than other informants and tended to be less moralistic, but agreed that sexual attitudes and behaviour changed significantly in this period. 'People were just having sex freely . . . young men would be brought in saying "I'm a man, I've got gonorrhoea."'[11] Elders' analysis of why behaviour had evolved in Ankole should perhaps be viewed with more caution than their memories of when that evolution had occurred. Compared to Ganda and Haya, Nkole were less likely to personalize their accounts of changing sexual patterns, while many of the issues that informants in all three societies referred to have been topics of public controversy and debate for several decades. For example, education as well as what was described as civilization or enlightenment were frequently identified, rather ruefully, by informants as the main factors leading to the liberalization of sexual morality in Ankole. More precisely, according to some women, female schooling and membership of clubs and societies had undermined the idea that husbands and wives should adopt different codes of moral behaviour. 'So then the wife, when her husband went out, she also would say "I too am going, we shall meet when you're back."' . . . Now a woman could tell you. 'If you don't fear me, then I also don't fear you.' 'If you bring, I shall also bring, and we shall meet at the same meeting place.' But some explanations were more time-specific and so appeared more convincing. For example,

[10] Kamugisha, 'Beliefs', p. 63; B. Mwesiga, 'Traditional marriage among the Banyankole' (unpublished BA Fine Arts dissertation, MUK, 1976–7), pp. 48–50; *Uganda Argus*, 19 July 1971, p. 4; FGD Male Kiyungu Shema, 21 Aug. 2004; Female FGD Kyenjenyi , 22 Aug. 2004.
[11] e.g. Int. JT, 16 Aug. 2004, Mbarara Hospital, F; Int. DCT, 20 Aug. 2004, Mbarara, M.

informants remembered the 1970s, until Amin's last years, as a period of prosperity, which accelerated the spread of the new forms of socializing that had emerged in the late 1950s and 1960s. During those years, one recalled, 'almost every weekend in the villages there would be a function during the harvest seasons. It was easy to end up indulging in sexual matters there. Where there is merry-making, definitely.' Meanwhile, in Mbarara town under Amin 'there were many bars so men would go there and have the barmaids . . . Those who had cars would pick up their friends and they would all go.'[12] Much of the local memory of sexual behaviour at this time is defined by a sense of growing freedom, but local mores were reportedly also reshaped by the unrestrained abuse of power by the agents of Amin and Obote II's militarized states. 'A soldier would put on his uniform, and take on any woman of his choice. He would even go ahead to rape and carry off girls . . . The soldiers were all over the place . . . It was risky to have a beautiful wife. They would kill you and then take your woman.' 'I had a bar; they would come, take alcohol without paying and grab girls.' 'The change in behaviour started during Amin's time. The 70s. It was started by soldiers who would give a woman good things and eventually take her. If she refused they would beat her. So every girl started becoming a *malaya* [prostitute].' 'During the *mafuta mingi* [a lot of fat—corruption] time, when Amin sent away the Indians, the Africans took over and they could get money. So they thought of having sex instead of using it to develop . . . It was not about affairs of friendship, but prostitution. Many women and girls came from the villages to the towns.' According to these informants, Amin's state allowed disrespect for parental concern for female virtue and marriage to become endemic in Ankole, undermining this society's relatively strict sexual codes.[13]

The issue which defined the new amorality of the 1970s, according to most informants, was the rise of prostitution. Some men remembered sex workers as being particularly beautiful and attractively dressed, and a few women made enough money to build houses for themselves, but overall prostitution and barmaiding were distinctly unglamorous.[14] Local narratives blamed poverty or parental neglect for pushing young women into prostitution. Most women who sold sex did so part-time, to supplement their income from bar work or beer brewing. According to some accounts sex workers sometimes even had images of dogs forcibly tattooed on their faces, as they were blamed for transmitting *kauzi*, an STD of supposedly canine origin,

[12] Male FGD Kyangyenyi/Kiyungu, 22 Aug. 2004; Female FGD Kyenjenyi, 22 Aug. 2004; Int. RNT, 9 Aug. 2004, Mbarara, M; Female FGD Nyamitanga, 19 Aug. 2004. Cf. Juliana Nkakibona, Letter, *Ageteraine*, 22 Sept. 1973.

[13] Male FGD Ruti, 19 Aug. 2004; Male FGD Namitanga, 19 Aug. 2004.

[14] Male FGD Namitanga, 19 Aug. 2004; Male FGD Ruti, 19 Aug. 2004.

which was most likely antibiotic-resistant gonorrhoea.[15] Amin's regime is credited in local memory with attacking prostitutes and with forcing them to attend weekly check-ups so they would receive treatment. Some men remembered that the presumed absence of STD infection was one of their main attractions in those years. But oral accounts make it clear that while sex work for cash perhaps declined in visibility in the 1970s, it became much more pervasive, taking root not only in small towns like Bushenyi and Kabwohe, but even in small trading centres by the end of the decade. Meanwhile village life too saw some women exchanging sex for material items. Moreover, the attempt to licence and monitor prostitutes and barmaids, like so many of Amin's decrees, was only sustained for a relatively short period.[16]

Buganda

Some oral interviewees and much of the literature identified the 1970s as the decade when sexual behaviour and attitudes in Buganda were radically transformed, creating the conditions in which HIV could spread rapidly. This perception is only partly true, for the changes of the 1970s were characterized more by the intensification of existing trends than the emergence of new forms of sexuality. Pre-marital sex, for example, seems to have become more common, as schooling became almost universal by the early 1970s and mixed-sex socializing as well as dating and courting became increasingly accepted.[17] In the 1980s a survey found that the average age of female sexual debut was 15.3, several years younger than the average age of first marriage.[18] No equivalent data are available from the early 1970s, but what evidence does exist suggests that early sexual experience was already the norm, in the Greater Kampala region at least. Mere Kisekka, a Ganda researcher, interviewed a number of secondary schoolchildren at the start of the decade and found that 97% of boys and 69% of girls claimed to have lost their virginity. Perhaps even more striking was the predominantly positive attitudes these adolescents had to pre-marital sex, with 77% of males and 54% of females describing it as

[15] 'Prostitution', *Ageteraine*, 22 February 1970; Int. JT, 16 Aug. 2004, Mbarara Hospital, F; Int. HM, 16 Aug. 2004, Mbarara District Hospital, F; Female FGD Ruti, 19 Aug. 2004; Kiyungi Female FGD 21 Aug. 2004.

[16] Int. RNT, 9 Aug. 2004, Mbarara, M; Male FGD Namitanga, 19 Aug. 2004; Female FGD Nyamitanga, 19 Aug. 2004; Kyenjenyi Female FGD 22 Aug. 2004; Int. EM, 27 Sept. 2001, Kampala, M; Male FGD Ruti, 19 Aug. 2004. Cf. M. Leopold, 'Sex, violence and history in the lives of Idi Amin: Postcolonial masculinity as masquerade', *Journal of Postcolonial Writing*, 45, 3 (2009), pp. 321–30.

[17] Male FGD Kitala, 1 Sept. 2004; Male FGD Kisubi Kiwulwe, 4 Sept. 2004; Int. IST, 21 August 2004, Kagezi village, Masaka, M.

[18] W. Agyei and E. Epema, 'Adolescent fertility in Kampala, Uganda: Knowledge, perceptions and practice', *Biology and Society*, 7, 4 (1990), pp. 203–4.

strengthening a relationship, exciting, or natural. A few years later another anthropologist, Christine Obbo, emphasized the ubiquity of pre-marital sex in Kampala, and recounted the story of how the news that a sixteen-year-old girl from Wabigalo was found to be a virgin at marriage 'was discussed for weeks'. A further study based on 1970s research that pre-dated Uganda's crisis reported that 'today an unmarried mother is no longer considered a great scandal for the parents, as the case was formerly.' One of the key characteristics of Ganda sexuality in this period was the complexity of sexual networks, which were not confined by class, ethnicity, residential area or, in this case, age. Young people in Buganda were sexually highly active not only with their peers, but also it seems with the older generation. Local schoolgirls' ideal sexual partner in 1970–71, before the era of the *mafuta mingi*, was supposedly one of the *Abamabenzi*, an owner of a Mercedes. Obbo in 1971–2 found that 'some young men attached themselves to older women so as to save. I knew students, clerks, and unemployed school dropouts who had no worry over accommodations, food and clothing. They enjoyed the financial comforts provided by older women, but liked to sleep with younger women whom they accused of being mean with their money.'[19] Equally importantly, sexual precocity seems to have been associated with high-risk sexual behaviour later in life. A survey of soldiers in the early 1980s found that men who had lost their virginity before the age of fifteen were significantly more likely to have been infected with an STD in the past year compared to those who had commenced sexual activity later.[20]

As was discussed in Chapter 4, post-marital sex was also already common in Buganda before 1970, though again it seems that it became more so during Amin's rule. It is unclear whether divorce became more prevalent during this period, though some sources suggest that it did, partly because men became less careful in concealing their affairs. Male infidelity, it was claimed, was generally accepted as being almost inevitable, but a lack of discretion was regarded as a sign of disrespect. The 'generation of fun and entertainment', as some informants termed those who came to maturity in the 1970s, at times

[19] M. Kisekka, 'Heterosexual relationships in Uganda' (unpublished PhD dissertation, University of Missouri, 1973), pp. 139–40, 158–9, 170; Obbo, 'Town', pp. 156–7; F.-X. Kyewalyanga, *Traditional Religion, Custom and Christianity in Uganda: As Illustrated by the Ganda with Some References to other African Cultures and Islam* (Freiburg: Klaus Renner, 1976), p. 208. Kisekka, like most sources on this region, focused almost entirely on heterosexual sex, but did mention that same-sex relationships were not uncommon in boarding schools, and to a lesser degree in Kampala.

[20] B. Ndahura, 'Sexually Transmitted Diseases in a military unit in Uganda' (unpublished DPH dissertation, MUK, 1984), p. 45. Cf. R. White, J. Cleland and M. Caraël, 'Links between premarital sexual behaviour and extramarital intercourse: a multi-site analysis', *AIDS*, 14 (2000), pp. 2323–31. Only a minority of these soldiers were Ganda, but most of the sample had local girlfriends or frequented local bars.

failed to heed local norms that affairs should not be conducted in public. Marriages were also thought to fail more often because of a growing incompatibility between male and female goals. While men generally still wished wives to remain submissive and dependent, according to Kisekka and Obbo, women increasingly sought to achieve economic independence, typically by purchasing land, as insurance against the failure of their marriage. Within elite groups the tensions were most explicit, with many men still aspiring to have multiple wives and large families, while women typically argued for monogamy and fertility control.[21] It certainly seems that women whose first relationship broke down became increasingly reluctant to remarry. Obbo reported that many of the women she interviewed regarded men as 'a nuisance', held that the status of having once been married secured sufficient respectability, and had few qualms about securing children outside wedlock. One survey found that in 1970 only 15% of divorced women in a community had remarried. The ability of divorcees, as well as widows and unmarried women, to sustain themselves in the absence of a marital relationship explains why female-headed households were so prominent in Buganda, making up between 17 and 52% of all households in various surveys in the 1970s.[22]

Paula Davis has argued that in the mid-1970s Uganda's deteriorating economic and political situation caused single women to be scapegoated by both military government and the general public. Yet the portrayal of 'town women' as sexually loose and immoral had begun to intensify in the late 1960s, long before Amin's coup, and the first presidential decrees that attempted to regulate women's physical appearance were issued in 1972, before Amin's popularity and Uganda's prosperity had significantly declined.[23]

[21] C. Obbo to A. Richards, 15 Feb. 1975, Richards papers, LSE, 6/25; Kisekka, 'Heterosexual relationships', pp. 44, 87, 127–8; Male FGD Kitala, 1 Sept. 2004; Obbo, 'Town', pp. 157, 175, 187, 216; Female FGD Bugiri Kiwulwe, 10 Sept. 2004. Cf. C. Ndugwa, 'There is no easy way to mature love', *Uganda Weekly News*, 9 Apr. 1978, p. 12; J. Opolot, 'Unmarriageable city women', *Uganda Weekly News*, 5 Feb. 1978, p. 13.

[22] Obbo, 'Town', pp. 140–56, 170–5; Kisekka, 'Heterosexual relationships', pp. 127–8; E. Mandeville, 'The formality of marriage: A Kampala case study', *Journal of Anthropological Research*, 31, 3 (1975), pp. 183–95; T. Kizito, 'A study of the demographic characteristics and environmental problems of the heads of family units in slums around Nakulabye' (unpublished DPH, Makerere University Kampala, 1980), p. 13. Obbo's survey, which recorded by far the lowest proportion of female-headed households, covered an area, the suburbs of Namuwongo and Wabigalo, which were well-known for their conservatism. Obbo emphasized that this was an area where sex workers remained out of sight, women generally behaved in traditional ways such as speaking softly to men and kneeling to greet them, where Nubi and Luo, ethnic groups whose menfolk were reputed to be especially sexually repressive, were unusually common, and where there was a notably religious atmosphere.

[23] P. Davis, 'On the sexuality of "town women" in Kampala', *Africa Today*, 47, 3/4 (2000), pp. 39–41; 'Venereal Diseases on the Increase', *The People*, 14 Jan. 1969, p. 5; 'War on minis in Uganda?', *The People*, 14 Jan. 1969; 'Opinions on minis: for and against', *The People*, 17 Jan. 1969, p. 9; D. Mabirizi-Busulwa, Letter to editor, *The People*, 14 Feb. 1969; C. Obang-Achere, Nsambya barracks, Letter to editor, *The People*, 17 Feb. 1969, p. 7.

At first Amin adopted a restrained position on issues of private morality, stating that it was parents' responsibility to determine how adolescent girls should dress. But the Field-Marshall's survival as head of state for eight years depended on his populism as well as his unrestrained use of force, and he quickly bowed to the clamour to 'abandon this democracy of nakedness', issuing a series of decrees against women wearing miniskirts, trousers, wigs, and make-up, and using skin-lightener. 'The President said women who use these creams to change the appearance of their faces and skin, lose their natural beauty and as a result they now look like monkeys or gorillas.' Amin went on to attack prostitution and finally in 1977 announced that people suspected of being infected with STDs in 'notorious areas' would be identified and forced to receive treatment. A number of women were beaten up and prosecuted for disobeying these laws in the months after they were passed, but, judging from photos and descriptions in local newspapers, women gradually reclaimed much of their wardrobe as the decade progressed. The association of Amin's regime with moral probity moreover declined in 1975 when the government newspaper published a nude photo supposedly of Elizabeth Bagaya, the former minister of foreign affairs and sometime model whose fall from grace was marked by the announcement that she had disgraced the nation by having sex in a Paris airport toilet. Overall there is little reason to think that Amin's hollow state made any significant impact on prostitution, the number or behaviour of unmarried women, or sexual morality more generally.[24]

Inconsistency, a lack of judgement, and the inability to ensure that policies were sustained also contributed to the collapse of the Ugandan economy under Amin. Uganda's GDP is estimated to have fallen by 30% in the 1970s, though official data probably exaggerate the scale of the decline, given that smuggling had become endemic by the end of the decade. Much of the decline occurred towards the end of the 1970s, when drought coincided with war. Even so, it is significant that, according to official data, exports of coffee, the major source of income for the peasantry in both Buganda and Ankole, declined much less sharply between 1970 and 1980 than those of any other major cash crop. The economic situation in Buganda then worsened rapidly during Milton Obote's second period in office, between 1980 and 1985, partly

[24] Y. Serwanga, Letter to editor, *Uganda Argus*, 10 Jan. 1972, p. 3; Y. Buregyeya, Letter to editor, *Uganda Argus*, 12 Jan. 1972, p. 4; 'President Amin bans use of skin makeup', *Voice of Uganda*, 6 May 1975, p. 1; P. Setel, M. Lewis, and M. Lyons (eds.), *Histories of Sexually Transmitted Diseases and HIV/AIDS in Sub-Saharan Africa*, p. 108; Obbo, 'Town', pp. 285–90; Female FGD Bugiri Kiwulwe, 10 Sept. 2004; J. Kakembo, 'A study of the prevalence and incidence of venereal diseases in the Uganda police community' (unpublished DPH dissertation, MUK, 1978), p. 34; Radio comment on Miss Bagaya, *Voice of Uganda*, 24 Jan. 1975, p. 1. Cf. Leopold, 'Amin'.

because of the devastating civil war in the Luwero Triangle, partly because the obstacles to free movement obstructed trade, so crucial to Buganda's prosperity.[25] There is no doubt that by the end of the 1970s poverty had become severe for a large proportion of the population. Some authors have argued that the *magendo* or black market economy in 1970s rural Buganda heightened women's economic insecurity and dependence on men for cash and consumer goods, worsening marital instability and pushing women into exchanging sexual favours for material rewards. Black marketeers, for example, reportedly found it easy to use their money to seduce women in isolated rural areas who had no other access to cash. Research into the epidemiology of HIV clearly demonstrated that for many women deep poverty and sexual vulnerability were indeed interrelated.[26] This though was not a new development of the 1970s and 1980s but an intensification of a well-established phenomenon. In the late 1960s Mandeville found that the majority of women in one of Kampala's poorer areas lived in all-female households and depended on presents from lovers to keep themselves and their children above the poverty line.[27]

But it would be mistaken to think that this is only a story of ever increasing victimization. Mandeville emphasized that the women she studied preferred their semi-autonomous state to marriage, while, according to Kisekka, some women achieved real wealth by manipulating a series of prosperous lovers. One of her informants, Maaso, had four children by three men. All were in boarding school, and she lived in a three-bedroomed apartment, employed two servants, and owned a television and a car. Her current

[25] B. Odonga Mwaka, 'Widowhood and property among the Baganda of Uganda: Uncovering the passive victim' (unpublished Phd dissertation in law, University of Warwick, 1998), p. 10; C. Dodge and P. Wiebe, 'Introduction' in C. Dodge and P. Wiebe (eds.), *Crisis in Uganda: The Breakdown of Health Services* (Oxford: Pergamon Press, 1985), p. 3; H. Welbourn, 'Uganda—end or beginning' (unpublished TS in possession of author, 1980). Cf. H. Hansen and M. Twaddle (eds)., *Uganda Now: Between Decay and Development* (Oxford: James Currey, 1988). It should be noted that in part the sustained enthusiasm for coffee production related to the relative ease and profit with which it could be smuggled, but this was very much a mixed blessing, given the close association between smuggling and early HIV infections.

[26] H. Welbourn, 'Uganda—end or beginning' (unpublished TS in possession of author, 1980); A. Southall, 'Social disorganisation in Uganda: Before, during, and after Amin', *The Journal of Modern African Studies*, 18, 4 (1980), p. 643; A. Barnett and P. Blaikie, *AIDS in Africa: Its Past and Future Impact* (New York: Guilford Press, 1992), pp. 72–8; J. Kuhanen, '"Balinsalamu embawo?" AIDS and the context of sexual behaviour adjustment in Rakai, Uganda, *c*. 1975–90', *Journal of Eastern African Studies*, 4, 1 (2010), pp. 20–43; J. McGrath et al., 'Cultural determinants of sexual risk behavior for AIDS among Baganda women', *Medical Anthropology Quarterly*, 6, 2 (1992), pp. 153–61.

[27] E. Mandeville, 'Poverty, work and the financing of single women in Kampala', *Africa*, 49, 1 (1979), pp. 49–50. P. Robertz, 'Sharing with adolescents' (unpublished research paper, Pastoral Institute of Eastern Africa, Gaba, *c*.1969) found that the majority of secondary schoolchildren in Kampala in the late 1960s lived in poverty.

lovers provided her with a higher standard of living than she thought was experienced by married women, 'whose husbands may squander the money on drinks and prostitutes . . . most of the time I feel happy and I like my independence.' Other studies meanwhile noted that Uganda's deteriorating economic situation encouraged many women to establish themselves in trade, while 'the position of working wives was strengthened in relation to their husbands', due to their earnings increasing in importance within the household. Moreover, the 1970s were remembered by informants not only as the decade of Amin's henchmen 'falling into things' and showering their ill-gotten wealth on multiple girlfriends, or black marketeers making and abusing easy money. 'In Amin's regime people would work hard and get a lot of money, and so have a lot of affairs.'[28]

Uganda's economic crisis was then clearly associated with patterns of sexual activity which facilitated the spread of HIV, but it is important to note that earlier chapters have indicated that the association between inequality and multiple sexual partners pre-dated Amin, and that focusing on black marketeers and vulnerable women only partially explains the shape of the epidemic in this region. This is not to downplay the role played by high-risk groups, but rather to try to distinguish between them, and shift the focus onto the interconnections between these groups and the wider society. The military have frequently been identified as a key accelerant in the spread of HIV in the Great Lakes, with a lack of discipline being blamed for the frequency with which soldiers raped women during the 1970s and early 1980s.[29] Many informants supported this thesis, emphasizing particularly the Tanzanian war as the time when coerced sex became particularly common.[30] But some claimed that rape was not used as much by Obote's men as Amin's and a number of interviewees made it clear that there had been no rapes by military in their areas.[31]

[28] Mandeville, 'Poverty', pp. 42–52; Kisekka, 'Heterosexual', p. 112; Andrew Mickleburgh, 'The relevance of marriage for Ganda women in Bwaise, Kampala, Uganda' (unpublished PhD dissertation, University of Cambridge, 1998), pp. 120–1; G. Kyomuhendo and M. McIntosh, *Women, Work and Domestic Virtue in Uganda, 1900–2003* (Oxford: James Currey, 2006), p. 152; 'Shopkeeper's friend', *Uganda Weekly News*, 10 Dec. 1978, p. 10; Female FGD Bugiri Kiwulwe, 10 Sept. 2004. Cf. J. Kuhanen, 'Sexualised space, sexual networking and the emergence of AIDS in Rakai, Uganda', *Health and Place*, 16, 2 (2010), pp. 226–35.

[29] See e.g. G. Bond and J. Vincent, 'Living on the edge: Changing social structures in the context of AIDS', in H. Hansen and M. Twaddle (eds.), *Changing Uganda* (London: James Currey, 1991), pp. 113–29; M. Kisekka, 'AIDS in Uganda as a gender issue', in E. Rothblum and E. Cole (eds.), *Women's Mental Health in Uganda* (London: Haworth, 1990), pp. 39–45.

[30] Male FGD Kisubi Kiwulwe, 4 Sept. 2004; Male FGD Kitala, 1 Sept. 2004; Int. CNSM, 28 Aug. 2004, Butanga, M; Int. HGN, 10 Sept. 2004, Kiiso, F.

[31] Int. AN, 25 Aug. 2004, Kagezi, F; Int. FN, 29 Aug. 2004, Butanga, F; Male FGD Kagezi village, 25 August 2004; Female FGD Kagezi village, 25 Aug. 2004; Int. NM, 28 Aug. 2004, Lugazi, Butanga, F; Int. MMA, 24 Aug. 2004, Kyanakase, F.

It seems then that the incidence of rape was relatively localized, but was certainly not insignificant. It should be further noted that none of my interviews were conducted in the Luwero Triangle, where Obote's troops are commonly believed to have used mass rape to undermine resistance in northern Buganda during the early 1980s.[32] It is necessary to consider also soldiers' non-coercive sexual activity. Soldiers' relative wealth made them appear particularly attractive lovers, according to Southall, while a 1984 study of Entebbe garrison found that 81% of soldiers had had extra-marital sex in the past six months, typically with women encountered at local bars. Twenty-eight percent had had three or more irregular sexual partners over this period. Only 22% had not had an STD in the past year. Perhaps unsurprisingly STDs were much less prevalent within the police than the army, but still 18% of those examined at a Kampala station in 1978 had suffered some form of sexually transmitted infection in the past six months. But in both groups lovers or casual contacts were much more likely to be identified as the source of STD infections than prostitutes or barmaids, indicating that high-risk behaviour was not confined to particular occupations. Indeed, policewomen had a strikingly high level of STD infection, which they unanimously blamed on their civilian husbands.[33]

In Buganda, as in many societies, the term prostitute has often been used indiscriminately to label all unmarried women, or all women who accept gifts for sex. Christine Obbo observed that in the 1970s new, more derogatory words were employed to supplant *malaya*, a term which had become so overused as to be almost meaningless. Women who sold sex were called *embalasasa*, after a sleek, brightly coloured lizard, popularly thought to have been sent by either Governor Cohen, Milton Obote, or Idi Amin to kill the Ganda, or *ningu* after a fish whose eyes remained permanently open, connoting brazenness. *Malaya* still continued to be used to refer to all kinds of women considered promiscuous, and it was and is recognized in Buganda that fully professional prostitutes occupy one end of a spectrum of behaviour. Ganda though would acknowledge that offering gifts to a lover was a normal part of any relationship. It was when women depended on such gifts, and viewed them as essential to the maintenance of their households, that they became vulnerable to accusations of playing *malaya*. Yet in Buganda true prostitution required a cash transaction, not the receipt of non-monetary gifts. Even this refinement of itself does not help narrow down the definition of the sex worker in Buganda, for many women sold sex to supplement their income

[32] Cf. e.g. J. Crisp, 'National security, human rights and population displacements Luwero district, Uganda', *Review of African Political Economy*, 10, 27–28 (1983), pp. 164–74.
[33] Southall, 'Social disorganisation', p. 643; Ndahura, 'Sexually Transmitted Diseases', pp. 39–53; Kakembo, 'A study', pp. 5–29.

from other sources. Barmaids, for example, were paid less than a living wage so it was considered inevitable that they would need also to earn cash from sex. Bar workers though claimed that they did not sell their bodies indiscriminately to a range of clients, but instead selected and played off several concurrent, often short-term, lovers. In interviews prostitutes were defined as women whose primary source of income derived from selling sex.[34]

Academic studies in the 1970s emphasized how many sex workers there were in Kampala, one source referring to them as innumerable, another suggesting there were hundreds, a third asserting that the city had 'a wealth' of streetwalkers and that 'open door prostitutes . . . are quite abundant'. Amin's attack on sex work seems to have had no enduring impact. In 1978 a study of STDs described prostitution as being out of control, and newspapers in the mid-1970s referred to streetwalkers as though they were a common sight in central Kampala. Most prostitution probably occurred relatively discreetly, away from the city centre, with women catering for local clients in their own homes. Sex workers in the slums in the early 1970s reported an income similar to those earned by clerks or bus drivers, sufficient to maintain a respectable standard of living.[35] Prostitution was already very common in Kampala before the 1970s, but, according to informants, the change that occurred during that decade was that sex work became much more prominent in major towns like Masaka, and in trading centres on main roads which catered for truck and bus drivers as well as local traders. 'A driver would stop in places like Mbiko, from there he stops in Ndeeba, then Lukaya, Lyantonde etc.'[36]

According to one source Ganda men preferred barmaids to sex workers, considering that the latter's role was to cater for foreigners' needs. This was not supported by male interviewees, however, who gave no indication that male Ganda had been particularly discriminating.[37] Nonetheless it is likely

[34] C. Bakwesegha, *Profiles of Urban Prostitution; A Case Study from Uganda* (Nairobi: EAPH, 1982); L. White, *Speaking with Vampires: Rumor and History in Colonial Africa* (Berkeley: University of California Press, 2000), pp. 41–3; C. Obbo, 'Dominant male ideology and female options: Three East African case studies', *Africa*, 46, 4 (1976), p. 388; Obbo, 'Town', p. 172; 'Workers in restaurants and bars need to be helped', *Taifa Empya*, 14 Dec. 1970, p. 1.

[35] A. Masawe, 'Syphilis in Uganda: The history, clinical features and cellular immunity' (unpublished MMed dissertation, Makerere University Kampala, 1971), pp. 47–8; P. Kilbride, 'Barmaiding as a deviant occupation among the Baganda of Uganda', *Ethos*, 7, 3 (1979), p. 246; Kakembo, 'A study', pp. 1–5; S. Opak, *Voice of Uganda*, 12 June 1976, p. 5; Obbo, 'Town', pp. 172, 266.

[36] Male FGD Bukoto, 24 Aug. 2004; Int. AN, 25 Aug. 2004, Kagezi, F; Int. MMA, 24 Aug. 2004, Kyanakase, F; Int. NPNK, 24 Aug. 2004, Kyanakase, F; H. Manyolo, 'Factors that predispose to the spread of sexually transmitted diseases (e.g. gonorrhoea) among Makerere University students' (unpublished Diploma in Nursing Administration dissertation, MUK, 1980–81), p. 5.

[37] Kilbride, 'Barmaiding', p. 246; Male FGD Bukoto, 24 Aug. 2004; Int. NNFW, 28 Aug. 2004, Kaswa, F; Int. AN, 25 Aug. 2004, Kagezi, F.

that most men who paid for sex in Buganda did so with a barmaid, simply because barworkers were so numerous and dispersed. The biggest bars in Kampala might employ thirty barmaids, while any sizable village it seems could sustain one or two. The communities that made up the Kasangati Defined Area near Kampala had twenty bars in 1978, each with an average of seven barmaids, catering for around 12,000 people.[38] Kilbride has argued that sex was a fundamental part of barmaiding. 'Many patrons . . . particularly married men, wish to attract a barmaid as a potential lover.' Barmaids therefore had to develop strategies for 'keeping all men interested but only a few satisfied. Expertise in sexual conversation (*okuwemula*), deception (*okulimba*), and other manipulatory verbal strategies are things that a barmaid must master.' Contemporary newspaper accounts repeatedly attacked barmaids for dressing provocatively and seducing men, but occasionally commentators noted that men selected their drinking places on the basis of the aesthetic qualities of the staff. One letter-writer in 1970 advised 'bar-owners in Kampala to maintain a clean environment, as well as to have good-looking and attractive waitresses.'[39] Barmaiding was a high-risk profession in general, but some drinking places were riskier than others. A 1977 study found that bars which sold bottled beer tended to employ particularly transient staff. Whereas sellers of banana beer tended to be relatively mature women, barmaids in bottle bars were predominantly young divorcees. In Kasangati two bottle bars employed sixteen staff who were found to have twenty separate STDs between them, a prevalence rate four times higher than that found in the more traditional bars.[40] It seems though that risk had little deterrent effect for some men. In the early 1970s, 215 out of 292 university students infected with an STD identified barmaids as their contact. Two-thirds of these men were infected more than once within eighteen months.[41]

In order to achieve a fuller understanding of the spread of STDs in this society it is necessary to move beyond this focus on the well-known high-risk groups, and analyse broader patterns of behaviour and Buganda's changing sexual culture. At the start of the 1970s, Kisekka, asserted that in terms of sexual attitudes there existed a clear distinction between her object of interest,

[38] Kilbride, 'Barmaiding', pp. 240–6; V. Ongom, 'A study of the prevalence of sexually transmitted diseases amongst bar attendants and a surveillance on their movements for a year in the Kasangati defined area', *Makerere Medical Journal* (Oct. 1978), pp. 9–13.

[39] Kilbride, 'Barmaiding', p. 242; S. Musisi-Mulindwa, Letter to the editor, *Taifa Empya*, 12 Jan. 1970; Samuel Kalwanyi, Letter to the editor, *Taifa Empya*, 13 Mar. 1970; Mr. S. Nsubuga, Letter to the editor, *Taifa Empya*, 21 Oct. 1970.

[40] Ongom, 'Study', pp. 1–12.

[41] O. Arya and C. Bosa, 'Treatment of gonorrhoea with three different penicillin schedules—a preliminary report', Uganda Medical Association Annual Scientific Conference, 19–20 Feb. 1972, pp. 1–4.

the urban, educated youth, and the wider population within Buganda. All of the young adults whom she interviewed in Kampala reported having been sexually unfaithful. Significantly, she found that the dividing line was between the generations rather than between the Ganda and immigrants, a sign of the growing homogenization of sexual patterns across the region.[42] But even within Buganda it would be wrong to exaggerate the marginality of Kisekka's subjects. In 1969, 60% of the population were under twenty-five, and around 80% of teenagers had some education. Elite groups, moreover, were intimately connected to the rest of society by ties of kinship, clientship and affection. For example, one of the most distinctive features of Buganda's social life, noted by academics and local journalists alike, was that its bars were not segregated by class. According to Robbins and Pollnac, 'People from different tribes, owners and tenants, neighbors, halfcastes, etc., normally drink in the same places. In fact, a major role of drinking in Kiganda society has been to narrow social distance and integrate people from various social positions in the society.' Moreover, in a rich analysis of sexual behaviour in 1980s Buganda, Christine Obbo demonstrated how regularly rural and urban networks interlinked. This theme had also featured prominently in her doctoral work in the early 1970s, when she identified *bakirerese*, rootless women who shuttled between lovers in town and countryside, as the key transmitters of urban norms into the villages. Obbo reported that rural men found *bakirerese* exciting to look at and talk to, due to their modernity, while rural women emulated them partly because they feared they would otherwise appear too dull to keep hold of their husbands, partly in order to ensure that men did not spend all their income on chasing 'town' women. 'Village women were demanding outings to bars where they could get bottled drinks even if it was Coke or Fanta, and dance to jukebox or band music.' Beyond the sphere of personal relationships Ganda society was also interconnected through networks of communication and fashion. A 1969 study of a community in rural Buddu county found that around a half of all adults went to the cinema and read magazines, 39% of households owned a radio, and 42% of women had straightened hair, one of the markers of the town woman. In addition bars in trading centres gave their customers 'access to the national culture through mass media (e.g. radio, TV, dress, music) and the exchange of information'.[43]

[42] Kisekka, 'Heterosexual', pp. 1–5.

[43] Uganda, *1969 Census*; M. Robbins and R. Pollnac, 'Drinking patterns and acculturation in rural Buganda', *American Anthropologist*, 71, 2 (1969), pp. 278–81; 'Man about town', *Uganda Argus*, 8 Jan. 1972, p. 4; C. Obbo, 'HIV transmission through social and geographical networks in Uganda', *Social Science and Medicine*, 36, 1 (1993), pp. 949–55; Obbo, 'Town', pp. 187–90. In Kampala in the 1960s though immigrants had often clustered in their own drinking places, preferring their own forms of beer to Ganda *mwenge*.

It is also important to note that East Africa became much more heavily urbanized as the 1970s progressed. Some studies have approached the relationship between urbanization and the spread of HIV by focusing only on the role of cities and major towns.[44] But in this region smaller urban centres were crucial to the diffusion of the epidemic. Kampala, it should be noted, grew much more slowly than any other East African city over this decade, primarily because of Amin's misrule, while for similar reasons the population of major garrison towns like Entebbe increased marginally or actually shrank in size between 1969 and 1980. Instead, the defining feature of urbanization in Buganda during the 1970s was the mushrooming of small towns and trading centres, particularly those located near borders and major routes. By 1980 then the relative decline of Uganda's major urban centres was countered by the eruption of new towns like Kyotera, which grew fat on the *magendo* black market economy, and which played a major role in dispersing urban sexual norms into the countryside and in connecting up localized sexual networks.[45]

Urban and rural society then seem to have been strikingly integrated in Buganda. Kisekka's assertion though that there existed a divide between modern liberal attitudes to sex and those more associated with tradition does seem to have some validity, at least initially. The periodic upwelling of moral outrage which characterized Uganda's newspapers through the colonial period and 1960s continued into the early 1970s, but then seems to have remained largely quiescent over the next decade. In 1971, for example, the media themselves came under attack when the cartoon character 'Ekanya' in the main national paper was considered to have crossed a moral boundary. In Ekanya's first incarnation he was used by the colonial state to educate Ugandans in the modern skills of agriculture, voting, and hygiene. Ekanya symbolized ignorant backwardness, and fully entered public consciousness when he featured in a campaign against intestinal worms, squatting in the long grass. In 1969 Ekanya was revived, but the crudity now was sexual, and his backwardness had been supplanted by the urbane craftiness of the middle-aged serial adulterer. Two years later Ekanya went further than merely chasing women. For the first time he was depicted in the act of adultery, having been caught by his wife in bed with a bare-breasted woman. Ekanya's response to his wife's tears, 'Stop looking so holy! You also cheat me . . . You cheated me at golf yesterday!', provoked particular condemnation from a number of

[44] e.g. R. Gray et al., 'Spatial phylodynamics of HIV-1 epidemic emergence in east Africa', *AIDS*, 23, 14 (2009), pp. 9–17.

[45] Uganda, *1969 Census*; Uganda Census office, *Report on the 1980 Population Census: Vol. 1 Provisional Results by Administrative Areas* (Kampala: Census Office, 1982); J. Iliffe, *The African AIDS Epidemic: A History* (Oxford: James Currey, 2006), p. 25. Two-thirds of barmaids in Lyantonde, a major truckstop, tested positive for HIV in 1986.

letter writers. But the paper defended itself on the grounds 'that such phenomena are quite common and that they are public knowledge. Ekanya only reflected what is real in our society.' 'The man we admire is the man who is crafty, reckless even satanic. He dangles a cigarette upon his lips, plays around with a car key, and can play off a dozen women friends . . . one against the other. It is a James Bond world in which individualism, not community life is triumphant.' The problem supposedly was that Ekanya publicized what people wanted to remain unspoken. The next month the *Uganda Argus* returned to this theme in response to Makerere University's vice-chancellor's call on the youth to no longer let 'the ethical decadence of developed countries corrupt what was most admirable in African society.' The editor, equating the search for true authenticity with retrogression, suggested instead that the need was 'to marry our past ethical codes with this secular world of drug addiction, sexual permissiveness, drunkardness and power corruptions'.[46] The challenge posed by evolving moral codes also featured prominently in Luganda love songs of the early 1970s. One began by asking the singer's loved one to 'walk in front of me so that I may watch your beautiful big legs' but then begged her to take him to her parents so that they could get married. A common theme was that while 'infidelity is natural', traditional rules governing unfaithfulness were no longer being observed. Some people considered themselves too modern to conceal their affairs, while others had lost all self-control. 'When he looks at another woman his mouth waters. When he is driving in a car and passes by one on foot, he almost has an accident . . . Why is your heart never content, but is instead always hungering after another. Those extra-marital affairs will cause diseases like gonorrhoea and syphilis which will in turn infect your wife.' In these songs, women, proposing a more companionate form of marriage, complained that their husbands no longer just strayed, they were almost permanently absent. 'I did not marry to eat alone, stay alone.'[47] By the mid-1970s though this musical style had declined in popularity, being overtaken by Zairois, disco and soul music, more sexualized genres that were less concerned with the need to uphold marriage. Similarly moral outrage featured rarely in Uganda's newspapers after 1973, so that a man's infidelity was only worthy of comment when he was beaten up by his wife.[48]

[46] *Uganda Argus*, 10 June 1971, p. 6; Dent Ocaya Lakidi, *Uganda Argus*, 3 July 1971, p. 2; 'Accent on Good Morals', *Uganda Argus*, 19 July 1971, p. 5; Viewpoint, *Uganda Argus*, 20 July 1971, p. 2.

[47] Kisekka, 'Heterosexual', pp. 78–93.

[48] S. Nannyonga-Tamusuza, *Baakisimba: Gender in the Music and Dance of the Baganda People of Uganda* (New York: Routledge, 2005), p. 127; 'Any day of the week you'll find young people dancing to band music', *Uganda Weekly News*, 7 May 1978, p. 11; 'Wife beats husband', *Munno*, 16 Feb. 1977.

The most visible sign of changing sexual norms was the new popularity of erotic imagery and writing. Around 1968 mainstream cinemas started to show films which veered between sex education and soft pornography. These proved so popular that by early 1972 *Love in our Time* [advertised as 'The facts about the couples'], *Helga and the Sexual Revolution* ['The art of love-making in colour'] and *Grimm's Fairy Tales for Adults* ['For mature audiences'] were all on extended release. No data on cinema attendance could be found for that year but in 1959 there were already 1,800,000 cinemagoers in Uganda. It is likely that the numbers would have increased over the following fifteen years. Presumably cinema attendance dropped as the economic crisis worsened but in the late 1970s pornography was still being shown in Uganda, though Blaxploitation films like *Superfly* commanded the biggest audiences, admired for the 'prime beef' on display, according to one review. Plays at the National Theatre in the late 1970s meanwhile focused heavily on themes of infidelity, young men's promiscuity in the city, prostitution, and incest. Pornographic magazines such as *Mayfair* and *Playboy* seem to have been popular in the 1970s, as was *Ekitabo ky'Ekyama* [The Book of Secrets about Sex], a series mostly in Luganda containing content copied from biology textbooks and western erotic magazines, information about the sexual customs of various ethnic groups, and letters to the editor. This publication was sold from markets and verandas in urban centres across Buganda and was reportedly read by a third of secondary schoolchildren surveyed in the early 1970s. The author, a self-trained sex therapist, claimed, presumably with some exaggeration, to receive hundred of letters a day on subjects such as 'How to seduce women?', 'Girlfriend's infidelity' and 'How can I detect a woman with any sexual diseases?'[49]

National newspapers too became increasingly sexualized as the decade progressed. In the early 1970s an article which observed that everyone knew which bars were the best for extramarital sex was a relative rarity. By 1976 it was not. One of many examples from that year was a travel piece which discussed the merits of red light districts around the world: 'do not forget in Addis Ababa to visit Mercato, and if ever you visit Hamburg do not miss Saint Pauli.' And from 1978, partly no doubt to fill space cheaply, the papers were increasingly dominated by serialized fictional accounts of the sexual lives of young people in the city. One of the most prominent themes of these serials was the materialization of sex. Elite foreign brands were fetishized as

[49] *Uganda Argus*, 7 Jan. 1972 and 24 Feb. 1972; J. Banfield, 'Film in East Africa: A report', Transition, 13 (1964), pp. 18–21; *Uganda Weekly News*, 5 Feb. 1978; *Uganda Weekly News*, 14 May 1978, p. 11; *Uganda Weekly News*, 3 Dec. 1978, p. 9; 'Ekivve', Theatre review by Judith Naluggya, *The Weekly Topic*, 21 January 1980, p. 10; Kisekka, 'Heterosexual', pp. 5, 94–6; *Uganda Argus*, 7 July 1971 p. 3; Manyolo, 'Factors', pp. 1–2. Ugandans also read *Drum* magazine, whose letters pages were a further source of information on new standards of morality.

objects of desire, with women stroking their hands along their lovers' Grundig hi-fi systems. The heroine of the longest-running of these series, 'Stella's weekend', could have been modelled on some of the women interviewed by Kisekka and Obbo at the start of the decade, though she perhaps lacked their sense of grand strategy. Stella had an office job, a suburban apartment, and a steady though unfaithful boyfriend, and seemingly unconsciously fell into a cycle of affairs with wealthy, older married men. In one typical episode Stella went out with her boyfriend and two female friends, was chatted up and left with another young man. He and his friends dressed 'in flabby flairs, and huge high-heeled platform shoes, with flamboyant shirts and gaudy jackets', and had two new Honda Accords outside. He seemed 'more modern in everything compared to Ronnie', her boyfriend. Even the horoscope for 5 February 1978 suggested that sexual norms of behaviour had changed. '*Aquarius*, 'Love—go out and have your nets stretched for a big catch . . . *Aries*—If you still want to be at peace, let alone the married and the students . . . *Taurus*—Love: be very careful about members of the opposite sex who want you for just one thing only! Money . . . *Virgo*—Love: try to be as loyal to your friend as you would like that person to be to you . . . *Scorpio*—Money: invest it rather in assets than in bottles of beer and sex.'[50]

A 1981 study of STDs among students reported that 41% blamed 'sexy novels and movies' for leading them astray. But equally striking was the strong association between heavy consumption of alcohol and high-risk sex. Heavy drinkers made up 70% of cases but only 15% of controls. Fifty-three percent of cases reported multiple sexual partners, and 31% reported casual, irregular sex. According to Robbins, drinking patterns in Buganda had changed by the 1970s with *nguli*, an illegally distilled spirit, displacing *mwenge*, the traditional beer, as the alcohol of choice. *Nguli* was described by villagers as being associated with youth, excitement and strength, but also with disinhibition and sexual aggression. Robbins found that rural adults drank the equivalent of

[50] 'Man about town', *Uganda Argus*, 8 Jan. 1972, p. 4; C. Byekwaso, 'Ah! But the girls in Saint Pauli and Mercato!', *Voice of Uganda*, 10 June 1976, p. 5; A. Kayizzi, 'Shackles of polygamy', *Uganda Weekly News*, 5 Feb. 1978, p. 10; P. Mayanja, 'Too young to die—Part III: A weekly fiction', *Uganda Weekly News*, 1 Jan. 1978; C. Ndugwa, 'There is no easy way to mature love', *Uganda Weekly News*, 9 Apr. 1978, p. 12; J. Opolot, 'Unmarriageable city women', *Uganda Weekly News*, 5 Feb. 1978, p. 13; 'Stella's weekend', *Uganda Weekly News*, 16 Apr. 1978, p. 10; 'Stella's weekend', *Uganda Weekly News*, 14 May 1978, p. 10; Obbo, 'Town', p. 5; Kisekka, 'Heterosexual', p. 112; 'Your stars this week', *Uganda Weekly News*, 5 Feb. 1978, p. 13. The particular horoscope quoted here was an extreme example, but the provision of romantic advice which emphasized the materiality of sex was not unusual. For a more contemporary study of sexualized serials in Uganda see M. Gysels, R. Pool and S. Nyanzi, 'The adventures of the Randy Professor and Angela the Sugar Mummy: Sex in fictional serials in Ugandan popular magazines', *AIDS Care*, 17, 8 (2005), pp. 967–77.

seventy grams of alcohol per week on average, not remarkably high by western standards, but three-fifths of their alcohol consumption was *nguli*.[51] Interviewees repeatedly associated a perceived increase in extra-marital sex in the 1970s with new forms of entertainment, identifying the cinema, bars, and nightclubs as the venues where affairs increasingly began. Bars and clubs were not new in 1970s Buganda but they seem to have become much more widely dispersed. Some sources suggested that the liberation from Amin's dictatorship reduced social controls on sexual behaviour still further. Certainly some descriptions of social life in Buganda in the early 1980s suggest a very high degree of sexual freedom.[52]

CHANGING MORTALITY TRENDS

The outbreak of AIDS in this region brought catastrophic levels of mortality. Some villages in southern Buganda and rural Buhaya lost almost an entire generation of young adults. In Kampala in the early 1990s one of the most visible signs of economic activity was the remarkable number of coffin makers along all the major roads. The contrast with the 1950s and 1960s when life expectancy soared in all three societies was tragic. But the emergence of HIV did not signal a sharp reversal of mortality trends in this region, in contrast to countries such as Botswana, Zimbabwe, or South Africa. For in Ankole, Buganda, and Buhaya the momentum of rising life expectancy had already stalled in the 1970s and early 1980s.

In general Tanzania was very successful in its efforts to reduce mortality levels before AIDS. Healthcare's share of national expenditure trebled in the early 1970s, the proportion of the medical budget that was devoted to preventive medicine increased from 2 to 10% over the 1970s, and the institutional focus shifted from urban hospitals to rural mother and child health and the creation of health posts to provide basic care in every village. Mass immunization started late in Tanzania, but by the early 1980s around half of all children were fully immunized. Uganda, once the model for tropical African

[51] Manyole, 'Factors', pp. 22–8; M. Robbins, 'Problem-drinking and the integration of alcohol in Buganda', *Medical Anthropology*, 1, 3 (1977), pp. 193–206.

[52] Male FGD Kitala, 1 Sept. 2004; Int. IST, 21 August 2004, Kagezi village, Masaka, M; Ndahura, 'Sexually Transmitted Diseases', p. 7. Attempts to control what were perceived as excessive displays of sexual promiscuity did not disappear after the early 1970s, but they do seem to have become relatively rare. A barmaid who was particularly indiscreet about where she had sex was dismissed in Kasangati in 1977, for example. Newspapers in 1984 called for moral reform, yet continued to contain highly sexualized material. Even the Luo Union, which had maintained strict control of female migrants' sexual behaviour in Kampala in the 1960s found that its disciplinary power was undermined in the early 1970s. Ongom, 'A study', p. 10; *The Star*, 2 Aug. 1984, p. 4; Editorial, *The Star*, 31 Aug. 1984, p. 2; Obbo, 'Town', p. 158.

healthcare, was rapidly overtaken, as three-quarters of Tanzanians gained easy access to medical attention, and the national infant mortality rate fell from 129 per 1,000 in 1970 to 106 in 1980. Some of Tanzania's policies proved unsuccessful, with village health posts failing due to a lack of supervision and support, and Tanzania's worsening economic situation caused severe shortages of drugs and equipment by the early 1980s even at Muhimbili, the country's flagship teaching hospital. Nonetheless, Tanzania demonstrated that ideological commitment could deliver improved standards of health at the national level. Unfortunately for Buhaya, TANU/CCM's commitment to equality had severe consequences west of Lake Victoria. President Nyerere's determination to uplift disadvantaged regions meant that areas like Buhaya suffered reverse discrimination in such fields as health provision and the allocation of government posts and secondary school and university places. Meanwhile the deliberate reduction of farmgate cashcrop prices hit Buhaya particularly hard, due to its geographic isolation and rapidly declining transport infrastructure. These factors also contributed to the rapid de-industrialization which occurred during the 1970s. Buhaya, once second only to the area around Kilimanjaro in terms of prosperity, educational attainment, and social services, now became one of Tanzania's poorest and least developed regions. Hunger, almost non-existent in colonial Buhaya, became commonplace in families with small landholdings and large numbers of children. The fragmentation of plots, declining soil fertility, worsening problems of crop disease, as well as falling incomes, contributed to this crisis. Levels of infant and child mortality among the Haya accordingly stagnated between the 1967 and 1988 censuses.[53]

By virtue of its political and geographic peripherality, Buhaya was largely ignored by medical researchers between the late 1960s and early 1980s, and no health records could be obtained there for this period. In Uganda, decline was much better recorded and explained, in the area around Kampala at least, even though most of the 1980 census questionnaires were stolen before they could be processed.[54] Perhaps what may seem most surprising about the

[53] F. Bennett, 'A comparison of community health in Uganda with its two East African neighbours in the period 1970–1979', in Dodge and Wiebe, *Crisis*, pp. 45–9; Iliffe, *East African Doctors*, pp. 200–12; J. Iliffe interview with S. Mwankemwa (TS, 25 July 1995), RHO, MSS Afr. s. 2261; K. Havnevik, 'A resource overlooked: crafts and small-scale industries', in J. Boesen, K. Havnevik, J. Koponen and R. Odgaard (eds.), *Tanzania: Crisis and Struggle for Survival* (Uppsala, 1986), p. 274; R. Henin and B. Egero, '1967 population census of Tanzania: a demographic analysis' (BRALUP Research Notes 19, UDSM, 1972); Tanzania, *1978 Population Census: Vol. 5, Fertility and mortality data for rural and urban areas of regions* (Dar es Salaam: Ministry of Planning and Economic Affairs, 1982); Tanzania, *1988 Population Census* (Dar es Salaam : Bureau of Statistics, 1992).

[54] Pers. Comm. J. Ntozi.

Ugandan experience during the 1970s was that mortality levels did not worsen far more than they appear to have done, given how severely the economy, infrastructure, and state services provision suffered in the later years of Amin's rule. It will be suggested that the demographic and medical impact of this mismanagement seems to have been less severe than would have been expected, because the informal economy was so vibrant, food security was relatively strong, the voluntary sector expanded, and the legacy of decades of medical provision and education meant that some beneficial health habits and high levels of vaccination in the older population prevented disease levels from becoming extreme.

National levels of infant mortality are estimated to have fallen from 118 per 1,000 in 1969 to 92 in 1975, before rising again to 114 in 1978–82 and 120 in 1985. One of the districts whose census records survived in 1980 was South Kampala, whose infant mortality rate (IMR) of 77 per 1,000 was only marginally worse than Kampala's overall rate of 75 in 1969. Mothers questioned in 1977 in a survey within Greater Kampala reported that 11.6% of their children had died, compared to 18.1% in an identical study in the late 1950s. Mortality between the ages of one and five in South Kampala in 1980 was, at 49 per 1,000, 13% lower than the Kampalan rate in 1969. A major 1980 survey of a slum area of north-west Kampala found that three in four parents had lost none of their children before the age of five, a reasonably impressive achievement, but indicating nonetheless that mortality levels among the poor were relatively high. Data on parental survival in South Kampala in 1980 meanwhile show that total adult mortality was around 8% lower than that reported in the 1969 census of the entire city. Yet young adults' mortality levels were higher in 1980, most likely because of the recent worsening of maternity services and security.[55] It seems then that life expectancy probably continued to improve into the mid-1970s, and only then did a significant reversal in mortality patterns begin. Figures from the early 1980s suggest that the situation in Ankole did not worsen so severely as in Buganda after Amin's overthrow. Estimates of infant mortality for Ankole in the mid-1980s ranged

[55] A. Kasozi, *The Social Origins of Violence in Uganda, 1964–1985* (Montreal: Queens University Press, 1994), p. 196; Uganda DHS, p. 54; W. Agyei and G. Nakintu-Kyeyune, 'Mortality estimates for south Kampala based on 1980 Uganda population census', *Journal of Biosocial Science*, 20 (1988), pp. 245–9; S. Kazibwe, 'The salient factors in the aetiology of kwashiorkor' (unpublished DPH dissertation, 1976–7, Makerere University Kampala), p. 43; H. Welbourn, 'Backgrounds and follow-up of children with kwashiorkor', *Journal of Tropical Paediatrics*, 5, 4 (1959), pp. 84–6; Kizito, 'A study', p. 13; Muhammad Semwogerere-Serunjogi, 'Population dynamics in Uganda for period 1959–1969', (unpublished PhD, University of London, 1980), p. 134. The prevalence of ante-natal provision seems to have been maintained at a surprisingly high level, largely no doubt because it was cheap and required few resources, even though obstetric care deteriorated. This, and the revival of breastfeeding due to the unavailability of weaning foods, is likely to have helped limit the worsening of infant mortality.

from 98 to 108 per 1,000, compared to 116 in 1969. Infant mortality in the Kasangati Defined Area, outside Kampala, by contrast, which had fallen to 22 per 1,000 in 1969 reached 97 per 1,000 by 1984, while the crude death rate trebled over the same period, in response to the almost complete collapse of the local health centre and a sharp rise in violence, with gunshot wounds constituting the second-largest cause of death in that year. The situation was even worse in the Luwero Triangle, north-central Buganda, where a guerrilla war against Milton Obote's regime resulted in the local IMR reaching 305 per 1,000.[56] Maternal mortality as recorded in Kampala's six hospitals rose from 1.14 per 1,000 in 1972 to 2.12 in 1980 and 3.77 in 1985. Understaffing and shortages of antibiotics and other essential supplies contributed significantly to this increase, as did the growing tendency for women to deliver at home due to insecurity and transport difficulties, only reaching hospital when complications ensued. A sharp reported rise in illegal abortions was also thought to have caused many deaths, but most striking was the increase in the proportion of maternal deaths attributed to sepsis from 4% in 1970 to 41% in the early 1980s. The systems of hygiene so carefully developed over several decades for hospital and home births had largely collapsed, as supplies of antiseptic, razor blades, and surgical gloves dried up.[57] The figures reported in these paragraph should be viewed with some caution, as the accuracy of mortality recording is likely to have declined as the efficacy of the state reduced. But the apparent trend, of falling mortality until the mid-1970s and then a reversal in the Amin regime's later years, which accelerated in the early 1980s, is supported by a range of sources, and should not be lightly dismissed.

According to Dodge and Wiebe, Uganda had the best medical system in 1960s tropical Africa. Healthcare was not a major developmental priority of Milton Obote's first government but still significant expansion occurred up to 1971. Amin's takeover at first had little impact on the level of medical funding or the quality of care, but his expulsion of the Asian community in 1972 deprived the health service of many doctors and technicians, and prompted the departure of other expatriate medical staff. It also triggered a downward economic spiral which accelerated after the collapse of the East African Community in 1977. Rapidly declining real earnings, restrictions on private medicine, and political threats caused many Ugandan clinicians to leave the country so that by the end of Amin's reign the number of doctors per capita had fallen back to the level of the 1950s. Informants complained bitterly

[56] Namboze and Hillman 1987:116; UNICEF, *Children and Women in Uganda: A Situation Analysis* (Kampala: UNICEF, 1989), p. 33; C. Dodge and P. Henderson, 'Recent health surveys: towards a morbidity and mortality baseline', in Dodge and Wiebe, *Crisis*, p. 211.

[57] UNICEF, *Children*, p. 45; Int. SMD, 1July 2003, Dublin, F; A. Kampikaho and L. Irwig, 'Incidence and causes of maternal mortality in five Kampala hospitals, 1980–1986', *East African Medical Journal*, 68, 8 (1991), pp. 624–31; Int. DPO, 28 June 2004, Kampala, M.

about the neglectfulness and corruption of medical staff in the late 1970s. Amin's government undermined structures of medical direction and supervision, while healthworkers were so underpaid that moonlighting and theft of supplies became endemic. These problems deepened in the early 1980s, with medical spending, which had declined rapidly under Amin, being cut by a further 9% between 1979 and 1985, by which point the real purchasing power of the health budget had fallen to just 6% of what it had been in 1968–9. A return busfare from Kampala city centre to Mulago Hospital cost three times a nurse's daily earnings by the early 1980s. At that point more than half of Mulago's paediatric wards lacked a thermometer, blood pressure monitor, or scales. The hospital also lacked such basic supplies as surgical alcohol, soap, and bandages, and frequently had no running water, electricity, or paraffin. From the mid-1970s it became standard to instruct patients at Kasangati Health Centre which drugs they should buy from a private pharmacist in Kampala because the clinic had none to dispense itself. Mulago in the early 1980s had neither penicillin nor tetracycline, while in 1983 a survey of thirteen health centres found that on average fewer than 10% of twenty-seven core drugs were in stock.[58]

Given such conditions it is remarkable that patients continued to attend health facilities in such large numbers. According to government reports, the trend seems to have been for outpatient attendance at government hospitals to have remained largely stable until 1977–8, when it fell by almost 30%. Reported attendance at health centres and dispensaries by contrast fell dramatically in 1973–4 and then again in 1977–8 by which time it was around a fifth of its peak. It is likely that rural units had weaker access to medical supplies and certainly had inferior diagnostic capability than hospitals so would have been especially disadvantaged by the crisis in funding. Mission hospital outpatient treatment by contrast seems to have expanded marginally through the 1970s, though at most only 12% of outpatients were seen by the voluntary sector. In terms of admissions the number of in-patients received at mission hospitals fell gradually from 1972, presumably due to their suffering particularly severely from the loss of Asian and expatriate staff, but then expanded again from 1975–6, it seems to compensate for the declining capacity of the

[58] Dodge and Wiebe, 'Introduction', p. 1; S. Scheyer and D. Dunlop, 'Health services and development in Uganda', in Dodge and Wiebe, *Crisis*, pp. 27–33; Male FGD Bukoto, 24 Aug. 2004; 'Notes on paediatric teaching at Makerere Medical School, Uganda. May 1980', H. Welbourn papers, RHO, MSS Afr. s. 1872.152; Mickleburgh, 'Relevance', p. 78; R. Rwakatonera, 'Factors affecting the quality of nursing care at Mulago', in Dodge and Wiebe, *Crisis*, pp. 70–3; Int. JN, 28 June 2004, Kampala, F; A. Enns, 'The clocks have stopped in Uganda', in Dodge and Wiebe, *Crisis*, p. 53; F. Mburu, 'Evaluation of government rural health centres and UNICEF essential drug input', in Dodge and Wiebe, *Crisis*, p. 92.

state sector whose admissions fell by 30% in the second half of the 1970s. By 1978 the voluntary sector admitted a third of all in-patients in Uganda.[59]

It should again be emphasized that medical statistics' reliability declined during the 1970s, with investigations revealing that many patients' diagnosis and treatment were never recorded, and several regions and mission hospitals in any particular year failing to submit returns. So the scale of the decline in medical attendance was exaggerated by the official record. No annual medical reports, meanwhile, were available for the crucial period of the late 1970s and early 1980s. The records of the mission hospital at Nsambya in Kampala, however, have been well maintained, and probably give a more reliable sense of trends in the voluntary sector than the centrally collated data. The number of outpatient attendances at Nsambya increased more than sixfold between 1971–2 and 1983–4, with the fastest increases occurring in the early 1970s and early 1980s. The number of inpatients doubled and that of ante-natal cases and deliveries trebled between 1971–2 and 1982–3. A doctor who worked at Nsambya from the late 1970s believed that Nsambya became busier as Mulago declined, in part because the mission hospital waived its fees for the increasing numbers of the very poor.[60] It may be though that mission hospitals that were not run by nuns had more difficulty in maintaining expatriate staffing levels, due to concerns about the safety of spouses and children, and thus suffered a greater decline in capacity.

When Hebe Welbourn returned to Uganda in 1980 to evaluate how far the medical system had deteriorated since the 1960s she emphasized the shortages of drugs and equipment, the lack of supervision of staff, and the difficulties experienced in securing effective treatment by those without money or connections. But her conclusion was that performance of the state sector was patchy, not hopeless, and had proven impressively resilient in very difficult circumstances.[61] Moreover, much of the slack left by the weakening of government medical institutions was picked up by those, such as Nsambya, run by religious organizations. In addition, the late 1970s saw an upsurge in private medical activity and, more dangerously, in self-medication.[62] The decline in the number of doctors was not catastrophic, she believed, while staffing levels of midwives and nurses remained stable. In health centres where medical assistants were absent, nurses took over responsibility for diagnosis and treatment, ensuring continuity in the provision though not the quality of

[59] Uganda, 'Ministry of Health Annual Reports 1970–78', Ministry of Health Library, Kampala; Int. HM, 16 Aug. 2004, Mbarara District Hospital, F.

[60] Nsambya Hospital Annual Reports, FMSA archives, Dundalk, Ireland; Int. DPO, 28 June 2004, Kampala, M.

[61] H. Welbourn, 'Uganda—end or beginning' (unpublished TS, 1980), pp. 2–3; Int. HW, Bristol, 31 July 2008.

[62] Iliffe, *East African Doctors*, pp. 148–53; Int. HM, 16 Aug. 2004, Mbarara District Hospital, F.

service. Official data indicate that the hospital death rate increased only marginally during the 1970s, but this seems highly unlikely, given that at Mulago by the end of the decade the supply of antibiotics was intermittent, the blood donor system had collapsed, and broken sewage pipes had leaked onto the floor of the main operating theatre. At Nsambya Hospital, which maintained a much higher standard of care, the death rate jumped from 1.3% in the first half of the 1970s to 7.6% in the second. Shortages and overwork would have accounted for much of this increase. Another factor must have been that the proportion of in-patients who required surgery rose steadily during the 1970s, more than doubling over this decade, an indication presumably of declining quality of basic healthcare pre-admission, and also of increasing violence.[63]

It seems from the patchy data that are available that mortality in hospitals may have worsened in part because the pattern of disease changed during the 1970s. The incidence of malaria at rural medical units in Buganda increased from 21 to 26% in the first half of the 1970s, perhaps due to a decline in mosquito control measures. But the proportion of inpatients admitted to hospital for malaria in Uganda increased much faster, from 6% in 1970 to 10% in 1981, most likely due to the severe shortages of chloraquine, the frontline treatment, across the country. The incidence of malnutrition more than doubled at rural units in southern Buganda between 1974–5 and 1977–8, as did diarrhoea. Dysentery as a cause of admission to hospital rose from 0.6% to 2.9% between 1970 and 1981. Over the same period hospital admissions for whooping cough and measles rose from 1% to 1.4% and from 4% to 12%. Just as significantly the case fatality rate for these childhood diseases more than doubled, probably due to worsening nutrition and complications due to other infections.[64]

The real crisis in Uganda was not so much in the declining quality of curative care, but in the weakening of systems of disease prevention. Uganda had made impressive progress towards comprehensive immunization in the 1960s and early 1970s, but these gains were lost by the early 1980s. In 1973, for example, over 70% of children were immunized against tuberculosis. By 1980, fewer than 10% were. In 1983 only 5% of Ugandan children were fully immunized. Poignantly, in Kasangati, the area where comprehensive immunization had begun, fewer than one in a hundred children were fully immunized in 1984. The most disastrous consequence was an epidemic of measles which broke out in Uganda in the early 1970s, and increased in intensity until the

[63] Scheyer and Dunlop, 'Health', p. 34; D. Alnwick, M. Stirling and G. Kyeyune, 'Morbidity and mortality in selected Ugandan hospitals, 1981–2', in Dodge and Wiebe, *Crisis*, p. 85; Uganda, 'Ministry of Health Annual Reports 1970–78', Ministry of Health Library, Kampala; Iliffe, *East African Doctors*, p. 147; Nsambya Hospital Annual Reports, FMSA archives, Dundalk, Ireland.
[64] Uganda, 'Ministry of Health Annual Reports 1970–78', Ministry of Health Library, Kampala; UNICEF, *Children and Women*, p. 36; Alnwick, Stirling and Kyeyune, 'Morbidity', pp. 81–5.

mid-1980s, by which time it caused 34% of paediatric deaths at Mulago.[65] The story of sanitation is very similar. By 1962, 85% of Ugandan households had a pit latrine, a proportion which is likely to have increased over the next decade, a period which also saw major investment in safe water supply. The collapse of preventive interventions which began in 1975 meant that by 1983 the proportion of Ugandan homes with latrines had fallen to 30%, and three-quarters of boreholes in Buganda were out of action due to a lack of maintenance. Meanwhile soap production within Uganda fell 91% between 1970 and 1978, while black market imports cost sixteen times more than the pre-crisis price, too much for most households. The need for urban residents to purchase water in jerrycans also reduced the frequency of washing. Yet while the squalor of outside space in Kampala was emphasized by commentators at the end of the decade, a visitor in 1980 noted that houses' interiors were 'amazingly brightly clean'. Kyomuhendo and McIntosh have argued that 'because women were aware that lack of soap . . . led to a decline in hygiene . . . they turned to local substitutes.' It seems that while the material components of sanitation deteriorated through the 1970s, the principles which had been inculcated through decades of health education survived reasonably intact, in part because the provision of female education appears to have declined only marginally. Disease levels associated with poor sanitation could have been much worse.[66]

Similarly, there seems to be little evidence that Ugandans' nutritional knowledge declined significantly over the 1970s. By 1971 the basic message that children needed to be fed a mixed diet with a high proportion of protein-rich foods had been disseminated through numerous sources for many years. The problem was more one of food supply. The price of key high-protein foods such as eggs, milk, and meat was twenty to thirty times higher in 1979 compared to 1971, so that marketed food 'was out of reach of most people', according to one researcher. This food-price hyperinflation, which probably was most severe after the collapse of the East African Community in 1977,

[65] C. Costello, 'Maternal and child health in rural Uganda: the role of nutrition' (unpublished PhD dissertation, University of Pennsylvania, 1986), p. 124; Scheyer and Dunlop, 'Health', p. 31; Int. DPO, 28 June 2004, Kampala, M; Male FGD Bukoto, 24 Aug. 2004; Iliffe, *East African Doctors*, p. 147; Dodge and Wiebe, 'Introduction', p. 5; Dodge and Henderson, 'Recent health surveys', p. 211; K. Wotton, 'Paediatric mortality in Mulago Hospital, June 1982 to July 1983', in Dodge and Wiebe, *Crisis*, p. 76.

[66] J. Hebert and S. Ssentamu, 'Water supply, sanitation and the effect on the healthcare delivery system', in Dodge and Wiebe, *Crisis*, p. 118; H. Welbourn, 'Uganda—end or beginning' (unpublished TS, 1980), p. 2; Kizito, 'A study', p. 36; Kyomuhendo and McIntosh, *Women*, p. 154; Dodge and Wiebe, 'Introduction', p. 6. For a comparative study of the remarkable demographic impact of maternal understanding of principles of hygiene in nineteenth-century USA see M. Tomes, *The Gospel of Germs: Men, Women and the Microbe in American Life* (Cambridge MA: Harvard University Press, 1999).

would have impacted more negatively on Buganda than Ankole, since a 1968 survey had found that the average diet in Buganda was at that time slightly superior to that in Ankole only because the Ganda purchased six times as much animal protein as the Nkole. Nkole's relative self-sufficiency seems to have protected them from the worst effects of Amin and Obote II's regimes. Nutritional surveys indicated that average weight for height declined very little in Ankole between 1971 and 1981. But in the latter year two and a half times as many children fell below the 80th percentile for weight for height in a Kampala slum as in rural western Ankole. Strikingly, a 1980 study had found that nutritional problems were even worse in rural northern Buganda, where 18% of children were below the 75th percentile for weight for age. Most importantly this study showed that almost as many five year olds were underweight as one to three year olds. Buganda's nutritional problems were no longer defined essentially by a poor selection of foodstuffs during the period of weaning, but now simply indicated an absolute food shortage.[67] This was shown particularly clearly by the changing pattern of birthweight of babies born in hospital in Buganda, a highly effective marker of maternal nutritional status. The average birthweight of babies with Ganda mothers had increased by 2% during the 1960s at Kampala's Nsambya hospital, remained stable through to 1974, but then fell 1% by 1979 and another 1% by 1984. The proportion of babies who weighed less than 2,500 grams and therefore were defined as low birthweight had fallen from 10% in 1959 to 5% in 1969 and then rose to 8.5% in 1984 (see Figures 7.11 and 7.12). Revealingly, Ganda babies born in 1979 at Nsambya's private ward weighed 3.5% more than their non-elite cousins, though even the wealthy seem to have been affected to some degree by the shortages. Babies born to mothers able to afford private healthcare weighed 0.6% less in 1979 compared to 1974. The same missionary order also provided a maternity service at Nkokonjeru Hospital, in a deeply rural community fifty kilometres from Kampala. In the 1960s Ganda babies here weighed 110 grams more than their urban counterparts, presumably because of the high purchase cost of the Ganda staple, plantains, in the city.

[67] J. Mugisha, 'Prevalence of malnutrition in Kayunga using weight for ages as the index' (unpublished DPH dissertation, Makerere University Kampala, 1980), pp. 20–33; Ministry of Planning and Economic Development, *Rural Food Consumption Survey, 1968, in Ankole, Busoga, Masaka and West Nile* (Entebbe: Government Printer, 1970), pp. 27–8; G. Imani, 'A survey of health problems among school children in Igara county, Bushenyi district, Uganda' (unpublished DPH dissertation, MUK, 1981), pp. 34–8; Costello, 'Maternal', pp. 230–50; UNICEF, *Children and Women*, p. 43; Scheyer and Dunlop, 'Health services', pp. 27–33. It should be noted that 1980 was a year of particularly poor rainfall in Uganda, and that the fall in average weight almost certainly was due to the declining availability of anti-helminthic drugs as well as of food. Moreover, expanding family size, a reduction in average landholding size, and declining soil fertility would also have contributed to worsening food security.

Nkokonjeru's average birthweight then rose by 4% by 1974, before falling by 3% by 1979 and 9% by 1984. It seems then that Ganda mothers were better fed in the countryside than the city until 1974. But rural Buganda suffered more during Amin's declining years and especially during the horrors of Obote II, as the distribution of high-value food to remote areas became extremely difficult. Deprivation was commonplace during these years, but more intense in some areas and for some social groups than others.[68]

SEXUALLY TRANSMITTED DISEASES: TRENDS AND CONTROL

It is commonly acknowledged that one of the reasons why HIV spread so fast in East Africa during the 1980s was because other STDs were already common in the region. Syphilis, chancroid, and other infections which caused open sores to form in the genital area enhanced the risk of HIV transmission during sex. Even non-ulcerative STDs such as gonorrhoea encouraged the concentration of CD4 cells in the genitalia, increasing receptivity to HIV, while people co-infected with an STD had higher levels of HIV in their sexual fluids.[69] However, it is not yet well known whether levels of STD infection were stable or rising in the late 1970s and early 1980s, the period when HIV transmission increased in rapidity. Only a tentative answer can be given to this question, due to the inadequacy of medical statistics in this era. The medical archives relating to these years remain largely closed. The centralized data that have been published declined in quality and geographical specificity over time, and were largely absent between 1978 and 1984 in Uganda. Buhaya formed such a small yet distinct part of the Tanzanian picture that national-level data there are essentially worthless. Diagnosis moreover was increasingly based on clinical signs and patients' histories as the number of facilities capable of conducting serological tests declined. The following discussion will attempt to identify broad trends from the various government reports, academic studies, and local medical records that are available, but these should be interpreted with caution.

[68] Nsambya Hospital Maternity Registers; Nkokonjeru Hospital Maternity Registers. Babies who were premature or twins were excluded from the birthweight calculation. Part of the decline in birthweight probably reflected the increasing population pressure on the land and the gradual decline of the plantain crop in Buganda, afflicted by banana weevil, nematodes, and Panama wilt. It would also have resulted, but only slightly, from the decline in average parity over this period, as higher parity women tended to have heavier babies.

[69] D. Fleming and J. Wasserheit, 'From epidemiological synergy to public health policy and practice: The contribution of other sexually transmitted diseases to sexual transmission of HIV infection', *Sexually Transmitted Infections*, 75 (1999), pp. 3–17; M. Lyons, 'Sexually transmitted diseases in the history of Uganda', *Genitourinary Medicine*, 70 (1994), pp. 143–4.

No records relating to STDs in Buhaya in the 1970s could be identified. The limited sources from the late 1960s indicated that levels of infection had declined rapidly due to the intensive campaign of mass treatment that had begun in the early 1950s. By 1987 though a random study of 2,307 adults in Buhaya found that 5.9% had active syphilis according to a generally reliable combination of the Venereal Disease Research Laboratory (VDRL) test and Treponema pallidum hemagglutination assay (TPHA) tests, which also indicated that 14.5% had suffered previous infection with the disease. The risk of infection increased strongly with the number of previous sexual partners. Most interesting of all, people in urban Buhaya had a significantly higher history of past syphilis infections compared to rural Haya, but a lower level of current infection. This may have been an early sign of behaviour change in response to Bukoba town's high HIV rate, or a consequence of the superior availability of STD treatment in urban over rural areas. Without doubt urban Bukoba was a high risk environment, given that in 1986, 38% of the town's barmaids had vaginal sores and discharge, and 55% of a small group of controls reported a previous STD infection. But rural and urban Buhaya were linked by complex networks of relationships, and in addition Haya villages continued to receive regular visits from the hundreds of sex workers who had migrated to more distant conurbations across the region. The potential of these women to disperse STDs when they returned to their rural homes was indicated by a 1989 study of a group of 105 Haya sex workers in the towns of Arusha and Moshi, which found that 53% were infected with gonorrhoea, 30% with syphilis, and 21% with chlamydia.[70]

A similar story of gains made in the 1950s and 1960s being reversed can also be told of Uganda. Here, the patchy statistics indicate though that the first signs of STD resurgence appeared in the late 1960s, but that a relative decline then followed before a second peak developed from the mid-1970s (see Figure 8.3). The incidence of gonorrhoea among outpatients at government hospitals, for example, rose steadily from 2.3% in 1965–6 to 4.1% in 1968–9, before falling back during the 1970s and then surging to 4.9% in 1981–2. Among mission hospital outpatients, gonorrhoea first peaked in 1967–8 at 3.3%, then fell relatively rapidly before climbing back to 2.8% in 1977–8. Urethral stricture among males, a common complication of advanced gonorrhoea was between four and eight times more commonly

[70] J. Killewo et al., 'Prevalence and incidence of syphilis infection and its association with HIV-1 infection among adults in the Kagera region of Tanzania: A population-based study', *International Journal of STD and AIDS*, 5 (1994), pp. 424–31; Forthal et al., 'AIDS', p. 6; W. Nkya et al., 'The role of self-proclaimed prostitutes in STD transmission in Tanzania', in Tanzania Public Health Association, *Epidemiology and Control of Communicable Diseases in Tanzania. Proceedings of the 8th Annual Scientific Conference, Dar es Salaam, 14–17 November 1989* (Dar es Salaam: Tanzania Public Health Association, 1991), pp. 12–40.

diagnosed at government hospitals in the decade after 1968 compared to the mid-1960s, though in mission hospitals a major increase was only noticeable in the late 1970s. The incidence of syphilis and other STDs such as chancroid among outpatients at state and voluntary institutions also rose briefly in the late 1960s before falling back and then increasing again from the mid-1970s.[71]

Below the national level, it seems that STDs were relatively common in Ankole in the 1970s, but more so in Buganda. Medical personnel who worked in Ankole during this period remember that STDs were frequently encountered, and that they increased significantly over time, especially following the 1979 war. A survey of several hundred rural Nkole in the early 1970s found that 4.2% of men and 2.4% of women tested positive for gonorrhoea. The only district-level STD data were derived from rural dispensaries and health centres, and thus of uncertain, but almost certainly deteriorating, accuracy. Nonetheless these showed clearly that the incidence of gonorrhoea was around twice as high in Buganda as Ankole for most of this period. Records of female outpatient diagnoses were found for Kitagata hospital in the far west of rural Ankole for 1976 and also for Masaka hospital in southern Buganda for 1979. These again suggest that while Ankole's sexual culture had come to imitate Buganda's in many ways by the end of our period, in more remote areas it remained significantly more conservative. In Kitagata only 0.4% of women were diagnosed with an STD and 0.6% with pelvic inflammatory disease (PID). By contrast in Masaka 2.6% of women had a confirmed STD, another 5.6% had a vaginal discharge, and a further 4.2% suffered from PID.[72]

Medical researchers in Buganda in the late 1970s emphasized the inadequacy of record-keeping in most institutions but observed that it was generally recognized that STDs were on the rise.[73] A number of studies certainly suggested that STDs were very common in Buganda. This, as would be expected, was especially the case among known high-risk groups. For example, 39% of barmaids surveyed in Kasangati in 1973 had trichomoniasis, 17.4% had gonorrhoea, and 6.5% had syphilis. A semi-random sample of Kampala's police in 1977 found that 2.5% of males and 23.7% of females had gonorrhoea, 28.8% of females had trichomoniasis, and 1.9% of males had nonspecific urethritis. Over the previous six months the police clinic had treated

[71] Uganda Medical Reports 1962–83, Ministry of Health Library, Kampala.

[72] Int. DCT, 20 Aug. 2004, Mbarara, M; Int. ML, 12 Aug. 2004, Mbarara, F; Int. HM, 16 Aug. 2004, Mbarara District Hospital, F; Int. JT, 16 Aug. 2004, Mbarara Hospital, F; O. Arya, S. Taber and H. Nsanze, 'Infertility and venereal disease in Uganda: A review' (unpublished TS, 1983; O. Arya, S. Taber and H. Nsanze, 'Gonorrhea and female infertility in rural Uganda', *American Journal of Obstetrics and Gynecology*, 138, 7 (1980), pp. 929–32; Uganda Medical Reports 1962–83, Ministry of Health Library, Kampala; Kitagata Hospital records store; Masaka Hospital records store.

almost 8,000 patients, 11.8% of whom attended with urethral discharge, and 2.8% with penile sores or bubo. Of those randomly surveyed, almost one in five said they had had an STD in the past six months. But even among the general public STDs were highly prevalent. Of Kampala women who were tested for STDs prior to being licenced to work as food handlers in 1976, 2% tested positive for syphilis, 9% for gonorrhoea. In 1980, 18% of women attending an ante-natal clinic in northern Buganda had trichomoniasis, the rate being almost four times higher among unmarried compared to married women.[74]

More usefully, several sources provide some sense of change over time. The prevalence of gonorrhoea among soldiers rose from 1.7% to 2.9% between 1970 and 1984, while non-specific urethritis increased still faster from 1% to 4.2%. It is, of course, problematic to compare military prevalence before and after two regime changes, though it is highly likely that the ethnic composition of the army during Obote's first and second regimes would have been rather similar. Meanwhile, the incidence of gonorrhoea in rural medical units in Buganda rose only slightly from around 4% through the 1970s to 5% in 1981–2. Southern Buganda, the centre of the region's smuggling economy, had consistently had a slightly higher incidence of gonorrhoea than the rest of the kingdom. In 1977–8, the last year in which the data were disaggregated, 8.3% of rural outpatients there were recorded as having gonorrhoea. This though was almost certainly an exaggeration, as only 3% of all cases were identified as malaria. In previous years malaria had contributed around a quarter of all disease in the area. If that was also the case in 1977–8 then gonorrhoea incidence would still have been over 6%, but little faith should be given to data of such demonstrable unreliability.[75]

A degree of mystery remains regarding STD trends in this crucial period, but it seems likely that they were moving upward in the later 1970s and early 1980s, but were not remarkably higher than they had been a generation earlier. Nor does there seem to have been major variation between urban and rural

[73] Kakembo, 'A study', p. 2; Manyolo, 'Factors', p. 13; Ndahura, 'Sexually Transmitted Diseases', p. 1.

[74] Ongom, 'A study', pp. 9–11; Kakembo, 'A study', pp. 8–36; V. Ongom et al., 'The prevalence of venereal diseases among food and liquor-handlers in public places in Kampala, Uganda.' *East African Medical Journal*, 53, 7 (1976), pp. 389–97; C. Zirabamuzaale, 'A study of sexually transmitted infections in pregnant women attending antenatal clinics in a rural health unit of Singo County, Kiboga hospital' (unpublished DPH dissertation, MUK, 1980), pp. 1–55.

[75] Ndahura, 'Sexually Transmitted Diseases', pp. 1–44; V. Ongom, 'Prevalence and incidence of venereal diseases in military communities in Uganda', East African Medical Journal, 47, 9 (1970), pp. 479–83; Uganda Medical Reports 1962–83, Ministry of Health Library, Kampala; M. Lubega, 'Knowledge, attitudes and prevalence of sexually-transmitted diseases among adolescents in Uganda' (unpublished MA dissertation, Makerere University Kampala, 1991), p. 76.

prevalence. The HIV epidemic then does not seem to have developed on the back of a sustained increase in STD levels after 1970. There were peaks and troughs during this period, and while it does seem that the overall trend was for STD levels to rise, the data suggest a return to the levels of the 1950s rather than anything unprecedented. The thesis that AIDS emerged out of the exceptional circumstances of the late 1970s and early 1980s seems not very well evidenced. The possibility remains that STD prevalence was increasing rapidly near the border between Buganda and Buhaya after 1970, but more local-level statistics will need to be found if that hypothesis is to be confirmed.

The higher-risk sexual practices discussed earlier in this chapter would have contributed to this rise in STD levels, but so too did the deteriorating quality of medical care in the region. STD specialists complained during the 1970s that drugs to which STDs were known to be resistant were commonly prescribed in many medical units. Worse still, in some units when no antibiotics were in stock, placebos were given. In 1979 only 15% of women with trichomoniasis in a rural area had received the appropriate treatment. Unsurprisingly illicit sales of antibiotics, already a problem in the 1950s, became extremely common in the 1970s. As well as involving the re-use of unsterilized needles, these black market treatments commonly underdosed sufferers, accelerating the development of drug-resistant strains of gonorrhoea and chancroid. One study told the story of a man in 1974 who:

> had contracted gonorrhoea from his brother's wife while his brother was on safari [travelling]. When advised to bring his consort for treatment, he informed the researcher that there was no need to worry on that score; his brother was regularly taking a capsule or two of tetracycline before and after intercourse with anyone, including his three wives because he did not trust women. He had the belief that the medicine secreted in his sperms during intercourse was curing his wives too.

The informant had himself recently bought hundreds of tetracycline capsules.[76] As testing became rare outside the major hospitals, the accuracy of diagnosis meanwhile must also have decreased, which perhaps contributed to the increasing prevalence of non-specific urethritis. The system of partner tracing, which had never worked perfectly, also seems to have reduced in effectiveness over the 1970s.[77] Meanwhile, although regulations in both

[76] Kakembo, 'A study', p. 36; Zirabamuzaale, 'A study', p. 68; B. Ndahura, 'Sexually Transmitted Diseases', pp. 11–13, 57; Manyolo, 'Factors', p. 3.

[77] Int. DPO, 28 June 2004, Kampala, M; C. Olayiwola Akerele, 'Review of present M.C.H. services in West Mengo' (unpublished DPH dissertation, MUK, 1971), p. 53; Int. JT, 16 Aug. 2004, Mbarara Hospital, F; Int. HM, 16 Aug. 2004, Mbarara District Hospital, F; Int. ML, 12 Aug. 2004, Mbarara, F; J. Owange-Iraka, 'Congenital syphilis as seen at Mulago hospital' (unpublished MMed. (Paediatrics) dissertation, MUK, 1976), p. 13; Ndahura, 'Sexually', p. 41.

Tanzania and Uganda required compulsory treatment of barmaids, this system was not sustained under Amin, and it seems operated only sporadically in Buhaya, given that in 1986 more than a third of Bukoba's female barstaff had an STD.[78] It seems moreover that health education through schools, the media, and other channels also suffered during the 1970s. It was striking how infrequently STDs were mentioned in the national newspapers during that decade. A 1980 study of Makerere University students, whose awareness should have been above average, was very telling. Only 29% had any knowledge of STDs and none knew how to avoid becoming infected. In 1968 by contrast all students had known about STDs and 24% had some understanding of prophylaxis. It seems that the medical information regarding STDs that had been provided in Uganda before 1970 had not embedded itself in popular consciousness, or was no longer passed on to the young.[79]

FERTILITY

Uganda is not one of the countries normally associated with fertility decline in Africa. As of 2009, its total fertility rate (TFR) was the highest on the continent, and had changed very little in almost half a century. Yet the national rate concealed sharp differentials between different areas, with Buganda and Kigezi having substantially lower TFRs than the rest of the country. Tanzania's fertility decline appears to have started in the early 1980s. By 2005 its TFR had fallen to 5.7, but in the Kagera Region within which Haya predominate the TFR was, at 7.3, the second highest in the country. The three case study areas had had an unusual fertility experience during the colonial period, with Ankole's birth rates rising early to an extremely high peak, while Buganda and Buhaya's remained particularly low before undergoing a sharp increase in the last years of empire. Fertility levels in all three societies converged at a high level in the 1970s. But then, while birth rates in Ankole and Buhaya continued to rise into the new millennium, in Buganda they took a different trajectory after 1980. It is remarkable that Buganda's escape from a pattern of low fertility lasted little more than a decade. Indeed, the first signs of fertility limitation emerged in and around Kampala in the 1950s, and were sustained

[78] Kakembo, 'A study', p. 78; *Uganda Argus*, 16 Feb. 1972, p. 3; Female FGD Nyamitanga, 19 Aug. 2004; Male FGD Ruti, 19 Aug. 2004; Int. ML, 12 Aug. 2004, Mbarara, F; Int. DCT, 20 Aug. 2004, Mbarara, M.

[79] Manyolo, 'Factors', p. 24; O. Arya and F. Bennett, 'Attitudes of college students in East Africa to sexual activity and venereal disease', *British Journal of Venereal Diseases*, 44 (1968), p. 162. The papers were not totally silent on the subject of STDs. See e.g. Law obeyer, Tororo, Letter to the editor, *Voice of Uganda*, 17 Mar. 1975; *Uganda Weekly News*, 4 June 1978, p. 10.

at a low level through the years of economic crisis, political insecurity, and social dislocation that followed. The story of fertility decline in central Buganda is just as remarkable as the speed with which birth rates had risen in the preceding decades.[80] That it has largely escaped academic attention is due to the decline in ideal and completed family size coinciding with a rapid reduction in levels of female infertility. The average woman may have wanted a smaller number of children, but far more women than before were able to have a family.

Early explanations of the decline in fertility levels in Africa were influenced by demographic transition theory, which held that birth rates would fall in response to improvements in living standards, life expectancy, and especially infant survival. Researchers at first concentrated on the role of education, the availability of contraception, and women's increasing involvement in the workplace in enabling reproductive decision-making to shift from the lineage to the individual.[81] More recent analysis, however, has challenged the assumption that fertility decline in Africa would follow the pattern set in other parts of the world. The decline in birth rates in many African societies coincided with the introduction of structural adjustment policies which brought worsening unemployment, urban poverty, and a weakening of state educational and medical systems. The exceptionally negative context within which fertility decline occurred in much of Africa has forced a reassessment of the motivations underlying fertility limitation, which has placed emphasis more on Africans' desire to maintain rather than enhance their living standards and children's life chances.[82] Moreover, the experience of Kenya, where the TFR fell rapidly during the 1980s and early 1990s but then stalled at a relatively high level of five births per woman, has challenged the assumption that demographic transition is irreversible. One influential outcome of this rethinking has been Caldwell, Orubuloye, and Caldwell's thesis that contraception would be utilized differently in Africa, due to the sustained power of

[80] Population Reference Bureau, *World Population Report 2009 Datasheet* http://www.prb.org/pdf09/09wpds_eng.pdf; UBOS and Macro International, *Uganda Demographic and Health Survey 2006* (Entebbe and Calverton MD: UBOS and Macro International, 2007), p. 54 http://www.measurehs.com/pubs/pdf/FR194/FR194.pdf; UBOS and Macro International, *Uganda Demographic and Health Survey 2000-01* (Entebbe and Calverton MD: UBOS and Macro International, 2001), p. 43; National Bureau of Statistics and ORC Macro, *Tanzania Demographic and Health Survey 2004-05: Key Findings* (Calverton, Maryland, USA: NBS and ORC Macro, 2005), p. 3. Fertility decline has not affected Buganda uniformly. Rakai in the southwest for example has relatively high marital fertility.

[81] Cf. S. Szreter, 'The idea of demographic transition and the study of fertility change: A critical intellectual history', *Population and Development Review*, 19, 4 (1993), pp. 659–701; K. Mason, 'Explaining fertility transitions', *Demography*, 34, 4 (1997), pp. 443–54.

[82] D. Potts and S. Marks, 'Fertility in Southern Africa: The quiet revolution', *Journal of Southern African Studies*, 27, 2 (2001), pp. 190–200.

pro-natalism and birth spacing traditions. Rather than being employed as a means of stopping further pregnancies once a desired number of children had been achieved, which is the pattern elsewhere in the world, contraception would be used by Africans as a culturally acceptable substitute for traditional birth spacing techniques. These scholars predicted therefore that African fertility decline would affect women of all ages and parities.[83] More recently the work of Victor Agadjanian, Jennifer Johnson-Hanks, Tom Moultrie, and Ian Timaeus among others has turned attention increasingly to the apparent frequency with which Africans have understood fertility limitation in terms of postponement until personal or social circumstances improve. Of course for many women, circumstances may never improve, but if the focus is placed on intention rather than reproductive outcome, then such behaviour should not be viewed as 'stopping'. The particular attraction of this theory is that it can help explain emerging patterns of fertility decline in particularly troubled situations, such as central Uganda in the 1970s and early 1980s.[84]

What survived of the 1980 census in Uganda had little to say about fertility. Not until 1988 with the publication of the country's first Demographic and Health Survey (DHS) did the first suggestive evidence of Buganda's fertility decline emerge. Whereas the DHS found that on average women aged 40–49 in Kampala had given birth to 7.8 children, it was calculated that the city's TFR was only 6.2 live births per woman between 1982 and 1984, and 5.9 between 1985 and 1988. Kampala's birth rates then seem to have peaked at a high level in the 1970s but had started to fall by the early 1980s. In the rest of Buganda fertility levels reached their maximum in the early 1980s and then started an uneven decline between 1985 and 1988.[85] It would be incorrect to assume from these data that Ganda suddenly became interested in fertility decline around 1980. Instead what seems to have happened is that a long-running struggle between factors favouring fertility limitation and those encouraging maximization finally turned in the former's favour. Fertility had risen rapidly from the 1950s for a number of reasons. Tolerance of extra-marital reproduction increased. The duration of breastfeeding fell rapidly in the late colonial period, partly because of the popularity of bottle-feeding.

[83] J. Caldwell, I. Orubuloye and P. Caldwell, 'Fertility decline in Africa: a new type of transition?', *Population and Development Review*, 18, 2 (1992), pp. 211–42.

[84] V. Agadjanian, 'Fraught with ambivalence: Reproductive intentions and contraceptive choices in a Sub-Saharan fertility transition', *Population Research and Policy Review*, 24, 6 (2005), pp. 617–45; J. Johnson-Hanks, 'The lesser shame: abortion among educated women in southern Cameroon', Social Science and Medicine, 55, 8 (2002), pp. 1337–49; I. Timaeus and T. Moultrie, 'On Postponement and Birth Intervals', *Population and Development Review*, 34, 3 (2008), pp. 483–510.

[85] UBOS and Macro International, *Uganda Demographic and Health Survey 1988* (Entebbe and Calverton MD: UBOS and Macro International, 1988), p. 19. Subsequent DHS reports confirmed this trend towards fertility decline.

Most importantly, women's reproductive health improved. The incidence of STDs was relatively low for much of this period. It is likely, moreover, that the impact of STD infections on female fecundity fell as treatment reduced their duration and severity. In addition, the medicalization of childbirth reduced pregnancy loss and post-partum complications. Accordingly, the proportion of women aged over twenty-five who were childless fell sharply from 14% in 1969 to below 5% in the early 1990s.[86]

Buganda's fertility then had seemingly increased from the 1950s primarily because of a shortening of birth intervals, a possible increase in the length of women's reproductive lives, and a decline in sterility. Yet this fertility increase coincided with the first signs of interest in fertility limitation. By 1955 'it was commonplace for women in Buganda to seek advice on family planning when bringing their offspring to infant welfare clinics.' The provision of advice and contraception improved from 1963 when the Family Planning Association of Uganda opened its first clinic in central Kampala. At first women who sought to control their fertility were criticized for wishing to imitate Europeans, for participating in a western plot to limit the numbers of Africans, or for seeking to have risk-free extra-marital sex. Male Ganda were particularly suspicious of any threat to their numerical predominance within the country, fearing in the 1950s that they were going to be swamped within their homeland by immigrants from more prolific ethnic groups, and in the 1960s, with a degree of paranoia, that the abolition of the Ganda monarchy would be followed by their enforced sterilization. Even Catholic Ganda clergy were on one occasion condemned for their personal failure to patriotically enlarge their kin-groups. By the early 1970s though media discussion of family planning was as likely to emphasize the difficulties of educating and securing employment for large numbers of children, as it was to worry about how the uncolonized lands of rural Uganda were to be filled.[87] Family planning expanded rapidly

[86] C. Crocker, 'A study of knowledge, attitudes, and practices of family planning in Uganda, East Africa', *Journal of Reproductive Medicine*, 7, 5 (1971), pp. 235–8; H. Welbourn, 'Notes on differences between Baganda and Luo children in Kampala', *East African Medical Journal*, 32, 7 (1955), pp. 291–98; H. Welbourn, 'Childhood in a changing world' (unpublished TS, n/d, Hebe Welbourn papers); J. Nabaitu, C. Bachengana and J. Seeley , 'Marital instability in a rural population in South-West Uganda: Implications for the spread of HIV-1 infection', *Africa*, 64, 2 (1994), p. 250.

[87] R. Hennessey, 'Personal reminiscences', RHO, MSS. Afr. s. 1872, Box XVIII; A. Nyika, 'A study to assess the effectiveness of counselling services provided by Family Planning Association of Uganda at Kampala Clinic between January 1991 and December 1991' (unpublished Diploma in Adult Education dissertation, MUK, 1992), p. 2; M. Southwold, 'The Baganda of central Uganda', in A. Molnos (ed.), *Cultural Source Materials for Population Planning in East Africa III* (Nairobi, University of Nairobi, 1973), pp. 172–3; R. Tanner, 'Rumour and the Buganda Emergency, 1966', *The Journal of Modern African Studies*, 16, 2 (1978), pp. 333–5; F. Meta, 'Birth control is elimination', *The People*, 5 Feb. 1969, p. 7; *Uganda Argus*, 7 Jan. 1972, p. 1; T. Knapman, 'All about women: Views about family planning', *Uganda Argus*, 7 July 1971, p. 3.

in Kampala in the 1960s, and was starting to make inroads beyond the city when Amin banned it in 1972. This decision was reversed in 1975, but some medical superintendents remained wary of such a self-evidently controversial service. Nonetheless by 1976 around 1% of Uganda's women were clients of the Family Planning Association of Uganda (FPAU), and it was believed that at least as many secured contraception from private sources. This is a very small proportion of the national population, but given the concentration of family planning provision in the capital, it is likely that the proportion of women who used fertility control within Kampala was much higher than the Ugandan average. A rough estimate would be that perhaps one in seven women in the Greater Kampala region used modern contraception at this point. Various sources indicate that many others were sterilized or aborted unwanted pregnancies, while abstinence, withdrawal, and the rhythm method were also commonly employed. In the late 1970s media coverage of the issue softened, and the Obote II regime's relative enthusiasm for family planning saw a large increase in attendance in the early 1980s. By 1984 the FPAU operated sixty-four clinics in Uganda, including thirty-seven in government hospitals, so that by 1988 a quarter of women in Kampala used family planning while in the rest of Buganda 5% used it and 49% wanted to.[88]

It is not at all surprising that a number of women adopted family planning around Kampala in the 1960s. The majority of women here had been to school, levels of female employment were high, and the infant mortality rate had fallen to around 75 per 1,000. What seems remarkable, on first sight, is that the number of family planning clients should have been ten times higher in 1976 than 1966, and rose rapidly in the grim years that followed. In fact though, as Blacker et al. have noted, such a pattern is far from unusual: 'a period of progressive affluence and education may help to create a climate of opinion favourable to family limitation. If this period of prosperity is then followed by a downturn in the economy such that people's aspirations and living standards are threatened by the increasing burden of a large family, the onset of the fertility transition may be triggered.' What was unusual about Kampala was how severe the contrast was between the good and bad times, and how early the shift occurred.[89] The early scholarly and popular perception

[88] Nyika, 'Study', pp. 1–12; T. Black, 'A survey of contraceptive markets in four African countries', *Journal of Biosocial Science*, 4 (1972), pp. 287–98; Editorial: 'Doctor's noble duties', *Voice of Uganda*, 10 June 1976, p. 4; 'Mother and child care', *Uganda Weekly News*, 19 Feb. 1978, p. 12; 'The seeds of family planning', *Uganda Weekly News*, 23 July 1978, p. 10; M. Okello, 'Family planning in difficult times', in Dodge and Wiebe, *Crisis*, pp. 235-8; FPAU, *The Story of the Family Planning Association of Uganda* (Kampala: FPAU, 2007), pp. 3–9; UBOS and Macro Int., *Uganda DHS 1988*, pp. 32–52.

[89] Uganda, *1969 Census*; FPAU, *Story*, pp. 1–9; J. Blacker et al., 'Fertility in Kenya and Uganda: A comparative study of trends and determinants', *Population Studies*, 59, 3 (2005), p. 365.

that family planning was only for the elite was not true on the whole in Buganda. What could be defined as classically rural attitudes still shaped the behaviour of many prosperous urbanites, especially those who were male, in the 1970s. In 1978 Thompson reported that desired family size among men in Kampala increased with income, an abundance of children being associated with high status, particularly within the kin-group. What Thompson defined as exposure to modernity did tend to lower family size, but a sense of relative deprivation was the crucial factor favouring family planning. 'The desire for a large family on the part of less affluent urbanites is incompatible with modern consumption aspirations.'[90] A 1971 study of 500 women attending a post-natal clinic at Mulago found that the average desired number of children was a relatively low 5.5, 60% wanted no more children, 45% had heard of family planning, and 9% had used an effective method, a very high proportion for this period in Africa. These were not elite women, for the mission hospitals provided a better standard of maternity care, and only 23% of these patients had had more than five years education. In 1977 among a group of women of predominantly modest education attending Mulago, a quarter stated that their ideal family size was one to four children, and a further 45% wanted no more than eight. The very fact that almost all women were prepared to put a precise number on their fertility aspirations was a marker of attitudinal change, for in Ankole in this period the standard response to such questions was that family size was in the hands of God, or that people should have as many children as they were capable of producing. Another 1977 study, this time in peri-urban Kasangati, found that six children were considered the ideal, knowledge of family planning was almost universal and two-thirds of women reported that they would agree to sterilization once their ideal family size had been reached. Highly educated women and the young were more favourable towards family planning, but support came from all social groups.[91]

It may be that it was the widely felt determination to maintain or strive for a desired standard of living that seems to have made stopping and postponing behaviour feature to some extent within the story of fertility control in central Buganda. In interviews all but one of the elderly informants who had

[90] R. Thompson, 'Fertility aspirations in urban Uganda', *Urban Anthropology*, 7, 2 (1978), pp. 164–6.

[91] C. Crocker, R. Trussell, H. Wallace and E. Gold, 'A study of knowledge, attitudes, and practices of family planning in Uganda, East Africa', *Journal of Reproductive Medicine*, 7, 5 (1971), pp. 235–8; Kazibwe, 'The salient', p. 42; J. Namboze and M. Kakande, 'Some aspects of knowledge and attitude towards family planning and sterilisation on the periurban area of Kampala, Uganda', in N. Mwaniki, M. Marash, J. Mati and M. Mwaniki (eds.), *Surgical Contraception in Sub-Saharan Africa: Proceedings of a Conference, Nyeri, Kenya, May 8–13, 1977* (Chestnut Hill, MA: Pathfinder Fund, 1979), pp. 74–84.

limited their fertility had done so once a desired family size had been reached. Some women wanted to cease childbearing for health reasons. A few did so because they were 'fed up with giving birth' or found it difficult to raise a large family if their husbands were away with work much of the time. But for most it was simple economic logic, whether in town or countryside. One man remembered that he had only wanted five children 'because it was useless having many who would just stay at home to look after my goats, without money to pay for themselves'. The highly monetized nature of Buganda's economy seems to have devalued children's labour value to an unusual degree. Sometimes men forced their wives to cease childbearing against their will: 'he felt it was increasing the burden on him'. But more often women emphasized that men made irrational decisions, wanting the status of a large family but being unprepared to take responsibility for the costs of childrearing. A number of women stated that they had decided to stop having children without informing their husbands. 'The problem was that my husband did not have enough money to look after all the children', as one remembered. Another recalled that 'after having my second girl, since the first two were boys, I decided to stop . . . We teachers do not earn a lot of money, so I thought we would best manage the few we had.' A third explained 'he wanted more children but I could not think of any way out when it came to educating them . . . it was my sole decision . . . you could not say anything about family planning to your husband those days.'[92] Once again, the life histories of Ganda women challenge the stereotype of their subjugation and submissiveness.

Some of the earliest statistical evidence which suggests that fertility trends were changing comes from the maternity records of Nsambya hospital in Kampala. These show that the average parity of mothers who delivered in this hospital peaked in 1969 at 4.1. In that year a remarkable 39.8% of deliveries were to grandmultiparous women, those who had five or more births. Average parity then fell steadily, reaching 3.6 by 1979, due to a sharp decline in the proportion of grandmultiparous mothers to 29% (see Figures 7.9 and 7.10). At Nkokonjeru hospital, in rural eastern Buganda, the peak in parity was higher, at 4.2, and later, occurring in 1974, and the decline in fertility thereafter was less precipitous than in the capital, but again it was

[92] Int. MGK, 26 Aug. 2004, Takajjunge, F; Int. TNN, 3 Aug. 2004, Kitala, F; Int. NNFW, 28 Aug. 2004, Kaswa, F; Int. EM, 28 Aug. 2004, Kyansi, M; Male FGD Bukoto, 24 Aug. 2004; Int. TNN, 3 Aug. 2004, Kitala, F; SKKG, Kabonera, Masaka District, 25 Aug. 2004, M; Female FGD 1 Kisaasi-Kampala, 2 Feb. 2008; Female FGD 2 Kisaasi-Kampala, 2 Feb. 2008. On reproductive decision making within families see E. Boserup, 'Economic and demographic interrelationships in sub-Saharan Africa', *Population and Development Review*, 11, 3 (1985), pp. 383–97; J. Caldwell, 'The population factor in African change', in A. Mafeje and S. Radwan (eds.), *Economic and Demographic Change in Africa* (Oxford: Clarendon Press, 1995), p. 25; Mickleburgh, 'The relevance', pp. 145, 183.

effected by a reduction in the number of grandmultiparous women who delivered in hospital. These data must of course be treated with caution, as it may be, for example, that the insecurity associated with the war of 1979 was most likely to discourage women of higher parities from giving birth in hospital, due to their greater experience of childbirth. Moreover, the decline in grandmultiparity could have been due to factors such as a sharp rise in secondary sterility or rapidly worsening female adult life expectancy, rather than spacing, postponing, or stopping behaviour. There is, however, no evidence of a drastic change in sterility or longevity during this period, and the reduction in grandmultiparity was already very visible in 1974 and continued through the 1980s.[93]

It seems significant that around Kampala the most common form of fertility control that was identified at the time was induced abortion, which is more likely to have been a technique used to postpone or stop reproduction, rather than to space births in a regular way. Most women who aborted had not yet married, it seems, which suggests postponement above all else. In the 1970s it was estimated, based on interviews by doctors, and medical records of treatment for post-abortion complications, that around a fifth of all pregnancies were terminated.[94] That a significant, but often unmet, demand for abortion may have existed among young women is indicated by the evidence reported by the 1988 DHS that, due to a sharp increase in female marriage age in the late 1970s, the median age at first birth was twenty-one months lower than the median age at first marriage in Kampala, and seven months higher in rural Buganda. Ganda attitudes towards pre-marital sex and conception had softened considerably by this time, but not all young women would have responded enthusiastically to the prospect of having a child before marriage.[95] The strongest evidence of support for stopping behaviour comes from a 1984 study which found that 65% of women wanted to be sterilized once they reached their ideal family size.[96]

The 1988 DHS showed that while spacing behaviour did contribute to the decline in fertility, among women in their late forties almost as many had

[93] Nsambya Hospital Maternity Registers; Nkokonjeru Hospital Maternity Registers.

[94] Nyika, 'Study', pp. 10–11; 'L'avortement en Afrique', *Afrique Medicale*, 13, 121 (1974), pp. 568–9; C. Lwanga, 'Abortion in Mulago Hospital, Kampala', *East African Medical Journal*, 54, 3 (1977), pp. 142–8; C. Rwabukwali, 'Adolescent fertility and sexuality in Uganda: determinants, consequences and management', (seminar paper, Arusha, 1987), p. 8; Agyei and Epema, 'Adolescent fertility', pp. 203–7.

[95] Uganda and Macro International, *Uganda DHS 1988*, p. 15.

[96] C. Lwanga, 'Interval tubal ligation', (unpublished paper presented at the Conference on Reproductive Health Management in Sub-Saharan Africa, Freetown, Sierra Leone, 5-9 Nov. 1984). Due to limited surgical capacity however, most of the demand for sterilization was unfulfilled at this time.

initially used contraception to postpone their first pregnancy as had used it after their first, second, or third child. More importantly, the majority of women over thirty who had ever used contraception only did so after having at least four children, which does not indicate that fertility control was equally significant at all parities, though it might reflect a cohort effect relating to increased availability of contraception at some point in the past.[97]

Evidence of apparent fertility decline was also found in the family reconstitution data from the semi-rural parish of Kisubi, situated between Kampala and Entebbe. Here average birth intervals, which had fallen consistently since the First World War rose from 26.1 months in the late 1960s to 27.1 months in the early 1970s, and 27.8 months between 1975 and 1979. But birth spacing rose fastest at high parities, with an increase of four months during the 1970s for women baptizing eight or more children. By contrast, birth intervals rose by only 1.1 months among women with five to seven children. Women of low parity, two to four children, who perhaps were focusing more on trying to maintain their careers, increased their birth intervals by 1.5 months. The outcome of this apparent revival of birth spacing was that the average number of children baptized per woman fell by about 5.5% from the late 1960s to the late 1970s. Most of this decline was the result of a reduction in grandmultiparity, with the frequency of women baptizing five or more children dropping from 17.9% to 14.2% (see Figures 7.4, 7.7, and 7.8).[98] Like all the results of the family reconstitutions used in this study, these parity data should be interpreted with some caution, given the limited scope for sample refinement. Moreover, it might be suspected that the unusual conditions of the 1970s might have affected the baptismal data, possibly by reducing adherence to church doctrines, or more likely by increasing population mobility. Given that the proportion of parishioners who married in church rose over the 1970s, then it would be risky to assume any decline in religiosity. But the fact that the average age at baptism rose substantially, while the absolute number of baptisms registered fell by 14%, comparing the 1970s with the 1960s, does suggest that the data became less comprehensive, which would have tended to artificially lengthen birth intervals. However, it is unclear why the effect of this underreporting might have been so much greater among women of parity 8 and above. In fact the largest increase in average age at baptism during the 1970s occurred at parity 5–7, which had the lowest increase in birth intervals.

[97] Uganda and Macro International, *Uganda DHS 1988*, pp. 32–5.

[98] Kisubi Parish Baptism Register. That overall fertility levels rose in the 1970s while the Kisubi and Nsambya data indicate a modest reduction in fertility rates is presumably explained by the sharp fall in infertility over this period. It is possible that the reduction in the number of children baptized was affected by greater population mobility during this period, though that is more likely to have been a factor during the conflict-ridden years of the early 1980s.

Moreover, it should be noted that Nyamitanga parish in Ankole also experienced a decline in the absolute number of baptisms during the 1970s, and a marked increase in the delay between birth and baptism, yet its birth interval results produced an entirely different trend from those of Kisubi, with much smaller variation by parity, and no increase in birth intervals at higher parities. The Kisubi data do not inspire absolute faith, but in combination with other evidence, do point to an unusual pattern of fertility change in this decade.

To some extent an increase in birth intervals in Buganda from the 1970s would not have been not the result of free choice, for the unaffordability and frequent unavailability of formula milk in this era caused the abandonment of bottle feeding, which had become extremely popular from the 1950s. The average duration of breastfeeding did not increase between the 1960s and the 1980s, but by 1982 all women surveyed in the Greater Kampala region breast-fed for at least six months, a remarkable return to traditional practices, albeit in curtailed form.[99] This factor, which was not a common feature of fertility decline elsewhere in Africa, would have tended to homogenize birth spacing across parities. This makes it all the more remarkable that Buganda appears to have experienced such an unusual pattern of fertility limitation, with some evidence of stopping behaviour, pre-marital prevention of pregnancy, and high parity birth spacing.[100] Four factors seem likely to explain this distinctiveness. One is the long-standing scepticism of many Ganda about the value of extremely large families which, when combined with Buganda's historic sub-fertility, seems to have underlain a common desire to have some but not necessarily very many children.[101] A second is the economic crisis in 1970s and early 1980s Uganda, which was more severe than that associated with

[99] C. Karamagi, 'Breast-feeding in and around Kampala', in Dodge and Wiebe, *Crisis*, p. 229; Semwogerere-Serunjogi, 'Population dynamics', p. 81; Welbourn, 'Baganda and Luo children', pp. 291–98; H. Welbourn, 'Childhood in a changing world' (unpublished TS, n/d, Hebe Welbourn papers).

[100] A number of studies have supported the thesis that contraception was used primarily for spacing at all parities. E. Van der Walle and F. van der Walle, 'Birthspacing and abstinence in sub-Saharan Africa', *International Family Planning Perspectives*, 14 (1988), pp. 25–6; C. Bledsoe, A. Hill, U. d'Alessandro and P. Langerock, 'Constructing natural fertility: The use of Western contraceptive technologies in rural Gambia', *Population and Development Review*, 20 (1994), pp. 81–113; D. Kirk and B. Pillet, 'Fertility levels, trends and differentials in sub-Saharan Africa in the 1980s and 1990s', *Studies in Family Planning*, 29 (1998), pp. 1–22. But see S. Walters, 'Fertility, mortality and marriage in northwest Tanzania, 1920–1970: A demographic study using parish registers' (unpublished PhD dissertation, University of Cambridge, 2008) for an important recent examination of historical data whose results seem also to indicate parity-specific fertility decline.

[101] M. Kisekka, 'The Baganda of central Uganda', in Molnos, *Cultural Source Materials II*, p. 167; Nabaitu, Bachengana and Seeley, 'Marital instability', p. 248. This was not unique to Buganda, characterizing some other societies in this region in the past, such as Buhaya.

structural adjustment during later fertility transitions elsewhere, and which made the possession of a large number of children particularly problematic. The third is the interruption in the provision of some family planning services during the 1970s, which seems to have encouraged interest in sterilization simply because ongoing contraception was so difficult to secure. The fourth is the gender politics of relationships and decision-making about fertility in Buganda. At first sight Buganda seems an exceptionally patriarchal society. It is not uncommon to see women kneel down to serve their husbands or male guests, or to adopt a soft, submissive tone of voice when speaking to them. Yet men, often correctly, suspect that this deference is frequently superficial and manipulative, and that Ganda women, especially as they mature, act more autonomously than gendered norms should permit.[102]

Ankole's reputation as a society characterized by high fertility is well deserved. In a 1985 survey the average TFR was 8.7. Yet in the late 1960s Mbarara had the highest usage of family planning per capita of all the clinics in Uganda. These early users were drawn from the town's elite, and also what were termed 'the desperate', women who had had a large number of children. On one level, the reason why Ankole's birth rates remained so high through to the 1990s was that the early investment in family planning was not sustained. The area's two clinics closed in the early 1970s, and while Mbarara Hospital's unit re-opened later in the decade it was relatively neglected by overworked medical staff whose energies were naturally focused on curative work. In 1985 the unit remained largely moribund. Surveys in the 1980s found that 85% of men knew of modern family planning methods, 65% approved of them, but only 10% of men or their wives had ever used them and less than 1% currently did so. The unavailability of modern methods of fertility control played a major role in sustaining Ankole's birth rates.[103]

Many female informants in Ankole complained that they had been unable to space their births as much as they wanted to, frequently falling pregnant while breastfeeding before they even realized their menstrual cycle had resumed. A number of women claimed that they had desired a relatively modest family size, but only a few had been able to achieve their limited goal. Some had been able to persuade their husbands to abstain from sex or practice withdrawal in order to maintain reasonable birth intervals. Others had been

[102] C. Obbo to A. Richards, 15 Feb. 1975, Richards papers, 6/25; Uganda and Macro International, *Uganda DHS 1988*, pp. 48–52.

[103] J. Ntozi, *The Role of Men in Determining Fertility among the Banyankore of Southwestern Uganda* (Kampala: Marianum Press, 1993), pp. 9, 42; Ntozi and Kabera, 'Marriage patterns', pp. 117–21; R. Turner, 'Ugandan women more familiar with traditional contraceptive methods than with modern ones', *International Family Planning Perspectives*, 17, 4 (1991), pp. 154–5; R. Cook, 'Child health in Ankole, Uganda: a Programme of immunization and health education and its evaluation' (unpublished DMed dissertation, University of Oxford, n/d [*c.*1968]), p. 175.

taught the rhythm method by the Mothers' Union.[104] But most informants had very large families, in large part, as James Ntozi has emphasized, because of the sustained power of Ankole's pro-natalist culture into the latter years of the twentieth century. Marriage for women remained almost universal, and remarriage following divorce or especially widowhood remained common. And Nkole typically continued to obey a host of ritual injunctions to have sex at particular moments in the calendar. The majority of informants expressed strongly natalist sentiments. 'For us we would produce until the eggs got over. Even if you told your wife we should stop, she would refuse, likewise your parents would reject the idea . . . There was no problem of land scarcity so having many children was imperative.' 'How do I know all these children will grow up. They might die. So if I have quite a number, and some pass away, I still will have some.' Nkole felt pressure to produce children of both sexes, but having a son was essential. 'My wife was in a risky situation. I had a tough mother who would always say, this women is not producing a boy, only girls, so send her away. But in 1977, she gave birth to a boy and she was saved.' Not only was the older generation more influential than in Buganda, but male demands for large families were even greater. Several women made comments about their husbands such as 'That man is unpredictable. I believe even sixty children wouldn't be enough for him.' There was no sign here of the secret attempts to limit family size seen among Ganda women.[105] But just as important was the low sterility rate among Nkole, with surveys in the 1970s finding that only 2% of ever married women had not been pregnant. Female age at marriage in church rose marginally in the 1970s (see Figure 7.6), age at first pregnancy remained stable at around nineteen, but almost all Nkole women had long reproductive lives.[106]

[104] Female FGD Kyenjenyi, 22 Aug. 2004; Female FGD Nyamitanga, 19 Aug. 2004; Female FGD Ruti, 19 Aug. 2004; Int. HM, 16 Aug. 2004, Mbarara District Hospital, F; A. Kamugisha, 'Beliefs and customs connected with childbirth among the Banyankole, with special reference to utilisation of modern medical services' (unpublished BA Social Work and Social Administration dissertation, Makerere University Kampala, 1980), pp. 43–4; Cook, 'Child health', pp. 94–123. Nyamitanga parish baptism registers show that birth intervals increased very slightly at parity three and four in the late 1970s but not enough to make any significant difference to overall fertility levels. Statements that informants had had many more children than they desired may of course have been conditioned by my presence, and what informants thought I would have wanted to hear about family planning, but it is unclear why my impact on the nature of testimonies would have been far greater in Ankole than Buganda and Buhaya. Moreover, informants were happy to criticize other aspects of western 'progress', such as human rights, the empowerment of women and the young, and freedom of movement across ethnic boundaries.

[105] J. Ntozi, *High Fertility in Rural Uganda: The Role of Socioeconomic and Biological Factors* (Kampala: Fountain, 1995), p. 7; Male FGD Ruti, 19 Aug. 2004; Male FGD Namitanga, 19 Aug. 2004; Female FGD Kyenjenyi, 22 Aug. 2004; Int. GK, 14 Aug. 2004, Mbarara, F.

[106] O. Arya and S. Taber, 'Maladies vénériennes et fécondité dans les régions rurales de l'Ouganda' (unpublished paper presented to the Medical Society for the Study of Venereal Diseases, Malta, April 1975); Ntozi and Kabera, 'Marriage patterns', p. 14; Mbarara Hospital Maternity Registers; Kitagata Hospital Maternity Registers.

Buhaya's transformation from having one of the lowest fertility rates in mainland Tanzania during the colonial period to having one of the highest by the 1990s is remarkable. In part the increase in birth rates reflected a wider, and just as dramatic, change in Haya society. Buhaya, once renowned for the frequency of divorce, had by the 1990s seen marriage become unusually stable and common. The proportion of women of reproductive age who were currently unmarried had already fallen significantly to 26.3% by 1973 and then fell to 22.7% in 1991. Again, high sterility rates, once a defining feature of Haya life, fell rapidly after the 1950s due to improving reproductive health, so that by 1984 southern Buhaya had the lowest levels of female infertility of seven districts surveyed in Tanzania, and by 1991 only 2% of ever married women in Kagera region were childless, the same proportion as in Ankole.[107] Buhaya's position as one of Tanzania's high fertility regions though also rested on its relative isolation, which meant that the Haya were relatively immune from some of the developments which affected much of the rest of the country after the 1960s. Buhaya's female age at first marriage remained low whereas the national trend was significantly upwards, while the duration of breastfeeding, which had been lower than the Tanzanian average in the 1970s, remained stubbornly stable through to the 1990s, in contrast to the situation in the rest of the country. By 1991 women in Kagera breastfed for a median length of twenty-five months, the second longest of any region in the country.[108] It was not long before the impact of the increase in fertility in Buhaya's densely settled eastern ridges was noticed. However, according to interviewees elders in this society were exceptionally antagonistic to the concept of fertility limitation:

[107] Henin, *National Demographic Survey*, p. 32; National Bureau of Statistics and ORC Macro, *Tanzania Demographic and Health Survey 1991–02* (Calverton, Maryland, USA: NBS and ORC Macro, 1993), pp. 53–8; L. Mtimavalye et al., 'Infertility among women in five rural and two urban districts of Tanzania', *Journal of Obstetric and Gynecology in East and Central Africa*, 3 (1984), pp. 125–9; U. Larsen, 'Primary and secondary infertility in Tanzania', *Journal of Health and Population in Developing Countries*, 3 (2003), pp. 1–15; U. Larsen, 'Childlessness, subfertility, and infertility in Tanzania', *Studies in Family Planning*; 27,1(1996), pp. 18–28. It is surprising that female sterility was so low in Buhaya in this period given this society's high incidence of STDs and large numbers of sex workers. It is likely that medical treatment limited the sterilizing complications associated with STD infection.

[108] Henin, *National Demographic Survey*, pp. 30–34; J. Lugalla et al., 'Social, cultural and sexual behavioral determinants of observed decline in HIV infection trends: Lessons from the Kagera Region, Tanzania', *Social Science and Medicine*, 59, 1 (2004), p. 186; A. Mturi, 'Patterns of fertility and contraceptive use in Tanzania' (unpublished PhD dissertation, University of Southampton, 1996), p. 119, Tanzania and Macro International, *Demographic and Health Survey 1991–92*, p. 103. Buhaya's low marriage age by the 1990s was in part however a response to AIDS.

> The older parents, they said that we did not have enough children. For example I was born alone, my mother she is the only daughter of her parents, so then when I said that I would like to have not more than six children, she said 'you see, if you will be blessed to have as many children as possible, I would be very happy indeed, because . . . you will have children who will replace those I would have borne.'

Pressure on young couples from the older generation to maximize reproduction after 1950 was particularly effective here because it derived not from tradition but from the trauma of societal sub-fertility. Parental influence over couples' reproductive decision-making declined with time, and some Haya did eventually utilize family planning 'because we were squeezed'. But most informants stated that the standard response when Haya could not sustain their growing families on their small farms was to migrate inland to Kianja, Missenyi, or Karagwe. Take-up of contraception in Buhaya was relatively low in 1991, yet the unmet need for family planning was no more than average. It seems that Haya overall were not desperate to reduce their family size, but those who did, or who stated that they wanted to, were much more likely to use contraceptive methods to seek to stop rather than space, perhaps because prolonged breastfeeding had been retained here, because of historic antagonism to extremely large families, or because Haya had a much more precise concept of how large a household could be sustained on their small landholdings than was typical of rural Tanzania.[109]

CONCLUSION

The sense that HIV in these societies emerged in a time of catastrophe is firmly entrenched in the literature. This chapter suggests that this perception

[109] Int. WR, 21 June 2000, Rubya, M; Int. AC, 9 Aug. 2000, Rubaa-Rubya, F; Int. MM B, 26 Aug. 1999, Katoma-Irogero, M; Int. FKK, 29 Aug. 1999, Kaishemarwa-Katoma, M; Int. MM, 7 Sept 1999, Rubale, M; Int. LK and SR, Bugandika, 1 Sept. 1999, M; Int. WK, 31 Aug. 1999, Igurati-Bugandika, M; Tanzania and Macro International, *Demographic and Health Survey 1991–92*, p. 66. Chrys Kamuzora's elderly informants told him that enthusiasm for large families had declined in Buhaya by the 1980s because the costs of having children had increased while the benefits had reduced due to the laziness and disobedience of the younger generation. It should be noted though that the expense of childrearing in Buhaya was presumably less than in most districts given that only 0.3% of primary graduates went on to secondary education here, while the labour value of children could not be defined as essential as adults devoted five hours a day to leisure, and six to economic activities. C. Kamuzora, 'High fertility and the demand for labour in peasant economies: The case of Bukoba District, Tanzania', *Development and Change*, 15, 1 (1984), pp. 105–24; C. Kamuzora, 'Formation of a low fertility culture in Kigarama village, Tanzania: Cultural materialism versus idealism', University of Dar es Salaam Department of Statistics Demographic Unit, Occasional Paper no. 9 (1997), pp. 184–98.

is only partly true. Without doubt poverty and inequality increased, as did urban squalor and the incidence of many childhood diseases. The quality of medical care and, in Uganda, the efficacy of government deteriorated significantly. But the immediate demographic impact of these problems appears to have been rather modest, and relatively few people in these societies seem to have been absolutely destitute. The evidence does not always provide chronological support for the catastrophe thesis. The worst period of economic collapse and political insecurity occurred after HIV had already become established. Sexual culture and behaviour had changed significantly over a period of decades prior to the 1970s, and it would be as easy to identify the late 1960s as marking a distinct shift in attitudes and practices as the mid- to late 1970s. Certainly the resurgence in STD incidence seems to have begun in the late 1960s, slowed somewhat thereafter and then risen again a decade later. The first signs of fertility decline in Buganda began before the period of economic decline started, but fertility control seems to have been sustained throughout the years of collapse, suggesting that parental ambition remained undimmed. Aspiration as much as desperation shaped attitudes to sex and reproduction in this period.

Conclusion and Epilogue: Aids and Demographic Change in Historical Context

The recent sexual and demographic history of the three societies examined in this study is one of extremes. Ankole has experienced one of the fastest population growth rates in recorded human history, whereas fertility levels were low for generations in Buganda and Buhaya until the period of independence when they appear to have almost doubled within a couple of decades. Buganda's period of high fertility was exceptionally brief, with the first signs of fertility limitation becoming visible even as birth rates moved towards their maximum. Meanwhile, in the early 1980s Africa's first mass rural AIDS epidemic broke out in southern Uganda and northwest Tanzania. Within a few years terrifyingly high prevalence rates were reported from the case study areas, but by the early 1990s evidence of a reduction in HIV infection levels had been discovered, associated primarily with a reduction in multiple partner sharing, especially among the young. The proportion of people with sexual experience by the age of nineteen, for example, fell from 72% to 49% in Uganda during this period.[1] The two most successful AIDS control programmes in Africa were to be found in Buganda and Buhaya.

This book aimed to contribute to understanding of two major issues. The first goal was to help explain the shape and timing of Africa's shift to rapid demographic expansion. The transition to population increase in this region seems to have been driven first by a reduction in child mortality rates from the First World War, quickly followed by an apparent shortening of birth intervals. A movement towards accelerating growth then became universal after the mid-colonial period due it seems to an enormous fall in levels of infertility

[1] J. Iliffe, *The African AIDS Epidemic: A History* (Oxford: James Currey, 2006), pp. 127–9; S. Ndeki, K. Klepp and G. Mliga, 'Knowledge, perceived risk of AIDS and sexual behavior among primary school children in two areas of Tanzania', *Health Education Research*, 9, 1 (1994), pp. 133–8; G. Kwesigabo et al., 'Monitoring of HIV-1 infection prevalence and trends in the general population using pregnant women as a sentinel population: Nine years experience from the Kagera Region of Tanzania', *Journal of Acquired Immune Deficiency Syndromes*, 23, 5 (2000), pp. 410–17.

and stillbirth, an increased incidence of extra-marital and post-marital reproduction, and dramatic declines in mortality affecting all age groups. With regard to the debate about the relative significance of fertility or mortality in causing Africa's modern population boom, the evidence from this study mostly supports those who emphasize falling morbidity and mortality. These conclusions are presented with some caution, given the inevitable weakness of the data from this period. In some ways the most reliable indicators of change are those which are comparative in nature. Thus the most striking aspect of demographic growth in this region is that it was fastest in Ankole, which had much lower levels of wealth, education, medical provision, or missionization than the other two societies. Ankole's experience indicates that in areas with relatively low malaria prevalence modest investment in preventive medicine could achieve impressive reductions in death rates surprisingly early. Buganda and Buhaya, by contrast, show that high levels of income and social provision in colonial Africa could have negative demographic consequences, primarily by undermining marriage.

After independence what is remarkable about Uganda's mortality trends is that life expectancy did not drop sharply during the disastrous regimes of Idi Amin and Obote II. The momentum of mortality decline was halted but not significantly reversed during fourteen years of conflict and declining healthcare provision, partly because of habits of hygiene and childcare that had been ingrained through decades of health education, partly because of the exceptional vigour of missionary medical care in Uganda. The greatest failure in Uganda was the inability to sustain levels of immunization coverage, a service which perhaps delivers maximum returns for the expenditure of limited resources of time and money, but which is exceptionally difficult to sustain in a context of insecurity, a lack of foreign exchange, and inadequate refrigeration due to an intermittent supply of electricity and paraffin.

The divergent trends in fertility in these three societies emphasize firstly the need to historicize the development of pro-natalist attitudes. In contrast to the theories posited by Jack Caldwell and his associates, the sources relating to the three societies examined for this study indicate that, in the nineteenth and early twentieth centuries, reproductive culture was not universally aimed at maximization in Africa.[2] Peoples in the Great Lakes region typically wanted some children, but what was viewed as excessive childbearing provoked disapproval in Buganda, and positive anxiety among Ankole's minority pastoralists. Ankole's cultivating majority, even though they shared the same language and many of the same beliefs as their cattle-keeping neighbours, were by contrast exceptionally enthusiastic about large family size. Meanwhile,

[2] J. Caldwell, P. Caldwell and P. Quiggan, 'The social context of AIDS in sub-Saharan Africa', *Population and Development Review*, 15, 2 (1989), pp. 185–234.

in Buhaya natalist attitudes in the 1960s and 1970s appear to have been largely shaped by the recent trauma of many decades of sub-fertility.

The second major finding of the historical examination of fertility trends in these societies is that the available evidence gave only limited support to neo-Marxist theories that the nature of the colonial economy in combination with growing demands for tax and labour pushed Africans into a higher fertility regime, primarily by facilitating earlier marriage for men, and by increasing the value of familial labour. The longitudinal data available for this study, however, show that no apparent trend towards significantly earlier marriage could be identified, and that while Ankole, the society most affected by labour migration, had the lowest male age at marriage of the three societies examined, the female age at first marriage, a much more important demographic indicator, was highest in Ankole. Moreover, most informants, particularly in Buganda and Buhaya dismissed the notion that economic pressures or opportunities in the colonial period had inflated ideal family size. Birth intervals did fall in all three societies, from as early as the 1920s in Buganda, but it seems that more important causes of rising fertility were an increase in the proportion of the population who ever married, the growing stability of marriage, an increased tolerance of pre- and post-marital reproduction, and, above all, a decline in female sterility.

The third finding of significance in relation to fertility change was that fertility decline appears to have been significant in central Buganda from a surprisingly early date, and in a context which was particularly unpropitious. Buganda before the 1970s was the kind of society where the early adoption of family planning might have been expected. It was prosperous, had excellent medical provision, enjoyed low infant mortality rates, and was characterized by high levels of female education. Sure enough, demand for fertility control was reasonably high in the 1950s and 1960s. What is so interesting is that the momentum of fertility decline was maintained and indeed increased in the exceptionally unpromising conditions of life under Idi Amin and Obote II. Women, it seems, desired smaller families because of their aspirations for material success and security. Even more distinctive is that there is some evidence that around Kampala, the strategies for achieving fertility limitation involved not only contraceptive-reliant spacing, but also postponing and stopping behaviour, through sterilization and high levels of abortion.

The other major goal of this study was to tell the pre-history of AIDS in this region. Primarily the focus was placed on the origins of the patterns of sexual behaviour and attitudes that enabled the disease to spread so fast from the late 1970s. Contrary to assumptions that sub-Saharan African societies shared a unified sexual culture in the pre-colonial period, this study found that beliefs and practices, especially with regard to pre-marital and socially legitimate extra-marital sex, varied radically across this relatively homogeneous region before 1900. Patterns of sexuality changed dramatically during the colonial period. Much of the sexual culture which facilitated the rapid transmission of HIV in the early 1980s was already in place by the 1960s. Previous research on sexual change has tended to focus on the 1970s, a time of instability and economic decline. This study set the developments associated with this decade in a longer context, noted that STD incidence data provide little sense of radical change during the 1970s, emphasized that aspiration as much as desperation fostered higher-risk sexual practices during these years of violence and black marketing, and was as concerned with the mechanisms which enabled HIV to disperse so rapidly among rural communities as it was with the emergence of the key high-risk groups which spread the disease so quickly in its early stages.

It is also worth considering to what extent the historical context helps explain the impressive though limited success of the HIV control efforts in these societies. It would be reasonable to assume that one of the reasons why people in this region were unusually receptive to AIDS prevention messages was that these societies had been some of the most medicalized in Africa before the 1970s. Most obviously, from the beginning of the twentieth century right through to the 1970s the historical record in both Buganda and Buhaya is littered with campaigns to improve public morality, by missionaries, indigenous church leaders, chiefly councils, colonial and post-colonial administrators, cooperatives, migrant groups, nationalist politicians, and public health workers. In a direct sense they achieved little obvious success, but this series of attempted reforms must have familiarized many Ganda, Haya, and Nkole to the concept of safer sex, and habituated them to external interventions in the most private aspects of their lives. One of the most striking aspects of these societies' response to HIV was their willingness to talk openly about the disease from an early date, and the compassion with which, on the whole, the sick were treated. The Ugandan and Tanzanian governments should take credit for the energy and directness with which they addressed the epidemic, but it seems clear that the role of large numbers of formal and informal self-help groups was also crucial. It is probable that the remarkable number of these groups, which created an ideal context for localized discussion of HIV and how it could be contained, was in part a consequence of the collapse of the state in Uganda, and the sense of relative neglect in Buhaya after independence. But the vitality of civil society in the 1980s and 1990s is likely to have been built in part on the legacy of the flowering of various civic associations within this region during the late colonial period. Cooperatives, the local branches of nationalist and ethnic political movements, old boys' and old girls' associations, the hundreds of community clubs and women's clubs, interest groups such as the Uganda Council of Women, and the myriad of religious organizations such as Catholic Action, the Legion of Mary, and the Mothers' Union accustomed Ganda, Haya, and Nkole to public discussion and mobilization. Given the huge membership of the cooperatives and religious bodies in particular, and the surprising frequency with which all of these associations debated issues of morality, it is likely that the majority of the population of this region were involved, actively or passively, in organized, more or less direct discussion of sexuality long before the emergence of HIV. Cultural norms in this region did not define sex as a suitable subject for public discussion, so the frankness which was so noticeable from the late 1980s needs to be explained. It may have been purely a reaction to AIDS mortality, but it seems likely that inhibitions had begun to be broken down decades previously.[3]

HIV prevalence in southern Uganda and northwest Tanzania fell from a peak of around 13% in the late 1980s to 4% in 2003, but then stagnated, before rising again gradually in Uganda, for reasons that have not yet been fully explained. Three of the key factors that have been identified though as obstructing further falls in prevalence are of some historical interest. The first is the persistence of long-established patterns of concurrent sexual partnerships. The second is an increasing generational tension, with young people reporting what they perceive to be an excess of criticism and a lack of constructive advice on sexuality and relationships from the older generation. The third is a decline in the transparency about sexual behaviour that was so striking in the 1980s and 1990s. It seems likely that these two latter developments are interrelated.[4]

[3] D. Low-Beer and R. Stoneburner, 'Behaviour and communication change in reducing HIV: Is Uganda unique', *African Journal of AIDS Research*, 1, 2 (2004), pp. 9–21; S. Wallman, *Kampala Women Getting By: Wellbeing in the Time of AIDS* (London: James Currey, 1996); J. Lugalla et al., 'Social, cultural and sexual behavioral determinants of observed decline in HIV infection trends: lessons from the Kagera Region, Tanzania', *Social Science and Medicine*, 59 (2004), pp. 185–98; Iliffe, *AIDS*, p. 129; V. Griffith, 'An enquiry into community development in Uganda' (unpublished UNESCO report, African Studies Centre, Cambridge, 1960); 'Women's advancing status in Uganda', June 1955 (ASC Cambridge, reprint from *The Times British Colonies Review*, Spring 1955): 'On tour in Uganda I have been astonished by the number of times I've been invited to a meeting of the local women's club. Even in remote places one can find groups of anything up to a hundred women collected at a meeting and anxious to learn subjects such as dressmaking, childcare, diet improvement and so on.'

[4] Iliffe, *AIDS*, p. 131–2; R. Swai et al., 'Surveillance of HIV and syphilis infections among antenatal clinic attendees in Tanzania, 2003–2004', *BMC Public Health*, 6 (2006), p. 91; Lugalla et al., 'Social', pp. 185–198; UAC, *Accelerating HIV Prevention: The Road Map Towards Universal Access to HIV Prevention in Uganda* (Kampala: UAC, 2007); S. Reddy, '"Its not as easy as ABC": Dynamics of intergenerational power and resistance within the context of HIV/AIDS', *Perspectives in Education*, 23, 3 (2005), pp. 11–19; S. Parikh, 'The political economy of marriage and HIV: The ABC approach, "safe" infidelity, and managing moral risk in Uganda', *American Journal of Public Health*, 97 (2007), pp. 1198–1208.

In recent years two major book-length analyses of the stagnation of Uganda's HIV control programme by Helen Epstein and Robert Thornton have independently identified the prevalence of medium-to-long-term sexual concurrency as a key factor which has obstructed the further decline of HIV rates since around 2000. They argue that the response to HIV focused on individual behaviour that was defined, by medical authorities and then by members of the public, as particularly high-risk. This reduced HIV infections substantially and rapidly, but self-evidently has not nearly brought the disease under control. This, they suggest, is because long-running, concurrent sexual relationships are so common, and, moreover, are generally but incorrectly regarded as lower risk. In fact, based on an epidemiological model developed by Morris and Kretzschmar, they believe that dense networks of interconnected concurrent sexual partnerships are much more likely to result in the transmission of HIV than serial monogamy, or even serial monogamy combined with occasional sex with prostitutes. This is because the average risk of HIV infection is low during any isolated sex act, and because HIV is particularly transmissible in the weeks after infection has taken hold. Where serial monogamy predominates infected individuals typically pass through the most contagious period before the inception of a new relationship.[5] Epstein asserts that Ugandans do not have more sexual partners over their lifetime than do people in western societies, but holds that the frequency with which their relationships overlap is highly dangerous in the era of AIDS. Her belief is that control messages which focus on condom usage or avoiding premarital sex will only ever have limited success in Uganda, because regular, extra-marital affairs or concubinage relationships are not confined to the unmarried, and tend to involve the use of condoms only until a sense of mutual trust is established. Epstein further argues that women involved in transactional affairs are particularly vulnerable, 'because they are more likely than other women to tolerate an unfaithful partner and also to seek out additional concurrent sexual relationships themselves'. And she notes that the development of an intricate web of indirectly related sexual partners required that women as well as men commonly maintained concurrent relationships.[6]

[5] H. Epstein, *The Invisible Cure: Africa, The West and the Fight against AIDS* (London: Viking, 2007); R. Thornton, *Unimagined Community: Sex, Networks and AIDS in Uganda and South Africa* (Berkeley: University of California Press, 2008); M. Morris and M. Kretzschmar, 'Concurrent partnerships and the spread of HIV', *AIDS*, 11 (1997), pp. 641–48. See also D. Halperin and H. Epstein, 'Concurrent sexual partnerships help to explain Africa's high HIV prevalence: implications for prevention', *Lancet*, 364, 9428 (2004), pp. 4–6; T. Mah and D. Halperin 'Concurrent sexual partnerships and the HIV epidemics in Africa: evidence to move forward', *AIDS and Behavior,* 14 (2010), pp. 11–14. The concurrency thesis is controversial. L. Sawers and E. Stillwaggon, 'Concurrent sexual partnerships do not explain the HIV epidemics in Africa: A systematic review of the evidence', *Journal of the International AIDS Society*, 13 (2010), 34.
[6] Epstein, *Invisible Cure*, pp. 54–79, 159–61, 173–96.

These are important theories, which it is important to historicize. The evidence presented in this book suggests that while concurrency is a long-established phenomenon in these societies, its frequency and nature changed somewhat over the past century. Socially legitimate extra-marital sex and polygamy seem to have declined in acceptability over the colonial period, but less regularized sexual affairs appear to have become more common and more tolerated, generally creating more open, longer-distance sexual networks. Female sexual autonomy increased markedly throughout the period covered by this book, as, it seems, did transactional and intergenerational sex. This all tends to reinforce Epstein's argument, but the story told in earlier chapters of this book indicates that her thesis could be adapted in at least two areas. The first is that her assertion that Ugandans had fewer sexual partners than Americans and Europeans is based on surveys conducted after behavioural change in response to HIV had begun. Earlier studies in Uganda, and also in Buhaya, suggested that a very high number of sexual partners had in fact been the norm.[7] The second is that sexual networks in this region, as they were described by researchers in the 1960s and 1970s, commonly linked together relatively stable concurrent relationships with often rather frequent shorter-term encounters between sex workers and barmaids and their customers.[8]

The second factor which relates to the stalling of HIV decline in this region is the strength of intergenerational tension regarding sexual propriety that can be seen in these societies. With a few exceptions the several hundred elderly informants interviewed for this book agreed, initially at least, that the sexual morality of the young in recent years was much worse than that of their own generation. Typical statements were 'When I was young it was rare

[7] For Uganda see O. Arya and F. Bennett, 'Venereal disease in an elite group (university students) in East Africa', *British Journal of Venereal Disease*, 43 (1967), pp. 275–9; H. Pickering et al., 'Sexual behaviour in a fishing community on Lake Victoria, Uganda', *Health Transition Review*, 7 (1997), pp. 13–20; Iliffe, *AIDS*, pp. 26–32; Ndahura, 'Sexually Transmitted Diseases', pp. 39–53; Kakembo, 'A study', pp. 5–29. For Buhaya see J. Killewo et al., 'Incidence of HIV-1 infection among adults in the Kagera Region of Tanzania', *International Journal of Epidemiology, 22 (*1993), pp. 528–36; D. Forthal et al., 'AIDS in Tanzania' (unpublished paper, Centers for Disease Control, Atlanta, 1986), p. 2; G. L. Dahlgren, J. Killewo and A. Sandstrom, 'AIDS epidemic in Kagera region, Tanzania: The experiences of local people', *AIDS Care*, 5, 3 (1993), pp. 352–7; J. Killewo, 'Epidemiology towards the control of HIV infection in Tanzania with special reference to the Kagera Region' (unpublished PhD dissertation, University of Umea, 1994), p. 49; J. Killewo et al., 'Incidence of HIV-1 infection among adults in the Kagera Region of Tanzania', *International Journal of Epidemiology, 22 (*1993), pp. 528–36.

[8] The significance of the latter factor was noted by Epstein towards the end of her study (p. 196). Its importance is noted in R. Anderson et al., 'The spread of HIV-1 in Africa: Sexual contact patterns and the predicted demographic impact of AIDS', *Nature*, 352, 6336 (1991), pp. 581–9; and C. Obbo, 'HIV transmission through social and geographical networks in Uganda', *Social Science and Medicine*, 36, 1 (1993), pp. 949–55.

to hear of the girl conceiving before marriage. But now a girl of thirteen already knows the shape of a man's genitals.' 'Today's young women are too free. No beating. A girl is free to have a long discussion with a boy in the street, with no one interfering with them. If you beat her, she takes you to court.' 'Now things are changing. Boys get girls to marry by themselves ... Some even meet them in bars, and from there, they take them home. [This started] when discos were introduced ... around 1975, but before that everything was OK.'[9] Yet the personal histories of these elders were rarely characterized by absolute propriety, especially in Buganda and Buhaya, the societies where criticism of the young is most intense. A number of interviewees had fathered children outside marriage, one having nine with a string of unmarried women. Another man was asked how many wives he had had, and answered two. On being corrected by a friend who was present, he clarified that he had had two proper wives, the other women he had lived with 'were just harlots'.[10] Elderly women too were often very frank about their extra-marital sex lives. One recounted 'People like money. If you have money someone can have an affair with you.' Another related that after her first marriage she did not want to marry again, but 'of course, I had several lovers'.[11] Very many old men and women admitted in a matter of fact way to having suffered STDs when they were younger.[12] This disjuncture between elders' frank confession of their own sexual immorality and their sharp condemnation of the sexual behaviour of the young seems to result from strongly entrenched perceptions about which kinds of misdemeanours were tolerable.

Elderly informants held that marriage was the marker of adulthood, the event that legitimized sexual activity. Adultery and having affairs as a widow or divorcee was immoral but not shocking, 'a mistake like other mistakes', 'a natural thing'. But to have sex before marriage was in Ankole and Buhaya 'an abomination' and in Buganda 'very wrong'—it threatened the honour of the

[9] e.g. Int. MM, 12 Aug. 2000, Kamachumu, F; Int. TM, 13 Aug. 2000, Busindi, F; Int. MM, 14 Aug. 2000, Ruhija, F; Male Focus Group Discussion (FGD) Kisubi Kiwulwe, 4 Sept. 2004; Male FGD Kitala, 1 Sept. 2004. One of the few who stated that sexual behaviour had changed little was Int. CM, 11 Aug. 2000, Rubya, F.

[10] e.g. Int. JBK, 11 Aug. 2000, Ijumbi, M; Male FGD Ruti, 19 Aug. 2004; Male FGD, Kisubi Kiwulwe, 4 Sept. 2004; Male FGD, Bukoto, 24 Aug. 2004; Int. RK, 26 Aug. 2002, Takajjunge, M; Int. FKW, 31 Aug. 2004, Kitala, M.

[11] e.g. FGD, 23 August 2000, F; Int. VPB, Busindi, 6, F, Aug. 2000; Int. MK, 16 Aug. 2000, Kikuku, F.

[12] e.g. Int. RMR, 13 Aug. 2000, Byabusha, Busindi, M; Int. VPB, 9 Aug. 2000, Busindi, F; Male FGD, Kisubi Kiwulwe, 4 Sept. 2004; Int. JS, 26 Aug. 2004, Takajjunge, Masaka, M; Int. LN, 19 Aug. 2000, Kikukwe, F; Int. MK, 16 Aug. 2000, Kikukwe, F; Int. MM, 17 Aug. 2000, Ibanga, F; Int. PB, 22 Aug. 2000, Maruku, F. Only in some cases was this lack of shame shown by those who believed the syphilis which they had suffered had been inherited rather than sexually transmitted.

family and reduced the likelihood of achieving a good marriage. Thus when they were young, as some elders explained, 'you had to be married to catch an STD.' It is not so much the age of the sexually active youth that offends the elders today—many of these old people were married in their teens—but their unmarried status.[13] Youths' sexuality appears uncontrolled, part of a syndrome of disrespectful autonomy that overrides the fact that young people in this part of Africa have responded to the rise of HIV by becoming much more sexually risk-averse than their parents and grandparents had been. One of the more disturbing aspects of elders' discourse on HIV is how negatively many regard some of the most successful aspects of the AIDS prevention campaign. Efforts to protect adolescent girls from the sexual advances of older men or to promote condom usage are interpreted by some as having encouraged the independence, and therefore the promiscuity, of the young. 'But today everything is done in broad daylight. Like me, an old man, when I look at you, I say the world has run mad ... You sing obscenities on radio? Dance naked in public! What shall we say? You brought your human rights. We are not happy!'[14]

The second factor that particularly offends elders is that the youth after independence flaunted their sexuality. Many elders, especially in Ankole and Buhaya, referred with venom to the notion of a girlfriend or boyfriend, the idea that the young should date, meet up unsupervised, and adorn themselves so as to look sexually attractive.[15] A number of informants emphasized that in the past affairs and visiting sex workers were very common, but they were done in secret, primarily so that the family and especially the spouse would not be dishonoured. Recent surveys of sexual behaviour and attitudes have shown that the young have in fact to some extent abandoned the openness about sexuality which so offended the elderly in the decades after independence. Epidemiologists have identified a growing disconnect between people's understanding of how they should behave to avoid HIV and how they actually behave. This region has been culturally dominated for so long by HIV

[13] Int. SK, 21 June 2000, Rubya, M; Int. JBK, 11 Aug. 2000, Ijumbi, M; Male FGD Kisubi Kiwulwe, 4 Sept. 2004. See also, e.g. *Weekend Magazine*, 3 Aug. 1990.

[14] Int. JS, 26 Aug. 2004, Takajjunge, Masaka, M; Male FGD, Kitala, 1 Sept. 2004; Male FGD, Bukoto, 24 Aug. 2004. Cf. 'Government downplays condoms', *New Vision*, 26 Nov. 2004.

[15] Male FGD, Takajjunge village, 26.08.04; Male FGD Ruti, 19 Aug. 2004; Female FGD Kyenjenyi, 22 Aug. 2004; Male FGD, Kitala, 1 Sept. 2004. Cf. S. Parikh, 'From Auntie to Disco: The bifurcation of risk and pleasure in sex education in Uganda', in V. Adams and S. Pigg (eds.), *Sex in Development: Science, Sexuality, and Morality* (Durham, NC: Duke University Press, 2005), pp. 125–58; B. Weiss, 'Northwestern Tanzania on a single shilling: Sociality, embodiment, valuation', *Cultural Anthropology*, 12, 3 (1997), p. 357; Iliffe, *AIDS*, p. 121. Of course many elders, especially in Buganda, had themselves chosen their own marriage partners through a process of courtship. Nonetheless some of these informants complained of the lack of discretion displayed by the young in recent decades in how they behaved in public.

prevention messages, and has become so influenced by charismatic forms of Christianity, that public intolerance of displays of sexuality and individual secrecy about sexual behaviour have grown together. It seems likely that the recent resurgence in HIV infection rates will continue so long as this persistent conflict between the old and the young in the field of sexual behaviour continues.[16]

It has become a truism that the responses to perceived crises of public health reveal as much about social and economic life in the societies affected as about disease itself.[17] Interviewees, in talking about their families' experiences, revealed that the HIV/AIDS epidemic, now part of the East African experience for a quarter of a century, has caused remarkable social change as well as immense mortality and misery. Ideas of the nature of disease and death have become both more scientific and more Christianized. Fear of witchcraft rose, fell then rose again. Concepts of human rights have become more accepted institutionally, and on the whole, despite some elders' complaints, within local society, with particular significance for the young and women. And the intimate relationship between fertility and mortality in Africa has become clearer. Some elderly informants indicated that the loss of a few relatives was less painful than in the past, because family sizes were larger. But where a man had lost all his children to AIDS, he might then start a new family, to maintain his line.[18] The story of sexuality and demography in this region remains one of rapid change.

[16] Male FGD, Bukoto, 24 Aug. 2004; Int. AN, 25 August 2004, Kagezi village, Masaka District, F; Int. MGK, 26 Aug. 2004, Takajjunge, F; C. Obbo, 'HIV transmission through social and geographical networks in Uganda', Social Science and Medicine, 36, 1 (1992), p. 953; J. Sadgrove, '"The condom culture is not the kingdom culture": Dissonant discourses and secret sex among born-again university students in Uganda' (unpublished PhD dissertation, School of Oriental and African Studies, 2007), pp. 3–8.

[17] Cf. e.g. T. Ranger and P. Slack (eds.), *Epidemics and Ideas: Essays on the Historical Perception of Pestilence* (Cambridge: Cambridge University Press, 1992).

[18] Male FGD, Takajjunge village, 26.08.04; Male F.G.D, Kagezi village, 25 August 2004; Int. RNT, 9 Aug. 2004, Mbarara, M; Int. SKKG, 25 Aug. 2004, Kabonera, Masaka District, M; Int. B, MM, 26 Aug. 1999, Katoma-Irogero, M, 1B. Cf. S. Doyle, '"The child of death": Personal names and parental attitudes towards mortality in Bunyoro, Western Uganda, 1900–2005', *Journal of African History*, 49, 3 (2008), pp. 361–82; Lugalla, 'Social', p. 195; J. Ntozi and S. Nakayiwa, 'AIDS in Uganda: How has the household coped with the epidemic?', in J. Caldwell, I. Orubuloye and J. Ntozi (eds.), *The Continuing African HIV/AIDS Epidemic* (Canberra: Health Transition Centre, 1999, pp. 155–81; J. Ntozi, 'Two decades of living with HIV/AIDS: The Uganda experience'. A Keynote Address on the World AIDS Day, 1st December 2004 to the Forum on International Cooperation (FIC), Concordia University, Montreal, Canada. Department of Population Studies Library, Makerere University, Kampala; Iliffe, *AIDS*, pp. 91–3, 156.

Bibliography

ARCHIVES

AFRICAN STUDIES CENTRE, CAMBRIDGE

Griffith, V., 'An enquiry into community development in Uganda' (unpublished UNESCO report, African Studies Centre, Cambridge, 1960).

Kamoga, F., 'School leaving as affected by separation of parents in Buganda' (unpublished TS, EAISR seminar paper 1963, African Studies Centre Library, Cambridge).

Uganda Council of Women, 'Memorandum to the commission of enquiry into marriage, divorce and the status of women in Uganda' (unpublished TS, African Studies Centre Library, Cambridge), n/d *c.*1961.

Uganda Protectorate Department of Agriculture, 'A report on nineteen surveys done in small agricultural areas in Uganda with a view to ascertaining the position with regard to soil deterioration' (Entebbe, *c.*1938, TS, ASC, Cambridge).

'Women's advancing status in Uganda', June 1955 (reprint from *The Times British Colonies Review*, Spring 1955).

BRITISH LIBRARY, LONDON

Uganda and Tanganyika annual medical reports.

BUKOBA ROMAN CATHOLIC PARISH OFFICE, TANZANIA

Bukoba parish baptism and marriage registers.

CAMBRIDGE UNIVERSITY LIBRARY

D. Stenning papers, ADD 7916

CHURCH MISSIONARY SOCIETY ARCHIVE, BIRMINGHAM

Anon. [A. Cook?], 'The treatment of ante-natal syphilis in Baganda women', a paper read before the Uganda branch of the British Medical Association, 22 Mar. 1929, CMS M/Y/A7 1931–5.

Cook, A., Annual letter 1923, CMS G3/AL/1917–1934.

Cook, A., Memorandum before the sub-committee on policy and the financial position of the hospital, Dec. 1933, and Albert to Jack Cook, 1 May 1932, CMS M/Y/A7 1931–5.

Cook, J., Interview with DMS Kauntze, n/d [1930s], CMS Acc. 318 Z4, G. Hewitt papers.

Mengo Maternity Records, CMS M59 Y A7 1955–6.

Mitchell to Colonial Office, 3 Dec. 1936, Native Marriage.

Parr, M., Governor of Equatoria Province, Sudan, Memorandum on the marriage and Divorce of native Christian members of African tribal communities, 2 Jan. 1938, and extract from the Annual Report on the Province of Buganda 1936.

Pearson to Mackay, 29 July 1880, CMS G3 A6/0 1881/22.
Pearson to Wright, 29 Sept. 1879, CMS CA6/019/13.
Taylor, J., 'Analysis of parishes', CMS Acc. 265 Z5.
Walker to Baylis, 1 Dec. 1907, CMS G3/A7/0/1907/190.

CHURCH OF UGANDA ARCHIVE, MUKONO, UGANDA
Mainly files from the following series:
Marriage 1931–45.
Marriage cases.
Marriage files.
Marriage questions: legal opinions and memoranda.
Marriage questions: the Uganda Council of Women, 1952–61.

ENTEBBE SECRETARIAT ARCHIVES, UGANDA
Mainly files from the A46 series, especially district annual reports.

FRANCISCAN MISSIONARY SISTERS ARCHIVE, DUNDALK, IRELAND
Nsambya Hospital Annual Reports.

H. WELBOURN PAPERS (IN THE POSSESSION OF H. WELBOURN)
Welbourn, H., 'Childhood in a changing world' (unpublished TS, n/d).
Welbourn, H., 'First impressions' (unpublished TS, 1946).
Welbourn, H., 'Uganda—end or beginning' (unpublished TS, 1980).

KISUBI ROMAN CATHOLIC PARISH OFFICE, UGANDA
Kisubi Parish baptism and marriage registers.

KITAGATA HOSPITAL RECORDS STORE, UGANDA
Kitagata Hospital Maternity Registers.

LONDON SCHOOL OF ECONOMICS ARCHIVE
Audrey Richards papers on Uganda.
J. Gorju, *Entre le Victoria, l'Albert et l'Edouard* (Rennes, 1920, translated by Ralph Butler, 1957, A. Richards papers, 6/23).

MAKERERE INSTITUTE OF SOCIAL RESEARCH LIBRARY, UGANDA
Reining, H., 'Village organisation in Buhaya' (unpublished conference paper, EAISR conference, June 1952).

DEPARTMENT OF POPULATION STUDIES LIBRARY, MAKERERE UNIVERSITY, UGANDA
Ntozi, J., 'Two decades of living with HIV/AIDS: The Uganda experience'. A Keynote Address on the World AIDS Day, 1st December 2004 to the Forum on International Cooperation (FIC), Concordia University, Montreal, Canada.

MAKERERE UNIVERSITY LIBRARY, UGANDA
Buganda Lukiiko Archives, 1894–1918.
Kaggwa, A., *Basekabaka be Buganda* (TS of English translation by S. Musoke).
Mutyaba, M. and P. Namukadde, 'Chwa II ne Muteesa II' (no date, *c.*1911).
Miti, J., 'A Short History of Buganda, Bunyoro, Busoga, Toro and Ankole' (trans. G. Rock, unpublished microfilm, n/d).

Robertz, P., 'Sharing with adolescents' (unpublished research paper, Pastoral Institute of Eastern Africa, Gaba, *c.*1969).
Zimbe, B., 'Buganda and the king: A royal history of Buganda' (TS, n/d, trans. Simon Musoke).

MASAKA HOSPITAL RECORDS STORE, UGANDA
Masaka Hospital Maternity Registers.

MBARARA HOSPITAL RECORDS STORE, UGANDA
Mbarara Hospital Maternity Registers.

MILL HILL FATHERS ARCHIVE, BISHOP'S HOUSE, JINJA, UGANDA
Marriage files.

MINISTRY OF HEALTH LIBRARY, KAMPALA, UGANDA
Ministry of Health, 'Medical Services Statistical Records, 1959' (unpublished TS).
Uganda Medical Reports 1962–83.

MWANZA PROVINCIAL ARCHIVES, TANZANIA
Mainly files relating to STDs, health, maternity and prostitution [F37, L5, M20 and MISS/DN/53 series].

NATIONAL ARCHIVES, LONDON
CO1018 series.
CO684 series.
CO685 series.
MRC files [FD series].
Uganda files, FO2 and CO536 series.

NKOKONJERU HOSPITAL RECORD STORE, UGANDA
Nkokonjeru Hospital Maternity Registers.

NSAMBYA HOSPITAL RECORDS STORE, KAMPALA, UGANDA
Nsambya Hospital Maternity, Ante-natal and Out-patient Registers.

NYAMITANGA ROMAN CATHOLIC PARISH OFFICE, UGANDA
Nyamitanga parish baptism and marriage registers.

RHODES HOUSE OXFORD
Alderdice, Dr. A. papers, RHO, MSS.Afr.s.1872 (3).
Barrett, R. papers, RHO, MSS.Afr.s.1879(9).
Bazley, W., 'Reminiscences as a district officer in Uganda, 1951–1953, 1958–1960', RHO, MSS Afr. s. 924.
Byrne, M. papers, RHO, MSS.Afr.s.1872 (23).
Connolly, D. papers, Judgements file (vol. II), RHO, MSS. Afr. s. 1678(2).
Elsden, E. papers, RHO, MSS.Afr.s.1872 (49).
Hennessey, R., 'Personal reminiscences', RHO, MSS. Afr. s. 1872, Box XVIII.
Hodges, A., Diaries, 1–3 Jan. 1905, MS, RHO, MSS. Afr. s. 1782.
Iliffe, J. interview with S. Mwankemwa (TS, 25 July 1995), RHO, MSS Afr. s. 2261.
Potts, C. papers, RHO, MSS. Afr. s. 590.
Stanton, H. papers, RHO, MSS. Afr. s. 2285.

Trant, H. papers, RHO, MSS.Afr. s.1872(143).
Welbourn, H. papers, RHO, MSS Afr. s. 1872. 152.
Williams, A. papers, RHO, Mss.Afr.s.1872/xxxix.
Willis, J., 'Reflections on Uganda' (TS, n/d), RHO, MSS. Afr. s. 1792 Box 38.
Yeld, E., 'Continuity and Change in Kiga patterns of marriage: An analysis of structural change in Kiga marriage in the 1930s and the 1960s' (UEA Social Science Conference, December 1966), RHO, MSS. Afr. s. 1792/48, 7/23.

ROYAL COMMONWEALTH SOCIETY ARCHIVE, CAMBRIDGE
Bell, H., Uganda papers.

RUBAGA ARCHIVES, KAMPALA, UGANDA
Brother Charles, 'Moral conditions in the schools', 904.1.
Files on marriage [49 series].
Michaud, E., 'Enquêtes sur les conditions morales dans le vicariat de l'Uganda, 1933', 904.1.
Survey of Catholic Dioceses, 1956, Rubaga archives, Kampala.

SIR ALBERT COOK ARCHIVE, MULAGO, KAMPALA, UGANDA
Annual Medical Report Mengo District 1958.
Arya, O. and S. Taber, 'Maladies vénériennes et fécondité dans les régions rurales de l'Ouganda', (unpublished paper presented to the Medical Society for the Study of Venereal Diseases, Malta, April 1975).
Arya. O. and C. Bosa, 'Treatment of gonorrhoea with three different penicillin schedules—a preliminary report', Uganda Medical Association Annual Scientific Conference, 19-20 Feb. 1972.
Bruce papers.
Cook papers.
Dean, R., 'Health education and protein-calorie malnutrition' (Report of a seminar 'Health education and the mother and child in East Africa', Makerere Medical School, Kampala, Nov. 1961).
Mengo Hospital Maternity Registers.
Mengo Hospital papers.
Rendle Short, C., 'Health education for the expectant mother' (Report of a seminar 'Health education and the mother and child in East Africa', Makerere Medical School, Kampala, Nov. 1961).
Report of the Lady Coryndon Maternity Training School, Namirembe, 1932.

SOAS ARCHIVE, LONDON
Melvin Perlman papers. List of civil cases at Buganda Provincial Appeal court 1943–61, File 22 Buganda and Kigezi, PPMS38/Perlman/Box 8, and Marriage files, GB 0102 PP MS 38.

TANZANIA NATIONAL ARCHIVES, DAR ES SALAAM
Mainly files from the G [German], 71 [Medical], 215 and 1733 [Bukoba district reports], 19153 [STD], 31732 [Yaws], 34929 and 36433 [Health] series.
Annual Medical Reports.
Bukoba District Book.

UNIVERSITY OF DAR ES SALAAM, TANZANIA

Bukoba: Official Correspondence relating to constitutional matters, politics and land, including notes and memoranda by Hans Cory, 1950-8, UDSM, EAF Cory 21.

Cory, H., 'The Haya tribe and the incidence of venereal disease, Bukoba 1938–48', TS, UDSM, EAF CORY 104.

Culwick, A., 'The population problem in the Bukoba district' (Bukoba, 1938, UDSM, EAF CORY 239).

Lwamgira, F., *Amakuru ka Kiziba na Abakama Bamu* (unpublished TS of English translation).

Rehse, H., *Kiziba: Land und Leute* (Stuttgart: Strecker und Schröder, 1910, translated by Mrs Donne, UDSM, CORY 369).

Richards, A. and P. Reining, 'Report on fertility surveys in Buganda and Buhaya, 1952' (UDSM, Cory 373).

WELLCOME ARCHIVE, LONDON

Dr. P. Evans' diary of 1953 visit to Uganda, A.3/1 PP/PRE.

Dr. W. Sheldon and Dr. P. Evans, 'Report to the Board of Governors of the Hospital for Sick Children, Great Ormond Street, of the visit to Uganda, 24.10.53–21.11.53', P. R. Evans papers, CMAC, PP/PRE A.1/2.

Frazer Committee meeting with the Ankole district team, 20 Sept. 1955, PP/CDW E.3/2.

Frazer Committee, Minutes of meeting, 30 Aug. 1955, PP/CDW E.3/2.

Uganda Frazer Committee agenda, 'Information concerning Mengo CMS hospital, Oct. 1955', PP/CDW E.3/1.

WHITE FATHERS ARCHIVE, ROME, ITALY

A. Achte to L. Livinhac, Rubaga, 7 Aug. 1898, no.87, 119.

Mission diaries of Kashozi, Kisubi, Nyamitanga and Rubaga.

H. Lapioche, 'Table d'enquête sur les moeurs et coutumes indigènes, Diocese de Bukoba', 1956.

P. Lefebre, 'Table d'enquête sur les moeurs et coutumes indigènes, Vicariat Apostolique de l'Ouganda: Tribu des Baganda', 1951.

P. Nicolet, 'Table d'enquête sur les moeurs et coutumes indigènes, Vicariat Apostolique de Rwenzori: Tribu des Hamites Abahima et Bantu Abairu de l'Ankole', 1951.

WOMEN'S LIBRARY, LONDON

AMSH files, Uganda 1908–54, Women's Library, London, 3AMS/D/49.

INTERVIEWS AND FOCUS GROUP DISCUSSIONS, REFERENCED IN THE TEXT

These interviews and focus group discussions were mostly conducted in the local vernacular by interpreters who used an evolving set of open-ended, non-leading questions. These interpreters then transcribed and translated informants' recorded testimonies verbatim. Working concurrently in three different ethnic groups meant that I could not conduct the interviews myself, but I could follow enough of what had been said to ask follow-up questions if interviewers had not sought clarification on particular points. Some highly educated informants, mainly medical personnel, were fluent in English and so were interviewed by myself. Between five and eight individuals participated in each focus group so overall almost 400 people contributed to this oral research. Not all interviews have been referenced, however, as some people were more revealing than others, and there was a great deal of local consensus on many issues. Only those interviews and focus groups which have been referenced in the text are detailed below. All the interview transcripts, however, are in the author's possession and are available for scholarly consultation. None of the interviewees asked that their testimonies be anonymised, but due to the sensitive nature of some statements, all interviews have been rendered anonymous. Informants' gender has been identified as M or F—male or female.

Int. AC, 9 Aug. 2000, Rubaa-Rubya, F
Int. AK, 8 Aug. 2000, Rubya, F
Int. AM, 11 Aug. 2000, Busindi, F
Int. AM, 14 June 2000, Isikila-Irungami, F
Int. AM, 24 June 2000, Kashambya, F
Int. AMA, 15 Aug. 2000, Rwagati, F
Int. AMR, 26 July 1998, Kenyana-Kilimilile, F
Int. AN, 25 Aug. 2004, Kagezi, F
Int. AR, 15 Aug. 2000, Ihagiro, F
Int. AS, 27 July 1998, Bukara, M
Int. BB, 2 Sept. 1999, Kenyana, M
Int. BK, 12 Aug. 2004, Mbarara, F
Int. BMJ, 29 Aug. 2004, Kyankoole, M
Int. CB, 13 Aug. 2000, Busindi, F
Int. CKM, 17 Aug. 2000, Kibanda, F
Int. CM, 11 Aug. 2000, Busindi, M
Int. CM, 11 Aug. 2000, Rubya, F
Int. CN, 12 Aug. 2000, Kanoni, F
Int. CNSM, 28 Aug. 2004, Butanga, M
Int. DCT, 20 Aug. 2004, Mbarara, M
Int. DPO, 28 June 2004, Kampala, M
Int. DT, 14 June 2000, Ntoma, F
Int. EB, 1 Sept. 1999, Bukoba, M
Int. EFC, 23 July 1998, Katongo, F
Int. EK, 7 Aug. 2000, Kanyangereko Nkimbo, F
Int. EM, 27 Sept. 2001, Kampala, M
Int. EM, 28 Aug. 2004, Kyansi, M
Int. FB, 9 Sept. 1999, Maruku, M
Int. FK, 16 Aug. 2000, Kikukwe, F
Int. FKK, 29 Aug. 1999, Kaishemarwa-Katoma, M
Int. FKW, 31 Aug. 2004, Kitala, M
Int. FM, 21 July 1998, Rubya, M
Int. FM, 21 June 2000, Rubya, F
Int. FN, 29 Aug. 2004, Butanga, F
Int. FNN, 28 Aug. 2004, Wekaaye, Kaswa, F
Int. FR, 27 June 2000, Rubya, M
Int. FR, 30 Aug. 1999, Kitobo, M

Int. GI, 30 Aug. 1999, Igurugati-Bugandika, M
Int. GK, 14 Aug. 2004, Mbarara, F
Int. GK, 21 Aug. 2000, Nkindo, F
Int. HGN, 10 Sept. 2004, Kiiso, F
Int. HL, 17 June 2000, Maruku, M
Int. HM, 16 Aug. 2004, Mbarara District Hospital, F
Int. HW, 31 July 2008, Bristol, F
Int. IST, 21 August 2004, Kagezi village, Masaka, M
Int. JH, 10 Aug. 2004, Mbarara, F
Int. JM, 12 Aug. 2000, Kanoni, M
Int. JM, 17 June 2000, Ntoma, F
Int. JN, 28 June 2004, Kampala, F
Int. JN, 29 Aug. 2004, Butanga, F
Int. JBK, 11 Aug. 2000, Ijumbi, M
Int. JR, 8 Aug. 2000, Rubya, F
Int. JS, 26 Aug. 2004, Takajjunge, Masaka, M
Int. JT, 16 Aug. 2004, Mbarara Hospital, F
Int. KJK, 31 Aug. 2004, Kitala, M
Int. KK, 15 June 2000, Bibanja, F
Int. KM, 18 Aug. 2000, Kikukwe-Kanyigo, F
Int. LK and SR, 1 Sept. 1999, Bugandika, M
Int. LLS, 21 Aug. 2004, Bukunda, Masaka, M
Int. LM, 12 Aug. 2000, Kanoni, F
Int. LM, 27 Aug. 1999, Katoma-Karwoshe, M
Int. LN, 19 Aug. 2000, Kikukwe, F
Int. MGK, 26 Aug. 2004, Takajjunge, F
Int. MK, 16 Aug. 2000, Kikukwe, F
Int. MK, 19 Aug. 2000, Kanyigo, M
Int. MK, 3 Sept. 1999, Rubafu, M
Int. ML, 12 Aug. 2004, Mbarara, F
Int. MM B, 26 Aug. 1999, Katoma-Irogero, M
Int. MM, 11 Aug. 2000, Ijumbi, F
Int. MM, 12 Aug. 2000, Kamachumu, F
Int. MM, 12 Aug. 2000, Kanoni, F
Int. MM, 14 Aug. 2000, Ruhija, F
Int. MM, 17 Aug. 2000, Ibanga, F
Int. MM, 20 June 2000, Karwoshe, M
Int. MM, 28 June 2004, Kampala, M
Int. MM, 7 Sept. 1999, Rubale, M
Int. MMA, 24 Aug. 2004, Kyanakase, F
Int. MMM, 12 Aug. 2000, Kanoni, F
Int. MPM, 10 Aug. 2000, Ibare, F
Int. MT, 24 July 1998, Igombe, F
Int. N, 23 July 1998, Katongo, M
Int. NM, 28 Aug. 2004, Lugazi, Butanga, F
Int. NNFW, 28 Aug. 2004, Kaswa, F
Int. NPNK, 24 Aug. 2004, Kyanakase, F
Int. PB, 22 Aug. 2000, Maruku, F

Int. PEK, 7 Aug. 2000, Nkimbo Bweramutima, F
Int. PK, 6 Sept. 1999, Rubafu, M
Int. PKK, 18 Aug. 2000, Mshumba-Byazi, F
Int. PLGS, 31 Aug. 2004, Kitala, Busiro, M
Int. PMJ, 9 Aug. 2000, Rubya, F
Int. RK, 16 June 2000, Kanyangereko, F
Int. RK, 26 Aug. 2002, Takajjunge, M
Int. RMR, 13 Aug. 2000, Byabusha, Busindi, M
Int. RNT, 9 Aug. 2004, Mbarara, M
Int. SG, 21 Aug. 2000, Nkindo, F
Int. SJ, 26 Aug. 2004, Takajunge, M
Int. SK, 21 June 2000, Rubya, M
Int. SKKG, 25 Aug. 2004, Kabonera, M
Int. SKN, 22 Aug. 2000, Maruku-Butailuka-Kasha, F
Int. SMD, 1 July 2003, Dublin, F
Int. SN, 25 Aug. 1999, Katoma, M
Int. SPM, 24 June 2000, Gera-Kashambya, M
Int. TM, 13 Aug. 2000, Busindi, F
Int. TNN, 3 Aug. 2004, Kitala, F
Int. VK, 27 June 2000, Bukoba, M
Int. VM, 16 June 2000, Kanyangereko, F
Int. VPB, 9 Aug. 2000, Busindi, F
Int. WBK, 27 July 1998, Bugabo, M
Int. WK, 31 Aug. 1999, Igurati-Bugandika, M
Int. WR, 21 June 2000, Rubya, M
Int. YK, 19 Aug. 2000, Kikukwe, F
Int. YS, 10 Aug. 2000, Bukoba, F
Int. YZ, 13 Aug. 2004, Mbarara, M
Int. ZMN, 28 Aug. 2004, Butanga, F
Int. ZR, 22 June 2000, Karwoshe, M

Female FGD Bugiri Kiwulwe, 10 Sept. 2004
Female FGD Bukoba, 23 Aug. 2000
Female FGD Bukoto, 24 Aug. 2004
Female FGD Bumbire (Bushenyi), 23 Aug. 2004
Female FGD Kagezi, 25 Aug. 2004
Female FGD Kisaasi-Kampala A, 2 Feb. 2008
Female FGD Kiyungi, 21 Aug. 2004
Female FGD Kyenjenyi, 22 Aug. 2004
Female FGD Nyamitanga, 19 Aug. 2004
Female FGD Ruti, 19 Aug. 2004
Female FGD Takajunge, 26 Aug. 2004

Male FGD Bukoto, 24 Aug. 2004
Male FGD Kagezi village, 25 Aug. 2004
Male FGD Kisubi Kiwulwe, 4 Sept. 2004
Male FGD Kitala, 1 Sept. 2004
Male FGD Kiyungu Shema, 21 Aug. 2004
Male FGD Kyangyenyi/Kiyungu, 22 Aug. 2004

Male FGD Nyamitanga, 19 Aug. 2004
Male FGD Ruti, 19 Aug. 2004
Male FGD Takajunge, 26 Aug. 2004

WEBSITES

http://myweb.tiscali.co.uk/petercooke/websiteDownloads/SSEMPEKE!pdf
http://www.unicef.org/infobycountry/botswana_statistics.html.
http://www.unicef.org/sowc03/tables/table9.html

UNPUBLISHED SEMINAR PAPERS

Arya, O., S. Taber and H. Nsanze, 'Infertility and venereal disease in Uganda: A review' (unpublished TS, 1983).

Colwell, S., 'Infant and child mortality on Kilimanjaro, 1894–1935' (unpublished paper, Harvard School of Public Health, 2001).

Forthal, D. et al. 'AIDS in Tanzania' (unpublished paper, Centers for Disease Control, Atlanta, 1986).

Lwanga, C., 'Interval tubal ligation', (unpublished paper presented at the Conference on Reproductive Health Management in Sub-Saharan Africa, Freetown, Sierra Leone, 5–9 Nov. 1984).

Maleche, A., 'Sociological and psychological factors favouring or hindering the education of African women in Uganda' (unpublished TS, EAISR seminar paper 1961, African Studies Centre Library, Cambridge).

Musisi, N., 'The journey of the first African female doctor through tropical medicine, international health and global health: Josephine Namboze of Uganda', (unpublished paper presented at the WHO Conference on African Health History, Nairobi, 6–8 Feb. 2007).

Peterson, D., 'Prostitution and patriotism in Northwestern Tanganyika' (unpublished seminar paper, African History Group, Cambridge, 30 October 2007).

Rwabukwali, C., 'Adolescent fertility and sexuality in Uganda: determinants, consequences and management' (unpublished seminar paper, Arusha, 1987).

NEWSPAPERS CONSULTED

Ageteraine
Daily News
Matalisi
Munno
New Vision
Obugagga bwa Uganda
Taifa Leo
Taifa Uganda Empya
The People
The Star
The Weekly Topic

Uganda Argus
Uganda Empya
Uganda Empya
Uganda Eyogera
Uganda Herald
Uganda Weekly News
Voice of Uganda
Weekend Magazine

BOOKS AND ARTICLES

Adeoba, A., 'Interpretation of positive serological tests for syphilis in pregnancy', *British Journal of Venereal Diseases*, 43 (1967), pp. 249–58.

Agadjanian, V., 'Fraught with ambivalence: Reproductive intentions and contraceptive choices in a Sub-Saharan fertility transition', *Population Research and Policy Review*, 24, 6 (2005), pp. 617–45.

Agyei, W. and E. Epema, 'Adolescent fertility in Kampala, Uganda: Knowledge, perceptions and practice', *Biology and Society*, 7, 4 (1990), pp. 203–14.

Agyei, W. and G. Nakintu-Kyeyune, 'Mortality estimates for south Kampala based on 1980 Uganda population census', *Journal of Biosocial Science*, 20 (1988), pp. 245–52.

Ahlberg, B., 'Is there a distinct African sexuality? A critical response to Caldwell', *Africa*, 64, 2 (1994), pp. 220–42.

Ainsworth, M., *Infancy in Uganda* (Baltimore: Johns Hopkins, 1967).

Akyeampong, E., '"Wo pe tam, won pe ba" ("You like cloth but you don't want children"): Urbanization, individualism and gender relations in colonial Ghana *c.* 1900–1939', in D. Anderson and R. Rathbone (eds.), *Africa's Urban Past* (Oxford: James Currey, 2000), pp. 222–34.

Akyeampong, E., 'Sexuality and prostitution among the Akan of the Gold Coast *c.* 1650–1950', *Past and Present,* 156 (1997), pp. 144–73.

Allbrook, D., 'Some problems associated with pelvic form and size in the Ganda of East Africa', *Journal of the Royal Anthropological Institute*, 42 (1962), pp. 102–14.

Allen, W., *The African Husbandman* (London: Oliver and Boyd, 1965).

Allman, J. and V. Tashjian, *"I Will Not Eat Stone": A Women's History of Colonial Asante* (Portsmouth NH: Heinemann, 2000).

Alnwick, D., M. Stirling and G. Kyeyune, 'Morbidity and mortality in selected Ugandan hospitals, 1981–2', in Dodge and Wiebe, *Crisis*, pp. 79–86.

Anderson, R. et al., 'The spread of HIV-1 in Africa: Sexual contact patterns and the predicted demographic impact of AIDS', *Nature*, 352, 6336 (1991), pp. 581–9.

Anon., 'L'avortement en Afrique', *Afrique Medicale*, 13, 121 (1974), pp. 568–9.

Anon., *The Native Laws of Buganda* (Kampala, 1947).

Arnfred, S., 'Introduction', in S. Arnfred (ed.), *Re-thinking Sexualities in Africa* (Uppsala: Nordic Africa Institute, 2004), pp. 7–34.

Arnold, D., *Colonizing the Body: State Medicine and Epidemic Disease in Nineteenth-Century India* (Berkeley: University of California Press, 1993).

Arnold, D., *Imperial Medicine and Indigenous Societies* (Manchester: Manchester University Press, 1988).

Arya, O. and F. Bennett, 'Attitudes of college students in East Africa to sexual activity and venereal disease', *British Journal of Venereal Diseases*, 44 (1968), pp. 160–6.
Arya, O. and F. Bennett, 'Role of the medical auxiliary in the control of sexually transmitted disease in a developing country', *British Journal of Venereal Diseases*, 52 (1976), pp. 116–21.
Arya, O. and F. Bennett, 'Venereal disease in an elite group (university students) in East Africa', *British Journal of Venereal Disease*, 43 (1967), pp. 275–9.
Arya, O. and F. Bennett, 'What do the educated want to know about VD? An analysis of the questions asked by university and college students in Uganda', *Uganda Medical Journal*, 2 (1973), pp. 91–103.
Arya, O. and I. Phillips, 'Antibiotic sensitivity of gonococci and treatment of gonorrhoea in Uganda', *British Journal of Venereal Diseases*, 46 (1970), pp. 149–52.
Arya, O., 'Changing patterns in the organization of the venereal diseases and treponematoses service in Uganda', *British Journal of Venereal Diseases*, 49 (1973), pp. 134–8.
Arya, O., C. Pearson, S. Rao and R. Blowers, 'Treatment of gonorrhoea with trimethoprim-sulphamethoxazole in Uganda', *British Journal of Venereal Diseases*, 46 (1970), pp. 214–6.
Arya, O., S. Taber and H. Nsanze, 'Gonorrhea and female infertility in rural Uganda', *American Journal of Obstetrics and Gynecology*, 138, 7 (1980), pp. 929–32.
Ashe, R., *Two Kings of Uganda* (London: Sampson, Low, 1889).
Austen, R., *Northwest Tanzania under German and British Rule: Colonial Policy and Tribal Politics, 1889–1939* (New Haven: Yale University Press, 1968).
Baijukya, F. and V. Mwita (eds.), 'Participatory planning and management: an agenda for equity and sustainable use of "Rweya" grassland in Kagera Region, Tanzania' in F. Baijukya and V. Mwita (eds.), *Proceedings of the 'Rweya' Workshop, Bukoba* (Bukoba: KAEMP, 2000), pp. 32–6.
Bakwesegha, C., *Profiles of Urban Prostitution*: A *Case Study from Uganda* (Nairobi: EAPH, 1982).
Banfield, J., 'Film in East Africa: A report', *Transition*, 13 (1964), pp. 18–21.
Barlow, D., *Sexually Transmitted Infections: the Facts* (Oxford: Oxford University Press, 2006).
Barnett, A. and P. Blaikie, *AIDS in Africa: Its Past and Future Impact* (New York: Guilford Press, 1992).
Barnett, A. and A. Whiteside, *AIDS in the Twenty-First Century: Disease and Globalisation* (Basingstoke: Palgrave, 2002).
Belsey, M., 'The epidemiology of infertility: a review with particular reference to sub-Saharan Africa', *Bulletin of the World Health Organization*, 54 (1976), pp. 319–41.
Bennett, F., 'A comparison of community health in Uganda with its two East African neighbours in the period 1970–1979', in Dodge and Wiebe, *Crisis*, pp. 43–52.
Bennett, F., 'Gonorrhoea: a rural pattern of transmission', *East African Medical Journal*, 41, 4 (1964), pp. 163–7.
Bennett, F., 'The social determinants of gonorrhoea in an East African town', *East African Medical Journal*, 39 (1962), pp. 332–42.
Berger, I., 'Fertility as power: Spirit mediums, priestesses and the pre-colonial state in interlacustrine east Africa', in D. Anderson and D. Johnson (eds.), *Revealing Prophets: Prophecy in Eastern African History* (London: James Currey, 1995) pp. 65–82.

Billington, R., *A Tune on Black and White Keys. Partnership in Healing: the Story of Mengo Hospital* (London: Janus, 1993).

Billington, W., 'Neurosyphilis in Uganda: a comparison of two five-year periods', *East African Medical Journal*, 43, 11 (1966), pp. 469–73.

Black, T., 'A survey of contraceptive markets in four African countries', *Journal of Biosocial Science*, 4 (1972), pp. 287–98.

Blacker, J. et al., 'Fertility in Kenya and Uganda: A comparative study of trends and determinants', *Population Studies*, 59, 3 (2005), pp. 355–73.

Bledsoe, C., A. Hill, U. d'Alessandro and P. Langerock, 'Constructing natural fertility: The use of Western contraceptive technologies in rural Gambia', *Population and Development Review*, 20 (1994), pp. 81–113.

Bledsoe, C. *Contingent Lives: Fertility, Time, and Aging in West Africa* (Chicago: University of Chicago Press, 2002).

Bond, G. and J. Vincent, 'Living on the edge: Changing social structures in the context of AIDS', in H. Hansen and M. Twaddle (eds.), *Changing Uganda* (London: James Currey, 1991), pp. 113–29.

Bongaarts, J. and J. Potter, *Fertility, Biology and Behavior: An Analysis of the Proximate Determinants* (New York: Academic Press, 1983).

Bongaarts, J., O. Frank and R. Lesthaeghe, 'The proximate determinants of fertility in Sub-Saharan Africa', *Population and Development Review*, 10, 3 (1984), pp. 511–37.

Boserup, E., 'Economic and demographic interrelationships in sub-Saharan Africa', *Population and Development Review,* 11, 3 (1985), pp. 383–97.

Brantlinger, P., *Dark Vanishings: Discourse on the Extinction of Primitive Races, 1800–1930* (Ithaca: Cornell UP, 2003).

Brass, W., 'The estimation of fertility rates from ratios of total to first births', *Population Studies*, 8, 1 (1954), pp. 74–87.

Brierley, J. and T. Spear, 'Mutesa, the missionaries, and Christian conversion in Buganda', *International Journal of African Historical Studies*, 21, 4 (1988), pp. 601–18.

Brockerhoff, M. and P. Hewett, 'Inequality of child mortality among ethnic groups in sub-Saharan Africa', *Bulletin of the World Health Organization*, 78, 1 (2000), pp. 30–41.

Bulkley, D., *Syphilis of the Innocent* (New York: Bailey and Fairchild, 1894).

Butler, J., 'Willingly to school: the day student in Uganda, *Transition*, 9 (1963), pp. 27–9.

Caldwell, J. and P. Caldwell, 'The demographic evidence for the incidence and cause of abnormally low fertility in tropical Africa', *World Health Statistics Quarterly*, 36, 1 (1983), pp. 2–34.

Caldwell, J. and P. McDonald, 'Influence of maternal education on infant and child mortality: Levels and causes', *Health Policy and Education*, 2, 3–4 (1982), pp. 251–67.

Caldwell, J. et al., 'The construction of adolescence in a changing world: implications for sexuality, reproduction, and marriage', *Studies in Family Planning*, 29, 2 (1998), pp. 137–53.

Caldwell, J., 'Rethinking the African AIDS epidemic', *Population and Development Review*, 26, 1 (2000), pp. 117–36.

Caldwell, J., 'Routes to low mortality in poor countries', *Population and Development Review*, 12, 2 (1986), pp. 171–220.
Caldwell, J., 'The population factor in African change', in A. Mafeje and S. Radwan (eds.), *Economic and Demographic Change in Africa* (Oxford: Clarendon Press, 1995), pp. 11–35.
Caldwell, J., 'The social repercussions of colonial rule: demographic aspects', in A. Adu Boahen (ed.), *UNESCO General History of Africa, VII* (London: Heinemann, 1985), pp. 458–80.
Caldwell, J., I. Orubuloye and P. Caldwell, 'Fertility decline in Africa: A new type of transition?', *Population and Development Review*, 18, 2 (1992), pp. 211–242.
Caldwell, J., P. Caldwell and P. Quiggan, 'The social context of AIDS in sub-Saharan Africa', *Population and Development Review*, 15, 2 (1989), pp. 185–234.
Caldwell, J., *Theory of Fertility Decline* (London: Academic Press, 1982).
Callahan, B., '"Veni, VD, Vici": Reassessing the Ila syphilis epidemic', *Journal of Southern African Studies* 23, 3 (1997), pp. 421–40.
Chambers, R. and B. Baitera, 'The anatomy of the urethral stricture', *British Journal of Urology* (1977), 49, pp. 545–51.
Chanock, M., *Law, Custom and Social Order: The Colonial Experience in Malawi and Zambia* (Cambridge: Cambridge University Press, 1985).
Chrétien, J.-P., 'The slave trade in Burundi and Rwanda at the beginning of German colonisation', in Médard and Doyle, *Slavery*, pp. 210–27.
Chrétien, J.-P., *The Great Lakes of Africa: Two Thousand Years of History* (New York: Zone, 2003, trans. S. Strauss).
Chwa, D., 'Education, civilization and foreignisation', in D. Low (ed.), *The Mind of Buganda: Documents of the Modern History of an African Kingdom* (Berkeley: University of California Press, 1971), pp. 104–8.
Cleland, J. and J. van Ginneken, 'Maternal education and child survival in developing countries: The search for pathways of influence'. *Social Science and Medicine*, 27, 12 (1988), pp. 1357–68.
Clyde, D., *History of the Medical Services of Tanganyika* (Dar es Salaam: Government Printer, 1962).
Cohen, D. and E. Atieno Odhiambo, *Burying SM: The Politics of Knowledge and the Sociology of Power in Africa* (London: James Currey, 1992).
Cook, A., 'A social purity campaign in Uganda', *Mercy and Truth*, 25 (1921), pp. 271–98.
Cook, A., 'An urgent need in Uganda', *Mercy and Truth*, 12 (1908), pp. 44–50.
Cook, A., 'Notes on the diseases met within Uganda, Central Africa', *Journal of Tropical Medicine*, 4 (1901), pp. 175–8.
Cook, A., 'Obstetric medicine in Uganda', *British Medical Journal*, 1, 2789 (1914), pp. 1281–3.
Cook, A., 'Syphilis in the Uganda Protectorate', *British Medical Journal*, 2, 2502 (1908), pp. 1780–1.
Cook, A., *A Medical Vocabulary and Phrase Book in Luganda* (Kampala: SPCK, 1921 [1903]).
Cook, A., *Uganda Memories, 1897–1940* (Kampala: Uganda Society, 1945).
Cordell, D. and J. Gregory, *African Population and Capitalism: Historical Perspectives* (Boulder, CO: Westview, 1987).

Cory, H. and M. Hartnoll, *The Customary Law of the Haya Tribe, Tanganyika Territory* (London: Routledge, 1971 [1945]).

Creinin, M. and H. Simhan, 'Can we communicate gravidity and parity better?', *Obstetrics and Gynecology*, 113, 3 (2009), pp. 709–11.

Crisp, J., 'National security, human rights and population displacements Luwero district, Uganda', *Review of African Political Economy*, 10, 27–28 (1983), pp. 164–74.

Crocker, C., R. Trussell, H. Wallace and E. Gold, 'A study of knowledge, attitudes, and practices of family planning in Uganda, East Africa', *Journal of Reproductive Medicine*, 7, 5 (1971), pp. 235–8.

Crozier, A., *Practising Colonial Medicine: The Colonial Medical Service in Colonial East Africa* (London: I.B. Tauris, 2007).

Culwick, A. and G. Culwick, edited by V. Berry, *The Culwick Papers 1934–1944: Population, Food and Health in Colonial Tanganika* (London: Academic Books, 1994).

Cunningham, J., *Uganda and its Peoples : Notes on the Protectorate of Uganda, Especially the Anthropology and Ethnology of its Indigenous Races* (London: Hutchinson, 1905).

Davies, J. et al., 'Cancer in an African community, 1897–1956: An analysis of the records of Mengo Hospital, Kampala, Uganda: Part I', *British Medical Journal*, 1, 5378 (1964), pp. 259–64.

Davies, J., 'A history of syphilis in Uganda', *Bulletin of the World Health Organisation*, 4 (1956), pp. 1042–59.

Davies, J., 'Causes of death in African children', *East African Medical Journal*, 25 (1948), pp. 228–35.

Davies, J., 'Pathology of central African natives: Mulago Hospital post mortem studies', *East African Medical Journal*, 24, 8 (1947), pp. 289–303.

Davis, P., 'On the sexuality of "town women" in Kampala', *Africa Today*, 47, 3/4, (2000), pp. 28–60.

Davis, P., 'Re-contextualizing the female-headed household: Culture and agency in Uganda', in S. Szreter, H. Sholkamy and A. Dharmalingam (eds.), *Categories and Contexts: Anthropological and Historical Studies in Critical Demography* (Oxford: Oxford University Press, 2004), pp. 295–321.

Dawson, M., 'Socioeconomic change and disease: smallpox in colonial Kenya, 1880–1920', in S. Feierman and J. Janzen, *The Social Basis of Health and Healing in Africa* (Berkeley: University of California Press, 1992), pp. 90–103.

Dodge, C. and P. Henderson, 'Recent health surveys: towards a morbidity and mortality baseline', in Dodge and Wiebe, *Crisis*, pp. 209–14.

Dodge, C. and P. Wiebe (eds.), *Crisis in Uganda: The Breakdown of Health Services* (Oxford: Pergamon Press, 1985).

Dodge, C. and P. Wiebe, 'Introduction' in *Crisis*, pp. 1–14.

Doornbos, M., 'Ethnicity, Christianity, and the development of social stratification in colonial Ankole, Uganda', *The International Journal of African Historical Studies*, 9, 4 (1976), pp. 555–75.

Doornbos, M., 'Images and reality of stratification in pre-colonial Nkore', *Canadian Journal of African Studies*, 7, 3 (1973), pp. 477–95.

Doyle, S., '"The child of death": Personal names and parental attitudes towards mortality in Bunyoro, Western Uganda, 1900–2005', *The Journal of African History,* 49, 1 (2008), pp. 361–382.

Doyle, S., 'Bunyoro and the demography of slavery debate: fertility, kinship and assimilation', in Médard and Doyle, *Slavery*, pp. 231–51.

Doyle, S., 'From Kitara to the Lost Counties: Genealogy, land and legitimacy in the kingdom of Bunyoro, Western Uganda', *Social Identities*, 12, 4 (2006), pp. 457–70.

Doyle, S., 'Immigrants and indigenes: the Lost Counties dispute and the evolution of ethnic identity in colonial Buganda', *Journal of Eastern African Studies*, 3, 2 (2009), pp. 284–302.

Doyle, S., 'Population decline and delayed recovery in Bunyoro, 1860–1960', *The Journal of African History*, 41 (2000), pp. 429–58.

Doyle, S., *Crisis and Decline in Bunyoro: Population and Environment in Western Uganda 1860–1955* (Oxford: James Currey, 2006).

Dunn, J. and F. Delange, 'Damaged reproduction: the most important consequence of iodine deficiency', *The Journal of Clinical Endocrinology and Metabolism*, 86, 6 (2001), pp. 2360–3.

East Africa High Commission, *African Population of Tanganyika Territory: Geographical and Tribal Studies* (Nairobi: East African Statistical Department, 1950).

East Africa High Commission, *Tanganyika African Population Census 1957: Analysis by Sex and Age for Province, District, and Territorial Census Areas* (East African Statistical Department, 1958).

East African High Commission, *General African Census, August 1957, Tribal Analysis: Tanganyika* (Nairobi: Government Printer, 1958).

East African Medical Survey, *Annual Report, 1951* (Nairobi: EAHC, 1952).

East African Medical Survey, *Annual Report, 1952* (Nairobi: EAHC, 1952).

East African Medical Survey, *Annual Report, 1953* (Nairobi: EAHC, 1954).

East African Medical Survey, *Annual Report, 1954* (Nairobi: EAHC, 1955).

East African Statistical Department, *African Population of Tanganyika Territory 1948: Geographical and Tribal Studies* (Nairobi: Government Printer, 1950).

East African Statistical Department, *African Population of the Uganda Protectorate 1948: Geographical and Tribal Studies* (Nairobi: Government Printer, 1950).

East African Statistical Department, *Uganda Census 1959* (Nairobi: Government Printer, 1961).

Eckart, W., 'Medical experiments at the colonial periphery: the fight against sleeping sickness in German East Africa and Togo', in V. Roelcke and G. Maio (eds.), *Twentieth Century Ethics of Human Subjects Research: Historical Perspectives on Values, Practices, and Regulations* (Stuttgart: Franz Steiner Verlag, 2004), pp. 65–82.

Edel, M., *The Chiga of Uganda* (New Brunswick, NJ: Transaction, 1996 [1957]).

Elam, Y., *The Social and Sexual Roles of Hima Women: A Study of Nomadic Cattle Breeders in Nyabushozi County, Ankole, Uganda* (Manchester: Manchester University Press, 1973).

Elkan, W., *Migrants and Proletarians: Urban Labour in the Economic Development of Uganda* (London: Oxford University Press, 1960).

Engelstein, L., *The Keys to Happiness: Sex and the Search for Modernity in Fin-de-siècle Russia* (Ithaca: Cornell University Press, 1992).

Enns, A., 'The clocks have stopped in Uganda', in Dodge and Wiebe, *Crisis*, pp. 53–6.

Epstein, H. *The Invisible Cure: Africa, The West and the Fight against AIDS* (London: Viking, 2007).

Evans, A. and H. Mitchell, 'Soil fertility studies in Tanganyika. Improvement of crop and grass production on a leached sandy soil in Bukoba', *East African Agricultural and Forestry Journal*, 27 (1962), pp. 189–96.

Everett, V., 'Causes of stillbirth in Mulago hospital, Kampala, and their prevention', *Uganda Medical Journal*, 1 (1972), pp. 45–7.

Felkin, R., 'Notes on the Waganda tribe of Central Africa', *Proceedings of the Royal Society of Edinburgh*, 13 (1885/86), pp. 699–770.

Fetter, B. (ed.), *Demography from Scanty Evidence: Central Africa in the Colonial Era* (Boulder: Lynne Rienner, 1990).

Fetter, B., 'Decoding and interpreting African census data: Vital evidence from an unsavory witness', *Cahiers d'études africaines*, 27, 105/106 (1987), pp. 83–105.

Fèvre, E., P. Coleman, S. Welburn and I. Maudlin, 'Reanalyzing the 1900–1920 sleeping sickness epidemic in *Uganda', Emerging Infectious Diseases*, 10, 4 (2004), pp. 567–73.

Fisher, K., *Birth Control, Sex, and Marriage in Britain 1918–1960* (Oxford: Oxford University Press, 2006).

Fleming, D. and J. Wasserheit, 'From epidemiological synergy to public health policy and practice: The contribution of other sexually transmitted diseases to sexual transmission of HIV infection', *Sexually Transmitted Infections*, 75 (1999), pp. 3–17.

Ford, J. and R. Hall, 'The history of Karagwe (Bukoba District', *Tanganyika Notes and Records*, 24 (1947), pp. 3–27.

Ford, J., *The Role of the Trypanosomiases in African Ecology* (Oxford: Oxford University Press, 1971).

Fosbrooke, K., 'The defensive measure of certain tribes in North-Eastern Tanganyika, Part 2', *Tanganyika Notes and Records*, 36 (1954) pp. 50–7.

Foster, W. and L. Kerchan, 'Biological false positive Wassermann reactions in Uganda', *British Journal of Venereal Disease*, 42 (1966), pp. 272–5.

Foster, W., *Sir Albert Cook: A Missionary Doctor in Uganda* (Newhaven: Newhaven Press, 1978).

Foster, W., *The Early History of Scientific Medicine in Uganda* (Nairobi: EALB, 1970).

FPAU, *The Story of the Family Planning Association of Uganda* (Kampala: FPAU, 2007).

Frank, O., 'Infertility in sub-Saharan Africa: Estimates and implications', *Population and Development Review*, 9, 1 (1983), pp. 137–44.

Frisch, R., 'The right weight: body fat, menarche and fertility', *Proceedings of the Nutrition Society*, 53 (1994), pp. 113–29.

Fyfe, C. and D. McMaster, 'Introduction', in C. Fyfe and D. McMaster (eds.), *African Historical Demography: II* (Edinburgh: Centre of African Studies, 1981), pp. 1–8.

Gilman, S., *Difference and Pathology: Stereotypes of Sexuality, Race, and Madness* (New York: Cornell UP, 1985).

Goering, P. et al., 'Toxicity assessment of mercury vapor from dental amalgams', *Fundamental and Applied Toxicology*, 19, (1992), pp. 319–29.

Goodall, J., 'The hospital care of East African children', *Journal of Tropical Paediatrics*, 18, 1 (1972), pp. 45–95.

Goody, J., *Production and Reproduction: A Comparative Study of the Domestic Domain* (Cambridge: Cambridge University Press, 1976).

Goulet, A., *Sur les bords du Victoria, chez les Baganda* (Toulouse: Librairie Missionnaire, 1949).
Government of Uganda, *Annual Reports of the Ministry of Health 1963–9* (Entebbe: Government Printer, 1964–70).
Gray, R. et al., 'Spatial phylodynamics of HIV-1 epidemic emergence in east Africa', *AIDS*, 23, 14 (2009), pp. 9–17.
Gray-Swain, M. and J. Peipert, 'Pelvic inflammatory disease in adolescents', *Current Opinion in Obstetrics and Gynecology*, 18, 5 (2006), pp. 503–10.
Grech, E., 'Review of the treatment of ruptured uterus and Mulago hospital, Kampala', *East African Medical Journal*, 45, 7 (1968), pp. 508–15.
Grech, E., 'Stillbirths in Uganda', *Obstetrics and Gynecology*, 29, 6 (1967), pp. 764–73.
Grech, E., J. Everett and F. Mukasa, 'Epidemiological aspects of acute pelvic inflammatory disease in Uganda', *Tropical Doctor*, 3, 3 (1973), pp. 123–7.
Grech, E., J. Galea and R. Trussell, 'Maternal mortality in Uganda', *International Journal of Gynaecology and Obstetrics*, 7, 6 (1969), pp. 263–7.
Greenhalgh, S., 'Anthropology theorizes reproduction: Integrating practice, political economic, and feminist perspectives', in S. Greenhalgh (ed.), *Situating Fertility: Anthropology and Demographic Inquiry* (Cambridge: Cambridge University Press, 1995), pp. 3–28.
Griffith, H., 'Infertility and gonorrhoea in Uganda', *Eugenics Review*, 55, 2 (1963), pp. 103–8.
Gutkind, P., 'A preliminary report of Mulago, Kampala, Uganda, 1954' (TS, ASC, Cambridge).
Gutkind, P., 'African urban family life: comment on and analysis of some rural-urban difference', *Cahiers d'études africaines*, 10 (1962), pp. 149–217.
Gutkind, P., 'African urban marriage and family life: a note on some social and demographic characteristics from Kampala, Uganda', *Bulletin de l'IFAN*, 25, 3 (1963), pp. 266–87.
Gutkind, P., 'Some problems of African urban family life', *Diogenes*, 10, 37 (1962), pp. 88–104.
Gutkind, P., *The Royal Capital of Buganda: A study of Internal Conflict and External Ambiguity* (The Hague: Mouton, 1963).
Gysels, M., R. Pool and S. Nyanzi, 'The adventures of the Randy Professor and Angela the Sugar Mummy: Sex in fictional serials in Ugandan popular magazines', *AIDS Care*, 17, 8 (2005), pp. 967–77.
Hackett, C., 'On the origin of the human treponematoses (pinta, yaws, endemic and venereal syphilis)', *Bulletin of the World Health Organization*, 29, 1 (1963), pp. 7–41.
Halperin, D. and H. Epstein, 'Concurrent sexual partnerships help to explain Africa's high HIV prevalence: implications for prevention', *Lancet*, 364, 9428 (2004), pp. 4–6.
Hansen, H. and M. Twaddle (eds), *Uganda Now: Between Decay and Development* (Oxford: James Currey, 1988).
Hansen, H., *Mission, Church and State in a Colonial Setting: Uganda 1890–1925* (New York: St. Martin's, 1984).
Hanson, H., *Landed Obligation: The Practice of Power in Buganda* (Portsmouth, NH: Heinemann, 2003).

Harris, T., *Donkey's Gratitude: Twenty-two Years in the Growth of a New African Nation—Tanzania* (Durham: Pentland Press, 1992).

Harrison. L. and T. Osmond, 'The uses and limitations of the serum tests for syphilis', *British Journal of Venereal Diseases*, 19 (1943), pp. 108–18.

Hartwig, G., 'Economic consequences of long-distance trade in East Africa: The disease factor', *African Studies Review*, 18, 2 (1975), pp. 63–75.

Hastings, A., *Christian Marriage in Africa, Being a Report Comissioned by the Archbishops of Cape Town, Central Africa, Kenya, Tanzania, and Uganda* (London: SPCK, 1973).

Havnevik, K., 'A resource overlooked: crafts and small-scale industries', in J. Boesen, K. Havnevik, J. Koponen and R. Odgaard (eds.), *Tanzania: Crisis and Struggle for Survival* (Uppsala: Scandinavia Institute of African Studies, 1986), pp. 269–91.

Haydon, E., *Law and Justice in Buganda* (London: Butterworths, 1960).

Heald, S., 'The power of sex: Some reflections on the Caldwells' "African sexuality" thesis', *Africa*, 65, 4 (1995), pp. 489–505.

Hebert, J. and S. Ssentamu, 'Water supply, sanitation and the effect on the healthcare delivery system', in Dodge and Wiebe, *Crisis*, pp. 117–26.

Henin, R. and B. Egero, '1967 population census of Tanzania: a demographic analysis' (BRALUP Research Notes 19, UDSM, 1972).

Henin, R., *National Demographic Survey of Tanzania, 1973: Volume II, Data for Socioeconomic Groups* (Dar es Salaam: Tanzania Bureau of Statistics, 1973).

Hill, K., 'Demographic estimation from deficient or defective data', in B. Fetter (ed.), *Demography from Scanty Evidence: Central Africa in the Colonial Era* (London: L. Rienner Publishers, 1990), pp. 133–42.

Horwitz, S., 'Migrancy and HIV/AIDS: A historical perspective', *South African Historical Journal* 45, 1 (2001), pp. 103–23.

Hunter, M., 'The materiality of everyday sex: Thinking beyond "prostitution"', *African Studies*, 61, 1 (2002), pp. 99–120.

Hutt, M. and A. Dulo, 'An analysis of diseases found in adults of the Baganda and Banyarwanda/Rundi tribes at autopsy in 1964', *Makerere Medical Journal*, 1 (1966), pp. 24–7.

Huxley, E., *The Sorcerer's Apprentice* (London: Chatto and Windus, 1948).

Hyden, G., *Political Development in Rural Tanzania: A West Lake Study* (Nairobi: East African Publishing House, 1969).

Iliffe, J., *A Modern History of Tanganyika* (Cambridge: Cambridge University Press, 1979).

Iliffe, J., *Africans: the History of a Continent* (Cambridge: Cambridge University Press, 2nd edn, 2007).

Iliffe, J., *Africans: The History of a Continent* (Cambridge: Cambridge University Press, 1995).

Iliffe, J., *East African Doctors* (Cambridge: Cambridge University Press, 1998).

Iliffe, J., *The African AIDS Epidemic: a History* (Oxford: James Currey, 2006).

Iliffe, J., *The African Poor: A History* (Cambridge: Cambridge University Press, 1987).

Ishumi, A., *Kiziba: The Cultural Heritage of an Old African Kingdom* (Syracuse: Maxwell School of Citizenship and Public Affairs, 1980).

Ivaska, A., *Cultured States: Youth, Gender and Modern Style in 1960s Dar es Salaam* (Durham, NC: Duke University Press, 2011).

Jean-Baptiste, R., '"These laws should be made by us": Customary marriage law, codification and political authority in twentieth-century colonial Gabon', *The Journal of African History,* 49, 2 (2008), pp. 217–40.

Jelliffe, D., 'Pediatrics in Uganda', *Clinical Pediatrics*, 5 (1965), pp. 55–61.

Jelliffe, D., 'Village level feeding of young children in developing tropical regions, with especial reference to Buganda', *Journal of the American Medical Women's Association*, 17, 5 (May 1962), pp. 409–18.

Jewsiewicki, B., 'Towards a historical sociology of population in Zaire: Proposals for the analysis of the demographic regime', in Cordell and Gregory, *African Population*, pp. 270–8.

Jochelson, K., *The Colour of Disease: Syphilis and Racism in South Africa, 1880–1950* (London: Palgrave Macmillan, 2001).

Johnson-Hanks, J., 'The lesser shame: abortion among educated women in southern Cameroon', *Social Science and Medicine*, 55, 8 (2002), pp. 1337–49.

Johnston, H., *The Uganda Protectorate* (London: Hutchinson, 1902).

Jokela, M., M. Elovainio and M. Kivimaki, 'Lower fertility associated with obesity and underweight: the US National Longitudinal Survey of Youth', *American Journal of Clinical Nutrition*, 88, 4 (2008), pp. 886–93.

Kagwa, A., *The Customs of the Baganda* (translated by E. Kalibala, edited by M. Edel, New York: Columbia University Press, 1934).

Kaijage, F., 'AIDS control and the burden of history in northwestern Tanzania', *Population and Environment*, 14, 3 (1999), pp. 279–300.

Kampikaho, A. and L. Irwig, 'Incidence and causes of maternal mortality in five Kampala hospitals, 1980–1986', *East African Medical Journal*, 68, 8 (1991), pp. 624–31.

Kamuzora, C., 'Formation of a low fertility culture in Kigarama village, Tanzania: cultual materialism versus idealism', (University of Dar es Salaam Department of Statistics Demographic Unit, Ocasional Paper no. 9, 1997).

Kamuzora, C., 'High fertility and the demand for labour in peasant economies: The case of Bukoba District, Tanzania', *Development and Change*, 15, 1 (1984), pp. 105–24.

Kanyadago, P., *Evangelizing Polygamous Families: Canonical and African Approaches* (Gaba: AMACEA, 1991).

Karamagi, C., 'Breast-feeding in and around Kampala', in Dodge and Wiebe, *Crisis*, pp. 227–32.

Karugire, S., *A History of the Kingdom of Nkore in Western Uganda to 1896* (London: Clarendon, 1971).

Kasozi, A., *The Social Origins of Violence in Uganda, 1964–1985* (Montreal: Queens University Press, 1994).

Katate, A. and L. Kamugungunu, *Abagabe b'Ankole* (Nairobi: EALB, 1967 [1947]).

Katoke, I., *The Karagwe Kingdom: A History of the Abanyambo of North-west Tanzania* (Nairobi: EAPH, 1975), pp. 70–104.

Kibukamusoke, J., 'Gonorrhoea and urethral stricture', *British Journal of Venereal Diseases*, 41 (1965), pp. 135–6.

Kibukamusoke, J., 'Venereal disease in East Africa', *Transactions of the Royal Society of Tropical Medicine and Hygiene*, 59, 6 (1965), pp. 642–8.

Kilbride, P., 'Barmaiding as a deviant occupation among the Baganda of Uganda', *Ethos*, 7, 3 (1979), pp. 232–54.

Killewo, J. et al., 'Incidence of HIV-1 infection among adults in the Kagera Region of Tanzania', *International Journal of Epidemiology, 22 (*1993), pp. 528–36.

Killewo, J. et al., 'Prevalence and incidence of syphilis infection and its association with HIV-1 infection among adults in the Kagera region of Tanzania: A population-based study', *International Journal of STD and AIDS*, 5 (1994), pp. 424–31.

Killewo, J. et al., 'Prevalence of HIV-1 infection in the Kagera region of Tanzania: a population-based study', *AIDS*, 4, 11 (1990), pp. 1081–6.

Killewo, J., L. Dahlgren and A. Sandström, 'Socio-geographical patterns of HIV-1 transmission in Kagera Region, Tanzania', *Social Science and Medicine*, 38, 1 (1994), pp. 129–34.

Kirk, D. and B. Pillet, 'Fertility levels, trends and differentials in sub-Saharan Africa in the 1980s and 1990s', *Studies in Family Planning*, 29 (1998), pp. 1–22.

Kisekka, M., 'AIDS in Uganda as a gender issue', in E. Rothblum and E. Cole (eds.), *Women's Mental Health in Uganda* (London: Haworth, 1990), pp. 39–45.

Kisekka, M., 'The Baganda of central Uganda', in Molnos, *Cultural Source Materials III*, pp. 148–162.

Kiwanuka, N. et al., 'HIV-1 viral subtype differences in the rate of CD4+ T-cell decline among HIV seroincident antiretroviral naive persons in Rakai district, Uganda', *Journal of Acquired Immune Deficiency Syndrome*, 54, 2 (2010), pp. 180–4.

Kitching, G., 'Proto-industrialisation and demographic change: A thesis and some possible African implications', *Journal of African History*, 24, 2 (1983), pp. 221–40.

Kiyimba, A., 'Gendering social destiny in the proverbs of the Baganda: Reflections on boys and girls becoming men and women', *Journal of African Cultural Studies*, 17, 2 (2005), pp. 253–70.

Kjekshus, H., *Ecology Control and Economic Development in East African history* (London: Heinemann, 1977).

Knodel, J., *Demographic Behaviour in the Past: a Study of Fourteen German Village Populations in the Eighteenth and Nineteenth Centuries* (Cambridge: Cambridge University Press, 1988).

Kodesh, N., *Beyond the Royal Gaze: Clanship and Public Healing in Buganda* (Charlottesville: University of Virginia Press, 2010).

Koerne, T., P. de Raadt and I. Maudlin, 'The Uganda sleeping sickness epidemic revisited: a case of mistaken identity?', *Parasitology Today,* 11, 8 (1995), pp. 303–306.

Kokole, O., 'The politics of fertility in Africa', *Population and Development Review,* 20 (1994), pp. 73–88.

Koku, M. and M. Ngaiza, 'The life history of a housewife: her life, work, income and property ownership', in M. Ngaiza and B. Koda (eds.), *Unsung Heroines: Women's Life Histories from Tanzania* (Dar es Salaam: WRDP, 1991), pp. 85–108.

Kollman, P., *The Victoria Nyanza: The Land, the Races and their Customs, with Specimens of some of the Dialects* (London: Swan Sonnenschein, 1899).

Kollmann, P., *Der Nordwesten unserer ostafrikanischen Kolonie* (Berlin: Schall, 1898).

Kuczynski, R., *Demographic Survey of the British Colonial Empire, Vol. II* (Oxford: Institute of International Affairs, 1949).

Kuhanen, J., '"Balinsalamu embawo?" AIDS and the context of sexual behaviour adjustment in Rakai, Uganda, *c.* 1975–90', *Journal of Eastern African Studies*, 4, 1 (2010), pp. 20–43.

Kuhanen, J., 'Sexualised space, sexual networking and the emergence of AIDS in Rakai, Uganda', *Health and Place*, 16, 2 (2010), pp. 226–35.

Kuhanen, J., 'The historiography of HIV and AIDS in Uganda', *History in Africa* 35 (2009), pp. 301–25.

Kuhanen, J., *Poverty, Health and Reproduction in Early Colonial Uganda* (Joensuun: Joensuun University Press, 2005).

Kwesigabo, G. et al., 'Monitoring of HIV-1 infection prevalence and trends in the general population using pregnant women as a sentinel population: Nine years experience from the Kagera Region of Tanzania', *Journal of Acquired Immune Deficiency Syndromes*, 23, 5 (2000), pp. 410–17.

Kyewalyanga, F.-X., *Traditional Religion, Custom and Christianity in Uganda: As Illustrated by the Ganda with Some References to other African Cultures and Islam* (Freiburg: Renner, 1976).

Kyomuhendo, G. and M. McIntosh, *Women, Work and Domestic Virtue in Uganda, 1900–2003* (Oxford: James Currey, 2006).

Lambkin, F., 'An outbreak of syphilis in a virgin soil: Notes on syphilis in the Uganda Protectorate', in D. Power and J. Murphy (eds.), *A System of Syphilis* (London: Oxford University Press, 1908), p. 339.

Lambkin, F., 'An outbreak of syphilis on virgin soil', *The Lancet* (1908), p. 1022.

Larsen, U., 'Childlessness, subfertility, and infertility in Tanzania', *Studies in Family Planning*, 27, 1 (1996), pp. 18–28.

Larsen, U., 'Primary and secondary infertility in Tanzania', *Journal of Health and Population in Developing Countries*, 3 (2003), pp. 1–15.

Larsen, U., 'Sterility in sub-Saharan Africa', *Population Studies,* 48, 3 (1994), pp. 459–74.

Larsson, B., *Conversion to Greater Freedom? Women, Church and Social Change in North-Western Tanzania under Colonial Rule* (Uppsala: University of Uppsala, 1991).

Laurie, W. and H. Trant, *East African Medical Survey, Monograph no. 2: A Health Survey in Bukoba District, Tanganyika* (Nairobi: EAHC, 1954).

Laurie, W., 'A pilot scheme of venereal disease control in East Africa', *British Journal of Venereal Diseases*, 34 (1958), pp. 16–21.

Le Blanc, M.-N., D. Meintel and V. Piché, 'The African sexual system: Comment on Caldwell et al.', *Population and Development Review*, 17, 3 (1991), pp. 497–505.

Lejju, B., P. Robertshaw and D. Taylor, 'Africa's earliest bananas?', *Journal of Archaeological Science*, 33, 1 (2006), pp. 102–13.

Leopold, M., 'Sex, violence and history in the lives of Idi Amin: Postcolonial masculinity as masquerade', *Journal of Postcolonial Writing*, 45, 3 (2009), pp. 321–30.

Lesthaeghe, R., 'Fertility and its proximate determinants in sub-Saharan Africa: The record of the 1960s and 1970s' (Interuniversity Programme in Demography, Working Paper 1984, Vrije Universiteit Brussels, Belgium).

Lesthaeghe, R., H. Page and O. Adegbola, 'Child spacing and fertility in Lagos', in H. Page and R. Lesthaeghe (eds.), *Child-spacing in Tropical Africa: Traditions and Change* (London: Heinemann, 1981), pp. 147–180.

Lockwood, M., *Fertility and Household Labour in Tanzania: Demography, Economy, and Society in Rufiji District, c.1870–1986* (Oxford: Oxford University Press, 1998).

Lonsdale, J., 'Kikuyu Christianities', *Journal of Religion in Africa*, 29, 2 (1999), pp. 215–25.

Low-Beer, D. and R. Stoneburner, 'Behaviour and communication change in reducing HIV: Is Uganda unique', *African Journal of AIDS Research*, 1, 2 (2004), pp. 9–21.

Lugalla, J. et al., 'Social, cultural and sexual behavioral determinants of observed decline in HIV infection trends: lessons from the Kagera Region, Tanzania', *Social Science and Medicine*, 59 (2004), pp. 185–98.

Lugard, F., *The Rise of Our East African Empire: Early efforts in Nyasaland and Uganda* (Edinburgh and London: William Blackwood and Sons, 1893).

Lwanga, C., 'Abortion in Mulago Hospital, Kampala', *East African Medical Journal*, 54, 3 (1977), pp. 142–8.

Lwihula, G., 'Sexuality and HIV transmission in Kagera Region, Tanzania', *International Conference on AIDS*, 5 (1989), p. 878.

Lwihula, G., L. Dahlgren, J. Killewo and A. Sandstrom, 'AIDS epidemic in Kagera region, Tanzania: The experiences of local people', *AIDS Care*, 5, 3 (1993), pp. 347–57.

Lyons, M., 'Medicine and morality: a review of responses to sexually transmitted diseases in Uganda in the twentieth century', in P. Setel, M. Lewis and M. Lyons (eds.), *Histories of Sexually Transmitted Diseases and HIV/AIDS in Sub-Saharan Africa* (London: Greenwood, 1999), pp. 97–117.

Lyons, M., 'Sexually-transmitted diseases in the history of Uganda', *Genitourinary Medicine*, 79 (1994), pp. 138–45.

Lyons, M., *The Colonial Disease: A Social History of Sleeping Sickness in Northern Zaire* (Cambridge: Cambridge University Press, 1992).

Mackay, G., *A Life of A. M. Mackay of Uganda* (London: Sunday School Union, 1893).

Mah, T. and D. Halperin 'Concurrent sexual partnerships and the HIV epidemics in Africa: evidence to move forward', *AIDS and Behavior,* 14 (2010), pp. 11–14.

Mair, L., *An African People in the Twentieth Century* (London: Routledge, 1934).

Mair, L., *Native Marriage in Buganda, International Institute of African Languages and Cultures Memorandum XIX* (Oxford: Oxford University Press, 1940).

Mandeville, E., 'Poverty, work and the financing of single women in Kampala', *Africa*, 49, 1 (1979), pp. 42–52.

Mandeville, E., 'The formality of marriage: A Kampala case study', *Journal of Anthropological Research*, 31, 3 (1975), pp. 183–95.

Manji, A., '"Her name is Kamundage": Rethinking women and property among the Haya of Tanzania', *Africa*, 70, 3 (2000), pp. 482–500.

Martin, C., 'Some estimates of the general age distribution, fertility and rate of natural increase of the African population of British East Africa', *Population Studies*, 7, 2 (1953), pp. 181–99.

Mason, K., 'Explaining fertility transitions', *Demography*, 34, 4 (1997), pp. 443–54.

Mason, K., *The Status of Women: A Review of its Relationships to Fertility and Mortality* (New York: Rockefeller, 1984).

Masters, K. and J. Iraka, 'The influence of custom and tradition on maternity care in Ankole district', *East African Medical Journal*, 47, 11 (1970), pp. 550–6.

Mburu, F., 'Evaluation of government rural health centres and UNICEF essential drug input', in Dodge and Wiebe, *Crisis*, pp. 86–92.

McClintock, A., *Imperial Leather: Race, Gender and Sexuality in the Colonial Contest* (London: Routledge, 1995).

McElligott, G., Venereal Diseases in the Tropics', *British Journal of Venereal Diseases*, 27 (1951), pp. 122–6.

McGrath, J. et al., 'Cultural determinants of sexual risk behavior for AIDS among Baganda women', *Medical Anthropology Quarterly*, 6, 2 (1992), pp. 153–61.

McKeown, T., *The Modern Rise of Population* (London: Arnold, 1976).

McMaster, D., 'Change of regional balance in the Bukoba district of Tanganyika', *Tanganyika Notes and Records*, 56 (1961), pp. 79–92.

Médard, H., 'Introduction' in Médard and Doyle *Slavery*, pp. 1–37.

Médard, H., 'La peste et les missionnaires: santé et syncrétisme médical au royaume du Buganda à la fin du 19ème siècle', *Outre-Mer Revue d'Histoire*, 346–347 (2005), pp. 79–102.

Médard, H., *Le royaume du Buganda au XIXe siècle. Mutations politiques et religieuses d'un grand état d'Afrique de l'Est* (Paris: Karthala, 2007).

Médard, H., 'L'homosexualité au Buganda, une acculturation peut en cacher une autre', *Hypothèse*, 1 (1999), pp. 47–52.

Médard, H. and S. D. Doyle (eds.), *Slavery in the Great Lakes Region of East Africa* (Oxford: James Currey, 2007).

Meldon, J., 'Notes on the Bahima of Ankole', *Journal of the Africa Society*, 6, 22 (1907), pp. 136–53, 234–49.

Messenger, J., 'Sex and repression in an Irish folk community', in D. Marshall and R. Suggs (eds.), *Human Sexual Behavior: Variations in the ethnographic spectrum* (New York: Basic Books, 1970).

Mettam, R., 'A short history of rinderpest with special reference to Africa', *Uganda Journal*, 5, 1 (1937), pp. 22–6.

Mills, D., 'Life on the hill: students and the social history of Makerere', *Africa*, 76, 2 (2006), pp. 247–66.

Milne, G., 'Bukoba: High and low fertility on a laterised soil', *The East African Agricultural Journal*, 4 (1938), pp. 1–21.

Mindel, A. and C. Estcourt, 'Syphilis', in Stanberry and Bernstein, *Sexually Transmitted Diseases*, pp. 387–420.

Ministry of Planning and Economic Development, *Rural Food Consumption Survey, 1968, in Ankole, Busoga, Masaka and West Nile* (Entebbe: Government Printer, 1970).

Moffat, R., 'Uganda Protectorate: Report for the year ending December 31, 1900', *Journal of Tropical Medicine and Hygiene*, 4 (1901), pp. 326–45.

Moller, M., 'Bahaya customs and beliefs in connection with pregnancy and childbirth', *Tanganyika Notes and Records*, 50, 1 (1958), pp. 112–7.

Molnos, A. (ed.), *Cultural Source Materials for Population Planning in East Africa: Innovation and Communication. Vol. II* (Nairobi: University of Nairobi, Institute of African Studies, 1972).

Molnos, A. (ed.), *Cultural Source Materials for Population Planning in East Africa: Beliefs and Practices. Vol. III* (Nairobi: University of Nairobi, Institute of African Studies, 1973).

Morris, K., 'The movement of sleeping sickness across central Africa', *The Journal of Tropical Medicine and Hygiene*, 66 (1963), pp. 59–76.

Morris, M. and M. Kretzschmar, 'Concurrent partnerships and the spread of HIV', *AIDS*, 11 (1997), pp. 641–48.

Mtimavalye, L. et al., 'Infertility among women in five rural and two urban districts of Tanzania', *Journal of Obstetric and Gynecology in East and Central Africa*, 3 (1984), pp. 125–9.

Mukwaya, A., *Land Tenure in Buganda: Present Day Tendencies* (Kampala: EAISR, 1953).

Mulokozi, M., 'The Nanga bards of Tanzania: are they epic artists?', *Research in African Literatures*, 14, 3 (1983), pp. 283–311.

Mushanga, M., 'The Nkole of South-Western Uganda', in Molnos *Cultural Source Materials III*, pp. 174–86.

Musisi, N., 'Colonial and missionary education: Women and domesticity in Uganda, 1900–1945', in K. Hansen (ed.), *African Encounters with Domesticity* (New Brunswick NJ: Rutgers University Press, 1992), pp. 172–94.

Musisi, N., 'Gender and the cultural construction of "bad women" in the development of Kampala-Kibuga, 1900–1962', in D. Hodgson and S. McCurdy (eds.), *'Wicked Women' and the Reconfiguration of Gender in Africa* (Oxford: James Currey, 2001), pp. 171–87.

Musisi, N., 'Morality as identity: The missionary moral agenda in Buganda,1877–1945', *Journal of Religious History* 23, 1 (1999), pp. 51–74.

Musisi, N., 'Women, "elite polygyny" and Buganda state formation', *Signs*, 16, 4, (1991), pp. 757–86.

Musoke, L., 'An analysis of admissions to the paediatric division, Mulago Hospital in 1959', *Archives of Disease in Childhood*, 36 (1961), pp. 305–15.

Muwazi, E., H. Trowell and J. Davies, 'Congenital syphilis in Uganda', *East African Medical Journal*, 24 (1947), pp. 152–70.

Nabaitu, J., C. Bachengana and J. Seeley, 'Marital instability in a rural population in south-west Uganda: Implications for the spread of HIV-1 infection', *Africa*, 64, 2 (1994), pp. 243–51.

Nair, P., 'Population aging in Botswana: Trends and implications', *Journal of African Studies and Development*, 2, 3 (2010), pp. 58–64.

Namboze, J. and M. Kakande, 'Some aspects of knowledge and attitude towards family planning and sterilisation on the periurban area of Kampala, Uganda', in N. Mwaniki, M. Marash, J. Mati and M. Mwaniki (eds.), *Surgical Contraception in Sub-Saharan Africa: Proceedings of a Conference, Nyeri, Kenya, May 8–13, 1977* (Chestnut Hill, MA: Pathfinder Fund, 1979), pp. 74–84.

Nannyonga-Tamusuza, S., *Baakisimba: Gender in the Music and Dance of the Baganda People of Uganda* (New York: Routledge, 2005).

National Bureau of Statistics and ORC Macro, *Tanzania Demographic and Health Survey 2004–05: Key Findings* (Calverton, Maryland, USA: NBS and ORC Macro, 2005).

National Bureau of Statistics and ORC Macro, *Tanzania Demographic and Health Survey 1991–02* (Calverton, Maryland, USA: NBS and ORC Macro, 1993).

Ndeki. S., K. Klepp and G. Mliga, 'Knowledge, perceived risk of AIDS and sexual behavior among primary school children in two areas of Tanzania', *Health Education Research*, 9, 1 (1994), pp. 133–8.

Nelson, N., '"Selling her kiosk": Kikuyu notions of sexuality and sex for sale in Mathare Calley, Kenya', in P. Caplan (ed.), *The Cultural Construction of Sexuality* (London: Tavistock, 1987), pp. 217–39.

Nkya, W. et al., 'Sexually transmitted diseases in prostitutes in Moshi and Arusha, Northern Tanzania', *International Journal of STD and AIDS*, 2, 6 (1991), pp. 432–5.

Nkya, W. et al., 'The role of self-proclaimed prostitutes in STD transmission in Tanzania', in Tanzania Public Health Association, Epidemiology and control of communicable diseases in Tanzania. Proceedings of the 8th Annual Scientific Conference, Dar es Salaam, 14–17 November 1989 (Dar es Salaam, 1991), pp. 12–40.

Notkola, V., I. Timaeus and H. Siiskonen, 'Mortality transition in the Ovamboland region of Namibia, 1930–1990', *Population Studies*, 54 (2000), pp. 153–67.

Ntozi, J. and J. Kabera, 'Marriage patterns in Ankole, South-Western Uganda' (African Demography Working Papers no.16, University of Pennsylvania, August 1988).

Ntozi, J. and S. Nakayiwa, 'AIDS in Uganda: How has the household coped with the epidemic?', in J. Caldwell, I. Orubuloye and J. Ntozi (eds.), *The Continuing African HIV/AIDS Epidemic* (Canberra: Health Transition Centre, 1999), pp. 155–81.

Ntozi, J. et al., 'The value of children as a major influence on fertility in Uganda: A case study of Ankole', *Fertility Determinants Research Notes*, 23 (1988), pp. 20–7.

Ntozi, J., *High Fertility in Rural Uganda: The Role of Socioeconomic and Biological Factors* (Kampala: Fountain, 1995).

Ntozi, J., *The Role of Men in Determining Fertility among the Banyankore of Southwestern Uganda* (Kampala: Marianum Press, 1993).

Nyakatura, J., *Anatomy of an African kingdom: a History of Bunyoro-Kitara* (edited by G. N. Uzoigwe (New York: NOK, 1973).

Nyanzi, S., J. Nassimbwa, V. Kayizzi and S. Kabanda, '"African sex is dangerous!" Renegotiating "ritual sex" in contemporary Masaka District', *Africa* 78, 4 (2008), pp. 518–39.

Obbo, C., 'Dominant male ideology and female options: Three East African case studies', *Africa*, 46, 4 (1976), pp. 371–89.

Obbo, C., 'HIV transmission through social and geographical networks in Uganda', *Social Science and Medicine*, 36, 1 (1993), pp. 949–55.

Obbo, C., 'HIV transmission: men are the solution', in S. James and A. Busia (eds.), *Theorizing Black Feminisms: The Visionary Pragmatism of Black Women* (London: Routledge, 1993), pp. 160–81.

Obbo, C., 'HIV transmission: Men are the solution', *Population and Environment*, 14, 3 (1993), pp. 211–43.

Obbo, C., *African Women: Their Struggle for Independence* (London: Zed Press, 1980).

Oberg, K., 'Analysis of the Bahima marriage ceremony', *Africa*, 19, 2 (1949), pp. 107–20.

Oberg, K., 'Kinship organization of the Banyankole', *Africa*, 11, 2 (1938), pp. 129–59.

Okello, M., 'Family planning in difficult times', in Dodge and Wiebe, *Crisis*, pp. 233–9.

Ongom, V. et al., 'The prevalence of venereal diseases among food and liquor-handlers in public places in Kampala, Uganda.' *East African Medical Journal*, 53, 7 (1976), pp. 389–97.

Ongom, V., 'A study of the prevalence of sexually transmitted diseases amongst bar attendants and a surveillance on their movements for a year in the Kasangati defined area', *Makerere Medical Journal* (Oct. 1978), pp. 9–13.

Ongom, V., 'Prevalence and incidence of venereal diseases in military communities in Uganda', *East African Medical Journal*, 47, 9 (1970), pp. 479–83.

Packard, R., 'Maize, cattle and mosquitoes: The political economy of malaria epidemics in colonial Swaziland', *The Journal of African History*, 25, 2 (1984), pp. 189–212.

Parikh, S., 'From Auntie to Disco: The bifurcation of risk and pleasure in sex education in Uganda', in V. Adams and S. Pigg (eds.), *Sex in Development: Science, Sexuality, and Morality* (Durham, NC: Duke University Press, 2005), pp. 125–58.

Parikh, S., 'The political economy of marriage and HIV: The ABC approach, "safe" infidelity, and managing moral risk in Uganda', *American Journal of Public Health*, 97 (2007), pp. 1198–1208.

Parkin, D., 'Types of urban African marriage in Kampala', *Africa*, 36, 3 (1966), pp. 269–85.

Parkin, D., *Neighbours and Nationals in an African City Ward* (London: Routledge, 1969).

Pepin, J., *The Origins of AIDS* (Cambridge: Cambridge University Press, 2011).

Peters, C., *New Light on Dark Africa* (London: Ward, Lock and Co., 1891).

Phillips, I., 'A guide to antibiotic treatment of gonorrhoea in Uganda', *Makerere Medical Journal*, 1, 3 (1968), pp. 103–9.

Pickering, H. et al., 'Sexual behaviour in a fishing community on Lake Victoria, Uganda', *Health Transition Review*, 7 (1997), pp. 13–20.

Piot, P. et al., 'Retrospective seroepidemiology of *AIDS* virus infection in Nairobi populations', *Journal of Infectious Diseases,* 155 (1987), pp. 1108–12.

Pison, G., J. Trape, M. Lefebvre and C. Enel, 'Rapid decline in child mortality in a rural area of Senegal', *International Journal of Epidemiology*, 22, 1 (1993), pp. 72–80.

Population Reference Bureau, *World Population Report 2009 Datasheet* http://www.prb.org/pdf09/09wpds_eng.pdf

Portal, G., *The British Mission to Uganda in 1893* (London: Arnold, 1893).

Potts, D. and S. Marks, 'Fertility in Southern Africa: The quiet revolution', *Journal of Southern African Studies*, 27, 2 (2001), pp. 189–205.

Raikes, P., *Coffee Production in West Lake Region, Tanzania* (Copenhagen: IDR, 1976).

Ranger, T. and P. Slack (eds.), *Epidemics and Ideas: Essays on the Historical Perception of Pestilence* (Cambridge: Cambridge University Press, 1992).

Reddy, S., '"Its not as easy as ABC": Dynamics of intergenerational power and resistance within the context of HIV/AIDS', *Perspectives in Education*, 23, 3 (2005), pp. 11–19.

Reid, R., *Political Power in Pre-colonial Buganda : Economy, Society and Warfare in the Nineteenth Century* (Oxford: James Currey, 2002).

Reining, P. and A. Richards, 'Report on fertility surveys in Buganda and Buhaya, 1952', in F. Lorimer et al. (eds.) *Culture and Human Fertility* (Paris: UNESCO, 1954), pp. 351–404.

Reining, P., 'Haya land tenure: landholding and tenancy', *Anthropological Quarterly*, 35, 2, (1962), pp. 58–73.

Reining, P., 'The Haya of north-western Tanzania', in Molnos *Cultural III*, pp. 215–23.

Reining, P., 'The Haya: The agrarian system of a sedentary people' (unpublished PhD dissertation, University of Chicago, 1965).

Rendle-Short, C., 'Causes of maternal death among Africans in Kampala, Uganda', *British Journal of Obstetrics and Gynaecology*, 68, 1 (1961), pp. 44–51.

Rendle-Short, C., 'Rupture of the gravid uterus in Uganda', *Obstetrics and Gynecology*, 79, 6 (1960), pp. 1114–20.

Republic of Uganda, *Report on the 1969 Population Census: Vol. III Additional Tables* (Entebbe: Statistics Division, 1973).

Retel-Laurentin, A., 'Sub-Fertility in Black Africa: The case of the Nzakara in Central African Republic', in B. Adadevoh (ed.), *Subfertility and Infertility in Africa* (Ibadan: Caxton Press, 1974), pp. 69–80.

Retel-Laurentin, A., *Causes de l'infécondité dans la Volta Noire* (Paris: INED, 1979).

Retel-Laurentin, A., *Un pays à la dérive: une société en régression démographique. Les Nzakara de l'est centrafricain* (Paris: Delarge, 1979).

Richards, A. (ed.), *Economic Development and Tribal Change: A Study of Immigrant Labour in Buganda*. (Cambridge: Heffer, 1954).

Richards, A., 'The assimilation of the immigrants', in A. Richards (ed.), *Economic Development and Tribal Change: A Study of Immigrant Labour in Buganda* (Cambridge: Heffer, 1952), pp. 161–93.

Richards, A., 'Traditional values and current political behavior', in L. Fallers (ed.), *All The King's Men: Leadership and Status in Buganda on the Eve of Independence* (London, 1964), pp. 294–335.

Robbins, M. and R. Pollnac, 'Drinking patterns and acculturation in rural Buganda', *American Anthropologist*, 71, 2 (1969), pp. 276–85.

Robbins, M., 'Problem-drinking and the integration of alcohol in Buganda', *Medical Anthropology*, 1, 3 (1977), pp. 193–206.

Robertson, D., A. McMillan and H. Young, *Clinical Practice in Sexually Transmissible Diseases* (Edinburgh: Churchill Livingstone, 1989).

Romaniuk, A., 'Increase in natural fertility during the early stages of modernization: Evidence from an African case study, Zaire', *Population Studies*, 34 (1980), pp. 293–310.

Roscoe, J., 'The Bahima: a cow tribe of Enkole in the Uganda Protectorate', *Journal of the Royal Anthropological Institute*, 37 (1907), pp. 93–108.

Roscoe, J., *The Baganda: An Account of Their Native Customs and Beliefs* (London: Macmillan, 1911).

Roscoe, J., *The Northern Bantu: An Account of some Central African Tribes of the Uganda Protectorate* (London: Cass, 1966 [1915]).

Roscoe, J., *The Soul of Central Africa: a General Account of the Mackie Ethnological Expedition* (New York: Negro University Press, 1969 [1922]).

Roscoe, J., *Twenty-Five Years in East Africa* (Cambridge: Cambridge University Press, 1921).

Rudengren, J., 'A methodological study of population density and distribution: A case study of West Lake Region', (BRALUP Research Report 7, University of Dar es Salaam, 1974).

Rutstein, S., 'Socio-economic differentials in infant and child mortality', *WFS Comparative Studies* 43 (London: World Fertility Survey, 1984).

Rwakatonera, R., 'Factors affecting the quality of nursing care at Mulago', in Dodge and Wiebe, *Crisis*, pp. 69–74.

Rwegelera, G., 'Tribal customs in infant feeding I: Among the Haya', *East Africa Medical Journal*, 40 (1963), pp. 366–9.

Rwiza, K., 'Natal customs in Bukoba', *Tanganyika Notes and Records*, 50, 1 (1958), pp. 104–17.

Sanderson, F., 'The development of labour migration from Nyasaland, 1891–1914', *Journal of African History*, 2, 2 (1961), pp. 259–71.

Sawers, L. and E. Stillwaggon, 'Concurrent sexual partnerships do not explain the HIV epidemics in Africa: A systematic review of the evidence', *Journal of the International AIDS Society,* 13 (2010), 34.

Schapera, I., *Migrant Labour and Tribal Life: A Study of Conditions in the Bechuanaland Protectorate* (London: Cambridge University Press, 1947).

Scheyer, S. and D. Dunlop, 'Health services and development in Uganda', in Dodge Wiebe, *Crisis*, pp. 25–42.

Schmidt, E., 'Patriarchy, capitalism, and the colonial state in Zimbabwe', *Signs*, 16, 4 (1991), pp. 732–56.

Schmidt, P., 'A new look at interpretations of the early iron age in East Africa', *History in Africa,* 2 (1975), pp. 127–36.

Schmidt, P., *Historical Archaeology: A Structural Approach in an African Culture* (Westport: Greenwood Press, 1978), pp. 280.

Schoenbrun, D., 'Cattle herds and banana gardens: The historical geography of the western Great Lakes region, ca AD 800–1500', *The African Archaeological Review*, 11 (1993), pp. 39–72.

Schoenbrun, D., *A Green Place, a Good Place: Agrarian Change, Gender, and Social Identity in the Great Lakes Region to the Fifteenth Century* (Portsmouth, NH: Heinemann, 1998).

Schweinfurth, G. et al. (eds.), *Emin Pasha in Central Africa: Being a Collection of His Letters and Journals* (London: George Philip, 1888).

Setel, P., M. Lewis, and M. Lyons (eds.), *Histories of Sexually Transmitted Diseases and HIV/AIDS in Sub-Saharan Africa* (London: Greenwood, 1999).

Shadle, B., *Girl Cases: Marriage and Colonialism in Gusiiland, Kenya, 1890–1970* (Portsmouth NH: Heinemann, 2006).

Sharp, P. and B. Hahn, 'Origins of HIV and the AIDS Pandemic', *Cold Spring Harbour Perspectives on Medicine* 1, 1 (2011), 15.

Shorter, A., *East African Societies* (London: Routledge and Kegan Paul, 1974).

Siiskonen, H., A. Taskinen and V. Notkola, 'Parish registers: A challenge for African historical demography', *History in Africa*, 32 (2005), pp. 385–402.

Southall, A. and P. Gutkind, *Townsmen in the Making: Kampala and Its Suburbs* (Kampala: EAISR, 1957).

Southall, A., 'Social disorganisation in Uganda: Before, during, and after Amin', *The Journal of Modern African Studies*, 18, 4 (1980), pp. 627–56.

Southwold, M., 'The Baganda of central Uganda', in Molnos, *Cultural Source Materials II*, pp. 171–80.

Southwold, M., 'The Baganda of Central Uganda' in Molnos, *Cultural Source Materials III*, pp. 163–73.

Southwold, M., 'The inheritance of land in Baganda', *Uganda Journal*, 10 (1956), pp. 88–96.

Speke, J., *Journal of the Discovery of the Source of the Nile* (London: Blackwood, 1863).

Stanberry, L. and D. Bernstein (eds.), *Sexually Transmitted Diseases: Vaccines, Prevention and Control* (Cambridge: Academic Press, 2000).

Stanley, H., *In Darkest Africa, or the Quest, Rescue, and Retreat of Emin, Governor of Equatoria* (London: Sampson Low, Marston, Searle and Rivington, 1890).

Stanley, H., *Through the Dark Continent* (London: Simpson Low, Marston, Searle, and Rivington, 1878).

Steiner, I., J. Thomas and M. Hutt, 'Aortopathies in Ugandan Africans', *Journal of Pathology*, 109, 4 (1973), pp. 295–305.

Steinhart, E., 'Slavery and other forms of social oppression in Ankole, 1890–1940', in Médard and Doyle *Slavery*, pp. 189–209.

Steinhart, E., *Conflict and Collaboration: The Kingdoms of Western Uganda, 1890–1907* (Princeton: Princeton University Press, 1977).

Stephens, R., 'Lineage and society in precolonial Uganda', *Journal of African History*, 50, 2 (2009), pp. 203–21.

Stevens, L., 'Bananas, babies, and women who buy their graves: Matrifocal values in a patrilineal Tanzanian society', *Canadian Journal of African Studies*, 29, 3 (1995), pp. 454–80.

Stewart, K., 'Toward a historical perspective on sexuality in Uganda: The reproductive lifeline technique for grandmothers and their daughters', *Africa Today* 47, 3/4 (2000), pp. 123–48.

Stuhlmann, F., *Mit Emin Pascha ins Herz von Afrika* (Berlin: Reimer, 1894).

Summers, C., 'Catholic Action and Ugandan radicalism: Political activism in Buganda, 1930–1950', *Journal of Religion in Africa*, 39, 1 (2009), pp. 60–90.

Summers, C., 'Grandfathers, grandsons, morality, and radical politics in late colonial Buganda', *The International Journal of African Historical Studies*, 38, 3 (2005), pp. 427–47.

Summers, C., 'Intimate colonialism: The imperial production of reproduction in Uganda, 1907–1925', *Signs*, 16, 4 (1991), pp. 787–807.

Summers, C., ' "Subterranean evil" and "tumultuous riot" in Buganda: Authority and alienation at King's College, Budo, 1942', *The Journal of African History*, 47, 1 (2006), pp 93–113.

Sundkler, B., 'Marriage problems in the church in Tanganyika', *International Review of Missions*, 34 (1945), pp. 253–66.

Sundkler, B., *Bara Bukoba: Church and Community in Tanzania* (London: Hurst, 1980).

Swai, R. et al., 'Surveillance of HIV and syphilis infections among antenatal clinic attendees in Tanzania, 2003–2004', *BMC Public Health*, 6, 91 (2006), pp. 1–10.

Swantz, M.-L., *Women in Development: a Creative Role Denied. The Case of Tanzania* (London: Hurst, 1985).

Swindell, K., 'Domestic production, labour mobility and population change in West Africa, 1900–80', in C. Fyfe and D. McMaster (eds.), *African Historical Demography, II* (Edinburgh: Centre of African Studies, 1981), pp. 675–83.

Swynnerton, A., *Report on the Control of Elephants in Uganda, 6 Nov. 1923* (Entebbe: Government Printer, 1924).

Szreter, S., ‘The idea of demographic transition and the study of fertility change: A critical intellectual history’, *Population and Development Review*, 19, 4 (1993), pp. 659–701.

Szreter, S. and K. Fisher, *Sex Before the Sexual Revolution: Intimate Life in England 1918–1963* (Cambridge, Cambridge University Press, 2010).

Tanganyika Territory, *Annual Medical report 1938* (Dar es Salaam: Government Printer, 1940).

Tanganyika Territory, *Annual Report of the Medical Department 1941* (Dar es Salaam: Government Printer, 1942).

Tanganyika Territory, *Annual Report of the Medical Department 1943* (Dar es Salaam: Government Printer, 1944).

Tanganyika Territory, *Department of Agriculture Annual Report, 1932* (Dar es Salaam: Government Printer, 1933).

Tanganyika Territory, *Ordinances Enacted during the Year 1923* (Dar es Salaam: Government Printer, 1924).

Tanganyika Territory, *Ordinances under the Tanganyika Order in Council, 1920* (London: HMSO, 1923).

Tanganyika Territory, *Post-war Development: Medical Department* (Dar es Salaam: Government Printer, 1947).

Tanner, R., ‘Rumour and the Buganda Emergency, 1966’, *The Journal of Modern African Studies*, 16, 2 (1978), pp. 329–38.

Tanzania, *1967 Population Census: Vol. II, Statistics for Urban Areas* (Dar es Salaam: Government Printer, 1970).

Tanzania, *1978 Population Census: Vol. 5, Fertility and mortality data for rural and urban areas of regions* (Dar es Salaam: Ministry of Planning and Economic Affairs, 1982).

Tanzania, *1988 Population Census* (Dar es Salaam: Bureau of Statistics, 1992).

Taylor, J., *The Growth of the Church in Buganda* (London: SCM, 1958).

Tejani, B., ‘Farewell Uganda’, *Transition*, No. 45. (1974), pp. 64–6.

Thibon, C., ‘Un siècle de croissance démographique au Burundi (1850–1950)’, *Cahiers d'études africaines*, 27, 105/106 (1987), pp. 61–81.

Thibon, C., *Histoire démographique du Burundi* (Paris: Karthala, 2004).

Thiel, P. van, *Multi-tribal Music of Ankole: an Ethnomusicological Study Including a Glossary of Musical Terms* (Tervuren: Musée royal de l'Afrique, 1977).

Thompson, L., J. Ryden and J. McGregor, ‘Vaginitis and sexually-transmitted diseases’, in J. Ryden and P. Blumenthal (eds.), *Practical Gynecology* (Philadelphia, PA: ACP, 2002).

Thompson, R., ‘Fertility aspirations in urban Uganda’, *Urban Anthropology*, 7, 2 (1978), pp. 155–70.

Thornton, R., *Unimagined Community: Sex, Networks and AIDS in Uganda and South Africa* (Berkeley: University of California Press, 2008).

Tilley, H., *Africa as a Living Laboratory: Empire, Development, and the Problem of Scientific Knowledge, 1870–1950* (Chicago: University of Chicago Press, 2011).

Timaeus, I. and T. Moultrie, ‘On postponement and birth intervals’, *Population and Development Review*, 34, 3 (2008), pp. 483–510.

Tomes, M., *The Gospel of Germs: Men, Women and the Microbe in American Life* (Cambridge MA: Harvard University Press, 1999).

Trowell, H., 'The beginning of the kwashiorkor story in Africa', in H. Trowell, J. Davies and R. Dean (eds.), *Kwashiorkor* (London: Arnold, 1982 [1954]), pp. i–xxiv.

Trussell, R., 'Pelvic inflammatory disease', *Proceedings of the Royal Society of Medicine*, 61 (1968), pp. 365–8.

Tuck, M. and J. Rowe, 'Phoenix from the ashes: Rediscovery of the lost Lukiiko archives', *History in Africa*, 32 (2005), pp. 403–14.

Tuck, M., 'Venereal disease, sexuality, and society in Uganda,' in R. Davidson and L. Hall (eds.), *Sex, Sin and Suffering: Venereal Disease and European Society since 1870* (London: Routledge, 2001), pp. 191–204.

Tuck, M., 'Women's experiences of enslavement and slavery in late nineteenth- and early twentieth-century Uganda', in Médard and Doyle, *Slavery*, pp. 174–86.

Tucker, A., *Eighteen Years in Uganda and East Africa* (Westport, CN, Negro Universities Press, 1970 [1911]).

Turner, R., 'Ugandan women more familiar with traditional contraceptive methods than with modern ones', *International Family Planning Perspectives*, 17, 4 (1991), pp. 154–5.

Turshen, M., 'Population growth and the deterioration of health, mainland Tanzania 1920–1960', in Cordell and Gregory, *African Population*, pp. 187–200.

Twaddle, M., *Kakungulu and the Creation of Uganda 1868–1928* (Athens, OH: Ohio University Press, 1993).

UAC, *Accelerating HIV Prevention: The Road Map Towards Universal Access to HIV Prevention in Uganda* (Kampala: UAC, 2007).

UBOS and Macro International, *Uganda Demographic and Health Survey 1988* (Entebbe and Calverton MD: UBOS and Macro International, 1988).

UBOS and Macro International, *Uganda Demographic and Health Survey 2006* (Entebbe and Calverton MD: UBOS and Macro International, 2007).

UBOS and Macro International, *Uganda Demographic and Health Survey 2000–01* (Entebbe and Calverton MD: UBOS and Macro International, 2001).

Uganda Bureau of Statistics, *The 2002 Uganda Population and Housing Census, Population Dynamics* (Kampala: UBOS, 2006).

Uganda Census office, *Report on the 1980 Population Census: Vol. 1 Provisional Results by Administrative Areas* (Kampala: Census Office, 1982).

Uganda Government Statistics Branch, *The Patterns of Income, Expenditure and Consumption of African Unskilled Workers in Kampala, February 1964* (Entebbe: Government Printer, 1966).

Uganda Government, *Report of the Commission on Marriage, Divorce and the Status of Women, 1965* (Entebbe: Government Printer, 1965).

Uganda Ministry of Health, *Annual Report 1967–8* (Entebbe: Government Printer, 1968).

Uganda Protectorate, *1911 Census Returns* (Entebbe: Government Printer, 1912).

Uganda Protectorate, *1921 Census Returns* (Entebbe: Government Printer, 1922).

Uganda Protectorate, *1931 Census Returns* (Entebbe: Government Printer, 1932).

Uganda Protectorate, *1946 Annual Medical Report* (Entebbe: Government Printer, 1947).

Uganda Protectorate, *1947 Annual Medical Report* (Entebbe: Government Printer, 1948).

Uganda Protectorate, *1948 Annual Medical Report* (Entebbe: Government Printer, 1949).

Uganda Protectorate, *1950 Annual Medical Report* (Entebbe: Government Printer, 1951).

Uganda Protectorate, *1951 Annual Medical Report* (Entebbe: Government Printer, 1952).

Uganda Protectorate, *1952 Annual Medical Report* (Entebbe: Government Printer, 1953).
Uganda Protectorate, *1955 Annual Medical Report* (Entebbe: Government Printer, 1956).
Uganda Protectorate, *1956 Annual Medical Report* (Entebbe: Government Printer, 1957).
Uganda Protectorate, *1957 Annual Medical Report* (Entebbe: Government Printer, 1958).
Uganda Protectorate, *1958 Annual Medical Report* (Entebbe: Government Printer, 1959).
Uganda Protectorate, *1960 Annual Medical Report* (Entebbe: Government Printer, 1961).
Uganda Protectorate, *1961 Annual Medical Report* (Entebbe: Government Printer, 1962).
Uganda Protectorate, *1962 Annual Medical Report* (Entebbe: Government Printer, 1963).
Uganda Protectorate, *African Population of Uganda Protectorate: Geographical and Tribal Studies* (Nairobi: EAHC, 1953).
Uganda Protectorate, *Annual Reports of the Veterinary Department 1950–59* (Entebbe: Government Printer, 1951–60).
Uganda Protectorate, *Laws of Uganda* (Entebbe: Government Printer, 1935).
Uganda Protectorate, *Medical Department and Statistical Office Annual Reports for 1959* (Entebbe: Government Printer, 1960).
Uganda Protectorate, *The Pattern of Income, Expenditure and Consumption of African Unskilled Workers in Kampala, September 1953* (Nairobi: EAHC, 1954).
Uganda Protectorate, *Uganda Census 1959: African Population* (Entebbe: Ministry of Economic Affairs, 1960).
Uganda, *Ministry of Health Annual Reports 1960–69* (Entebbe: Government Printer, 1961–70).
Uganda, *Report on the 1969 Population Census* (Entebbe: Ministry of Planning and Economic Development, 1971).
UN Fertility Data, http://data.un.org/Data.aspx?d=PopDiv&f=variableID%3a54.
UNICEF, *Children and Women in Uganda: A Situation Analysis* (Kampala: UNICEF, 1989).
Van de Walle, E. and F. Van de Walle, 'Post-partum abstinence in tropical Africa' in R. Gray, H. Leridon and A. Spira (eds.), *Biomedical and Demographic Determinants of Reproduction* (Oxford: Oxford University Press, 1993), pp. 446–60.
Van der Walle, E. and F. van der Walle, 'Birthspacing and abstinence in sub-Saharan Africa', *International Family Planning Perspectives*, 14 (1988), pp. 25–6.
Varkevisser, C., 'The Sukuma of northern Tanzania', in Molnos, *Cultural Source Materials III*, pp. 234–51.
Vaughan, M., *Curing Their Ills: Colonial Power and African Illness* (Cambridge: Polity Press, 1991).
Vimard, P., 'The decrease in infant mortality on the Dayes plateau, 1930–76' in Fyfe and McMaster, *African Historical Demography II*, pp. 763–70.
Wallman, S., *Kampala Women Getting By: Wellbeing in the Time of AIDS* (London: James Currey, 1996).
Walser, F., *Luganda Proverbs* (Berlin: Reimer, 1982).
Ward, K., '"Obedient rebels": The relationship between the early "Balokole" and the Church of Uganda: The Mukono crisis of 1941', *Journal of Religion in Africa*, 19, 3 (1989), pp. 194–227.
Weiss, B., 'Good-for-nothing Haya names: powers of recollection in Northwest Tanzania', *Ethnos*, 64, 3 (1999), pp. 397–420.
Weiss, B., 'Northwestern Tanzania on a single shilling: Sociality, embodiment, valuation', *Cultural Anthropology*, 12, 3 (1997), pp. 335–61.

Weiss, B., *Sacred Trees, Bitter Harvests: Globalizing Coffee in Northwest Tanzania* (Heinemann: Portsmouth, NH, 2003).
Weiss, B., *The Making and Unmaking of the Haya Lived World: Consumption, Commoditization and Everyday Practice* (Durham, NC: Duke University Press, 1996).
Weiss, M., *Die Völkerstämme im Norden Deutsch Ost Afrikas* (Berlin: Carl Marschner, 1910).
Welbourn, H. and G. De Beer, 'Trial of a kit for artificial feeding in tropical village homes', *Journal of Tropical Medicine and Hygiene*, 67 (1964), pp. 155–9.
Welbourn, H. for Uganda Council of Women, *Our Children* (Kampala, n/d *c.*1960).
Welbourn, H., 'A comparison between children attending child welfare clinics in 1950 and in 1955', *East African Medical Journal*, 34, 2 (1957), pp. 47–54.
Welbourn, H., 'Backgrounds and follow-up of children with kwashiorkor', *Journal of Tropical Paediatrics*, 5, 4 (1959), pp. 84–95.
Welbourn, H., 'Notes on differences between Baganda and Luo children in Kampala', *East African Medical Journal*, 32, 7 (1955), pp. 291–8.
Welbourn, H., 'Weaning among the Baganda', *Journal of Tropical Pediatrics*, 9, 1 (1963), pp. 14–24.
White, L., *Speaking with Vampires: Rumor and History in Colonial Africa* (Berkeley: University of California Press, 2000).
White, L., '"They could make their victims dull": Genders and genres, fantasies and cures in colonial southern Uganda', *American Historical Review*, 100, 5 (1995), pp. 1379–1402.
White, L., *The Comforts of Home: Prostitution in Colonial Nairobi* (Chicago: University of Chicago Press, 1990).
White, R., J. Cleland and M. Caraël, 'Links between premarital sexual behaviour and extramarital intercourse: a multi-site analysis', *AIDS*, 14 (2000), pp. 2323–31.
Willis, J., 'Clan and history in western Uganda: a new perspective on the origins of pastoral dominance', *The International Journal of African Historical Studies,* 30, 3 (1997), pp. 583–600.
Willis, J., *Mengo Notes*, 2, 7 (1901), p. 88.
Wilson, C. and R. Felkin, *Uganda and the Egyptian Soudan* (London: Sampson Low, 1882).
Wotton, K., 'Paediatric mortality in Mulago Hospital, June 1982 to July 1983', in Dodge and Wiebe, *Crisis*, pp. 75–8.
Wrigley, C., *Kingship and State: The Buganda Dynasty* (Cambridge: Cambridge University Press, 1996).
Wrigley, E. and R. Schofield, *The Population History of England 1541–1871: a Reconstruction* (Cambridge: Cambridge University Press, 1981).
Wrigley, E., R. Davies, J. Oeppen and R. Schofield, *English Population History from Family Reconstitution, 1560–1837* (Cambridge: Cambridge University Press, 1997).
Young, W., 'Extra-urethritic cases in an African venereal diseases hospital', *The British Journal of Venereal Diseases*, 20 (1944), pp. 141–54.
Zenilman, J. and C. Deal, 'Gonorrhea: epidemiology, control and prevention', in Stanberry and Bernstein, *Sexually Transmitted Diseases*, pp. 369–86.
Zivanovic, S., 'The anthropological characteristics of the Ganda pelvis', *East African Medical Journal*, 45, 2 (Feb. 1968), pp. 68–70.

PRIMARY SOURCES

UNPUBLISHED DISSERTATIONS

Akerele, C. Olayiwola, 'Review of present M.C.H. services in West Mengo' (unpublished DPH dissertation, Makerere University Kampala [MUK], 1971).

Akingbehin, P., 'Causes of naeonatal morbidity and mortality in New Mulago Hospital' (unpublished DPH dissertation, MUK, 1970).

Bader, Z., 'Women, private property and production in Bukoba district' (unpublished MA dissertation, University of Dar es Salaam [UDSM], 1975).

Billington, R., 'Neurosyphilis in natives of East Africa' (unpublished dissertation, University of Cambridge, 1945).

Bisase, F., 'The story of marriage in Buganda' (unpublished BA Fine Arts dissertation, MUK, 1976).

Byaruhanga, C., 'Divorce in Uganda sociologically viewed' (unpublished Thesis ad lauream, Pontifical Gregorian University, 1954).

Chipadza, E., 'The correlation of socio-economic and educational levels, cultural factors and malnutrition among the Banyankole tribesmen of Uganda' (unpublished PhD dissertation, United States International University, 1982).

Cook, R., 'Child health in Ankole, Uganda: a programme of immunization and health education and its evaluation' (unpublished DMed dissertation, University of Oxford, n/d [*c.*1968]).

Costello, C., 'Maternal and child health in rural Uganda: the role of nutrition' (unpublished PhD dissertation, University of Pennsylvania, 1986).

Curtis, K., 'Capitalism fettered: state, merchant and peasant in northwestern Tanzania, 1917–1960' (unpublished PhD thesis, University of Wisconsin-Madison, 1989).

Gateley, I., 'The traditional education of women and girls in Uganda' (unpublished PhD dissertation, University of London, 1968).

Gbejuade, H., 'Review of the problems of a rural health centre in Uganda' (unpublished DPH dissertation, MUK, 1969).

Imani, G., 'A survey of health problems among school children in Igara county, Bushenyi district, Uganda' (unpublished DPH dissertation, MUK, 1981).

Kabwoto, E., 'Cases of decline in major crop production in Bukoba: banana, coffee and tea' (unpublished MA dissertation, 1976, UDSM).

Kachuchuru, S., 'A historical survey of Banyambo economy in Karagwe district, 1860–1960' (unpublished MA (History) dissertation, UDSM, 1975).

Kagume, A., 'Church and society in Ankole, Uganda: an analysis of the impact of evangelical African Christianity on ethnic and gender relations in Ankole, 1901–1961 (unpublished PhD dissertation, University of Bristol, 1993).

Kakembo, J., 'A study of the prevalence and incidence of venereal diseases in the Uganda police community' (unpublished DPH dissertation, MUK, 1978).

Kamugisha, A., 'Beliefs and customs connected with childbirth among the Banyankole, with special reference to utilisation of modern medical services' (unpublished BA Social Work and Social Administration dissertation, MUK, 1980).

Kazibwe, S., 'The salient factors in the aetiology of kwashiorkor' (unpublished DPH dissertation, 1976–7, MUK).

Kiguli, S., 'Oral poetry and popular song in post-Apartheid South Africa and post-civil war Uganda: A comparative study of contemporary performance' (unpublished PhD dissertation, University of Leeds, 2004).

Killewo, J., 'Epidemiology towards the control of HIV infection in Tanzania with special reference to the Kagera Region' (unpublished PhD dissertation, University of Umea, 1994).

Kisekka, M., 'Heterosexual relationships in Uganda' (unpublished PhD dissertation, University of Missouri, 1973).

Kizito, T., 'A study of the demographic characteristics and environmental problems of the heads of family units in slums around Nakulabye' (unpublished DPH, MUK, 1980).

Kodesh, N., 'Beyond the royal gaze: Ganda clans and the construction of an African methistory' (unpublished PhD dissertation, Northwestern University, 2005).

Lubega, M., 'Knowledge, attitudes and prevalence of sexually-transmitted diseases among adolescents in Uganda' (unpublished MA dissertation, MUK, 1991).

Manyolo, H., 'Factors that predispose to the spread of sexually transmitted diseases (eg gonorrhoea) among Makerere University students' (unpublished Diploma in Nursing Administration dissertation, MUK, 1980–81).

Marasha, B., 'Causation and prevention of stillbirths and postnatal deaths at Mulago hospital, 1970–71' (unpublished DPH dissertation, MUK, 1972–3).

Masawe, A., 'Syphilis in Uganda: The history, clinical features and cellular immunity' (unpublished MMed dissertation, MUK, 1971).

Médard, H., 'Croissance et crises de la royauté du Buganda au XIXe siècle' (unpublished PhD thesis, University of Paris 1, 2001).

Mickleburgh, A., 'The relevance of marriage for Ganda women in Bwaise, Kampala, Uganda' (unpublished PhD dissertation, University of Cambridge, 1998).

Morrow, O., 'Sexual cultures and vulnerability to HIV infection among Baganda youth in Mpigi' (unpublished PhD dissertation, Johns Hopkins University, 2000).

Mturi, A., 'Patterns of fertility and contraceptive use in Tanzania' (unpublished PhD dissertation, University of Southampton, 1996).

Mugisha, J., 'Prevalence of malnutrition in Kayunga using weight for ages as the index' (unpublished DPH dissertation, MUK, 1980).

Musisi, N., 'Transformations of Baganda women: from the earliest times to the demise of the kingdom in 1966' (unpublished PhD dissertation, University of Toronto, 1991).

Mwaka, B. Odonga, 'Widowhood and property among the Baganda of Uganda: Uncovering the passive victim' (unpublished Phd dissertation in Law, University of Warwick, 1998).

Mwesiga, B., 'Traditional marriage among the Banyankole' (unpublished BA Fine Arts dissertation, MUK, 1976–7).

Ndahura, B., 'Sexually Transmitted Diseases in a military unit in Uganda' (unpublished DPH dissertation, MUK, 1984).

Nyika, A., 'A study to assess the effectiveness of counselling services provided by Family Planning Association of Uganda at Kampala Clinic between January 1991 and December 1991' (unpublished Diploma in Adult Education dissertation, MUK, 1992).

Obbo, C., 'Town migration is not for women' (unpublished PhD dissertation, University of Wisconsin-Madison, 1977).

Owange-Iraka, J., 'Congenital syphilis as seen at Mulago hospital' (unpublished MMed. (Paediatrics) dissertation, MUK, 1976).

Rubega-Baryakere, F., 'A study of divorce rate in Igara county, Bushenyi district' (unpublished BA Dip. Ed. dissertation, MUK, 1995).

Sadgrove, J., ' "The condom culture is not the kingdom culture": Dissonant discourses and secret sex among born-again university students in Uganda' (unpublished PhD dissertation, School of Oriental and African Studies, 2007).

Schmidt, P., 'An investigation of early and late iron age cultures through oral tradition and archaeology: an interdisciplinary case study in Buhaya, Tanzania' (unpublished PhD dissertation, Northwestern University, 1974).

Sembajwe, I., 'Impact of urbanization on fertility and child mortality. The case studies of Tanzania and Uganda' (unpublished MA dissertation, UDSM, 1973).

Sempungu, D., 'Punishment of sin in Baganda traditional religion and in Christianity: an anthropological and biblico-moral study' (unpublished PhD dissertation, Lateran University, Rome, 1985).

Semwogerere-Serunjogi, M., 'Population dynamics in Uganda for period 1959–1969', (unpublished PhD dissertation, University of London, 1980).

Sheku, B., 'Pathological determinants of sterility in rural Uganda' (unpublished PhD dissertation, University of Pennsylvania, 1987).

Smith, C., 'The commoditization of African agriculture and changed social relations: The case of the Haya of Tanzania' (unpublished PhD dissertation, University of Essex, 1985).

Soff, H., 'A history of sleeping sickness in Uganda: administrative responses, 1900–1970' (unpublished PhD dissertation, Syracuse University, 1971).

Stephens, R., 'A history of motherhood, food procurement and politics in east-central Uganda to the nineteenth century' (unpublished PhD dissertation, Northwestern University, 2007).

Tuck, M., 'Syphilis, sexuality, and social control: A history of venereal disease in colonial Uganda' (unpublished PhD dissertation, Northwestern University, 1997).

Waliggo, J., 'The Catholic Church in the Buddu Province of Buganda, 1879–1925' (unpublished PhD dissertation, University of Cambridge, 1976).

Walters, S., 'Fertility, mortality and marriage in northwest Tanzania, 1920–1970: A demographic study using parish registers' (unpublished PhD dissertation, University of Cambridge, 2008).

Watts, T., 'Some observations on birth weights and nutritional changes during pregnancy: a prospective study of a self-selected group of mothers at an ante-natal clinic in West Mengo District Uganda' (unpublished DPH dissertation, MUK, 1969).

Zeller, D., 'The establishment of western medicine in Buganda' (unpublished PhD dissertation, Columbia University, 1972).

Zirabamuzaale, C., 'A study of sexually transmitted infections in pregnant women attending antenatal clinics in a rural health unit of Singo County, Kiboga hospital' (unpublished DPH dissertation, MUK, 1980).

Index